P9-BZG-942

Eckhert

The Nazi Doctors

Other Books by Robert Jay Lifton

The Broken Connection: On Death and the Continuity of Life

In a Dark Time (with Nicholas Humphrey)

Indefensible Weapons: The Political and
Psychological Case against Nuclearism (with Richard Falk)

Six Lives/Six Deaths: Portraits from Modern Japan
(with Shuichi Kato and Michael Reich)

The Life of the Self: Toward a New Psychology

Living and Dying (with Eric Olson)

Home from the War: Vietnam Veterans—
Neither Victims nor Executioners

History and Human Survival

Boundaries: Psychological Man in Revolution

Revolutionary Immortality: Mao Tse-tung and
the Chinese Cultural Revolution

Death in Life: Survivors of Hiroshima

Thought Reform and the Psychology of Totalism:
A Study of "Brainwashing" in China

THE NAZI DOCTORS

Medical Killing
and the
Psychology of Genocide

ROBERT JAY LIFTON

Basic Books, Inc., Publishers   New York

Library of Congress Cataloging-in-Publication Data

Lifton, Robert Jay, 1926–
   The Nazi doctors.

   Includes Index.
   1. Human experimentation in medicine—Germany—
Psychological aspects.   2. Medical scientists—Germany—
Psychology.   3. Holocaust, Jewish (1939–1945—Germany—
Psychological aspects.   4. World War, 1939–1945—Atrocities
—Psychological aspects.   I. Title.
R853.H8L54   1986   940.54'05   85-73874
ISBN   0-465-04904-4

Copyright © 1986 by Robert Jay Lifton
Printed in the United States of America
Designed by Vincent Torre
86 87 88 89 HC 9 8 7 6 5 4 3 2 1

To the victims of the Nazis.

To those who survived.

And to those who continue to struggle
against the forces of mass murder and genocide.

Speak, you also,
speak as the last,
have your say. . . .

Look around:
look how it all leaps alive—
where death is! Alive!

—PAUL CELAN

I swear by Apollo Physician, by Asclepius, by Health, by Panacea, and by all the gods and goddesses, making them my witnesses, that I will carry out, according to my ability and judgment, this oath and this indenture. . . . I will use treatment to help the sick according to my ability and judgment, but never with a view to injury and wrongdoing. I will keep pure and holy both my life and my art. In whatsoever houses I enter, I will enter to help the sick, and I will abstain from all intentional wrongdoing and harm. . . . Now if I carry out this oath, and break it not, may I gain forever reputation among all men for my life and for my art; but if I transgress it and forswear myself, may the opposite befall me.

—Oath of Hippocrates

Contents

PART III
THE PSYCHOLOGY OF GENOCIDE

Foreword

Soon after I completed my earlier study of atomic bomb survivors, a rabbi friend visited me and in the course of our conversation declared, "Hiroshima is your path, as a Jew, to the Holocaust." The comment made me uneasy, and I thought it a bit pontifical, even for a rabbi.

Yet from that time (the late 1960s) I had my own strong sense that I would, before too long, attempt some form of study of Nazi genocide. All of the work I had done on "extreme situations"—situations of massive violence to bodies and minds—seemed to point, professionally and personally, to such a study. Friends and students provided affectionate prodding, and without any clear plan, the idea took on for me a certain inevitability.

At several conferences on the Holocaust I made presentations on the psychology of the survivor, but came to the conviction that what was now most needed was a study of perpetrators. No wonder, then, that I was more than ready when I received a call from an editor (who had worked with me on my Hiroshima book) asking whether I would like to look over some documents he had been sent on Josef Mengele and Auschwitz medical practices. From those documents, and an immersion into related writings, I began to realize the extraordinary importance of doctors in general for the Nazi killing project. While the work was to extend far beyond those first materials, it was for me already under way.

Though I had little hesitation in proceeding, a few people I talked to expressed certain misgivings. "I hope you have a strong stomach!" was a comment I frequently heard. Some went on to make a compelling case for leaving the whole subject alone. Their argument was that Nazi evil should merely be recognized and isolated: rather than make it an object of study, one should simply condemn it. Psychological study in particular, it was feared, ran the risk of replacing condemnation with "insights." Those misgivings gave me pause and forced me to look at some difficult personal and philosophical issues.

I had no doubt about the reality of Nazi evil. But I could now be more clear that the purpose of my psychological project was to learn more about, rather than replace, precisely that evil. To avoid probing the sources of that evil seemed to me, in the end, a refusal to call forth our capacity to engage and combat it. Such avoidance contains not only fear of contagion but an assumption that Nazi or any other evil has no relationship whatsoever to the rest of us—to more general human capacities. While Nazi mass murder and brutality tempts one toward such an assumption, it is nonetheless false and even dangerous. As for the strong stomach, I was by no means without fear about what I was getting into; but decisions of that kind, in my experience, are made from one's deepest intuition about oneself, about what is appropriate and right for one to do. That inner inclination to go ahead did not, however, relieve me of painful awareness that whatever I did would be considerably less than full moral and intellectual justice to the subject.

As I pursued the work, it became clear that the Nazis were not the only ones to involve doctors in evil. One need only look at the role of Soviet psychiatrists in diagnosing dissenters as mentally ill and incarcerating them in mental hospitals; of doctors in Chile (as documented by Amnesty International) serving as torturers; of Japanese doctors performing medical experiments and vivisection on prisoners during the Second World War; of white South African doctors falsifying medical reports of blacks tortured or killed in prison; of American physicians and psychologists employed by the Central Intelligence Agency in the recent past for unethical medical and psychological experiments involving drugs and mind manipulation; and of the "idealistic" young physician-member of the People's Temple cult in Guyana preparing the poison (a mixture of cyanide and Kool-Aid) for the combined murder-suicide in 1978 of almost a thousand people. Doctors in general, it would seem, can all too readily take part in the efforts of fanatical, demagogic, or surreptitious groups to control matters of thought and feeling, and of living and dying. I have had professional or personal concern with all of these examples, and they bear some relationship to destructive patterns of the "medicalization" I will discuss.

But I found that Nazi doctors differed significantly from these other groups, not so much in their human experimentation but in their central role in genocidal projects—projects based on biological visions that justified genocide as a means of national and racial healing. (Perhaps Turkish doctors, in their participation in genocide against the Armenians, come closest, as I shall later suggest.) For this and many other reasons, Nazi doctors require a study of their own, and although I deal more broadly with patterns of genocide in the last section, this book is mainly about them.

Yet I make no claim to a comprehensive historical study of all Nazi doctors, or of the medical profession in general during the Third Reich. I often wished I had had access to such a study, as it would have greatly lessened the extensive digging into archives and trial documents in various parts of the world that my assistants and I had to undertake. What I have emphasized is the relationship of specific groups of Nazi doctors, and particular individuals, to mass murder—as well as the broader "healing" claim of the regime. This reversal of healing and killing became an organizing principle of the work, and I came to suspect the relevance of that reversal for other genocidal projects.

Much has been said about relationships of perpetrators and victims, and such relationships had considerable importance in Auschwitz and elsewhere. But I have found it essential to make the sharpest differentiation between the moral and psychological situation of members of the two groups. Whatever the behavior of either, prisoners were in the situation of being threatened inmates while Nazi doctors were threatening victimizers. This clear distinction must be the beginning of any evaluation of medical behavior in Auschwitz. Jews were the main object of Nazi genocide and therefore the main victims of Nazi doctors. But my concerns in this book also include non-Jewish Auschwitz inmates such as Poles and political prisoners and Russian prisoners of war; and also mental patients in Germany and occupied areas victimized even more directly by Nazi doctors.

As I reached the end of this work, many people asked me what it had done to me. My answer usually has been, "A great deal," followed by a change of subject. The truth is that it is still a little early to tell. One cannot expect to emerge from a study of this kind spiritually unscathed, all the more so when one's own self is the instrument for taking in forms of experience one would have preferred not to have known about. But the other side of the enterprise for me has been the nourishing human network, extending throughout much of the world, within which I worked. Survivors were at the heart of it, and they provided a kind of anchoring. But the network included colleagues, students of Nazi genocide, Germans committed to confronting the Nazi era, young assistants —some of whom I have known over years, and others I met for the first time—so many in all of these categories that I must list them at the end of the volume. Sharing an enterprise such as this vivifies old friendships and, in the most immediate and powerful ways, creates new ones. A compensation perhaps for my very limited knowledge of languages involved (German, Hebrew, Yiddish, Polish, and French) was the breadth of this nourishing network that took shape.

I have been aware for decades of Albert Camus's insistence that we be neither victims nor executioners, that we avoid institutions and actions in which these two categories come into being. But I have a new understanding of what he meant. Camus in fact learned his original lesson from participating in the anti-Nazi underground. It is hardly necessary to point out how often the advice is ignored. But I would at the same time insist that we are capable of acting on it, however imperfectly—capable of learning from carefully examined past evil. I undertook this study, and now offer it, in that spirit of hope.

The Nazi Doctors

I have used pseudonyms consisting of a first name and last initial for the people I interviewed for this book and a few others. In addition, I have altered certain identifying details that do not affect the substance of the interviews, and in a few cases refrained from specific citations.

Introduction

"This World Is Not This World"

Approaching Auschwitz

I gained an important perspective on Auschwitz from an Israeli dentist who had spent three years in that camp. We were completing a long interview, during which he had told me about many things, including details of SS dentists' supervision of prisoners' removal of gold fillings from the teeth of fellow Jews killed in the gas chambers. He looked about the comfortable room in his house with its beautiful view of Haifa, sighed deeply, and said, "This world is not this world." What I think he meant was that, after Auschwitz, the ordinary rhythms and appearances of life, however innocuous or pleasant, were far from the truth of human existence. Underneath those rhythms and appearances lay darkness and menace.

The comment also raises the question of our capacity to approach Auschwitz. From the beginning there has been enormous resistance on the part of virtually everyone to knowledge of what the Nazis were doing and have done there. That resistance has hardly abated, whatever the current interest in what we call "the Holocaust." Nor have more recent episodes of mass slaughter done much to overcome it. For to permit one's imagination to enter into the Nazi killing machine—to begin to experience that killing machine—is to alter one's relationship to the entire human project. One does not want to learn about such things.

Psychologically speaking, nothing is darker or more menacing, or harder to accept, than the participation of physicians in mass murder. However technicized or commercial the modern physician may have become, he or she is still supposed to be a healer—and one responsible to a tradition of healing, which all cultures revere and depend upon. Knowledge that the doctor has joined the killers adds a grotesque dimension to the perception that "this world is not this world." During my work I gained the impression that, among Germans and many others, this involvement of physicians was viewed as the most shameful of all Nazi behavior.

When we think of the crimes of Nazi doctors, what come to mind are their cruel and sometimes fatal human experiments. Those experiments, in their precise and absolute violation of the Hippocratic oath, mock and subvert the very idea of the ethical physician, of the physician dedicated to the well-being of patients. I shall examine those human experiments from the standpoint of the regime's medical and political ideology.

Yet when we turn to the Nazi doctor's role in Auschwitz, it was not the experiments that were most significant. Rather it was his participation in the killing process—indeed his supervision of Auschwitz mass murder from beginning to end. This aspect of Nazi medical behavior has escaped full recognition—even though we are familiar with photographs of Nazi doctors standing at the ramp and performing their notorious "selections" of arriving Jews, determining which were to go directly to the gas chamber and which were to live, at least temporarily, and work in the camp. Yet this medicalized killing had a logic that was not only deeply significant for Nazi theory and behavior but holds for other expressions of genocide as well.

In this book I will examine both the broad Nazi "biomedical vision" as a central psychohistorical principle of the regime, and the psychological behavior of individual Nazi doctors. We need to look at both dimensions if we are to understand more about how Nazi doctors—and Nazis in general—came to do what they did.

The very extremity of Auschwitz and related Nazi murder renders it close to unreality. A distinguished European physician, who had struggled with Nazi brutality for forty years—first as an inmate of Auschwitz and other camps and then as an authority on medical consequences of that incarceration—said to me very quietly at the end of a long interview, "You know, I still can't really believe that it happened—that a group of people would round up all of the Jews in Europe and send them to a special place to kill them." He was saying that the Auschwitz "other world" is beyond belief. The wonder is that there is not an even greater tendency than actually exists to accept the directly false contention that Nazi mass murder did not take place.

Also at issue for us here is the relationship of Nazi doctors to the human species. Another Auschwitz survivor who knew something about them asked me, "Were they *beasts* when they did what they did? Or were they *human beings*?" He was not surprised by my answer: they were and are men, which is my justification for studying them; and their behavior—Auschwitz itself—was a product of specifically *human* ingenuity and cruelty.

I went on to tell this survivor of the ordinariness of most Nazi doctors I had interviewed. Neither brilliant nor stupid, neither inherently evil nor particularly ethically sensitive, they were by no means the demonic figures—sadistic, fanatic, lusting to kill—people have often thought them to be. My friend replied, "But it is *demonic* that they were *not* demonic." He could then raise his second question, really the one he had in mind in the first place: "How did they become killers?" That question can be addressed, and this book is in the way of an answer.

What my survivor friend was struggling with—what I have struggled with throughout this study—is the disturbing psychological truth that participation in mass murder need not require emotions as extreme or demonic as would seem appropriate for such a malignant project. Or to put the matter another way, ordinary people can commit demonic acts.

But that did not mean that Nazi doctors were faceless bureaucratic cogs or automatons. As human beings, they were actors and participants who manifested certain kinds of behavior for which they were responsible, and which we can begin to identify.

There are several dimensions, then, to the work. At its heart is the transformation of the physician—of the medical enterprise itself—from healer to killer. That transformation requires us to examine the interaction of Nazi political ideology and biomedical ideology in their effects on individual and collective behavior. That in turn takes us to the significance of medicalized killing for Nazi mass murder in general—and for large-scale killing and genocide on the part of others. Finally, the work has relevance for broad questions of human control over life and death —for physicians everywhere, for science and scientists and other professionals in general, for institutions of various kinds—and also for concepts of human nature and ultimate human values. I can no more than touch on most of these general issues, having made a decision to focus on Nazi doctors and medicalized killing, and then on issues of mass murder. But my hope is that others will find here experience that might help them explore any of the searing moral issues implicit in this study.

That hope raises the important question of specificity and generality. I believe that one must stress the specificity of the Nazi killing project, especially concerning Jews: its unique characteristics, and the particular forces that shaped it. But having done that, one must also search for larger *principles* suggested by that unique project. No other event or institution can or should be equated with Auschwitz; but nor should we deny ourselves the opportunity to explore its general relevance for genocide and for situations of a very different order in which psychological and moral questions may be considerably more ambiguous.

The sequence of this book will be as follows. In the remainder of this introductory section, I say something about my overall psychological approach, interviews, and accompanying moral questions; and then I introduce the general Nazi theory and practice of medicalized killing. Part I examines the sequence from forcible sterilization to direct medical killing—or "euthanasia," as it was falsely named—made possible by the Nazification of the German medical profession, and culminating in an extension of "euthanasia" to the concentration camps. Part II, the longest segment of the book, concerns Auschwitz: its evolution as an institution; the large selections performed by Nazi doctors at the ramp and the smaller ones within the camp, especially on the medical blocks; the socialization of Nazi doctors to the killing project; the struggles of prisoner doctors to survive and remain healers despite dependency upon Nazi doctors; the use of phenol injections for killing; and the experiments done on Auschwitz inmates and the relation of these experiments to Nazi biomedical principles. Finally, this section includes three studies of individual Nazi doctors: one, that of Ernst B., revealing the ambiguity of Nazi decency; and the other two charting respectively the psychological behavior of Josef Mengele as an ideological fanatic and of Eduard Wirths as a formerly "good man" who set up the entire medical killing machinery of Auschwitz.

In part III, I explore psychological principles drawn directly from Nazi doctors, notably that of "doubling": the formation of a second, relatively autonomous self, which enables one to participate in evil. Then I turn to more general principles of Nazi genocide as they may apply to other and possibly all forms of genocide. The book closes with a somewhat personal afterword.

The Interviews

My assumption from the beginning, in keeping with my twenty-five years of research, was that the best way to learn about Nazi doctors was to talk to them; interviews became the pragmatic core of the study. But I knew that, even more than in earlier work, I would have to supplement the interviews with extensive reading in and probing of all related issues—having to do not only with observations by others on Nazi medical behavior but with the Nazi era in general, as well as with German culture and history and with overall patterns of victimization in general and anti-Jewishness in particular.

From the beginning I sought counsel from authorities on every aspect of the era—historians, social scientists, novelists and playwrights (some themselves survivors of camps)—about ways of understanding the regime and its behavior; about readings, libraries, trial documents, and other sources; and about other people to talk to. With the help of foundation grants I began to travel: preliminary trips to Germany in January 1978 and to Israel and Poland in May and June of that year. I lived in Munich from September 1978 through April 1979, during which time I did the greater part of the interviews, mostly in Germany and Austria, but also again in Poland and Israel, as well as in France, England, Norway, and Denmark. In January 1980, I did more work in Israel and Germany; and in March of that year, I interviewed three Auschwitz survivors in Australia. I have never been so intense a traveler nor so engrossed or pained a psychological investigator.

I interviewed three groups of people. The central group consisted of twenty-nine men who had been significantly involved at high levels with Nazi medicine, twenty-eight of them physicians and one a pharmacist. Of that group of twenty-eight doctors, five had worked in concentration camps (three in Auschwitz) either as SS physicians assigned there or in connection with medical experiments; six had some association with the "euthanasia" (direct medical killing) program; eight were engaged in medical policy making and in developing and implementing Nazi medical-ideological theory; six held other important medical positions which involved them in tainted behavior and ideological conflict; and three were engaged mainly in military medicine which brought them in contact with (or led them to seek distance from) massive Nazi killing of Jews behind the lines in Eastern Europe.

I interviewed a second group of twelve former Nazi nonmedical professionals of some prominence: as lawyers, judges, economists, teachers, architects, administrators, and Party officials. My purpose here was to probe the experiences of professionals in general under the Nazis and their relationship to ideology as well as to obtain background information about medical and related policies.

Very different was the third group I interviewed: eighty former Auschwitz prisoners who had worked on medical blocks, more than half of them doctors. The majority were Jewish (interviewed in the United States, Israel, Western Europe, and Australia); but they included two non-Jewish groups, Poles (interviewed in Krakow, Warsaw, and London) and former political prisoners (interviewed mostly in various parts of Western Europe, notably Vienna). I focused on their encounters with and observations of Nazi doctors and Auschwitz medical policies in general.

Concerning the two groups of former Nazis, especially the doctors, arrangements were never simple. It seemed clear from the beginning that I could best approach them through introductions from Germans of some standing in their society who were sympathetic to my research. The process was enhanced by a formal appointment I was given as a fellow at the Max Planck Institute for Research in Psychopathology and Psychotherapy, directed by Dr. Paul Matussek. My first task was to locate former Nazi doctors of standing in the regime—which I did with the help of assistants, through books, knowledgeable scholars, hearsay, and intensive address searches. When a name and address had been uncovered, Professor Matussek would send a form letter, which he and I had carefully constructed, to that person. The letter described me as a prominent American psychiatric researcher who was conducting a study of the "stresses and conflicts" of German physicians under National Socialism; mentioned my earlier work on Hiroshima and Vietnam; emphasized my commitment to confidentiality; and urged the person in question to cooperate fully with me. In the case of positive replies, I wrote a brief letter mentioning my desire to understand events of that time as accurately as possible.

The recipients of those letters undoubtedly understood that "stresses and conflicts" were euphemisms for more sinister matters. But for varying psychological reasons of their own, about 70 percent of those approached agreed to see me. Some felt they should show this courtesy to a "colleague" from abroad introduced to them by a person of great medical standing in their country. The amount of time that had passed since the Nazi period permitted some of them to look upon it as something they could now begin to talk about. Indeed to do so could afford them an opportunity to affirm a post-Nazi identity. I had the impression that many of these former Nazi doctors retained pockets of guilt and shame, to which they did not have access—that is, unconscious or numbed forms of quiet self-condemnation. Those unacknowledged feelings were consistent with a need to talk.

But their way of dealing with those feelings was frequently the opposite of self-confrontation: rather, the dominant tendency among these Nazi doctors was to present themselves to me as decent people who tried to make the best of a bad situation. And they wanted a confirmation from me of this view of themselves. Moreover, as elderly men—the youngest were in their late fifties, most were in their late sixties or older, and one was ninety-one—they were at the stage of life when one likes to "review" one's past in order to assert its meaning and affirm its legacy beyond impending death.

Some part of these men wished to be heard: they had things to say that most of them had never said before, least of all to people around them. Yet none of them—not a single former Nazi doctor I spoke to—arrived at a clear ethical evaluation of what he had done, and what he had been part of. They could examine events in considerable detail, even look at feelings and speak generally with surprising candor—but almost in the manner of a third person. The narrator, morally speaking, was not quite present.

I had to consider many levels of truth and untruth. I tried to learn all I could about each Nazi doctor before seeing him, and afterward to compare and cross-check details and interpretations with those available from other sources: from interviews with other former Nazi doctors and with nonmedical professionals; from interviews with former inmates and victims, especially those who had been physicians at Auschwitz; from written accounts of all forms of Nazi medical behavior, especially those writings that appeared relatively soon after the war; and from a great variety of books and documents, including trial records as well as diaries and letters when available. All this additional information was necessary for evaluation not only of willful falsehood or (more often) distortion but of questions of memory as well. We were discussing events that had occurred thirty or forty or more years before; persistent forgetting and manifestations of psychic numbing could blend with self-serving distortion. Yet I also encountered vivid and accurate recall, along with surprising candor and self-revelation. I had to combine all of this information in making interpretive judgments; but in the end, I felt I had learned much about the Nazi doctors I interviewed, and about Nazi doctors in general.

I spent four or more hours with the majority of Nazi doctors, usually during two or more interviews. But arrangements varied greatly according to their availability and their importance to the work. I saw some only once, and one terminated the interview after just half an hour. But I saw others for much longer periods, several for a total of twenty to thirty hours in a series of day-long meetings. The great majority of interviews had to be interpreted. As in past work, I was able to train a few regular assistants to interpret in a fashion that permitted quick and relatively direct exchange. Whatever its limitations, the presence of an interpreter in several cases provided a certain advantage: a buffer that enabled Nazi doctors, when uncomfortable and conflicted, to deal more freely with highly charged matters than they might have been able to do in direct, and therefore more threatening, exchange. The intensity that developed in these interviews was no less than that in those relatively few interviews I was able to conduct in English (because of the fluency of the interviewee). In both of those situations, with no exception, these German doctors agreed to my tape-recording the interviews, so that I had a precise record of what was said and was able to work later from the original German.

An ironic element in the approach was the requirement (made by the Yale University Committee on Research with Human Subjects, and generally followed in American research) that I obtain "informed consent" from the Nazi doctors. The requirement itself stemmed from the Nuremberg Medical Trial, and was therefore a consequence of the misbehavior of the very doctors I was interviewing or their associates. That touch of humanity seemed exactly right. Therefore, in correspondence with these doctors before our meeting, I reaffirmed the principles of confidentiality and of their right to raise any issues or questions they wished as well as to cease to participate in a particular interview or the research in general at any time. These principles were stated in written forms I asked each doctor to sign, sometimes at the beginning or the end of the first interview and at other times during the second meeting or through the mail (depending upon my estimate of whether introducing the form at a particular time would intensify an already stressful situation and thereby interfere with the work).

Among the doctors I interviewed, two were in the midst of trials stemming from their Nazi activities. Another had served a long jail sentence. And many of them had been held for periods of up to several years after the war without formal trial. On the whole, however, they were not the most identifiable criminal group of the doctors: members of that group had either been put to death at Nuremberg and subsequent trials or else died of natural causes years before, having been for the most part relatively senior at the time of their crimes. But the ones I did see, as I shall describe, were hardly free of evil, sometimes murderous, behavior.

I decided not to mention my Jewishness in preliminary correspondence with these doctors. Some undoubtedly suspected I was Jewish, though none asked me directly. On the one occasion when the matter came up specifically, the doctor concerned (during an interview near the end of the work) referred to an article in *Time* magazine describing the research and mentioning the fact that I was Jewish. His unctuous reference to the "tragic history" of our two peoples tended to confirm my impression that, had I emphasized my Jewishness from the beginning, this information would have colored and limited responses during the interviews and caused a much higher percentage of former Nazi doctors to refuse to see me. Whether talked about or not, however, my Jewishness was in some way significantly present in every interview, surely in my approach and probably in perceptions at some level of consciousness on the part of the German doctors.

Concerning the interview sequence, I first described briefly the purpose, method, and ground rules of the research, including a casual reference to my policy of recording interviews. Upon obtaining a doctor's agreement to proceed, I asked a few factual questions about his immediate situation, but essentially began by asking him to trace his educational, especially medical, background. Because those experiences were relatively less emotionally loaded than subsequent ones, he could establish a pattern of fairly free discourse along with a kind of medical dialogue with me. It would also usually require him to describe the impact of the early Nazi period on his medical study and work and on his life in general. I would then usually ask more about the man's family and cultural background, before examining in detail what he did and experienced during the Nazi years. The doctors knew that this was what I had come for, and many plunged energetically into those experiences. They tended to be less ready for detailed questions about feelings and conflicts—and about images and dreams, aspirations and self-judgments. But over the course of the interviews, the doctors came to reveal a great deal in these areas as well. With a little encouragement, these doctors—like other people I have interviewed in different research—entered readily into the interview's combined pattern of focused explorations on the one hand, and spontaneous associations on the other.

The atmosphere tended to vary from uneasy to cordial. There could be periods of genuine rapport, usually alternating with tensions, various forms of distancing, and reassertion on the part of both the Nazi doctor and myself of our essentially antithetical existences. I shall have more to say later about the worldviews these doctors expressed; but generally most adopted a rather characteristic post–Second World War, conservative political and social stance which included criticism of Nazi excesses but support for relatively authoritarian elements in German society and a certain uneasiness about what the young might be up to. Every once in a while there would be a flash of nostalgia for the Nazi times, for an era when life had intensity and meaning, whatever the conflicts engendered.

I never quite got over the sense of strangeness I experienced at sitting face to face with men I considered to be on the opposite side of the victimizing barricade, so to speak. Nor did I cease to feel a certain embarrassment and shame over my efforts to enter their psychological world. These feelings could be compounded when, as in a few cases, I found things to like about a man, and felt myself engaging his humanity. My central conflict, then, had to do with my usual sense of the psychological interview as an essentially friendly procedure, and my considerably less than friendly feelings toward these interviewees. I worked always within that conflict. I frequently had the impulse to divest myself of the conflict by means of aggressive moral confrontation. For the most part, I resisted that impulse—though my psychological probing could resemble such confrontation and certainly left little doubt concerning my perspective. But it was necessary to maintain that distinction; and the psychological probing, rather than moral confrontation, was required for eliciting the kind of behavioral and motivational information I sought. That distinction was also necessary, I later realized, for maintaining something important to me, my own professional identity in doing the work. So much so that it would probably be accurate to say that for me psychological probing *was* a form of moral confrontation. Yet I must add that there were moments when I wanted not only to confront but to accuse—indeed in some way attack—the man sitting opposite me. With it all, I experienced, and still experience, an obligation to be *fair* to these former Nazi doctors—that is, to make as accurate and profound an overall assessment as I am able.

With Auschwitz survivors the atmosphere of the interviews was entirely different. Just about all of them (with the exception of one who felt too upset by these matters to talk to me) involved themselves immediately in a common effort toward understanding Nazi doctors and what they did in the camp and elsewhere. The former inmates proved to be invaluable observers on both counts. Not surprisingly, my closest personal identification was with Jewish survivor physicians. In many cases they had come from families and social and ethnic backgrounds not too different from my own, and from areas close to my grandparents' original homes. I could not help contrasting their ordeal with my own privileged existence, and would come from these interviews literally reeling, sometimes close to tears. But I also had moving interviews with non-Jewish doctors from Poland and various other parts of Europe, many of whom had been sent to Auschwitz because of having tried to help Jews. An exception to this fundamental sympathy was one painful but revealing interview with an anti-Semitic Polish doctor who had worked closely with the Nazis and whom I shall discuss later in the book.

The interviews I conducted were unlike any I had previously attempted. Over their course I experienced every kind of emotion—from rage to anxiety to revulsion, and (with survivors) to admiration, shared pain, guilt, and helplessness—and now and then the wish that I had never begun the whole enterprise. I had nightmares about Auschwitz, sometimes involving my wife and children. When I mentioned these to my survivor friend just after I had begun the research, when they were most frequent, he looked at me without particular sympathy but perhaps with a glimmer of approval, and said softly, "Good. Now you can do the work." That helped me.

Yet, whatever the pain involved, I was not for the most part depressed or extremely distraught, and in fact experienced considerable energy in carrying out the study. I was immersed in its active requirements—the elaborate arrangements in organizing and carrying out the interviews and the general sense of a task that had to be completed. The pain hit me a bit harder when I returned to the United States in the spring of 1979 and sat down alone in my study to contemplate and begin to order what I had learned. Now I was no longer in motion, my only task was to imagine myself into Auschwitz and other killing centers, as I have been attempting to do ever since. Of course, one moves imaginatively in and out of such places—one cannot stay in them too long. Contributing to my well-being in the recent part of the work was the very struggle to bring form to the material. Over the course of such an enterprise, self-discipline is made possible by the anticipation of combating an evil and those responsible for it, of having one's say.

The Limits of Psychological Explanation

Psychological research is always a moral enterprise, just as moral judgments inevitably include psychological assumptions. Consider, for instance, Hannah Arendt's celebrated judgment on Adolf Eichmann and the "banality of evil."[1] That phrase has emerged as a general characterization of the entire Nazi project. What I have noted about the ordinariness of Nazi doctors as men would seem to be further evidence of her thesis. But not quite. Nazi doctors were banal, but what they did was not. Repeatedly in this study, I describe banal men performing demonic acts. In doing so—or in *order* to do so—the men themselves changed; and in carrying out their actions, they themselves were no longer banal. By combining psychological and moral considerations, one can better understand the nature of the evil and the motivations of the men.

My goal in this study is to uncover psychological conditions conducive to evil. To make use of psychology in that way, one must try to avoid specific pitfalls. Every discipline courts illusions of understanding that which is not understood; depth psychology, with its tenuous and often defensive relationship to science, may be especially vulnerable to that illusion. Here I recall the cautionary words of a French-speaking, Eastern European survivor physician: "The professor would like to understand what is not understandable. We ourselves who were there, and who have always asked ourselves the question and will ask it until the end of our lives, we will never understand it, because it cannot be understood."

More than being merely humbling, this passage suggests an important principle: that certain events elude our full understanding, and we do best to acknowledge that a partial grasp, a direction of understanding, is the best to be expected of any approach. It is an eloquent rejection of psychological reductionism: the collapsing of complex events into single, all-embracing explanations, in ways that sweep away rather than illuminate the interlocking structures and motivations behind those events. In that kind of reductionism, one can sacrifice psychological accuracy no less than moral sensitivity.

Another pitfall, even in the absence of reductionism, has to do with "understanding" as a replacement for moral judgment: with the principle contained in the frequently invoked French aphorism *Tout comprendre c'est tout pardonner.* But here I would say that if such full understanding were to include a grasp of moral as well as psychological issues, the second part of the aphorism—"forgiving all"—would not follow. The danger has to be recognized, and it can be overcome only by one's remaining aware of the moral context of psychological work.

Partly to address some of these moral questions in connection with social and historical experience, the early psychoanalyst Otto Rank called his last major work *Beyond Psychology* (1941).[2] Rank had long been preoccupied with ethical principles he believed Freud and others had excluded from psychological work, largely because psychology itself was entrapped in its own scientific ideology. By implication, that kind of scientific-psychological ideology could reduce Auschwitz, or its SS medical practitioners, to a particular mechanism or set of mechanisms. The question of evil would then not be raised. In that sense we may say that, to address moral issues one need not remain entirely *beyond* psychology, but must constantly look at matters that most psychology has ignored. Even then we do well to acknowledge, as Rank did, that psychology can explain just so much. Concerning Auschwitz and Nazi genocide, there is a great deal about which we will remain in ignorance, but we must learn what we can.

Of considerable importance here is one's psychological model or paradigm. My own departs from the classic Freudian model of instinct and defense and stresses life continuity, or the symbolization of life and death.[3] The paradigm includes both an immediate and an ultimate dimension. The immediate dimension—our direct psychological involvement—includes struggles with connection and separation, integrity and disintegration, movement and stasis. Separation, disintegration, and stasis are death equivalents, images that relate to concerns about death; while the experiences of connection, integrity, and movement are associated with a sense of vitality and with symbolizations of life. The ultimate dimension addresses larger human involvements, the sense of being connected to those who have gone before and to those who will follow our own limited life span. We thus seek a *sense* of immortality, of living on in our children, works, human influences, religious principles, or in what we look upon as eternal nature. This sense can also be achieved by the experience of transcendence: of a special psychic state so intense that within it time and death disappear—the classic experience of mystics.

One must address this ultimate dimension—what Otto Rank called "immortality systems"[4]—if one is to begin to grasp the force of the Nazi projection of the "Thousand Year Reich." The same is true of the Nazi concept of the *Volk*—a term not only denoting "people" but conveying for many German thinkers "the union of a group of people with a tran-scendental 'essence'. . . [which] might be called 'nature' or 'cosmos' or 'mythos,' but in each instance . . . was fused to man's innermost nature, and represented the source of his creativity, his depth of feeling, his individuality, and his unity with other members of the *Volk*."[5] Here we may say that *Volk* came to embody an immortalizing connection with eternal racial and cultural substance. And that connection begins to put us in touch with the Nazi version of "revolutionary immortality."[6]

The paradigm also delimits the researcher's combined attitude of ad-vocacy and detachment: articulating one's inevitable moral advocacies, rather than bootlegging them in via a claim to absolute moral neutrality; and, at the same time, maintaining sufficient detachment to apply the technical and scientific principles of one's discipline. My own advocacies include those related to my being an American, a physician, a psychiatrist, a Jew, and a human being concerned with forces of destruction in our world—and to my generally critical stance on ethical, social, and political questions.

The balance sought in dealing with these staggering experiences, how-ever difficult to maintain, is what Martin Buber described as one of "distance and relation."

Medicalized Killing

In Nazi mass murder, we can say that a barrier was removed, a boundary crossed: that boundary between violent imagery and periodic killing of victims (as of Jews in pogroms) on the one hand, and systematic genocide in Auschwitz and elsewhere on the other. My argument in this study is that the medicalization of killing—the imagery of killing in the name of healing—was crucial to that terrible step. At the heart of the Nazi enter-prise, then, is the destruction of the boundary between healing and killing.

Early descriptions of Auschwitz and other death camps focused on the sadism and viciousness of Nazi guards, officers, and physicians. But subsequent students of the process realized that sadism and viciousness alone could not account for the killing of millions of people. The emphasis then shifted to the bureaucracy of killing: the faceless, detached bureaucratic function originally described by Max Weber, now applied to mass murder.[7] This focus on numbed violence is enormously important, and is consistent with what we shall observe to be the routinization of all Auschwitz function.

Yet these emphases are not sufficient in themselves. They must be seen in relation to the visionary motivations associated with ideology, along with the specific individual-psychological mechanisms enabling people to kill. What I call "medicalized killing" addresses these motivational principles and psychological mechanisms, and permits us to understand the Auschwitz victimizers—notably Nazi doctors—both as part of a bureaucracy of killing and as individual participants whose attitudes and behavior can be examined.

Medicalized killing can be understood in two wider perspectives. The first is the "surgical" method of killing large numbers of people by means of a controlled technology making use of highly poisonous gas; the method employed became a means of maintaining distance between killers and victims. This distancing had considerable importance for the Nazis in alleviating the psychological problems experienced (as attested over and over by Nazi documents) by the *Einsatzgruppen* troops who carried out face-to-face shooting of Jews in Eastern Europe (see pages 159–60)—problems that did not prevent those troops from murdering 1,400,000 Jews.[8]

I was able to obtain direct evidence on this matter during an interview with a former *Wehrmacht* neuropsychiatrist who had treated large numbers of *Einsatzgruppen* personnel for psychological disorders. He told me that these disorders resembled combat reactions of ordinary troops: severe anxiety, nightmares, tremors, and numerous bodily complaints. But in these "killer troops," as he called them, the symptoms tended to last longer and to be more severe. He estimated that 20 percent of those doing the actual killing experienced these symptoms of psychological decompensation. About half of that 20 percent associated their symptoms mainly with the "unpleasantness" of what they had to do, while the other half seemed to have moral questions about shooting people in that way. The men had greatest psychological difficulty concerning shooting women and children, especially children. Many experienced a sense of guilt in their dreams, which could include various forms of punishment or retribution. Such psychological difficulty led the Nazis to seek a more "surgical" method of killing.

But there is another perspective on medicalized killing that I believe to be insufficiently recognized: *killing as a therapeutic imperative.* That kind of motivation was revealed in the words of a Nazi doctor quoted by the distinguished survivor physician Dr. Ella Lingens-Reiner. Pointing to the chimneys in the distance, she asked a Nazi doctor, Fritz Klein, "How can you reconcile that with your [Hippocratic] oath as a doctor?" His answer was, "Of course I am a doctor and I want to preserve life. And out of respect for human life, I would remove a gangrenous appendix from a diseased body. The Jew is the gangrenous appendix in the body of mankind."[9]

The medical imagery was still broader. Just as Turkey during the nineteenth century (because of the extreme decline of the Ottoman empire) was known as the "sick man of Europe," so did pre-Hitler ideologues and Hitler himself interpret Germany's post–First World War chaos and demoralization as an "illness," especially of the Aryan race. Hitler wrote in *Mein Kampf,* in the mid–1920s, that *"anyone who wants to cure this era, which is inwardly sick and rotten, must first of all summon up the courage to make clear the causes of this disease."*[10] The diagnosis was racial. The only genuine "culture-creating" race, the Aryans, had permitted themselves to be weakened to the point of endangered survival by the "destroyers of culture," characterized as "the Jew." The Jews were agents of "racial pollution" and "racial tuberculosis," as well as parasites and bacteria causing sickness, deterioration, and death in the host peoples they infested. They were the "eternal bloodsucker," "vampire," "germ carrier," "peoples' parasite," and "maggot in a rotting corpse."[11] The cure had to be radical: that is (as one scholar put it), by "cutting out the 'canker of decay,' propagating the worthwhile elements and letting the less valuable wither away, . . . [and] 'the extirpation of all those categories of people considered to be worthless or dangerous.' "[12]

Medical metaphor blended with concrete biomedical ideology in the Nazi sequence from coercive sterilization to direct medical killing to the death camps. The unifying principle of the biomedical ideology was that of a deadly racial disease, the sickness of the Aryan race; the cure, the killing of all Jews.

Thus, for Hans Frank, jurist and General Governor of Poland during the Nazi occupation, "the Jews were a lower species of life, a kind of vermin, which upon contact infected the German people with deadly diseases." When the Jews in the area he ruled had been killed, he declared that "now a sick Europe would become healthy again."[13] It was a religion of the will—the will as "an all-encompassing metaphysical principle";[14] and what the Nazis "willed" was nothing less than total control over life and death. While this view is often referred to as "social Darwinism," the term applies only loosely, mostly to the Nazi stress on natural "struggle" and on "survival of the fittest." The regime actually rejected much of Darwinism; since evolutionary theory is more or less democratic in its assumption of a common beginning for all races, it is therefore at odds with the Nazi principle of inherent Aryan racial virtue.[15]

Even more specific to the biomedical vision was the crude genetic imagery, combined with still cruder eugenic visions (see pages 23–24). Here Heinrich Himmler, as high priest, spoke of the leadership's task as being "like the plant-breeding specialist who, when he wants to breed a pure new strain from a well-tried species that has been exhausted by too much cross-breeding, first goes over the field to cull the unwanted plants."[16]

The Nazi project, then, was not so much Darwinian or social Darwinist as a vision of absolute control over the evolutionary process, over the biological human future. Making widespread use of the Darwinian term "selection," the Nazis sought to take over the functions of nature (natural selection) and God (the Lord giveth and the Lord taketh away) in orchestrating their own "selections," their own version of human evolution.

In these visions the Nazis embraced not only versions of medieval mystical anti-Semitism but also a newer (nineteenth- and twentieth-century) claim to "scientific racism." Dangerous Jewish characteristics could be linked with alleged data of scientific disciplines, so that a "mainstream of racism" formed from "the fusion of anthropology, eugenics, and social thought."[17] The resulting "racial and social biology" could make vicious forms of anti-Semitism seem intellectually respectable to learned men and women.

One can speak of the Nazi state as a "biocracy." The model here is a theocracy, a system of rule by priests of a sacred order under the claim of divine prerogative. In the case of the Nazi biocracy, the divine prerogative was that of cure through purification and revitalization of the Aryan race: "From a dead mechanism which only lays claim to existence for its own sake, there must be formed a living organism with the exclusive aim of serving a higher idea." Just as in a theocracy, the state itself is no more than a vehicle for the divine purpose, so in the Nazi biocracy was the state no more than a means to achieve *"a mission of the German people on earth":* that of *"assembling and preserving the most valuable stocks of basic racial elements in this* [Aryan] *people . . .* [and] *. . . raising them to a dominant position."*[18] The Nazi biocracy differed from a classical theocracy in that the biological priests did not actually rule. The clear rulers were Adolf Hitler and his circle, not biological theorists and certainly not the doctors. (The difference, however, is far from absolute: even in a theocracy, highly politicized rulers may make varying claims to priestly authority.) In any case, Nazi ruling authority was maintained in the name of the higher biological principle.

Among the biological authorities called forth to articulate and implement "scientific racism"—including physical anthropologists, geneticists, and racial theorists of every variety—doctors inevitably found a unique place. It is they who work at the border of life and death, who are most associated with the awesome, death-defying, and sometimes death-dealing aura of the primitive shaman and medicine man. As bearers of this shamanistic legacy and contemporary practitioners of mysterious healing arts, it is they who are likely to be called upon to become biological activists.

I have mentioned my primary interest in Nazi doctors' participation in medicalized or biologized killing. We shall view their human experiments as related to the killing process and to the overall Nazi biomedical vision.

At Nuremberg, doctors were tried only limitedly for their involvement in killing, partly because its full significance was not yet understood.[19]

In Auschwitz, Nazi doctors presided over the murder of most of the one million victims of that camp. Doctors performed selections—both on the ramp among arriving transports of prisoners and later in the camps and on the medical blocks. Doctors supervised the killing in the gas chambers and decided when the victims were dead. Doctors conducted a murderous epidemiology, sending to the gas chamber groups of people with contagious diseases and sometimes including everyone else who might be on the medical block. Doctors ordered and supervised, and at times carried out, direct killing of debilitated patients on the medical blocks by means of phenol injections into the bloodstream or the heart. In connection with all of these killings, doctors kept up a pretense of medical legitimacy: for deaths of Auschwitz prisoners and of outsiders brought there to be killed, they signed false death certificates listing spurious illnesses. Doctors consulted actively on how best to keep selections running smoothly; on how many people to permit to remain alive to fill the slave labor requirements of the I. G. Farben enterprise at Auschwitz; and on how to burn the enormous numbers of bodies that strained the facilities of the crematoria.

In sum, we may say that doctors were given much of the responsibility for the murderous ecology of Auschwitz—the choosing of victims, the carrying through of the physical and psychological mechanics of killing, and the balancing of killing and work functions in the camp. While doctors by no means ran Auschwitz, they did lend it a perverse medical aura. As one survivor who closely observed the process put the matter, "Auschwitz was like a medical operation," and "the killing program was led by doctors from beginning to end."

We may say that the doctor standing at the ramp represented a kind of omega point, a mythical gatekeeper between the worlds of the dead and the living, a final common pathway of the Nazi vision of therapy via mass murder.

PART I

"LIFE UNWORTHY
OF LIFE":
THE GENETIC CURE

Introduction to Part I

Prior to Auschwitz and the other death camps, the Nazis established a policy of direct medical killing: that is, killing arranged within medical channels, by means of medical decisions, and carried out by doctors and their assistants. The Nazis called this program "euthanasia." Since, for them, this term camouflaged mass murder, I have throughout this book enclosed it within quotation marks when referring to that program.

The Nazis based their justification for direct medical killing on the simple concept of "life unworthy of life" *(lebensunwertes Leben)*. While the Nazis did not originate this concept, they carried it to its ultimate biological, racial, and "therapeutic" extreme.

Of the five identifiable steps by which the Nazis carried out the principle of "life unworthy of life," coercive sterilization was the first. There followed the killing of "impaired" children in hospitals; and then the killing of "impaired" adults, mostly collected from mental hospitals, in centers especially equipped with carbon monoxide gas. This project was extended (in the same killing centers) to "impaired" inmates of concentration and extermination camps and, finally, to mass killings, mostly of Jews, in the extermination camps themselves. In part I, I discuss the first four steps, in relation to the Nazis' overall biomedical vision and as a prelude to Auschwitz and the other death camps.

Chapter 1

Sterilization and the Nazi Biomedical Vision

The Führer holds the cleansing of the medical profession far more important than, for example, that
of the bureaucracy, since in his opinion the duty of
the physician is or should be one of racial leadership.

—Martin Bormann

The *völkisch* state must see to it that only the
healthy beget children. . . . Here the state must act
as the guardian of a millennial future. . . . It must
put the most modern medical means in the service
of this knowledge. It must declare unfit for propagation all who are in any way visibly sick or who
have inherited a disease and can therefore pass it
on.

—Adolf Hitler

First Steps: Policies and the Courts

Only in Nazi Germany was sterilization a forerunner of mass murder.
Programs of coercive sterilization were not peculiar to Nazi Germany.
They have existed in much of the Western world, including the United
States, which has a history of coercive and sometimes illegal sterilization
applied mostly to the underclass of our society. It was in the United States
that a relatively simple form of vasectomy was developed at a penal
institution around the turn of the century. This procedure, together with
a rising interest in eugenics, led, by 1920, to the enactment of laws in
twenty-five states providing for compulsory sterilization of the criminally
insane and other people considered genetically inferior.

No wonder that Fritz Lenz, a German physician-geneticist advocate of sterilization (later a leading ideologue in the Nazi program of "racial hygiene"), could, in 1923, berate his countrymen for their backwardness in the domain of sterilization as compared with the United States. Lenz complained that provisions in the Weimar Constitution (prohibiting the infliction of bodily alterations on human beings) prevented widespread use of vasectomy techniques; that Germany had nothing to match the eugenics research institutions in England and the United States (for instance, that at Cold Spring Harbor, New York, led by Charles B. Davenport and funded by the Carnegie Institution in Washington and by Mary Harriman); and that Germany had no equivalent to the American laws prohibiting marriage both for people suffering from such conditions as epilepsy or mental retardation, and between people of different races. Lenz criticized America only for focusing too generally on preserving the "white race" instead of specifically on the "Nordic race"—yet was convinced that "the next round in the thousand year fight for the life of the Nordic race will probably be fought in America."[1]* That single reservation suggests the early German focus on a specific racial entity, the "Nordic" or "Aryan race," however unsupported by existing knowledge.

There had been plenty of racial-eugenic passion in the United States, impulses to sterilize large numbers of criminals and mental patients out of fear of "national degeneration" and of threat to the health of "the civilized races," who were seen to be "biologically plunging downward." Associated with the American eugenics movement was a biomedical vision whose extent is suggested by the following quotation from a 1923 book by A. E. Wiggam: "The first warning which biology gives to statesmanship is that the advanced races of mankind are going backward; . . . that civilization, as you have so far administered it, is self-destructive; that civilization always destroys the man that builds it; that your vast efforts to improve man's lot, instead of improving man, are hastening the hour of his destruction."[3]†

(A clear distinction must be made between genetics and eugenics. Genetics was, and is, a legitimate science, though one with limited development at the time [it began as a science with the recognition of Mendel's laws in 1900]; its principles were crudely, often falsely, applied by the

---

*Lenz did not at this point infer anti-Semitism from his belief in racial differences. Citing him, among others, George L. Mosse has argued that "there is no warrant for the claim to see in the . . . doctrine of 'racial biology and hygiene' an immediate forerunner of the Nazi policy against the Jews."[2] But once the Jews came to be viewed as a race, the connection was readily made.

†In a 1932 study of the sterilization movement in the United States, J. P. Landman spoke of "alarmist eugenics" and of "over zealous and over ardent eugenicists" who "regard the socially inadequate persons, i.e., the feeble-minded, the epileptics, the mentally diseased, the blind, the deformed and the criminals as inimical to the human race . . . [because] these peoples perpetuate their deficiencies and thus threaten the quality of the ensuing generations. It should be our aim to exterminate these undesirables, they contend, since a nation must defend itself against national degeneration as much as against the external foreign enemy."[4]

Nazis. "Eugenics" is a term coined by Francis Galton in 1883 to denote the principle of strengthening a biological group on the basis of ostensible hereditary worth; despite its evolutionary claims and later reference to genetic laws, eugenics has no scientific standing.)

But the German version of eugenics had a characteristic tone of romantic excess, as in Lenz's earlier (1917) declaration, in a thesis written for his professor, Alfred Ploetz (a social-Darwinist and the founder, in 1904, of the German Society for Racial Hygiene), that "race was the criterion of value" and "the State is not there to see that the individual gets his rights, but to serve the race." Lenz understood his advocacy to be one of "organic socialism" and feared that, without a radical eugenics project, "our [Nordic] race is doomed to extinction."[5]

For Germans like Lenz in the 1920s, establishing widespread compulsory sterilization became a sacred mission—a mission that led them to embrace National Socialism, with its similar commitment. While American and British advocates of eugenics sometimes approached this German romantic excess, the political systems in the two countries allowed for open criticism and for legal redress. In Britain there was continual legal resistance to coercive sterilization; and in the United States, legal questions could be raised concerning individual rights and limited knowledge about heredity, which eventually led to the rescinding or inactivation of sterilization laws in the states where they had been passed.* In Nazi Germany, on the other hand, the genetic romanticism of an extreme biomedical vision combined with a totalistic political structure to enable the nation to carry out relentlessly, and without legal interference, a more extensive program of compulsory sterilization than had ever previously been attempted. Indeed, the entire Nazi regime was built on a biomedical vision that *required* the kind of racial purification that would progress from sterilization to extensive killing.†

As early as his publication of *Mein Kampf* between 1924 and 1926, Hitler had declared the sacred racial mission of the German people to be "assembling and preserving the most valuable stocks of basic racial elements [and] . . . slowly and surely raising them to a dominant position." He was specific about the necessity for sterilization (*"the most modern medical means"*) on behalf of an immortalizing vision of the state-mediated race (*"a millennial future"*). And for him the stakes were absolute: *"If the power to fight for one's own health is no longer present, the right to live in this world of struggle ends."*[9]

---

*In observing Nazi sterilization policies, the *Journal of the American Medical Association* did not so much express outrage as it contrasted America's "more gradual evolution of practice and principles" regarding sterilization.[6] Ardent American sterilizers, such as Dr. Joseph S. De Jarnette of Virginia, could even complain: "The Germans are beating us at our own game."[7]

†Thus Daniel J. Kevles reports: "Within three years, German authorities had sterilized some two hundred and twenty-five thousand people, almost ten times the number so treated in the previous thirty years in America."[8]

Once in power—Hitler took the oath of office as Chancellor of the Third Reich on 30 January 1933—the Nazi regime made sterilization the first application of the biomedical imagination to this issue of collective life or death. On 22 June, Wilhelm Frick, the minister of the interior, introduced the early sterilization law with a declaration that Germany was in grave danger of *Volkstod* ("death of the people" [or "nation" or "race"]) and that harsh and sweeping measures were therefore imperative. The law was implemented three weeks later, less than six months after Hitler had become chancellor, and was extended by amendation later that year. It became basic sterilization doctrine and set the tone for the regime's medicalized approach to "life unworthy of life." Included among the "hereditarily sick" who were to be surgically sterilized were the categories of congenital feeblemindedness (now called mental deficiency), an estimated 200,000; schizophrenia, 80,000; manic depressive insanity, 20,000; epilepsy, 60,000; Huntington's chorea (a hereditary brain disorder), 600; hereditary blindness, 4,000; hereditary deafness, 16,000; grave bodily malformation, 20,000; and hereditary alcoholism, 10,000. The projected total of 410,000 was considered only preliminary, drawn mostly from people already in institutions; it was assumed that much greater numbers of people would eventually be identified and sterilized.

Special "Hereditary Health Courts" were set up to make decisions on sterilization, their composition reflecting the desired combination of medicalization and Nazi Party influence. Of the three members, two were physicians—one an administrative health officer likely to have close Party ties and the other ostensibly knowledgeable about issues of hereditary health; the third was a district judge, also likely to be close to the regime, who served as chairman and coordinator. There were also appeals courts, which made final decisions in contested cases and on which some of the regime's most recognized medical leaders served. All physicians were legally required to report to health officers anyone they encountered in their practice or elsewhere who fell into any of the preceding categories for sterilization, and also to give testimony on such matters unrestricted by the principle of patient-doctor confidentiality. Physicians also performed the surgical procedures. The entire process was backed up by law and police power.[10]

On 18 October 1935, a major ordinance regulating sterilization and the issuing of marriage licenses followed directly upon the notorious Nuremberg Laws (15 September), which prohibited marriage or any sexual contact between Jews and non-Jews. The Nuremberg lawmakers described themselves as "permeated with the knowledge that the purity of the German blood is a precondition for the continued existence of the German people, and filled with the inflexible determination to make the German nation secure for all future time."[11]

There were revealing discussions of method. The favored surgical procedures were ligation of the vas deferens in men and of the ovarian tubes in women. Professor G. A. Wagner, director of the University of Berlin's Women's Clinic, advocated that the law provide an option for removing the entire uterus in mentally deficient women. His convoluted argument was based on the principle of "hereditary health": mentally deficient women, after being sterilized, were especially likely to attract the opposite sex (who need not worry about impregnating them) and therefore to develop gonorrhea, which is most resistant to treatment when it affects the uterine cervix; the men who would then contract gonorrhea from these women would, in turn, infect other women with desirable hereditary traits and render them sterile. Other medical commentators, making a less genetic and more specifically moralistic argument, favored removal of the uterus in those candidates for sterilization who showed tendencies to promiscuity.* Still more foreboding was an official edict permitting sterilization by irradiation (X rays or radium) in certain specified cases "on the basis of scientific experiments."[13] These experiments, ostensibly in the service of improving medical procedures for specific cases, were a preliminary step toward later X-ray sterilization experiments conducted extensively, harmfully, and sometimes fatally on Jewish men and women in Auschwitz and elsewhere.

Directors of institutions of various kinds had a strong impulse to sterilize in order to eliminate the possible hereditary influence of a wide variety of conditions—blindness, deafness, congenital defects, and such "crippled" states as clubfoot, harelip, and cleft palate.[14] The genetically dominated worldview demanded of physicians led to discussions of the advisability of sterilizing not only the weak and impaired but their relatives, anyone who might be a "carrier" of these defects. Not surprisingly, Fritz Lenz carried the concept farthest in suggesting the advisability of sterilizing people with only slight signs of mental disease, though he recognized that a radical application of this principle would lead to the sterilization of 20 percent of the total German population—something on the order of twenty million people![15]

In that atmosphere, humane efforts were likely to take the form of pleas for restriction and exemption: for example, the recommendation by the distinguished anti-Nazi Berlin psychiatrist Karl Bonhoeffer that people who combined hereditary defects with unusual qualities or talents should not be sterilized; and the Munich psychiatrist Dr. Oswald Bumke's recommendation against sterilizing people who were schizoid rather than schizophrenic, along with his cautionary statement that schizophrenia itself could not be eliminated by sterilization because of the complexity of hereditary influences.[16] (The eugenics courts sometimes did make exceptions for the artistically gifted.)

But the regime discouraged qualifications and employed a rhetoric of

---

*There was, indeed, concern that degenerate individuals might seek sterilization to pursue "unrestrained sexual gratification."[12]

medical emergency: "dangerous patients" and "urgent cases" were people with hereditary taints still in the prime of life. Among "urgent cases" were mentally deficient but physically healthy men and women between the ages of sixteen and forty, schizophrenic and manic-depressive patients in remission, epileptics and alcoholics under the age of fifty, etc.[17] Once a petition was heard before a sterilization court, the die was pretty well cast. More than 90 percent of petitions taken before the special courts in 1934 resulted in sterilization (though a screening process eliminated some before they got to court); and fewer than 5 percent of appeals against sterilization, made to higher courts, were upheld.[18] But the principle of legality was nonetheless extremely important, and the strict secrecy surrounding court deliberations lent power and mystery to this expression of medicalized authority.

The legal structure cloaked considerable chaos and arbitrariness in criteria for sterilization (especially concerning mental conditions, which resulted in the greatest number of sterilizations) and concerning alleged hereditary factors. Inevitably, too, political considerations affected diagnoses and decisions—as was made clear by a directive from Martin Bormann, Hitler's private secretary and close associate, instructing that the moral and political behavior of a person be considered in making a diagnosis of feeblemindedness. The clear implication was that one could be quick to label "feebleminded" a person seen as hostile to the Nazis, but that one should be cautious indeed about so labeling an ideologically enthusiastic Party member. Political currents and whims also affected the project in various ways; and, despite its high priority, there were undoubtedly periods of diminished enthusiasm for sterilization. No one really knows how many people were actually sterilized; reliable estimates are generally between 200,000 and 350,000.[19]

In association with the sterilization laws, and as a further expression of racial policy, steps were taken to establish a national card index of people with hereditary taints. Special research institutes for hereditary biology and racial hygiene were set up at universities—for example, the institute established by Otmar von Verschuer, a professor at Frankfurt. These institutes sought genetic information about individuals extending back over several generations, and made use of hospitals, courts, and local and national health institutions. The physician, as genetic counselor and policeman, could be the vigilant "protector of the family that is free from hereditary defects."[20] In other words, sterilization was the medical fulcrum of the Nazi biocracy.

Fanatical Genetics: The Role of Ernst Rüdin

The predominant medical presence in the Nazi sterilization program was Dr. Ernst Rüdin, a Swiss-born psychiatrist of international renown. Originally a student of Emil Kraepelin, the great classical psychiatrist,

Rüdin became a close associate of Alfred Ploetz in establishing the German Society for Racial Hygiene. Rüdin was an indefatigable researcher and saw as his mission the application of Mendelian laws and eugenic principles to psychiatry. A former student and associate of his told me that "the aim of his life" was to establish the genetic basis for psychiatric conditions, and that "he was not so much a fanatical Nazi as a fanatical geneticist."

But a Nazi Rüdin did become, joining the Party in 1937 at the age of sixty. From his prestigious position as director of the Research Institute for Psychiatry of the Kaiser Wilhelm Society in Munich, Rüdin worked closely with a regime whose commitment to genetic principles he applauded, and was one of the principle architects of the sterilization laws. He became a significant source of scientific legitimation for the regime's racial policies (including consultations with Hans F. K. Günther, the leading Nazi anthropologist-publicist on racial matters, whose intellectual repute was generally held to be very low). Rüdin was not involved in the direct medical killing of the "euthanasia" program; but a younger associate to whom I spoke had the impression that his teacher, though not without doubts about the program, could well have favored a version of it with careful medical control.

In a special 1943 issue of his journal, *Archive für Rassen-und Gesellschaftsbiologie* (Archive of Racial and Social Biology), celebrating ten years of National Socialist rule, Rüdin extolled Hitler and the movement for its "decisive . . . path-breaking step toward making racial hygiene a fact among the German people . . . and inhibiting the propagation of the congenitally ill and inferior." He praised both the Nuremberg Laws for "preventing the further penetration of the German gene pool by Jewish blood," and the SS for "its ultimate goal, the creation of a special group of medically superior and healthy people of the German Nordic type."[21]

A close relative, also a physician, told me that Rüdin felt it "necessary" to write those things and, in response to my question whether he had meant them at the time, answered, "Well, half and half." While Rüdin apparently did eventually become disillusioned with the regime, he could never (according to a former colleague) bring himself to resign his positions but sought always to work from within.*

No one I spoke to thought Rüdin a cruel person; to the contrary, he was seen as decent and dedicated to his work. Yet he not only served the regime but, in his person and scientific reputation, did much to effect the medicalization of racial policies—not quite those of killing but of suppressing in specific groups the continuity of life. He also demonstrates,

*Rüdin's defenders later claimed that he contested the "euthanasia" program from within. This is unlikely, as efforts in 1940 of two psychiatrists to enlist Rüdin, and through him the German Psychiatric Society, for opposition to the killing met with no success (see pages 88–89). Rüdin received two high awards from Hitler as the "pathfinder in the field of hereditary hygiene."[22]

in extreme form, the attraction of the Nazi biomedical vision for a certain kind of biologically and genetically oriented scientist.

Opposition to Sterilization

There did not seem to be much opposition to sterilization. The Catholic Church disapproved of it, but avoided confronting the issue and did little more than press for the exemption of Catholic judges and doctors from enforcing the law. One judge on a Hereditary Health Appeals Court raised the interesting question of the "burden of unusual responsibility" placed on doctors required to perform operations that "serve no therapeutic purpose." But Gerhard Wagner—then the leading Nazi medical authority and a zealous advocate of sterilization—denied any such moral conflict in doctors; and a Party newspaper ran a column with the significant heading "Life or Death," which made the simple point that the life of the nation took precedence over "dogma and conflicts of conscience," and also that opposition to the government's program would be met with strong retaliation.[23]

The great majority of the doctors I interviewed told me that they approved of the sterilization laws at the time. They believed the laws to be consistent with prevailing medical and genetic knowledge concerning the prevention of hereditary defects, though a few of these doctors had some hesitation about the laws' compulsory features. The doctors all stressed their absolute distinction between those sterilization policies and later "euthanasia."

Decisions about sterilization were affected by bureaucratic struggles both between doctors and lawyers and between extremely ardent and less ardent advocates of the procedure. One doctor I interviewed, Johann S., who had been a leading organizer and high-level participant in Nazi medical programs including sterilization, thought that "the law was totally messed up by the legal people." He and his medical colleagues believed strongly that "it would have been more appropriate to leave this decision [about whom and when to sterilize] to a doctors' team." While psychiatrists later emphasized their restraint, Dr. S. related incidents in which they had to be restrained from sterilizing people with relatively benign psychological difficulties such as treatable depressions. He told how even Gerhard Wagner (whom he tended to glorify) had restrained a physician-health officer with the admonition, "This is not a rabbit hunt." While Dr. S. recognized that excessive zeal was widespread, he tended to excuse it as a product of the idealism of that time: "The great enthusiasm that carried through the developments between 1933 and 1939 cannot be denied. Everybody wanted to contribute. One of the first National Socialist laws to be enacted was the law on [hereditary] health. Thus the [state] health officers demonstrated their ambition to have as many people as possible sterilized."

The Nazification of Medicine

Nazification of the medical profession—a key aspect of the transition from sterilization to direct medical killing—was achieved by a combination of ideological enthusiasm and systematic terror. An influential manual by Rudolf Ramm of the medical faculty of the University of Berlin proposed that each doctor was to be no longer merely a caretaker of the sick but was to become a "cultivator of the genes," a "physician to the *Volk*," and a "biological soldier." While Ramm harked back to traditional forms of medical idealism ("inner calling, high ethics, profound knowledge . . . sacrifice and dedication"), he favored abandoning the old "liberal-materialistic spirit" (associated especially with the harmful influence of Jews in the profession) and acquiring instead "the idealistic *Weltanschauung* of National Socialism." Thus, the physician could carry out what Gerhard Wagner identified as the task of his Public Health Office: the "promotion and perfection of the health of the German people . . . to ensure that the people realize the full potential of their racial and genetic endowment."[24] Ramm went on to speak of "breakthroughs in biological thinking" under National Socialism that enabled medical leaders to take an important part in projects to reverse racial decay such as the Nuremberg Laws and the sterilization program. To carry these programs out properly, the individual physician must become a "genetics doctor" *(Erbarzt)*. He could then become a "caretaker of the race" and a "politician of population." By following "public care" functions of preventing "bastardization through the propagation of unworthy and racially alien elements . . . and maintaining and increasing those of sound heredity," he could attain the national goal of "keeping our blood pure."[25]

Ramm also discussed the virtues of sterilization and labeled "erroneous" the widespread belief that a doctor should under no circumstances take a patient's life, since for the incurably sick and insane, "euthanasia" was the most "merciful treatment" and "an obligation to the *Volk*." That obligation was always central. The physician was to be concerned with the health of the *Volk* even more than with individual disease and was to teach them to overcome the old individualistic principle of "the right to one's own body" and to embrace instead the "duty to be healthy."[26] Thus, Johann S. spoke to me with pride about the principle of being "doctor to the *Volkskörper* ['national body' or 'people's body']" and of "our duty . . . to the collectivity."

Ramm's manual also specified that a doctor was to be a biological militant, "an alert biological soldier" living under "the great idea of the National Socialist biological state structure" (see also page 130). For it claimed that "National Socialism, unlike any other political philosophy or Party program, is in accord with the natural history and biology of man."[27]

Physicians could thrill to that message. Dr. S., for instance, described joining the Party immediately after hearing Deputy Party Leader Rudolf Hess say, at a mass meeting in 1934, "National Socialism is nothing but applied biology." And in his work of Nazi medical organizing, this doctor saw himself as primarily spreading a biological message: "We wanted to put into effect the laws of life, which are biological laws." His medical faction was disdainful of any politics that did not follow that principle: "We understood National Socialism from the biological side—we introduced biological considerations into [Party] policies." He stressed the conviction that physicians alone possess the necessary combination of theoretical knowledge and direct human experience to serve as the authentic biological evangelists: "Every practitioner has much more knowledge about biology than a philosopher or what have you, because he has seen it."

At the same time, it was claimed that the desired identity of the Nazi physician evolved naturally from medical tradition—a tradition that now required "Germanizing" and "eugenicizing." One lavishly illustrated volume by two medical historians was entitled *The Face of the Germanic Doctor over Four Centuries*. It featured Paracelsus, the great sixteenth-century Swiss-German physician-alchemist, and praised him for both his scientific empiricism and his nationalism. He was quoted as saying, "Each country developed its own sickness, medicine, and its own doctor." More recent German scientists, especially Carl Correns who did pioneering work in plant genetics, were hailed as having "created the foundation for the eugenic and racial-biological measures of the National Socialist people's state." The authors' SS ranks are included;* and the introduction by Ernst Robert von Grawitz, chief physician of the SS, puts forward the concept of the physician, past and present, as the "protector of life" who "knows himself to be deeply obligated to the future of our *Volk*."[28]†

Another such introduction to a volume on medical ethics was written by Joachim Mrugowsky, a high-ranking SS doctor who became head of the Hygienic Institute, which was responsible for maintaining and dis-

---

*The SS (*Schutzstaffel*, or defense squadron) began as Hitler's personal guard unit. Particularly after 1929, under the control of Heinrich Himmler, it advertised itself as an élite corps whose members fit the ideal Aryan model. As such, it attracted considerable support from the aristocracy and professional classes, including physicians. The SS grew in power and influence by purging the less disciplined and lower-class SA in 1934, then by its assumption of control over all police forces during the late 1930s. Himmler purportedly modeled the SS on the Jesuits, with absolute obedience sworn to Hitler. The SS came to be divided into a number of units, including the SD (*Sicherheitsdienst*, or Security Service), the Office of Race and Settlement, and the WVHA (Wirtschafts-und Verwaltungshauptamt, or Economic and Administrative Department), which administered the concentration camps. The Waffen-SS, or armed SS, amounted to a separate army, indeed existed in rivalry with the regular *Reichswehr*. Its units participated heavily in the atrocities of the *Einsatzgruppen* during the early part of the war. During the war the Waffen-SS became increasingly independent and acted more as a regular military force. Utilizing relatively large numbers of "ethnic" Germans from outside the Reich from the outset, after 1942 it depended upon conscription to maintain its forces.

†The concept of "Germanic" physicians included Austrians, Dutch, Belgians, and Scandinavians.

tributing the Zyklon-B gas used at Auschwitz. Mrugowsky was put to death at Nuremberg in 1948 for his extensive involvement in fatal medical experiments. The book he introduced had been written a hundred years earlier by Christoph Wilhelm Hufeland, one of Germany's great modern physician-humanists. In his introduction, Mrugowsky focused upon the doctor's function as "the priest of the holy flame of life" (in Hufeland's words), and on the "art of healing" as the doctor's "divine mission." Partially anticipating his own future, he spoke of the National Socialist breakdown of the distinction between research and healing, since the results of the work of the researcher are for the benefit of the *Volk*. [29]

Inevitably, the Nazi medical ideal went back to Hippocrates and related itself to the Hippocratic oath. The claim was that medicine had been "despiritualized" mainly by what Gerhard Wagner identified as the "mechanically oriented spirit" of Jewish teachers. There was thus a need to "return to the ethics and high moral status of an earlier generation . . . which stood on [the] solid philosophical ground" of the Hippocratic oath.[30] Finally, the *Reichsführer* of the SS and overall head of the Nazi police system, Henrich Himmler himself embraced Hippocrates as a model for SS physicians. In a brief introduction to a series of short books for SS doctors under the overall title "Eternal Doctors," Himmler spoke of "the great Greek doctor Hippocrates," of the "unity of character and accomplishment" of his life, which "proclaims a morality, the strengths of which are still undiminished today and shall continue to determine medical action and thought in the future." The series was edited by Grawitz and possessed the ultimate imprimatur in being "authorized" by none other than Hitler himself.[31] In testimony at the Nuremberg Medical Trial, a witness referred to the Nazi embrace of Hippocratic principles as "an ironical joke of world history."[32] But this ultimate absurdity had an internal logic: the sense of recasting the medical profession—and the entire German nation—in the service of larger healing.

There was one area in which the Nazis did insist upon a clear break with medical tradition. They mounted a consistent attack upon what they viewed as exaggerated Christian compassion for the weak individual instead of tending to the health of the group, of the *Volk*. This partly Nietzschean position, as articulated by Ramm, included a rejection of the Christian principle of *caritas* or charity, and of the Church's "commandment to attend to the incurably ill person and render him medical aid unto his death."[33] The same position was expressed in the Nazi Party medical outlet *Ziel und Weg* (Aim and Road) from the time of its founding in 1931. The matter was put strongly by Dr. Arthur Guett, a high-ranking health official, who declared that "the ill-conceived 'love of thy neighbor' has to disappear. . . . It is the supreme duty of the . . . state to grant life and livelihood only to the healthy and hereditarily sound portion of the population in order to secure . . . a hereditarily sound and racially pure folk [Volk] for all eternity." He added the visionary-idealistic principle that "the life of the individual has meaning only in the light of that ultimate aim."[34] The doctor, like everyone in Nazi Germany, was expected to become "hardened," to adopt what Hitler himself called the "ice-cold logic" of the necessary.

The keynote of the Nazi policy was transformation, in Ramm's words: "a change in the attitude of each and every doctor, and a spiritual and mental regeneration of the entire medical profession." The true physician, moreover, "must not only be a Party member on the outside, but rather must be convinced in his heart of hearts of the biological laws that form the center of his life." He was also to be a "preacher for these laws."[35] Dr. S. believed that Nazi medicine had achieved some of this transformation: that is, it had overcome the exaggerated stress on "technical things," reversed the prior tendency to "know only cases and not people," and "put in the foreground the questions of the psyche that had been neglected."

But the Nazis sought something more than mere psychosomatic inclusiveness or "holistic" medicine: their quest had the quality of *biological and medical mysticism.* Mrugowsky, for instance, wrote, in the introduction mentioned earlier, that "today the [German] *Volk* is holy to us." Of the physician's relationship to the *Volk*, or "community of fate," Mrugowsky added that "only in the art of healing does he find the myth of life."[36] Other writers had viewed the Third Reich as "immanent in all German history, which strives toward that moment when the *Volk* becomes the vessel of God."[37] But in the vision I am describing, the physician-biologists saw themselves as the core of the mystical body of the *Volk.*

There had to develop, as one Nazi doctor put it, "a totality of the physicians' community, with physicians having total dedication to the *Volk.*" This doctor's term for his biological mysticism was "biological socialism." The Nazis, he insisted, had been able to bring together nationalism and socialism because of their "recognition of the natural phenomena of life." Thus, "for the first time, the mind begins to understand that there are powerful forces over it which it must acknowledge"; that "the human being becomes . . . a working member in the kingdom of the living; and that his powers will be fulfilled when working within the balanced interplay of natural forces." We may say that mysticism, especially communal mysticism, was given a biological and medical face. (In chapter 5, I discuss this kind of biological romanticism at greater length.)

Medical Gleichschaltung

This Nazi medical ethos, though embraced by most doctors only in part, became the basis for reorganizing the profession. The reorganization process was known as *Gleichschaltung,* which means "coordination" or "synchronization" and also connotes the mechanical idea of shifting gears. Hitler had anticipated the principle of *Gleichschaltung* when he declared in *Mein Kampf* that "all future institutions of this state must grow out of the movement itself"[38]: that is, all political, social, and cultural institutions were to be totally ideologized and controlled by trusted Nazis. *Gleichschaltung* could be a euphemism for eliminating all possible opposition, whether by exclusion, threat, or violence. Certainly for anyone looked upon with disfavor by the regime, *Gleichschaltung* was experienced as persecution. But it also expressed the vision of absolute unity, of the totalized community *(Gemeinschaft)*, of making all things and people one.

Gleichschaltung, then, was the metaphor uniting visionary idealism and terror. And the expectation of *Gleichschaltung*, once the process was initiated, created everywhere—in government, universities, and all other institutions and professions—the expectation of coercive unification according to Nazi ideological requirements. In medicine as elsewhere there was widespread "voluntary *Gleichschaltung*"—one might even say anticipatory *Gleichschaltung*—by people who embraced Nazi ideology in varying degrees.

The *Gleichschaltung* of the medical profession was accomplished via the Nazi-dominated Reich Physicians' Chamber *(Reichsärztekammer)* and its various local branches, to which all practicing physicians had to belong. Pre-Nazi medical societies were either disbanded or "coordinated" into the Reich Physicians' Chamber, whose leaders were drawn from the "old medical fighters" who had marched and fought in the streets in the early days. The latter had formed the National Socialist German Physicians' League *(Nationalsozialistischer Deutscher Ärztebund)* at a Party rally in 1929 and were involved as well in medical infighting with such rival groups as the Socialist League of Doctors.

In medicine, as in other professions, there was perpetual conflict between "old fighters" emerging from the early Nazi movement, who tended to be militant and ideological, and the newer bureaucrats, who tended to be concerned with questions of organization and of integration of the existing medical profession.[39] This conflict, implicit in the dual authority of Party and government bureaucracy, plagued the Nazi regime throughout its existence. This vanguard of medical leadership, more notable for Nazi militance than scientific attainment, was nonetheless effective in pressuring its medical betters to fall in line with Nazi policies. And fall in line they did, to the extent that doctors had one of the highest ratios of Party members of any profession: 45 percent. Moreover, their ratio in the SA and SS was respectively two and seven times that of teachers.[40]* This medical movement toward the Nazis and toward self-*Gleichschaltung* was related both to strongly authoritarian and nationalistic tendencies within the medical profession, including "the underestimation of politics and the overestimation of order";[42] and to their special attraction as a group to the Nazi stress on biology and on a biomedical vision of national cure.

*But according to Michael Kater, their enthusiasm seems to have lessened after 1935 and again after the war began, and declined thereafter.[41]

Much of the spirit of Nazi medicine emerged from the politicized doctors of the Party's original Physicians' League, whose leading figure became Gerhard Wagner. As chief physician of the Reich, Wagner headed both the Reich Physicians' Chamber and the Party medical structures and favored a visionary ideological medicine that was highly racist, socially and clinically oriented (the Nazi version of a "people's medicine"), and distrustful of academic medicine and pure science. Wagner was active in formulating and explaining the sterilization program, and it was to him that Hitler first (in 1935) told his plans for extensive "euthanasia" killings; indeed, Wagner was considered by some Germans to have been the "godfather of the euthanasia programme."[43] When he died in 1939, he was replaced by Leonardo Conti, a more bureaucratic figure who held a health post in the Interior Ministry, though also possessing the credentials of an "old medical fighter." Eventually, Karl Brandt, a younger man and an ardent second-generation Nazi, emerged from more distinguished university connections to become the dominant medical figure.

"The Jews Are Our Misfortune"

Systematic persecution of Jewish doctors was bound up with the Nazi biomedical vision. Through victimization of their Jewish colleagues, German doctors could combine their own "scientific racism" and anti-Semitism with their professional and economic incentive of ridding themselves of formidable rivals. In their part in this solution to what was called the "Jewish problem," those German doctors were the heirs to a long-standing intellectual-professional anti-Semitism having to do with extraordinary German anxiety over the perceived threat of Jewish otherness to German society and to the German race and state.

A key image here is that of the leading late-nineteenth-century historian Heinrich von Treitschke: "The Jews are our misfortune." Expressed in 1879, that image reverberated over generations; a few decades later, a leading anti-Semite could write that it "became a part of my body and soul when I was twenty years old."[44]* Indeed, several of the doctors I interviewed referred uneasily, and usually somewhat noncommittally, to Treitschke's famous phrase. For that image of Jewish-caused German "misfortune" encouraged every level of anti-Semitism from the medieval-mystical kind to modern "scientific racism" to the seemingly milder, even "reflective" approach favored by educated Germans: namely, that there was indeed a serious "Jewish problem" which Germans had to engage.

*Although Treitschke was originally a liberal sympathetic to John Stuart Mill and the American Declaration of Independence, his fierce nationalism went even beyond that customary for the "National Liberals" among whom he initially belonged. Treitschke gave intellectual legitimation to the anti-Semitic movement of his time, and insisted (probably correctly) that his belief in the Jews as Germany's misfortune would be shared by "men who would scornfully reject every notion of clerical intolerance or national arrogance."[45]

Treitschke's stress was on the "intrusion" of Judaism into what had to be a "Christian-German state," and on the danger that the children of these alien people from the East (that is, eastern Europe) "would one day dominate" Germany's institutions, especially the economy and the press.[46] That fear of Jewish "domination" seemed to many German doctors to have been borne out in their profession. In large cities, Jewish doctors could constitute as much as 50 percent of all physicians. And although they made up about 13 percent of physicians in Germany in general, even that far exceeded their general percentage of the population.[47] Beyond their numbers, many German-Jewish physicians had achieved great prominence and worldwide fame as a result of their scientific accomplishments. The situation was especially intolerable to the Nazis, who were relying on the profession to articulate and carry out their bold and malignant biomedical vision. That expectation of "racial leadership" was what led Hitler to lay particular stress on "the cleansing of the medical profession."[48]

The essential violence in hard-core Nazi doctors' attitudes toward Jewish colleagues in the new Third Reich was expressed, within two months of Hitler's becoming chancellor, during an anti-Jewish boycott campaign. In Berlin, on 1 April 1933, they used such tactics as contacting Jewish colleagues for ostensible consultations and having them picked up by car (sometimes supplied by the same German doctors), in which they were taken to remote places and beaten and left bleeding—or else threatened and humiliated them by making them run the gauntlet, hitting them with sticks, and exposing them to the sound of rifle fire.[49] At early professional conferences, there were indications of what was to come, as doctors in the chair spoke of "a foreign invasion . . . from the East [that] constitutes a menace to the German race," and of the "imperative necessity that this menace be . . . suppressed and eliminated."[50]

Official measures against Jews also began in early 1933: prohibition—at first with exceptions, which were gradually eliminated—of Jewish doctors from joining (and eventually from continuing earlier association with) the important national health insurance panels; step-by-step limitations on Jewish medical practice—early prohibition of all Jewish medical practice would have decimated German medical care—until, on 3 August 1939, as a "fourth amendment" to the Nuremberg Laws, the medical licenses of all Jewish doctors were nullified. There were characteristically legalistic definitions of who was a "non-Aryan" or Jew; and prohibitions, during periods when Jewish doctors were allowed to practice or to see non-Jewish patients, and parallel discouragement and subsequent prohibition of Aryan doctors from seeing Jewish patients. Eventually, Jewish doctors were not permitted to be referred to as physicians but only as "treaters of the sick," and Jewish surgeons as "specialized treaters in surgery." Before being forced to leave, or being incarcerated or killed, Jews had to be divested of their membership in the anointed fraternity of physician-healers.[51]

In addition, German doctors were discouraged from making reference in their scientific papers to work by Jewish doctors. When necessary to refer to such work, they were required to prepare a separate reference list for Jewish sources—as if to "keep the races separate" and thereby protect Aryan medicine from the Jewish taint in this ultimate form of scientific-literary segregation. In all these ways, given the German shortage of doctors over much of this period, pragmatic need was overruled by ideological requirement. Indeed, Nazi medical leaders conveyed the sense that only after this purification of their profession could they begin to call upon that profession for the realization of the biomedical vision.

Academic Medicine

Academic medicine, as part of the overall university structure, was an important focus for Nazi organizational therapy. The "disease" to be cured was what Josef Goebbels, Hitler's propaganda minister, called "flabby intellectualism," and what the education and culture minister, Bernhard Rust, called "disastrous concepts of liberty and equality," or what one educational reformer identified as "any autonomy and freedom of the teacher." Even before the Nazis, German universities had been bastions of conservative or reactionary political thought which tended to deify the concept of the state. But the Nazis made clear that they wanted something more. As Bavarian professors were told by their new minister of culture: "From now on, it will not be your job to determine whether something is true, but whether it is in the spirit of National Socialist revolution." Universities were to become (in the words of one historian) "intellectual frontier fortresses" and "bodies of troops"; professors were to develop "trooplike cooperation."[52]

Again, with their combination of visionary idealism and terror, the Nazis attracted considerable support from leading German professors: for example, 960 prominent German educators signed a public vow to support Adolf Hitler and the Nazi regime, which was published in the fall of 1933. Among the notable figures in that list were the philosopher Martin Heidegger and the world-famous Berlin University–Charité Hospital surgeon Ferdinand Sauerbruch.*

The coercive side of *Gleichschaltung* from above stressed what was called the *"Führer* principle" (*Führer* meaning "leader" in general), appointing reliable Nazis of dubious professional attainment as rectors and deans, so that they became in effect extensions of the regime's similarly directed Education Ministry. The ministry set overall policies concerning subjects taught (for example, more stress on racial biology and ideologized Ger-

---

*Sauerbruch's ardor for the regime subsequently diminished, and he was ultimately relatively even-handed in making use of his power within medical circles. Eventually, through contacts with Karl Bonhoeffer and Hans von Dohnanyi, he became tangentially involved in resistance to Hitler (see page 91).

man-centered history), regulations for faculty (getting rid of Jews and the ideologically recalcitrant and promoting faculty members who manifested Nazi enthusiasm), as well as student and admission policies (excluding Jews and Social Democrats and favoring stellar members of the Hitler Youth, the SA, or the SS).[53]

Equally important was *Gleichschaltung* from below: militant behavior on the part of the National Socialist Student League, which organized early, soon came to dominate or replace traditional student groups and formed an arrogant subculture with intense camaraderie and more than a tinge of violence. Its members broke up lectures that displeased them, and understood their task as opposing all teaching that was not rooted in National Socialist doctrine. When the Education Ministry found it necessary to tone down the students, it passed the mantle of *Gleichschaltung* from below to the Nazi League of University Instructors, whose leader understood his organization to be "the appointed trustee of the National Socialist Party at the universities to see that universities and scholarship are not only painted brown [the Nazi color] but really made over to fit the pattern of National Socialism."[54]

Medical students were told that they required "the synthesis of the marching boot and the book": that is, concrete involvement in military or paramilitary training as students and commitment to an all-out "war" against alleged enemies of Germany or National Socialism. Becoming a biological soldier, then, meant placing one's body and mind in the service of the militarized and ideologized authority of the state.

The Nazis sought to combine their radical alterations of universities with the claim to be part of ennobling tradition. A dramatic effort at this legitimation was the elaborately staged 550-year jubilee celebration at the University of Heidelberg in June and July of 1936. The rector of the university stressed "the devotion of the new Germany to the task of universal civilization and its sponsorship of high intellectual achievement in all fields of learning." Delegations came from all over the world, including representatives from eight universities in the United States. Among the Americans who received honorary degrees were Harry H. Laughlin, Davenport's assistant at Cold Spring Harbor and a tireless polemicist against immigrant groups he considered biologically inferior; and Foster Kennedy, a physician advocate of putting to death "the utterly unfit" among young retarded children.[55]* Both men were sympathetic to the Nazi sterilization laws.

In addition to purges of Jews and the politically unacceptable, medical faculties de-emphasized basic research, shortened the time of medical study to produce more doctors for the state, and modified the classical

*At the celebration, Harvard University delegates invited German universities to send representatives to their two-hundredth anniversary celebration later that year. British universities showed greater ethical sensitivity in refusing to send delegates to Heidelberg, after an exchange of correspondence in the London *Times* in which it was declared that "Heidelberg stands in the forefront" of German persecution of professors and lecturers for racial, religious, and political reasons.[56]

curriculum to give greater stress to military medicine, population politics, and racial biology.[57]

Resistance to these changes within medical faculties was extremely limited. One notable example of courageous intellectual opposition was that of Karl Saller, a prominent anthropologist who, even prior to the Nazi regime, had been critical of concepts of a Nordic race as a fixed biological entity. In his writing he had the temerity to insist that in all races there was a continually changing gene pool, a constant state of flux, and that the German race had become entwined with many others and contained extensive Slavic influences. That thesis questioned the very basis of the Nazi biomedical vision; and no less a personage than the Gestapo chief Reinhard Heydrich initiated an order prohibiting Saller from teaching, which forced him to leave his chair at the University of Munich. At his farewell lecture, he repeated his scientific views and stated that his love of truth and sense of honor prevented him from renouncing them. A handful of other anthropologists were slowly forced to leave university positions, but Saller was notable in speaking out so forthrightly. While many anthropologists, as well as biologists and physicians, must have agreed with his views, they tended to remain silent, and he found himself generally rejected and avoided by former colleagues and friends.[58]

Occasionally, during lectures, physicians reasserted intellectual and ethical positions at odds with the regime's practices. One anti-Nazi doctor I spoke to told how one of his teachers, Professor Karl Kleist, had refused to serve on a "euthanasia" commission and had declared to his students, "Just imagine, they want to have me, an old doctor, commit a crime with my own hands." The professor was said to have been denounced on the spot by student activists, though he was subjected to no punitive measures, possibly because of his seniority. Most anti-Nazi physicians during lectures tended to speak cautiously, more by innuendo. It is possible that Professor Kleist did so as well but that his former student, to whom he was a hero, wishes to remember him as having been even bolder than he was.

Perhaps the most moving of all expressions of opposition in Nazi Germany involved three medical students and a few additional students from other faculties at the University of Munich, in the dramatic White Rose resistance group. Over several months during 1942 to 1943, the group issued bold leaflets denouncing the Nazi regime and its immoral behavior ("For Hitler and his followers there can be no punishment on this earth which will expiate their crimes"), and calling for the German people to overthrow the regime and restore their good name. The leaflets also declared: "We will not be silent. We are your bad conscience. The White Rose will give you no rest." The students were eventually discovered and condemned by a Nazi "people's court"; most were beheaded. Significantly, one of the group's leading figures, Hans Scholl, had been inspired by a sermon of Bishop Clemens von Galen of Münster, condemning the "euthanasia" program, and is said to have responded, "At last somebody has had the courage to speak out."[59]

The Regime as a Healing Movement

Medical *Gleichschaltung* attempted to combine Nazification policies with a claim to continuity with older traditions of medical healing. Thus, even while investing administrative medical authority in recognizable professional mediocrities, the Nazis courted, often successfully, doctors with high professional reputations. And while the Nazis terrorized potential medical opponents, they also exhibited a certain élan in extending various forms of medical care to the entire German population. And at the same time that they developed a policy of sterilizing or killing people considered unfit for a society of the strong, the Nazis boasted of spectacular operative results and humane employment arrangements for people who had lost hands or limbs, especially in combat. In these ways, most doctors could continue to view themselves as authentic physicians, whatever the degree of Nazification of their profession.

At advanced six-week training programs for future medical leaders, doctors were instructed in both Nazi biomedical principles and German public health needs. And ordinary doctors were required to take three-week courses every five years on recent medical developments. The medical true believers, such as Professor Franz Hamburger of Vienna, considered National Socialism to mean "a revolution in every sphere of our civilization and culture," including "a real renaissance of medical science, on Nazi foundations."[60] The Nazi regime sought international medical prestige and proudly sponsored international conferences, but at the same time turned inward, covered over things they did not want seen by physicians elsewhere in the world, and had a policy against doctors accepting Nobel Prizes out of fear that these might be given to Jews or Social Democrats and also because anything "international" rather than *völkisch* was suspect.

Perhaps the most severe conflict between the Nazi biomedical vision and the traditional medical profession was in relation to nonmedical healers, known as "healing practitioners" (*Heilpraktiker*) and "healers" (*Heilkundiger*). These groups generally stressed the outdoor life, natural foods, and overall reorientation in living; they often flouted established medical practice and sometimes treated serious diseases with dubious therapies. Long active in Germany, these healers appealed to the regime's biological romanticism and mysticism and found their strongest supporter in Deputy Party Leader Rudolf Hess, the most intense biological mystic in the Nazi inner circle. Gerhard Wagner praised their "biological insights" and repeatedly sought a "synthesis of the one-sided old school medicine and the nature cure methods" as consistent with the National Socialist concept of "natural and biological laws controlling all events."[61] With that kind of sponsorship, joint conferences of the healing practitioners and traditional medical groups were held and various forms of integration were projected. But these were resisted by traditional medical-academic groups; Wagner was forced to retreat from his integrative efforts, and his successor had considerably less sympathy for the healing practitioners.

The regime's fundamental conflict here could never be resolved: on the one hand, its attraction to these healers, seemingly consistent with the visionary National Socialist claim to harmony with nature and biology; on the other hand, its equal claim to continuity with scientific and medical tradition and its pragmatic commitment to mobilizing physicians for its medicalized approach to race and society. Clearly, traditional medicine won out, but the regime's continuing relationship to healing practitioners and their massive numbers of clients contributed to its aura as a "healing" movement.[62]*

Jewish Doctors as Anti-Healers

This claim to special healing power on the part of the "new German medicine" depended upon not only excluding Jews but rendering Jewish doctors a special medical antitype. In one cartoon (originally printed in the notorious journal *Der Stürmer*), there appeared caricatures of evil Jewish doctors performing abortions on young Aryan women and thereby subverting the Nazi campaign to create pure Aryan children. In another cartoon sequence, with the legend "What happened to Inge when she went to a Jewish doctor," little Inge is warned by the Nazi Girls League against going to him but does anyhow and encounters a frightening creature threatening to attack her. While claiming to be a healer, that is, the Jewish doctor threatened innocent Aryan girls with physical harm, rape, or abortion, undermined pure German womanhood, and was the enemy of Aryan racial revitalization.[63]

Moreover, these vulgar images were legitimated in writings by physicians. An article purporting to be a professional overview of the history of Jews in medicine went back to the time of Moses to focus on the Jewish *Volk,* on its policy of "preservation of purity" and refusal of "contamination" by intermarriage. The Germans were therefore correct in "holding them to this law" and in "guarding against mixing of our blood with Jews." The medical author then associated Jewish doctors with corrupt commercialism, socialism, and Marxism, self-serving networks of mutual referral, and atomization of medicine in which one focuses on chemistry and physics and "treats sicknesses and not sick people" while "forgetting

---

* In 1939, as a lasting expression of its relationship to the "nature movement," the Nazis opened a new hospital outside Munich that was to epitomize many of the principles of the "new German medicine": for example, common dining halls, outdoor bathing pools, special indoor physical-therapy centers, and recreation centers. These features would aid physical and mental rehabilitation, prevent "diseases of civilization," and strengthen "natural forces of resistance" to diseases that were both physical and psychological. Not a "hospital," it was a "house of health" *(Gesundungshaus).*

the patient." More than that, Jewish obsession with sexology and defense of homosexuality, along with the creation of Freudian psychoanalysis—all these were aspects of "sexual degeneration, a breakdown of the family and loss of all that is decent," and ultimately the destruction of the German *Volk*. [64]

Beyond the ordinary Jewish menace, the Jewish doctor became a more formidable threat to the German *Volk,* the embodiment of the anti-healer who must be dealt with if medicine was to join in the great national healing mission, and the advance image of what Nazi doctors were actually to become: the healer turned killer.

Positive and Negative Eugenics

Sterilization policies were always associated with the therapeutic and regenerative principles of the biomedical vision: with the "purification of the national body" and the "eradication of morbid hereditary dispositions." Sterilization was considered part of "negative eugenics": subsequent ordinances also prohibited the issuance of marriage licenses in situations where either party suffered from contagious disease, had been placed under a legal guardian, was afflicted with significant mental disturbance, or fell into any of the categories of hereditary disease listed in sterilization ordinances. These restrictions were "balanced" by programs of "positive eugenics"—encouraging large families and constructive health practices among Aryan couples, etc.—because "generations may come and go, but the German people shall live on forever."[65]

Always at issue for the medical profession was its role in protecting and revitalizing the genetic health of the *Volk.* Doctors were given special status on commissions created to approve marriages on the basis of Nuremberg racial statutes, even as the profession expanded its role in social programs and preventive work; at the same time, doctors continued to engage in private practice and to maintain their high earning power, aided by the elimination of Jewish medical competition. The 1935 Physicians' Law formalized the authority structure and its special status in the regime, reaffirming its "vocation" of preserving and improving the "good heredity," "racial stock," and general health of the German *Volk.* Subsequent laws, far from not diminishing this status, increased the requirements of physicians as "public servants" and "biological state officers," restricting such things as their traditional professional confidentiality with patients should the regime require information.[66]

This commitment to "positive eugenics"—or "the battle for births," as it was sometimes called—was inseparable from "negative eugenics"—sterilization and, eventually, "euthanasia." Abortions were prohibited, but sterilization courts could rule that pregnancy could be interrupted for eugenic reasons in a "racial emergency" situation: that is, if the future child was likely to inherit certain defects or (in all probability) had mixed (Jewish and non-Jewish) parentage.

The story of Carl Clauberg reveals the inseparability of the Nazi concepts of positive and negative genetics. A gynecologist who became a professor, Clauberg's early research on female hormones in collaboration with the Schering-Kahlbaum Pharmaceutical Company produced, during the late 1920s and early 1930s, the preparations known as Progynon and Proluton, for the treatment of infertility. After being introduced to Himmler in 1940, Clauberg began to concentrate his research on the development of nonsurgical methods of mass sterilization, eventuating in the notorious Auschwitz sterilization experiments which will be discussed in chapter 15. And as late as the latter part of 1944, Clauberg was back at research on sterility and reproduction as chief of a new institution known as the "City of Mothers."[67]

In another expression of positive eugenics, doctors were active in research on people viewed as hereditarily gifted, and in helping to enlist the medical profession for what was called the "fostering of talent."

They were also active in a criminal aspect of positive eugenics known as *Lebensborn,* or "Spring of Life." Heinrich Himmler had created this institution as part of his plan "to breed the SS into a biological élite, . . . [a] racial nucleus from which Germany could replenish an Aryan inheritance now dangerously diluted through generations of race-mixing." *Lebensborn* administered welfare assistance to SS families in the service of "racially valuable" children, and extended maternity and child-care facilities to married and unmarried mothers. But *Lebensborn* also engaged in the kidnaping of "biologically valuable" children (those who met Nordic criteria) in occupied areas, some of them fathered by German occupiers. The policy was explained plainly on one occasion by Himmler himself: "I really intend to take German blood from wherever it is to be found in the world, to rob it and steal it wherever I can."[68]

Doctors were central to *Lebensborn*; its medical director, Gregor Ebner, was an "old medical fighter" said to have been personally close to Himmler. Ebner was solicitous of his Nordic babies (once boasting that "in thirty years' time we shall have 600 extra regiments"); he applauded the kidnapings, signed orders for sterilizing "nonvaluable" (insufficiently Nordic) children, and supervised a "medical" sequence in which some of those children judged "nonvaluable" were shipped to their deaths in concentration camps.[69]

While it has been estimated that only about 350 doctors "committed medical crimes," that figure represents a vast wave of criminality, as Alexander Mitscherlich has written,[70] and was perhaps only "the tip of the iceberg" as he told me. Nor does that figure include the legions of German doctors who slandered and extruded their Jewish colleagues; or who perpetrated and acted upon vulgar and discriminatory racial concepts.

Thus, while a few doctors resisted, and large numbers had little sympathy for the Nazis, *as a profession* German physicians offered themselves to the regime. So also did most other professions; but with doctors, that gift included using their intellectual authority to justify and carry out medicalized killing. Doctors promoted the idea that collective German existence was a medical matter, and many succumbed to the temptation articulated as early as 1922 by the popular writer Ernst Mann.* Mann, in defending direct medical killing, considered illness "a disgrace to be managed by health control." His principle was that "misery can only be removed from the world by painless extermination of the miserable!" The entire process, moreover, was to be taken over by the physician—at which point, "doctors could be the true saviors of mankind."[71]

---

*Ernst Mann was a pseudonym for Gerhard Hoffman, a critic of mass culture and an interpreter of science.

Chapter 2

"Euthanasia": Direct Medical Killing

The state organism . . . [is] a whole with its own laws and rights, much like one self-contained human organism . . . which, in the interest of the welfare of the whole, also—as we doctors know— abandons and rejects parts or particles that have become worthless or dangerous.

—ALFRED HOCHE

Either one is a doctor or one is not.

—A former Nazi doctor

For a doctor, there is a large step from ligating spermatic cords or ovarian tubes, or even removing uteri, to killing or designating for death one's own patients. Medical *Gleichschaltung* made that step possible. The Nazis could combine active participation by a broad spectrum of German physicians, especially psychiatrists, with a secret plan emanating from the highest Party authority. The characteristic mixture of terror and idealism could now concretize the principle of "life unworthy of life" and authorize the killing of both children and adults.

The Background

There was considerable advocacy elsewhere of "mercy killing," including its recommendation in the United States by the same Foster Kennedy who was honored at the Heidelberg jubilee.[1] And anyone trained in American medicine has personal experience of doctors, nurses, and medical attendants colluding in the death of patients, usually children, who have been extremely impaired physically and mentally. But those practices have been restrained by legal limits and strong public reaction, and have not developed into a systematic program of killing those designated as unworthy of living.

In Germany, however, such a project had been discussed from the time of the impact of "scientific racism" in intellectual circles during the last decade of the nineteenth century. Central to that development was the stress upon the integrity of the organic *body* of the *Volk*—the collectivity, people, or nation as embodiment of racial-cultural substance. That kind of focus, as with any intense nationalism, takes on a biological cast. One views one's group as an "organism" whose "life" one must preserve, and whose "death" one must combat, in ways that transcend individual fate.

One such theorist, Adolf Jost, issued an early call for direct medical killing in a book published in 1895 and significantly entitled "The Right to Death" *(Das Recht auf den Tod)*. Jost argued that control over the death of the individual must ultimately belong to the social organism, the state. This concept is in direct opposition to the Anglo-American tradition of euthanasia, which emphasizes the *individual's* "right to die" or "right to death" or "right to his or her own death," as the ultimate human claim. In contrast, Jost was pointing to the state's right to kill. While he spoke of compassion and relief of suffering of the incurably ill, his focus was mainly on the health of the *Volk* and the state. He pointed out that the state already exercises those "rights" in war, where thousands of individuals are sacrificed for the good of the state. Ultimately the argument was biological: "The rights to death [are] the key to the fitness of life." The state must own death—must kill—in order to keep the social organism alive and healthy.[2]*

The crucial work—"The Permission to Destroy Life Unworthy of Life" *(Die Freigabe der Vernichtung lebensunwerten Lebens)*—was published in 1920 and written jointly by two distinguished German professors: the jurist Karl Binding, retired after forty years at the University of Leipzig, and Alfred Hoche, professor of psychiatry at the University of Freiburg. Carefully argued in the numbered-paragraph form of the traditional philosophical treatise, the book included as "unworthy life" not only the incurably ill but large segments of the mentally ill, the feebleminded, and retarded and deformed children. More than that, the authors professionalized and medicalized the entire concept. And they stressed the *therapeutic* goal of that concept: destroying life unworthy of life is "purely a healing treatment" and a "healing work."[3]

---

*The principle was disseminated by several influential writers. Implicit in some of Nietzsche's works, it was embraced by a circle of early "scientific" racists in Munich, led by the anthropologist Alfred Ploetz and including the publisher J. F. Lehmann, whose press brought out most of the group's pamphlets and books.

Binding's section explored the doctor's legal responsibility in "death assistance" *(Sterbehilfe)* and the "killing of the consenting participant," and in the killing of "incurable idiots" unable to consent. He advocated a carefully controlled juridical process, with applications for killing evaluated by a three-person panel (a general physician, a psychiatrist, and a lawyer). A patient who had given his consent to be killed would have the right to withdraw that consent at any time, but there was also an emphasis on the legal protection of physicians involved in the killing process.[4]

Hoche, in his section, insisted that such a policy of killing was compassionate and consistent with medical ethics; he pointed to situations in which doctors were obliged to destroy life (such as killing a live baby at the moment of birth, or interrupting a pregnancy to save the mother). He went on to invoke a concept of "mental death" in various forms of psychiatric disturbance, brain damage, and retardation. He characterized these people as "human ballast" *(Ballastexistenzen)* and "empty shells of human beings"—terms that were to reverberate in Nazi Germany. Putting such people to death, Hoche wrote, "is *not* to be equated with other types of killing . . . but [is] an *allowable, useful act. "* He was saying that these people are *already* dead.[5]

Hoche referred to the tremendous economic burden such people cause society to bear; especially those who are young, mentally deficient, and otherwise healthy and who would require a lifetime of institutionalization. He specifically medicalized the organic concept of the state by his insistence that "single less valuable members have to be abandoned and pushed out." He added a striking note of medical hubris in insisting that "the physician has no doubt about the hundred-percent certainty of correct selection" and "proven scientific criteria" to establish the *"impossibility of improvement* of a mentally dead person." But he ultimately revealed himself to be a biological visionary: "A new age will come which, from the standpoint of a higher morality, will no longer heed the demands of an inflated concept of humanity and an overestimation of the value of life as such."[6]

The Binding-Hoche study reflects the general German mood during the period following the First World War. Hoche was considered a leading humanitarian and, in a 1917 article, had rejected medical killing. Shortly afterward, his son was killed in the war, and he was said to have been deeply affected by both his personal loss and the German defeat. Like many Germans then, he felt himself experiencing the darkest of times, and the book was an expression of personal mission and a call to national revitalization. Indeed, from the time of Jost, war had been invoked by advocates of direct medical killing. The argument went that the best young men died in war, causing a loss to the *Volk* (or to any society) of the best available genes. The genes of those who did not fight (the worst genes) then proliferated freely, accelerating biological and cultural degeneration.

"Euthanasia" Consciousness

Binding and Hoche turned out to be the prophets of direct medical killing. While there were subsequent papers and discussions by German psychiatrists of the Hoche-Binding thesis, it is probably fair to say that, during the years prior to the Nazi assumption of power, their thesis was by no means a majority view in German psychiatry and medicine.[7] Under the Nazis, there was increasing discussion of the possibility of mercy killings, of the Hoche concept of the "mentally dead," and of the enormous economic drain on German society caused by the large number of these impaired people. A mathematics text asked the student to calculate how many government loans to newly married couples could be granted for the amount of money it cost the state to care for "the crippled, the criminal, and the insane."[8]

Moreover, the extensive public and medical discussion of the sterilization project tended always to suggest that more radical measures were necessary. In an August 1933 speech at the opening ceremony for a state medical academy in Munich, the Bavarian commissioner of health, Professor Walter Schultze, declared that sterilization was insufficient: psychopaths, the mentally retarded, and other inferior persons must be isolated and killed. He noted, "This policy has already been initiated in our concentration camps."[9] On all sides there took shape the principle that the practice of extermination was part of the legitimate business of government.

Mental hospitals became an important center for the developing "euthanasia" consciousness. From 1934, these hospitals were encouraged to neglect their patients; each year funds were reduced and state inspections of standards were either made perfunctory or suspended altogether. Especially important were courses held in psychiatric institutions for leading government officials and functionaries—courses featuring grotesque "demonstrations" orchestrated to display the most repulsive behavior of regressed patients—of "life unworthy of life." After 1938, these courses were systematically extended to include members of the SS, political leaders of the Party, the police, prison officials, and the press. In the process, the medical profession itself was made ready for the extraordinary tasks it was to be assigned.[10]

The Nazis exploited film for the same purpose, and doctors played a large role here as well. Early films, such as "The Inheritance" (*Das Erbe,* 1935), were mainly didactic and ostensibly scientific in depicting medical and social consequences of hereditary impairment. A subsequent film, "The Victim of the Past" (*Opfer der Vergangenheit,* 1937), covered the same ground and went much further: it not only contrasted "healthy German citizens" (girls doing gymnastics, etc.) with regressed occupants of back wards, but spoke of Jewish mental patients and of the "frightening transgression" of the law of natural selection, which must be reinstated "by humane methods." "The Victim of the Past" was ceremonially introduced by Gerhard Wagner at a Berlin film showcase and was shown widely throughout Germany's 5,300 cinema houses.

The third film, "I Accuse" (*Ich klage an,* 1941), was unique in that it dealt specifically with medical killing and, in fact, emerged from a suggestion by Karl Brandt, the early medical leader of that project, that a film be made to persuade the German public to accept the idea of "euthanasia." A related purpose was to test public opinion about whether there was sufficient support to legalize the program and bring it out into the open. The film was based on the novel *Mission and Conscience* by a physician-writer, Helmut Unger, a Berlin ophthalmologist who also served as a consultant of the child "euthanasia" program and as Dr. Wagner's press representative. "I Accuse" was clearly a falsification of the actual Nazi policy: the Nazis murdered mental patients against their will; the film depicts a physician giving a lethal injection to his incurably ill wife in response to her desperate plea that he do so to relieve her of her terrible pain and suffering. Indeed, a sympathetic member of the jury before whom the physician is eventually tried states categorically that "the most important precondition is always that the patient wants it." The film's real message is more or less subliminal—a reference, in the midst of ostensibly thoughtful discussion, that an exception to that voluntary principle should be made for the mentally ill, where "the state *must* take over the responsibility."[11]

But "I Accuse" is of respectable artistic quality; and after viewing portions of it, I could understand why doctors I interviewed still felt its impact and remembered the extensive discussion it stimulated among their colleagues and fellow students about the morality of a doctor's aiding incurable patients to achieve the death they long for.

These doctors' response was confirmed by a research report prepared by the SS Security Service (the *Sicherheitsdienst,* or SD), which stated that the film had "aroused great interest" throughout the Reich and had been "favorably received and discussed," and that the majority of the German population accepted its argument in principle, with some reservations concerning possible abuse and questions of consent. These reservations could generally be overcome by the "convening of a *medical committee* in the presence of the family doctor" for declaring a patient incurable: that is, by keeping the procedure medicalized. Doctors polled also had "a mostly positive response." Doubts were raised, especially by older physicians, concerning accuracy of diagnoses and other medical arrangements; but the investigators had the impression that the medical profession was ready to take on or at least go along with such a project.[12]* The project that doctors and others saw themselves approving, however, was essentially voluntary dying with careful medical supervision and built-in arrangements to prevent any possible abuse. It is unlikely that many respondents

---

*These SD "reports from the Reich" were, according to Heinz Hohne, based on "a sort of secret Gallup poll," and were thought to be rather accurate, although often impressionistic in content.

knew that a very different kind of killing had long been under way and had in fact already ended, at least officially, by the time the film was shown.

Hitler's Involvement—The First "Mercy Killing"

Hitler had an intense interest in direct medical killing. His first known expression of intention to eliminate the "incurably ill" was made to Dr. Gerhard Wagner at the Nuremberg Party rally of 1935. Karl Brandt, who overheard that remark, later testified that Hitler thought that the demands and upheavals of war would mute expected religious opposition and enable such a project to be implemented smoothly. Hitler was also said to have stated that a war effort requires a very healthy people, and that the generally diminished sense of the value of human life during war made it "the best time for the elimination of the incurably ill." And he was reportedly affected by the burden imposed by the mentally ill not only on relatives and the general population but on the medical profession. In 1936, Wagner held discussions with "a small circle of friends" (specifically, high-ranking officials, some of them doctors) about killing "idiotic children" and "mentally ill" people, and making films in "asylums and idiot homes" to demonstrate the misery of their lives. This theoretical and tactical linking of war to direct medical killing was maintained throughout.[13]

By 1938, the process had gone much further. Discussions moved beyond high-level political circles; and at a national meeting of leading government psychiatrists and administrators, an SS officer gave a talk in which he stated that "the solution of the problem of the mentally ill becomes easy if one eliminates these people."[14]

Toward the end of 1938, the Nazi regime was receiving requests from relatives of newborns or very young infants with severe deformities and brain damage for the granting of a mercy killing.[15] These requests had obviously been encouraged, and were channeled directly to the Chancellery—that is, to Hitler's personal office. Whatever the plans for using war as a cover, the program for killing children was well under way by the time the war began. And from the beginning, this program circumvented ordinary administrative channels and was associated directly with Hitler himself.

The occasion for initiating the actual killing of children, and of the entire "euthanasia" project, was the petition for the "mercy killing" (*Gnadentod*, really "mercy death") of an infant named Knauer, born blind, with one leg and part of one arm missing, and apparently an "idiot." Subsequent recollections varied concerning who had made the petition and the extent of the deformity, as the case quickly became mythologized.*

---

*Hans Hefelmann, chief of the responsible Chancellery office, remembered that the child lacked three limbs and that its grandmother made the request. Brandt made the father the petitioner.

In late 1938 or early 1939, Hitler ordered Karl Brandt, his personal physician and close confidant, to go to the clinic at the University of Leipzig, where the child was hospitalized, in order to determine whether the information submitted was accurate and to consult with physicians there: "If the facts given by the father were correct, I was to inform the physicians in [Hitler's] name that they could carry out euthanasia." Brandt was also empowered to tell those physicians that any legal proceedings against them would be quashed by order of Hitler.[16]

Brandt reported that the doctors were of the opinion "that there was no justification for keeping [such a child] alive"; and he added (in his testimony at the Nuremberg Medical Trial) that "it was pointed out [presumably by the doctors he spoke to] that in maternity wards in some circumstances it is quite natural for the doctors themselves to perform euthanasia in such a case without anything further being said about it." The doctor with whom he mainly consulted was Professor Werner Catel, head of the Leipzig pediatrics clinic and a man who was soon to assume a leading role in the project. All was to be understood as a responsible medical process, so that—as Brandt claimed was Hitler's concern—"the parents should not have the impression that they themselves were responsible for the death of this child."[17] (See pages 115–16 for the child's father's recollection of Brandt.) On returning to Berlin, Brandt was authorized by Hitler, who did not want to be publicly identified with the project, to proceed in the same way in similar cases: that is, to formalize a program with the help of the high-ranking Reich leader Philip Bouhler, chief of Hitler's Chancellery. This "test case" was pivotal for the two killing programs—of children and of adults.

The two programs were conducted separately, though they overlapped considerably in personnel and in other ways.

The Killing of Children

It seemed easier—perhaps more "natural" and at least less "unnatural" —to begin with the very young: first, newborns; then, children up to three and four; then, older ones. Similarly, the authorization—at first, oral and secret and to be "kept in a very narrow scope, and cover only the most serious cases"—was later to become loose, extensive, and increasingly known. A small group of doctors and Chancellery officials held discussions in which they laid out some of the ground rules for the project. Then a group of medical consultants known to have a "positive" attitude to the project was assembled, including administrators, pediatricians, and psychiatrists.[18]

The sequence was typical: the order to implement the biomedical vision came from the political leadership (in this case Hitler himself); the order was conveyed to a leading doctor within the regime, who combined with high-ranking administrators to organize a structure for the project; and prominent academic administrative doctors sympathetic to the regime were called in to maintain and administer this *medicalized* structure. It was decided that the program was to be secretly run from the Chancellery, though the health division of the Reich Interior Ministry was to help administer it. And for that purpose an organization was created: the Reich Committee for the Scientific Registration of Serious Hereditary and Congenital Diseases *(Reichsausschuss zur wissenschaftlichen Erfassung von erb- und anlagebedingten schweren Leiden)*. The name conveyed the sense of a formidable medical-scientific registry board, although its leader, Hans Hefelmann, had his degree in agricultural economics. That impression was maintained in a strictly confidential directive (of 18 August 1939) by the minister of the interior to non-Prussian state governments. The directive stated that, "for the clarification of scientific questions in the field of congenital malformation and mental retardation, the earliest possible registration" was required of all children under three years of age in whom any of the following "serious hereditary diseases" were "suspected": idiocy and mongolism (especially when associated with blindness and deafness); microcephaly; hydrocephaly; malformations of all kinds, especially of limbs, head, and spinal column; and paralysis, including spastic conditions.[19]

Midwives were required to make these reports at the time of birth (with a portion of the report filled in by a doctor, if present), and doctors themselves were to report all such children up to the age of three. District medical officers were responsible for the accuracy of the reports, and chief physicians of maternity clinics and wards were all notified that such reports were required.[20] The reports took the form of questionnaires that originated in the Reich Health Ministry. At first simple, they were expanded considerably in June 1940 by participating doctors to go beyond specific illness or condition and to include: details about the birth; elements of family history, especially concerning hereditary illness and such things as excessive use of alcohol, nicotine, or drugs; a further evaluation of the condition (by a physician) indicating possibilities for improvement, life expectancy, prior institutional observation and treatment, details of physical and mental development, and descriptions of convulsions and related phenomena.[21] The wording of the questionnaire and the essential absence of a traditional medical history and record led many physicians and district medical officers to assume, at least at first, that affected children would merely be registered for statistical purposes. (Hefelmann later testified that the diseases were broadly described in order to disguise the reason for the duty to report.)[22]

Three central medical experts* were then required to make their

---

*The medical experts consisted of four outside consultants and two members of the "euthanasia" bureaucracy. The consultants were Werner Catel, the professor of psychiatry at the Leipzig clinic where the Knauer child had been treated; Professor Hans Heinze, head of the state institution at Görden near Brandenburg, which had a large children's division;

either-or judgments without examining the children or even reading their medical records, but solely on the basis of the questionnaire. They recorded their decisions on a small form with the names of the three experts printed on the left side; on the right side, under the word "treatment" (*Behandlung*), were three columns, making a small space available parallel to each individual expert's name. If an expert decided upon "treatment" —meaning the killing of the child—he put a plus sign (+) in the left column. If he decided against killing the child, he put a minus sign (−) in the middle column. If he thought a definite decision should not yet be made, he wrote in the right-hand column the phrase "temporary postponement" or the word "observation" and then initialed this opinion. The same form was passed in sequence to the three experts, so that the second one receiving it would know the opinion of the first, and the third would know the opinion of the first two. A unanimous opinion was necessary for a child to be killed—an outcome favored by the reporting arrangement.

Where a decision for or against killing was not unanimous, there was initially a policy of requesting additional information from the responsible local medical officer. But this policy was soon abandoned, probably because of its further threat to the program's secrecy (which in any case gradually eroded, but which authorities tried nonetheless to maintain), and possibly also because of the administrative delays entailed. Instead, these children, along with those for whom observation or postponement was specifically recommended, were sent for further observation to the same children's units where the killing was done. After a specified time, the consultants received additional information on the children, along with the original questionnaires, as a basis for a final decision. This arrangement also strongly favored a decision for killing. But the process was referred to as a means of obtaining "expert opinion." The units where the killing was done were parts of children's institutions whose chiefs and prominent doctors were known to be politically reliable and "positive" toward the goals of the Reich Committee. These centers were grandly referred to as "Reich Committee Institutions," "Children's Specialty Institutions (or Departments)," or even "Therapeutic Convalescent Institutions." Actually no such separate institutions existed. The children marked for death were usually dispersed among ordinary pediatric patients; some were kept in separate wards of their own.23*

The first Children's Specialty Department was established in the state institution at Görden and was referred to publicly as a "Special Psychiat-

---

the pediatric psychiatrist Ernst Wentzler of Berlin, and the ophthalmologist-author Helmut Unger. The institutions led by three of these men eventually became part of the child-"euthanasia" network; indeed Görden was its first and most important establishment. The representatives of the "euthanasia" bureaucracy were Brandt and Linden.

*According to Hefelmann's testimony, children were already being sent to Görden in October 1939, the committee wanting particularly "to put newborns to sleep as soon as possible," to prevent "closer bonds between mothers and their children."24

ric Youth Department." Görden and a few other centers were exceptional in their degree of specialization. Since Görden was considered to be scientifically advanced and its psychiatrist head Dr. Heinze had special credentials in that area, a grotesque half-truth reinforced the deception in the announcement by the minister of the interior on 1 July 1940 that at Görden "under the direction of specialists, all therapeutic possibilities will be administered according to the latest scientific knowledge."[25] Eventually a network of some thirty killing areas within existing institutions was set up throughout Germany and in Austria and Poland. They could thus handle the volume of children designated for killing and at the same time provide the service close to the homes of the families involved —a saving in money and transportation and a means of rendering parents more amenable to accepting the necessary transfers. The heads of all these institutions were fully informed and worked closely with the Reich Committee. In various correspondence concerning transfers, it was announced that "the child would receive the best and most modern therapy available."[26]

Medical "As If"

All of this falsification, then, was in the service of medical claim. Everyone proceeded *as if* these children were to receive the blessings of medical science, were to be healed rather than killed. The falsification was clearly intended to deceive—the children's families, the children themselves when old enough, and the general public. But it also served psychological needs of the killers in literally expressing the Nazi reversal of healing and killing. For example, a doctor could tell a parent that "it might be necessary to perform a surgical operation that could possibly have an unfavorable result," or explain that "the ordinary therapy employed until now could no longer help their child so that extraordinary therapeutic measures have to be taken." Dr. Heinze, who used such phrases with parents, explained in court testimony that there had been truth to what he said: "A very excitable child . . . completely idiotic . . . could not be kept quiet with the normal dose of sedatives," so that "an overdose . . . had to be used in order to . . . avoid endangering itself through its own restlessness." At the same time, "we physicians know that such an overdose of a sedative, for children usually luminal . . . could cause pneumonia, . . . and that this is virtually incurable."[27] It is quite possible that Dr. Heinze not *only* was consciously lying, but was enabled by the medicalization of the murders partly to deceive himself: to come to believe, at least at moments, that the children were being given some form of therapy, and that their deaths were due to their own abnormality.

In the same spirit, the policy was to gain "consent" from the parents for the transfer. Those who showed reluctance to give that consent received letters emphasizing the seriousness and permanence of their child's disability, telling them that they "should be grateful" that there were available for children thus affected by fate facilities where "the best and most efficacious treatment is available," and then declaring that "neither a delay nor a cancellation of the transfer is possible." Should the parents continue to oppose it, "further steps, such as withdrawal of your guardianship, will have to be taken."[28] This threat to take away legal guardianship usually sufficed, but if it did not there could be the further threat of calling a parent up for special labor duty. The coercion here was in the service not only of the killing policy itself but also of maintaining its medical structure.

That structure served to diffuse individual responsibility. In the entire sequence—from the reporting of cases by midwives or doctors, to the supervision of such reporting by institutional heads, to expert opinions rendered by central consultants, to coordination of the marked forms by Health Ministry officials, to the appearance of the child at the Reich Committee institution for killing—there was at no point a sense of personal responsibility for, or even involvement in, the murder of another human being. Each participant could feel like no more than a small cog in a vast, officially sanctioned, medical machine.

Before being killed, children were generally kept for a few weeks in the institution in order to convey the impression that they were being given some form of medical therapy. The killing was usually arranged by the director of the institution or by another doctor working under him, frequently by innuendo rather than specific order. It was generally done by means of luminal tablets dissolved in liquid, such as tea, given to the child to drink. This sedative was given repeatedly—often in the morning and at night—over two or three days, until the child lapsed into continuous sleep. The luminal dose could be increased until the child went into coma and died. For children who had difficulty drinking, luminal was sometimes injected. If the luminal did not kill the child quickly enough—as happened with excitable children who developed considerable tolerance for the drug because of having been given so much of it—a fatal morphine-scopolamine injection was given. The cause of death was listed as a more or less ordinary disease such as pneumonia, which could even have the kind of kernel of truth we have noted.[29]

The institutional doctor, then, was at the killing edge of the medical structure, whatever the regime's assurance that the state took full responsibility. Yet he developed—in fact, cultivated—the sense that, as an agent of the state, he was powerless: from his vantage point, as one such doctor reported, "these children were already marked for killing on their transfer reports," so that "I did not even bother to examine them." Indeed, whatever examination he performed was no more than a formality, since he did not have the authority to question the definitive judgment of the three-man panel of experts.

Yet later, program administrators countered with the insistence that "the if, when, and how of carrying out a mercy death is up to the judgment of the doctor in charge, who voluntarily and out of conviction agrees to euthanasia and its implementation. It is a 'can' and not a 'must' order."[30] They even claimed that, in some situations, there were no expert opinions at all and the decision about whether to kill a child was left to the discretion of the institutional doctor. To be sure, this kind of later legal testimony was put forward by the program's organizers in order to deny or minimize their own responsibility. But that evasion of responsibility from the top can be said to have been built into the project: the institutional doctor's role as triggerman was a way of investing the actual killing with a "medical responsibility" that was at least partially his. And the contradictory legal status of the "euthanasia" program—a *de facto* law that was not a law—added to the confusion and contradiction surrounding the question of anyone's responsibility.

Inevitably, there was great slippage in whatever discipline originally prevailed—broadening the killing net and fulfilling the regime's ultimate purposes. As the age limit of children included moved upward, it came to include a large number of older children and adolescents and even at times overlapped with the adult killing project. Conditions considered a basis for killing also expanded and came to include mongolism (not listed at the beginning) as well as various borderline or limited impairments in children of different ages, culminating in the killing of those designated as juvenile delinquents. Jewish children could be placed in the net primarily because they were Jewish; and at one of the institutions, a special department was set up for "minor Jewish-Aryan half-breeds *(Mischlinge)*.

After 1941, the year Hitler officially ordered the general "euthanasia" project terminated, the killing of children continued, indeed probably increased, and was conducted still more haphazardly. It is estimated that five thousand children were killed—but the total was probably much higher if we include the "wild euthanasia" period (see chapter 4).[31]

The resistance to children's euthanasia came mostly from families of children killed or threatened with death, later from Catholic and Protestant clergy, and to a lesser extent from within certain medical circles, all of which I will discuss in chapter 3. But certain forms of resistance from within the children's project are worth mentioning here, if only because they were so limited. There were many attempts—it is hard to say how many—on the part of doctors either to avoid diagnoses on children that they knew would lead directly to death, or to arrange to release children from institutions before they were swallowed up by the killing machinery. A Dr. Möckel at Wiesloch is reported to have refused an appointment as chief of a children's section because he claimed to be "too weak" for the implementation of the Reich Committee's program. And there were other reports of high-ranking doctors in certain areas responsible for appointments to these institutions holding back on those appointments because of the claim that candidates were too young and inexperienced. One doctor who had been extremely active as an expert consultant in the adult program refused to kill nine of the twelve children sent to the children's unit he became chief of because, as he put it, "a therapeutic and nursing institution is not the right place for such measures." And there is a report of a nurse who refused to take part in killings of children because she felt herself becoming "hysterical" from the "mental strain."[32] In general, there was probably considerably less medical resistance to the killing of children than to the killing of adults.

"Not Murder [but] a Putting-to-Sleep"

Precisely that impression was vividly conveyed to me by a doctor I interviewed who had been immediately involved in the killing project: "According to the thinking of that time, in the case of children killing seemed somehow justifiable . . . whereas in the case of the adult mentally ill, that was definitely pure murder." Hans F. went on to tell how severely impaired the children were when they arrived ("My God . . . such high-grade imbeciles!"), that they had been insufficiently fed and were "in terrible condition," and how events were arranged so that the killing was not *quite* killing. The head of the institution told one of the two or three nurses colluding in the program to give the designated children luminal in their food—an order that, if not examined closely, could seem routine for impaired restless children:

> Those who were cleared for killing had prescribed for them much higher doses of luminal. . . . Those were children who were spastic, . . . had cerebral polio, . . . were idiots, . . . were unable to speak or to walk. And as one says today, all right, give them a sedative because they have been screaming. And with these sedatives . . . the child sleeps. If one does not know what is going on, he [the child] is sleeping. One really has to be let in on it to know that . . . he really is being killed and not sedated.

While Dr. F. admitted that one might wonder about a child, "Why is he sleeping so much?," he insisted (quite erroneously) that one could ignore that inner question because "the death rate [of those killed] wasn't much above the regular death rate with such children." He stressed the absence of either a direct command ("If I get the order to kill . . . I don't know but I [think I] would refuse . . . but certainly there was no such order . . . for us") or of manifest homicide ("I mean if you had directed a nurse to go from bed to bed shooting these children . . . that would not have worked"). As a result, "there was no killing, strictly speaking. . . . People felt this is not murder, it is a putting-to-sleep."

Of course Dr. F. sought by this kind of emphasis to justify and exonerate himself. Indeed, the exact extent of his culpability is not clear. He had been imprisoned for some years while awaiting trial, had been convicted partly on testimony that he had ordered that a child be given a fatal dose, but his case had been appealed and eventually dismissed, apparently for political reasons, at a time of considerable laxity in trying former Nazis.

Whether he ordered the drugs that killed that particular infant, he was certainly implicated in the killing project. He had responsibility for the false records, and admitted filling out many forms that resulted in children's deaths, and signing large numbers of false death certificates. He is widely suspected of having done much more: for a period of months during his work at the institution when there was no head doctor, children continued to die in ways considered suspicious. To me he clearly sought to explain his involvement in such a way as to minimize his responsibility. But I believe he also conveyed accurately the deliberate ambiguity that facilitated his actions and limited his sense of guilt about whatever he did in connection with the killing. This "as if" situation is characteristic of direct medical killing and, to a considerable extent, of indirect medicalized killing as well.

F.'s youthful embrace of the Nazi movement in Bavaria also had great bearing on his perceptions and actions. Having been an unusually enthusiastic member of the Hitler Youth and a Party member since he was eighteen, he was deeply troubled by rumors he heard, while working in psychiatric hospitals during the early 1940s, of the killing of the mentally ill. He at first denounced these rumors as "vicious propaganda against the regime"; and when they could no longer be denied, he still "tried to see all of this somehow in connection with the idealism of National Socialism." He had the need, that is, to seek, on the one hand, some justification of the killing within the biomedical vision; and, on the other hand, to continue to call forth defenses of denial and psychic numbing, helped by the bureaucratic medicalization of the program, in order to convince himself that "these forms [which he filled out] were absolutely harmless," and that even the policy of killing deformed children "was not a command but a regulation giving the authorization so that the children *could* be killed."

He described an interaction between the child-victim without ordinary human feelings ("whom one cannot speak to, who does not laugh, who is affectively unapproachable") and the physician-killer with the same malady ("Such an executioner does not have that bad feeling [that one has in directly killing a person]. . . . There is a lack of the affective tension, the emotional participation . . . and that can turn any human being into a murderer"). He spoke of the Hoche-Binding study as having provided "mental preparation" for that kind of attitude, and could say of the later killing of children: "One cannot call it a National Socialist program." Like many doctors and scientists, he combined professional advocacy within the biomedical vision with ideological embrace of National Socialism in the name of the greater German racial community: "One could not attack one's own people from behind [*dem eigenen Volk nicht in den Rücken fallen*]." He also spoke of the influence of the war: how "people feared that through events of the war they themselves would be killed" and "did not have much concern left over for the sufferings of other people—let's

say, sick people." Here he expressed both the Nazi view of the unaccepta-
bility of the wartime burden created by mental patients as well as the
actual death anxiety he and other doctors experienced at the time. The
situation was aggravated by his strong personal conflict about whether to
leave work in a mental hospital in order to rejoin the military at a time
of war, a conflict that could lead to profound fear and guilt either way—
over what he was doing and avoiding if he stayed with the mental hospital,
and over what he was leaving and what he was facing if he rejoined the
military, as he eventually did. For a time, he had been protected from
military duty because his work in "euthanasia" placed him in the category
of "indispensable."

Despite some control over that decision, he felt himself essentially in
a closed system of authority and policy: his chief called the doctors together and told them of the Hitler decree on "euthanasia" and the work
of the "medical commission" in making final decisions about children, all
of which, it was emphasized, constituted "a secret matter of the Reich
[*Geheime Reichssache*]." Both chiefs he worked under were part of that
closed system and "were convinced that it [the killing project] was right";
and that was a time when, unlike today, "one was afraid to do something
not in accord with the chief." Nor was there any communication between
colleagues about the policy, once it was initiated: "It was only the chain
of command from high to low, but no discussion," because it was "taboo"
to talk about the program to anyone. As an inexperienced doctor and
human being in his mid-twenties, he felt alone and anxious and experienced stirrings of disillusionment ("I did not believe it possible that
a Reich I had wished for . . . was capable of ordering something like
that"), along with a sense of there being "no exit." His way of coping was
to comply, to do what was expected of him.

One of his means of adapting was to throw himself into medical work.
He spent twelve to fourteen hours a day on the wards "trying to grasp
the whole thing, at least scientifically, . . . to examine . . . all factors that
were . . . important for the development of the condition, . . . to examine
the relatives, the whole family, . . . working with the patients, examining
them precisely." This permitted "the physician to break through," but it
also helped him solidify for himself his own medical "as if" situation: that
is, helped him maintain a partial illusion of medical authenticity.

But he was also aware that he was involved in something dirty, in the
killing of children—as when he asked himself why a particular child was
sleeping so much ("*That* one did indeed think")—and aware also that it
was "not the legal way" for orders to come from above concerning what
doctors should do. Dr. F. was later to admit publicly that the chief doctor
told him of the order to kill the children, and that he (F.) was aware that
the forms he filled out led directly to killing. He frequently spoke of the
deceptions as "diabolical" and added, with retrospective wisdom, of
course, but with significance for his feelings at the time as well: "Either

one is a physician or one is not." And: "The physician, regardless of his ideology or age, all these years he has been educated to help the sick, to heal the sick and not to kill the sick."

Doctors in Hans F.'s situation had to have some awareness of the reversal of healing and killing, but did not necessarily experience sufficient guilt to prevent them from participating. In this doctor's case, residual feelings of shame and guilt were later intensified by the knowledge that, among the doctors he worked closely with, one had served a five-year prison term, while the other, his former chief, had been sentenced to death at a trial held soon after the war. Our interviews could also have stimulated his guilt feelings: he later expressed publicly a sense of greater culpability and the conviction that he should have told Nazi leaders at the time that the program was "crazy" and was making doctors into monsters. Highly revealing was his rage—perhaps the only rage he expressed during our interviews—toward those who gave orders from above for people like him below to do the killing:

> Well, there is an enormous difference if one says the patients who fall under these provisions are unworthy of life, that they should be killed—that is still a *provision,* you know—but the actual carrying it out, that is the big problem, see. Who will do this thing? I believe those gentlemen who engaged in such theoretical reflections never reflected on *that.* . . . No judge who gave the verdict of death has ever hanged anyone, you see. . . . I can say a hundred times, "He [a patient] is such a mental defective that he can never develop at all," . . . etc., etc., but that does not enable me to kill him [*umzubringen;* literally, "put [him] away"].

He identified his former chief as one of those "desk criminals" (*Schreibtischtäter*)—a term used widely about the Nazis during the postwar period—who caused others, such as nurses and lower-ranked doctors, to do the dirty work and to be caught between the desk criminal and the victim. Dr. F. implied that he included himself in that latter, entrapped group.

His moral confusions were expressed in still another significant form: his attitude toward the specimens taken from the dead children. Autopsies were performed at the time of the killings by a pathologist in Dr. F.'s institution, and he himself would sometimes examine brains of his own former patients. He did that, he explained,

> not only because one could perhaps, so to speak, lighten one's conscience but because one is interested in finding out what was wrong with the person: What is going on there, why is he sick? What's the matter with him? . . . Why is this child an imbecile? Why is it paralyzed? There was a high scientific interest present—I must point that out.

In other words, he and other doctors could follow a pattern that recurs throughout this study: the immersion of themselves in "medical science" as a means of avoiding awareness of, and guilt over, their participation in a murderous project.

Moreover, some years after the war Hans F. returned to the same institutional complex and began to make more systematic studies of this "pathological material." As he explained to me, all brains of autopsied children, whether they were killed in the "euthanasia" project or not, were kept at the institute, and "among them were some of scientific interest." He compared his decision to study those brains to that of any contemporary medical scientist: "So just like today, when a patient dies, where I say, 'Yes, this is an interesting illness,' . . . I should like to know what was going on there and then I have the brain kept and I receive it for examination. Just like it was back then, right."

When I asked him whether, when doing these later dissections, he had any thoughts about what had happened to children during that earlier time, his answer was equivocal. He admitted "some . . . thoughts . . . about individual cases one remembered—that was this or that child." While he denied that one could tell whether the brain came from a child who had been killed, he did acknowledge that "one could assume that with severe cases that were, let's say, diagnostically and prognostically in the range of the ['euthanasia'] program, that some of these cases of course did suffer a forcible death."

Dr. F.'s political and biomedical ideology, together with his relationship to specific political and medical authority, contributed crucially to his psychological responses and, ultimately, to his participation in the killing program. Contributing also to his behavior was the prevailing stance of German—and not only German—psychiatry of that time toward mental patients in general and radically impaired children in particular, a stance of great distance and a limited perception of these patients as human beings. More than distance, former child patients later described a cruel, even sadistic institutional environment, including corporal punishment for misbehavior and electric shocks for bed wetting, all of which was undoubtedly intensified by the institution's killing function. Dr. F. was especially susceptible to this ultimate medical corruption because of the intensity of his relationship to the regime, but other doctors less involved with Nazi ideology did similar things within a structure that maximized whatever psychological potential one possessed for joining in the reversal of healing and killing.

"The Most Simple Method": Hermann Pfannmüller

Finally, there were the extremes in the killing of children. The following is a description by a nonmedical visitor, in the fall of 1939, to an important Reich Committee institution at Eglfing-Haar, where the director, Dr. Hermann Pfannmüller, developed a policy of starving the designated children to death rather than wasting medication on them:

I remember the gist of the following general remarks by Pfannmüller: These creatures (he meant the children) naturally represent for me as a National Socialist only a burden for the healthy body of our *Volk*. We do not kill (he could have here used a euphemistic expression for this word kill) with poison, injections, etc.; then the foreign press and certain gentlemen in Switzerland would only have new inflammatory material. No, our method is much simpler and more natural, as you see. With these words, he pulled, with the help of a . . . nurse, a child from its little bed. While he then exhibited the child like a dead rabbit, he asserted with a knowing expression and a cynical grin: For this one it will take two to three more days. The picture of this fat, grinning man, in his fleshy hand the whimpering skeleton, surrounded by other starving children, is still vivid in my mind. The murderer explained further then, that sudden withdrawal of food was not employed, rather gradual decrease of the rations. A lady who was also part of the tour asked—her outrage suppressed with difficulty—whether a quicker death with injections, etc., would not at least be more merciful. Pfannmüller then praised his methods again as more practical in view of the foreign press. The openness with which Pfannmüller announced the above-mentioned method of treatment is explicable to me only as a result of cynicism or clumsiness [*Tölpelhaftigkeit*]. Pfannmüller also did not hide the fact that among the children to be murdered . . . were also children who were not mentally ill, namely children of Jewish parents.[33]

The Killing of Adults

Extending the project from children to adults meant rendering medical killing an official overall policy—a policy Hitler enunciated in his "Führer decree" of October 1939. A few months earlier, he had called in Leonardo Conti, secretary for health in the Interior Ministry, as well as the head of the Reich Chancellery, Hans Lammers, and told them (as recalled by the latter) that "he considered it to be proper that the 'life unworthy of life' of severely mentally ill persons be eliminated by actions [*Eingriffe*] that bring about death." Hitler went on to cite "as examples . . . cases in which the mentally ill could only be bedded on sand or sawdust because they continually befouled themselves," and in which "patients put their own excrement into their mouths, eating it and so on." Hitler pointed out that in this way "a certain saving in hospitals, doctors, and nursing personnel could be brought about."[34] The caricatured mentally ill would come to symbolize all that threatened the purity of the *Volk*.

The decree itself was brief:

Reich Leader Bouhler and Dr. Brandt* are charged with the responsibility for expanding the authority of physicians, to be designated by name, to the end that patients considered incurable according to the best available human judgment [*menschlichem Ermessen*] of their state of health, can be granted a mercy death [*Gnadentod*].[35]†

Actually issued in October, the decree was backdated to 1 September, so that it could relate directly to the day of the outbreak of the Second World War. While the backdating is usually attributed to Hitler's conviction that a wartime atmosphere would render the German population more amenable to such a project, there was a deeper psychological relationship between "euthanasia" and war. As the fanatical Dr. Pfannmüller in the Nazi program put it: "The idea is unbearable to me that the best, the flower of our youth must lose its life at the front in order that feebleminded and irresponsible asocial elements can have a secure existence in the asylum."[37]

The Nazis viewed their biomedical vision as having a heroic status parallel to that of war. Hitler's concept that the state in itself was nothing, and existed only to serve the well-being of the *Volk* and the race, applied also to the major enterprises of the state, especially its transcendent enterprise of war. Rather than medical killing being subsumed to war, the war itself was subsumed to the vast biomedical vision of which "euthanasia" was a part. Or, to put the matter another way, the deepest impulses behind the war had to do with the sequence of sterilization, direct medical killing, and genocide.

Yet Hitler and other Nazi leaders were aware that they were embarking on a draconian, though in their eyes necessary, measure for which the German public and even the official state bureaucracy were not quite ready. Hence, the decree was written on Hitler's private stationery, as though he "considered the death of many thousands of sick persons as his private matter, not . . . a decision of the head of state."[38] Or, we may say, he understood himself to be a prophet whose racial vision outdistanced the state's structure, making it necessary for him to avoid the bureaucratic apparatus and proceed directly to the matter at hand.

His way of doing that was to go straight to the doctors. Inevitably, he ended up creating an elaborate new bureaucracy, one that was both medical and murderous. In his decision to turn the program over to Karl Brandt rather than to Conti (who, as health minister and Reich Health Leader, was the logical person to run it), Hitler was choosing his own

---

*Conti and Lammers were soon replaced as heads of the "euthanasia" program by Philip Bouhler and Karl Brandt.

†There was apparently some disagreement about the wording. The final draft was probably written by Dr. Max de Crinis, whose role will be discussed later. Note the broadened "incurable" criteria in this decree: Brandt later claimed that Hitler substituted "best available human judgment" for "nearly certain possibility."[36]

"escort physician and close confidant." Probably similar personal reasons determined his selection of Philip Bouhler, chief of Hitler's Chancellery and considered absolutely loyal to him, to run the program with Brandt. An additional reason for this arrangement was said to be the fear that radical district leaders *(Gauleiter)* might otherwise, "ruthlessly and without medical consultation," take over much of the control of the project —as they indeed eventually did.[39] For Hitler, this was a conscious choice of "party discipline" over a state apparatus that still made some demands for legal procedure and fiscal accountability; it was also a choice of procedure most protective of secrecy. Above all, these arrangements suggest how far the impulse toward killing mental patients had already taken hold among Nazi leaders, and their determination to keep the project in medical channels.

Not only Brandt and Bouhler, but also Dr. Herbert Linden of the Health Ministry and Dr. Grawitz, chief physician of the SS, were active in choosing doctors for leadership roles. Their criteria included the closeness of these doctors to the regime, high recognition in the profession, and known sympathy for "euthanasia" or at least a radical approach to eugenics, probably in about that order. Included were several doctors who had been associated with the children's program (Unger, Heinze, and Pfannmüller), but also a group of psychiatrists of some prominence in academic circles, notably Professor Werner Heyde of Würzburg, Professor Carl Schneider of Heidelberg, Professor Max de Crinis of Berlin, and Professor Paul Nitsche from the Sonnenstein state institution. Others, like Friedrich Mennecke, were primarily Nazified psychiatrists. Heyde became Brandt's representative and directed the program, with Nitsche his assistant and eventual replacement.[40]

At these early meetings, Brandt was introduced as the medical leader of the project, and Hitler's decree was read and sometimes displayed ("I believe I saw Adolf Hitler's signature on it," Mennecke later testified). It was carefully explained that there was no official law, because Hitler thought such a law could only feed enemy propaganda; that the authorization to Bouhler and Brandt in the Hitler decree was the equivalent of a law; and that doctors participating would be immune from legal consequences.* One participant later insisted that the emphasis was on killing

---

*Because of various forms of resistance, along with pressure from legal authorities, a law to legitimate the program was seriously considered, and at least two elaborate drafts were written. Those drafts, combined with the original Hitler decree, contributed to a *legal* "as if" situation—the assumption that such a law had actually been implemented. It was an assumption easily made because of the authority of the original decree. Hitler was thought to fear that an official "euthanasia" law would give a propaganda advantage to Germany's enemies, and also that it would increase German (especially Catholic) resistance, as well as psychiatric patients' resistance to entering hospitals (as several "euthanasia" leaders pointed out). From this experience, it is thought that the Nazis learned that, as a later authority explained, "illegal mass killing could not be carried through in the *Altreich* ["Old Reich," or Germany proper], where the net of normal working justice and administrative machinery was much too tight, but rather had to be transferred to the occupied areas [*Ostgebiete*] where the executive apparatus of the SS could work with less encumbrance and less trouble."[41]

only hopeless mental patients: "Those cases . . . we in psychiatry know as burned-out ruins *(ausgebrannte Ruinen)*."[42] But many of those present knew of Hitler's views on eliminating genetically inferior people in general. Although the phrase "life unworthy of life" was liberally invoked, another doctor could feel "not quite clear on where the line was to be drawn."[43] There was stress on constructing a careful medical sequence of evaluation before any patient would be put to death. And the entire project was to be "unconditionally kept secret." In those important early meetings, just one doctor—Max de Crinis—refused (and only for tactical reasons [see pages 120–22]) to participate fully. The general response was that "nobody mentioned any misgivings."[44]

What was secret was the actual killing project, not the idea. Some months earlier (April 1939), an article had appeared in a semi-official Nazi magazine, estimating that it would probably be desirable to exterminate one million people.[45]

Organizing for Killing

Unlike the children's "euthanasia" program, the T4 program, with its focus on adult chronic patients, involved virtually the entire German psychiatric community and related portions of the general medical community. The camouflage organization created for the medical killing was the Reich Work Group of Sanatoriums and Nursing Homes *(Reichsarbeitsgemeinschaft Heil- und Pflegeanstalten,* or RAG) operating from the Berlin Chancellery at its Tiergarten 4 address—hence, the overall code name "T4" for the adult project. Questionnaires were worked out by the leadership group of psychiatrists and administrators and distributed, with the help of the Health Ministry, not only to psychiatric institutions but to all hospitals and homes for chronic patients. The limited space provided for biographical and symptomatic categories, as well as the covering letter, gave the impression that a statistical survey was being undertaken for administrative and possibly scientific purposes. All the more so because the questionnaire for patients was accompanied by an institutional questionnaire, which focused on such matters as annual budget, number of beds, and number of doctors and nurses. But the sinister truth was suggested by the great stress put on a "precise description" of the working ability of the patients, as well as by the juxtaposition of the following four categories:

1. Patients suffering from specified diseases who are not employable or are employable only in simple mechanical work. The diseases were schizophrenia, epilepsy, senile diseases, therapy-resistant paralysis and other syphilitic sequelae, feeblemindedness from any cause, encephalitis, Huntington's chorea, and other neurological conditions of a terminal nature.

2. Patients who have been continually institutionalized for at least five years.

3. Patients who are in custody as criminally insane.

4. Patients who are not German citizens, or are not of German or kindred blood, giving race and nationality.

There are added instructions about filling in the section on work, including that of noting "patients in the higher diet categories [who] perform no work though they might be able to do so." (The original questionnaire, translated, is reproduced on pages 68–69.) By mid-1940, these report forms were required not only on patients who came under the four categories but on all inmates of these institutions.[46]

The process was haphazard from the start. It was required that forms be returned quickly, and one institutional doctor had to fill out fifteen hundred questionnaires in two weeks. Early confusion about the purpose of the form led some doctors to exaggerate the severity of patients' conditions, as a way of protecting them from what was assumed to be a plan to release them from institutions in order to send them to work. The extent to which psychiatrists could continue to disbelieve what was happening—especially when they did not *want* to believe it—is suggested by a leading professor of psychiatry's later description of his response to a rumor he had heard that patients were being "euthanized":

> I considered the rumor completely unbelievable. . . . Thinking that the questionnaire did not give the slightest cause to suppose such an action, . . . I imagined the intended action was a way of separating the curable patients, or those able to work, from those who were incurable, in order to provide better food for the first group and to provide the second group . . . only the amount of food necessary to keep them alive. . . . [My staff] was persuaded by my argument, and we all worked innocently on the questionnaire project.[47]*

The "expert evaluation" differed from the children's program in that the three medical (usually psychiatric) authorities, drawn from among the leaders of the project, did their reviewing independently. Of every questionnaire collected, four or five photocopies were made in the Reich Interior Ministry, one for each of these three "experts" (*Gutachter*), the other one or two for the later death procedure, with the original usually kept in the central files. Each of the experts wrote in a special thick black frame at the lower left-hand corner of the form, "+" in red pencil, meaning death; "−" in blue pencil, meaning life; or "?," sometimes with a comment, which was most often "worker." He then initialed the mark. If anything, their work was even more mercurial and superficial than the initial filling out of the forms. Each doctor was sent at least 100 photocopied questionnaires at a time; during one seventeen-

---

*This statement is especially significant as having been made by Dr. Gottfried Ewald who, as I discuss in chapter 3, became one of the very few significant psychiatric voices of dissent. His initial disbelief could have been due partly to his then ardent Nazi sympathies.

day period, Pfannmüller was required to complete 2,109 such evaluations. And once more they did no examinations, had no access to medical histories, and made their decision solely on the basis of the questionnaire. Their occasional disagreements had only to do with definitions and policy principles, and the pressure was always toward death. One expert remembered the general principle that "in doubtful or borderline cases . . . action should be requested," and recalled that Brack's injunctions "exceeded the . . . medically defensible standpoint." Another expert recalled the similar principle that "one should not be petty . . . but instead, liberal in the sense of a positive [killing] judgment."[48] These same "experts" served at times on special Physicians' Commissions, which had the ostensible purpose of providing further medical control but tended to be a medical cover for pressing ahead with the legal machinery of the project, especially where there had been any suggestion of recalcitrance or resistance or even pleas of insufficient time and personnel for the paperwork.

For example, there was the case of the Neuendettelsauer Nursing Homes in Bavaria, a scattered group of institutions asked to fill out fifteen hundred forms in four weeks. After the denial of a request for a delay to permit the chief doctor of the hospital to return from a trip, the commission appeared on less than a day's notice; it consisted of one expert and sixteen young men and women, about half of whom were medical students and the other half typists. The medical students filled in the forms, making use of material from the files to dig out damning information, even when no longer applicable, and working entirely independently of the institutional doctors. These students sometimes questioned nurses about patients in a perfunctory way, ignoring answers that conveyed favorable information and sometimes reversing in their report what was actually told them by the nurses. When it was pointed out to the "commissioner" (the expert) that the students had assumed that all cases of mental impairment were equally severe because all were listed in the files as "idiocy" (according to an earlier terminology), he agreed to take account of the fact in the future—but several hundred questionnaires had already been filled out in accordance with the students' misconception. It is estimated that during the week the commission members spent at the hospital, they brought about the death of more than a thousand patients.[49]

The marked questionnaires were then sent for a final review by a "senior expert" *(Obergutachter),* a function served at first only by Heyde but later by Nitsche and possibly Linden as well. At this level, there was no "?"; nor was this ultimate expert bound in any way by the earlier judgments. While this signature was *pro forma,* it carried with it the full authority not only of the project but usually of German academic psychiatry as well, since the signatory tended to be a distinguished professor. As far as is known, no formal written guidelines were provided for either level of these "expert reviews."[50]

Questionnaire 1

Case no. ....

      Name of Institution: ....

      in: ....

First and family name of patient: .... maiden name: ....

Date of birth:.......... City: .... District: ....

Last residence:.......................... District: ....

Unmarr., marr., wid., div.: Relig:.. Race[a] .... Natlty: ....

Address of nearest relative: ....

....

Regular visits and by whom (address): ....

....

Guardian or Care-Giver (name, address): ....

....

Cost-bearer:.... How long in this inst.: ....

In other Institutions, when and how long: ....

How long sick:.. From where and when transferred: ....

Twin $^{yes}_{no}$ ... Mentally ill blood relatives: ....

Diagnosis: ....

....

Primary symptoms: ....

....

Mainly bedridden? $^{yes}_{no}$ ... Very restless? $^{yes}_{no}$ ..... Confined? $^{yes}_{no}$ ....

Incurable phys. illness: $^{yes}_{no}$ ...... War casualty: $^{yes}_{no}$ ....

      For schizophrenia: Recent case ...... Final stage .. good remission ...

      For retardation: Debility: .... Imbecile: .... Idiot: ....

      For epilepsy: Psych. changes .... Average freq. of attacks ....

      For senile disorders: Very confused .... Soils self ....

Therapy (Insulin, Cardiazol, Malaria, Salvarsan, etc.):. Lasting effect: $^{yes}_{no}$ ......

Referred on the basis of §51, §42b Crim. Code, etc. .... By ....

Crime: ... Earlier criminal acts: ....

Type of Occupation: (Most exact description of work and *productivity,* e.g. Fieldwork, does not do much.—Locksmith's shop, good skilled worker.—No vague answers, such as housework, rather precise: cleaning room, etc. Always indicate also, whether constantly, frequently or only occasionally occupied)

....

....

Release expected soon:..

[a]German or related blood (German-blooded), Jew, Jewish *Mischling* [half-breed] 1st or 2nd degree, Negro *(Mischling),* Gypsy *(Mischling),* etc.

Remarks: ....

Do not mark in this space.

```
.........................
.........................
.........................
.........................
```

..... Place, Date ....

....

(Signature of medical director or his representative)

INSTRUCTION SHEET
To be followed in filling out the questionnaires

All patients are to be reported who

1. suffer from the diseases enumerated below and who within the institution can be occupied not at all or only at the most mechanical work (picking, etc.):

   Schizophrenia,

   Epilepsy (indicate if exogenous, war-related or other causes),

   Senile disorders,

   Therapy-resistant paralysis and other Lues [syphilitic] diseases,

   Retardation from whatever cause,

   Encephalitis,

   Huntington's chorea and other terminal neurological conditions;

   or

2. have been continuously in institutions for at least 5 years;

   or

3. are in custody as criminally insane;

   or

4. do not possess German citizenship or are not of German or related blood, giving/designating race[b] and nationality.

The questionnaires, to be filled out individually for each patient, are to be given serial numbers.

The questionnaires are to be filled out by typewriter whenever possible.

Due on ....

In the case of patients sent to this institution from outside the evacuation area, a (V) is to be placed behind the name.

In case the number of Questionnaire 1 forms sent are not sufficient, please order the number needed through my office.

   [b]German or related blood (German-blooded), Jew, Jewish *Mischling* 1st or 2nd class, Negro, Negro *Mischling*, Gypsy, Gypsy *Mischling*, etc.

SOURCE: Questionnaire translated from Judgment in Hadamar Trial, Frankfurt/M., February–March 1947 (4 KLS 7/47), Landgericht Frankfurt. Instruction sheet from Heyde Trial Documents, pp. 210–11. Questionnaire and instruction sheet translated by Amy Hackett.

Psychiatric Transfer: "White Coats and SS Boots"

Transportation arrangements were a caricature of psychiatric transfer. The organization created for this function, the Common Welfare Ambulance Service Ltd. (*Gemeinnützige Krankentransport,* or *Gekrat*),* sent out "transport lists" to the hospitals from which it was to collect patients; issued instructions that patients were to be accompanied by their case histories and personal possessions as well as lists of valuables held for them; and specified that those patients for whom lengthy transport could be dangerous to their lives should not be transferred (a show of medical propriety and an actual means of avoiding the awkward situation of a patient dying en route).

SS personnel manned the buses, frequently wearing white uniforms or white coats in order to appear to be doctors, nurses, or medical attendants. There were reports of "men with white coats and SS boots," the combination that epitomized much of the "euthanasia" project in general.[51]

To hide patients from the public, bus windows were covered with dark paint or fixed curtains or blinds. The destination of the buses was specifically kept secret from the medical staff of the institution from which they were loaded, and of course from the patients themselves. SS guards on the buses carried special documents enabling them to pass unchallenged through all checkpoints. The initial practice of taking patients directly to the killing centers was after some time discontinued in favor of "observation institutions" or "transit institutions"—often large state hospitals near killing centers—where patients spent brief periods before being sent to their deaths. These observation institutions, which were suggested by Heyde and may have enhanced scheduling arrangements, provided an aura of medical check against mistakes, while in fact no real examination or observation was made.[52] In addition, they seemed to have been part of an impulse toward bureaucratic mystification that further impaired the autonomous existence and the traceability of a patient and, to a considerable extent, of his or her family as well.

The bureaucratic mystification was furthered by letters sent to the family: first, notification of transfer "because of important war-related measures"; and then a second letter upon the patient's reaching the killing center announcing his or her "safe" arrival, and adding that "at this time . . . Reich defense reasons" and "the shortage of personnel brought about by the war" made visits or inquiries of any kind impossible, although the family would "immediately" be informed of changes in a patient's condition or in the visiting policy. The second letter was signed, with a false name, by either the killing doctor or the chief of the killing center. The third letter, sent—under a false name by the Condolence-Letter Department—just days or perhaps weeks later, was a notification of the patient's death.[53]

---

*A related Common Welfare Foundation for Institutional Care handled financial arrangements.

"The Syringe Belongs in the Hand of a Physician"

That death generally occurred within twenty-four hours of the patient's arrival at the killing center. Under T4 policy, a doctor had to do the actual killing, in accordance with the motto enunciated by Dr. Viktor Brack, head of the Chancellery's "Euthanasia" Department II: "The syringe belongs in the hand of a physician."[54] Rather than a syringe, however, it was usually a matter of opening a gas cock.

There were six main killing centers—Hartheim, Sonnenstein, Grafeneck, Bernburg, Brandenburg, and Hadamar. Typically they were converted mental hospitals or nursing homes; at least one had been a prison. They were in isolated areas and had high walls—some had originally been old castles—so that what happened within could not be readily observed from without. "The unloading of the buses could be done in a way [so that] neither the screams of the patients nor any other occurrences could penetrate to the outside world."[55]

Hitler himself is said to have decided upon the use of carbon monoxide gas as the killing method, on the so-called medical advice of Dr. Heyde. The decision followed upon an experiment conducted in early 1940 at Brandenburg, then being converted from a prison into a killing center. Killing by injection (using various combinations of morphine, scopolomine, curare, and prussic acid [cyanide]) was directly compared with killing by means of carbon monoxide gas. Karl Brandt, "a very conscientious man [who] took his responsibility very seriously," requested the experiment; and he and Conti administered the injections themselves "as a symbolic action in which the most responsible physicians in the Reich subjected themselves to the practical carrying through of the Führer's order."[56]

The four or six injected patients ("six at the most") "died only slowly," and some had to be injected again. In contrast, the gas worked perfectly. The first Nazi gas chamber had been constructed under the supervision of Christian Wirth, of the SS Criminal Police, lent to the T4 staff. The arrangement included a fake shower room with benches, the gas being inserted from the outside into water pipes with small holes through which the carbon monoxide could escape. Present were two SS chemists with doctoral degrees, one of whom operated the gas. The other, August Becker, told how eighteen to twenty people were led naked into the "shower room": through a peephole he observed that very quickly "people toppled over, or lay on the benches"—all without "scenes or commotion." The room was ventilated within five minutes; SS men then used special stretchers which mechanically shoved the corpses into crematory ovens without contact. The technical demonstration was performed before a select audience of the inner circle of physicians and administrators of the medical killing project. Having been shown the technique, Dr. Irmfried Eberl, newly appointed head of the Brandenburg institution, took over "by himself and on his own responsibility." Both Brack and

Brandt expressed their satisfaction with the experiment, the latter stressing that "only doctors should carry out the gassings."[57]

I have referred to those initial gassings as both experiments and demonstrations, since later testimony—for instance, Brandt's remarkable statements at the Nuremberg Medical Trial—make clear that they were both. Brandt said that the original plan was to kill people by injecting narcotics, until it was realized that these would cause loss of consciousness but that death would not occur for some time. An alternative suggestion was made by a psychiatrist (presumably Heyde) to use carbon monoxide gas (which, in turn, led to the demonstration just described). Brandt recalled not liking the idea because he felt that "this whole question can only be looked at from a medical point of view," and that "in my medical imagination carbon monoxide had never played a part." Killing by gas, that is, made it much more difficult to maintain a medical aura. Brandt was able to change his mind when he recalled a personal experience of carbon monoxide poisoning in which he lost consciousness "without feeling anything," and realized that carbon monoxide "would be the most humane form of death." Yet he remained troubled because that method required "a whole change in medical conception," and gave the matter extensive thought "in order to put my own conscience right." He brought up to Hitler the difference of opinion about the two methods, and later remembered the Führer asking, "Which is the more humane way?" "My answer was clear," Brandt testified—and other leading physicians in the program agreed. Brandt concluded this segment of testimony with a meditation on medical breakthrough:

> This is just one example of [what happens] when major advances in medical history are being made. There are cases of an operation being looked on at first with contempt, but then later on one learned it and carried it out. Here the task required by state authority was added to the medical conception of this problem, and it was necessary to find with good conscience a basic method that could do justice to both of these elements.[58]

Allowing for self-serving elements and for retrospective father-son mythology in his early relationship to Hitler, Brandt's description takes us to the heart of the doctors' embrace of medicalized killing.

The Bureaucracy of Medical Deception

Throughout the "euthanasia" project, the pattern was for senior doctors to make policy and render decisions, to serve as high consultants and experts, while younger doctors did the actual killing. That was the message from Dr. Hans F. in connection with the killing of children, even if somewhat older chief doctors provided either orders or deadly innuendos. The pattern was still more true in regard to adult patients. Where senior doctors were involved in killing, they soon gave way to younger men, and some of the young doctors were quickly elevated to senior status. Killing doctors came to be chosen apparently for their combination of inexperience and political enthusiasm.[59]

At Brandenburg, for instance, Dr. Eberl was twenty-nine years old when he learned to operate the gassing mechanism. The man later assigned to assist him, Dr. Aquilin Ullrich, was only twenty-six. Ullrich testified that his duties hardly required medical knowledge. He and Eberl did no more than make a "superficial inspection" of the naked patients in the anteroom of the gas chamber, which at the time he found "inexplicable"; subsequently he came to realize that "the presence of the physician at that moment was used to calm the mentally ill and camouflage the killing process."[60]

Another doctor, who first worked as an assistant at a killing center, was informed by his immediate superior that "a physician, according to the law, had the last say, and he therefore had to re-examine the arrivals." Later he was informed by Dr. Nitsche, one of the "senior experts," that these *pro forma* " 'examinations' before the death chamber served mainly to calm the conscience of the doctor who has to carry out the killing."[61] The Nazis were clearly aware of the psychological importance of the medical "as if" situation to the *doctors* involved.

For the most part, the "examination" consisted of the doctor simply checking on the fact that patient and chart coincided—the right person was being killed—and using the occasion to help decide which false diagnosis would be appropriate (consistent with the patient's record and appearance) for the death certificates soon to be issued. Reversing a decision about a patient's death at that point was extremely rare, probably limited only to a few discovered to have been war casualties of some kind.[62]* The fundamental significance of that pseudo examination was medical legitimation of murder.

Many of these patients were apparently deceived. A man who worked at the Hadamar killing center told how a patient he had known for many years said to him on the way to the gas chamber, "We will have a real bath now and get other clothes."[63] When patients were not deceived and did resist, they were quickly subdued by physical force, though even this could resemble ordinary treatment of psychiatric patients. What happened next makes clear the doctor's responsibility for the entire killing sequence:

> After doors were closed, the air was sucked out of the gas chamber through a ventilator by the same doctor who carried out the earlier "examination." Then for about ten minutes, carbon monoxide was let in [by that doctor] and its effect observed through a small window. As soon as he thought that those shut in had died, he had the gas chamber

*In Württemberg, only twenty-nine patients, mostly war veterans, were saved.

emptied. First fresh air was introduced through the ventilator, and the gas was forced out. From the beginning of the gassing until the reopening of the gas chamber took about one hour. The corpses that were to be dissected were removed to a special room. However the great majority of corpses were immediately taken to the ovens and burned there.[64]*

Concerning the "humanity" of this form of killing claimed by Brandt, another man who worked at Hadamar and looked into the gas chamber through a side window spoke of "a horrible sight when the patients gradually collapsed and fell over one another," and added, "I shall never get this picture out of my mind."[66]

We shall find this sequence, including the doctor's central role in it, to be strikingly similar to the killing sequence in Auschwitz.

Given the medical cover-up of killing, *every death certificate had to be falsified.* The key principle employed in choosing the false cause of death was medical credibility: assigning a disease consistent with a patient's prior physical and mental state, a disease that he or she *could* have contracted. Designated causes of death could include almost anything— infectious diseases, pneumonia, diseases of the heart, lung, brain, or other major organs. Skill at this falsification process was an important part of the "medical experience" of the killing doctors, and younger ones learned it during their "training" with their medical superiors and predecessors. To help them, they were given written guides specifying important details necessary for consistency.

One such guide, for instance, focused upon septicemia (bacteria in the bloodstream) as a cause of death, referred to bacterial infection of the skin as a possible source, and listed the sequence of symptoms and therapy to be mentioned. The document included additional useful tips: unclean mental patients often have boils which they scratch; and, "It is most expedient to figure four days for the basic illness [bacterial infection of skin] and five days for the resultant sepsis"; and, this diagnosis "should not be used with patients who are meticulously clean" but "is preferable for young strong patients who smear readily," but in that case "seven to eight days have to be allowed for the illness to take effect, since their circulation is relatively more resistant."[67]

It is no exaggeration to say that the primary—perhaps the only—*medical* function of the killing doctors was to determine the most believable falsification of each patient-victim's death certificate.

Maintaining these medical illusions required an extensive bureaucracy of deception. Every falsification in this "bloated apparatus" had to be

---

*In addition, as part of the scientific orientation of the program, "euthanasia" victims were photographed nude before they were killed. Dr. Friedrich Mennecke (see pages 139–42) had special training in "the photographic representation of types" during his T4 education in Heidelberg.[65] In some centers, the brain was removed for later study before the corpse was cremated.

"covered by two more." For instance, at each killing center, there was a "Special Registry Office," which had a subdivision whose specific task it was to determine a suitable death date for each patient. On the death certificate prepared by the doctor, the date of death was always omitted, to be provided by this department. On the basis of its "timecards" and "death files," it could prevent the recording of large numbers of deaths at a particular place during a particular time sequence.[68]

The bureaucracy of deception extended—logically, one might say—to the ashes of cremated patients, which were haphazardly mixed together so that the urn received by the family of a dead patient contained ashes that were not their relative's. (Families were told that quick cremation was necessary, especially during wartime, for public health reasons.) One of the program's leaders later said that he objected vehemently "for reasons of piety" when the policy had to be implemented because of a directive that corpses no longer be cremated individually. He claimed to have said to the administrator responsible for the order: "Even if the German people forgive you everything, they will never forgive you this."[69] While one must be skeptical about any such remembered conversation, it could suggest the existence, even then, of a glimmer of awareness of the desecration in this final medical falsification.

Inevitably, there were slip-ups in the bureaucracy of deception: a family receiving two urns; or being told that a patient, whose appendix had been removed earlier, had died of appendicitis; or being notified of the death of a patient who had not actually been killed and was alive and physically well. Or people learned (especially as church groups with national contacts began to look into the matter) of the suspicious deaths of a group of patients sent out together from the same mental hospital; or of letters received by families, at the same time in various parts of Germany, announcing the deaths of patients who were known to be physically healthy shortly after their arrival at a particular institution.

In addition, people working at killing centers would drink heavily at nearby bars and sometimes reveal aspects of what they were doing. Local people employed in "euthanasia" station kitchens and laundries also spread the word. Sometimes transfer procedures were conducted where they could be seen—even on occasion in a town marketplace—so that many people witnessed the force used on some recalcitrant victims.

And there was direct sensory evidence of the killing that no bureaucratic deception could eliminate: "The heavy smoke from the crematory building is said to be visible over Hadamar every day." And: "At full capacity . . . [the chimneys at Hartheim] smoked day and night. Locks of hair went up through the chimneys and landed in the street." These bureaucratic oversights were mentioned in Nazi documents critical of the way the program was run and urging that "more sensitivity be exercised in carrying out these activities."[70] But the "mistakes" were partly a product of the regime's own conflicts and contradictions about its principle of secrecy. In spite of the elaborate cover-up at every level and the pledge to eternal secrecy taken by all involved in the killing, at several of the killing centers outsiders—for example, the local *Gauleiter* (district leader) and other prominent Nazi personages at Hartheim—were received and, on some occasions, permitted to witness the killing of patients.

There were inconsistencies concerning who was permitted to know everything and who was not. While the nature of the medical killing project was not openly discussed, it was not completely withheld either. Courses consistent with the "euthanasia" program were given at large mental hospitals such as Eglfing-Haar, not an official killing center but a place where mental patients were nonetheless killed. An estimated twenty thousand Nazi military and civilian leaders and SS men were thus exposed to films* and "case demonstrations" of highly regressed patients, especially Jewish patients, as "life unworthy of life": recall Dr. Pfannmüller's demonstration of the "most simple method" of starving a child to death.[72]

These and other bureaucratic contradictions had to do with uncertainty concerning the official view of the program as necessary but difficult for the population to accept—that view accompanied by the sense that the program was on the one hand dirty, ugly, and unacceptable (to be hidden at all costs) and on the other a liberating therapy for the race (and therefore openly demonstrable). It is quite possible that the Nazi doctors and their companions in the bureaucracy of deception held all three images at once.

New Technology and the Killing of Jews: T4 in Poland and the Final Solution

From the beginning of the T4 operation, Jewish patients were viewed as a group apart. They were, before long, caught up in broader Nazi extermination policies. That was the time (late 1939 to early 1940) when the doctrine of "elimination [in the sense of removal] of Judaism as a whole" was being developed. Soon after Poland was overrun by German armies (September 1939), Heydrich formulated a plan to build a "Jewish reservation" in Lublin. Although this plan never materialized, deportation trains left for Poland during the winter of 1939–40, carrying Jews (who were not mental patients) from Austria, Bohemia, and Moravia.[73]†

Though the Madagascar Plan (for the use of that island as a "reservation" for Jews) was still being given some consideration, there was in Party circles increasing talk of a "radical solution" (*Radikalerlösung*) for

*One such film was "Existence without Life" (*Dasein ohne Leben*), which was intended not for the general public but rather for the education of T4 personnel and trusted circles. [71]

†In all talk of resettlement, whether of Jewish inmates or of Jews in general, the anti-Semitic attitude of the Polish population—the possibility of stimulating Poles to pogroms or the like—was frequently mentioned.

the "Jewish problem" which developed into the so-called Final Solution (*Endlösung*).[74]

Under T4, Jewish inmates of institutions in Germany did not have to meet the ordinary criteria for medical killing (mental deficiency or schizophrenia, length of hospitalization, capacity to work, etc.). For them, "no special consultations or discussions . . . were necessary": "The total extermination of this group of asylum inmates was the logical consequence of the 'radical solution' of the Jewish problem being embarked upon."[75]

Only at this point does direct medical killing provide an *exact* prefiguring of the Final Solution: Jews were to be killed—to the last man, woman, and child—simply because they were Jews. For the Nazis, Jewish mental patients were unique among all Nazi victims in that they could embody both "dangerous genes" in an individual medical sense, and "racial poison" in a collective ethnic sense.

Systematic T4 treatment of German Jews began in April 1940, with a proclamation from the Reich Interior Ministry that, within three weeks, all Jewish patients were to be inventoried. In June, the first gassings of Jews took place, as two hundred men, women, and children died in the Brandenburg facility, having been transported there in six *Gekrat* buses from the Berlin-Buch mental institution. There were more killings in July. On 30 August, another directive from the Interior Ministry ordered that Jews were to be transferred to various centers, depending on their geographic location. It was explained that employees and relatives of Aryan patients had complained about being treated and housed with Jews.[76]

The Bavarian collection center was Eglfing-Haar, where Dr. Pfannmüller had once declared proudly: "No Jews are allowed in my institution!"[77] Now the Jews transferred in were placed in two special houses (where they were separated by sex rather than degree of illness) and thrust into propaganda-film roles depicting them as "typical Jews" and "the scum of humanity." This segregation reflected the general policy that, in Schmidt's ironic words, " 'Aryan' mental patients could not be expected to die together with Jewish patients, much less live together."[78]

In the fall of 1940, Jewish patients began to be transported to Nazi-occupied Poland as part of the policy of removing all Jews from Germany. In December, it was announced that henceforth Jewish patients would be transferred to a facility for mentally impaired children in Bendorf near Neuwied in the Rhineland. This was a privately owned Jewish institution going back to 1869. Beginning in the spring of 1942, Bendorf patients were sent to Poland, in trains with sixty to seventy patients sealed in each freight car, trains that carried ordinary Jewish citizens as well. The Bendorf hospital was supposed to be used for soldiers, but never was. The director, a "privileged Jew" (married to an Aryan), stayed on to act as caretaker in the empty facility.[79]

Once the Jewish patients were herded into trains, the pretense of medicalized treatment ended. The trains arrived in Lublin, an area where Polish Jews were being concentrated and where Jewish confiscated goods were processed with slave labor. The precise fate of these patients is unknown and probably varied, except for the final outcome—their extermination in such camps as Sobibór and Belzec.[80]

The T4 office set up a Jewish camouflage operation: on "Cholm Insane Asylum" letterheads, statements of condolence and death certificates were sent out. Couriers took the mail to Chelm (the Polish spelling), near Lublin, where they were mailed with the proper postmark. As far as can be determined, the "Cholm Insane Asylum" was a fiction.[81]

From September 1939, when the war began, with German troops pushing eastward, the SS began to shoot inmates (of whatever race or nationality) of mental hospitals to empty them for the use of soldiers. For example, a hospital in Stralsund, an eastern German city on the Baltic Sea, was emptied by December 1939, and its patients were taken to Danzig to be shot. Their bodies were buried by Polish prisoners, who themselves were then shot. In Chelm-Lubielski, in the General Government of Poland, patients were shot *en masse* by SS troops, sometimes after having been chased through the asylum, and then buried in mass graves. Once Germany invaded Russia, in June 1941, *Einsatzgruppen* under Heydrich liquidated hospital patients as well as Jews, Gypsies, and Communist functionaries. Reports from the field mentioned the need for beds for injured soldiers, as well as "the German view" that these were lives unworthy of life.[82]

More closely related to T4, the Germans set up two psychiatric extermination facilities at Meseritz-Obrawalde and Tiegenhof, both in the old Prussian territory of Pomerania. The policy was first to massacre Polish patients, then bring German patients into the emptied facility, and finally to kill them as well by such methods as shooting, gassing, injection, starvation, or drugs given with food. Standard T4 letters of condolence were sent to families. There is some evidence that physically or mentally impaired German soldiers were also given "euthanasia" in both institutions.[83]

Concerning the technology of murder, there was diminished reliance on shooting because of psychological trauma to *Einsatzgruppen* troops. Explosives were tried—as in Russia, in September 1941, when mental patients were blown up. This method proved ineffective in that too much cleaning up was required and more than one charge was sometimes necessary. Gas was clearly preferable.

Carbon monoxide gas was increasingly resorted to—first in canisters (which became ever more expensive to bring from Germany as the troops moved east), and then, after further technological innovation, from the exhaust of vans. During two weeks in May and June of 1940, 1,558 mental patients from East Prussia were gassed in vans at a transit camp in Soldau. The killings were carried out by "the itinerant euthanasia squad known as Sonderkommando Lange [its commander]," and represented an early blending of three elements of the Final Solution: the "euthanasia" program, laboratory science and SS technology (contributing to innovations in gassing), and *Einsatzgruppen* units (here working with the new gassing technology). In October 1941, Brack and Eichmann decided to use these vans for Jews in general who were "incapable of working." Three were installed at the first pure extermination camp at Chelmno/Kulmhof (using personnel from Soldau), where they killed mainly Jews, but also Gypsies, typhus victims, Soviet POWs, and the insane. In a replica of the T4 procedure, victims were told they would shower while their clothing was being disinfected. SS officers wore white coats and carried stethoscopes. Prisoners had their valuables registered, then followed a "To the Bath" sign, up a ramp and into the van. When no more noise was audible from the van, it was driven to the woods nearby where Jewish *Kommandos* unloaded the corpses into mass graves. (Because of noxious gases, a crematorium was later installed.) Chelmno/Kulmhof, in reclaimed German territory, was the first of the extermination camps in the General Government, followed by Belzec, Sobibór, and Treblinka, all of which still more closely resembled "euthanasia" killing centers in the use of stationary gas chambers and T4 personnel.[84] (See chapter 7 and pages 142–44.)

Chapter 3

Resistance to Direct Medical Killing

There is strange talk in Munich about the fate of mental patients.

How come he died so fast? I enclose a stamp so that you will tell me about his last hours.

Why was my brother's body burned? I would like to have buried him in a grave.

We have to reproach you about not having given us a chance to say goodbye. . . . We are really bitter and do not understand your measures. I expect you will tell me your reasons for such behavior.

—Excerpts from letters of family members of patients killed in the "euthanasia" program

Resistance within Psychiatry

Some psychiatrists resisted medical killing—but mostly in limited, isolated, and indirect ways. Though insufficient, that resistance was not without significance.

What was undoubtedly the most widespread form of resistance is the most difficult to evaluate: the "silent resistance" in the form of actions taken by individual psychiatrists to enable patients to evade the lethal bureaucracy.[1] These measures included diagnosing patients as severely neurotic rather than schizophrenic, or minimizing mentally deficient patients' inability to work; releasing patients to their families or keeping them in university clinics or on general medical services, rather than transferring them to state hospitals; and generally emphasizing patients' potential capacity for improvement, work, and eventual contribution to society. There could be unspoken cooperation among colleagues in these maneuvers, sometimes with the help of medical, psychiatric, and non-medical administrators who were not fully enthusiastic about the program. Psychiatrists engaging in these attempts at evasion varied in their attitudes from ambivalence toward the program to strong condemnation, and their evasions tended to be accompanied by what they considered necessary cooperation with the project.

Nurses and ward workers could also contribute to evasive maneuvers, either by warning patients to leave the hospital before it was too late, or even on occasion helping them to hide. A former patient in a church-run institution told of how fearful she and other patients were upon hearing that cars were coming to take them to their deaths:

> We went through the forest, ran around, because we did not know where to go. . . . When the sisters [nurses] came to fetch them, many [patients] started to run again. . . . We hid in barns a few times. . . . One was safe nowhere. . . . As soon as a car came, the head nurse called: "Get up, march, hide yourself. If someone comes, don't stand still."[2]

These nurses and hospital workers could, like the doctors, express such resistance at one moment and carry out their part in the killing at another.

Expressions of discomfort could come from psychiatrists who wanted things to be more forthright and more legal. "If the government actually wishes to carry out the extermination of these patients . . . should not a clearly formulated law be proclaimed— . . . as in the case of the [Sterilization] Law," was the way the head of a mental hospital expressed his view to the Ministry of Justice.[3]

Crucial to whatever psychiatric resistance existed was the influence of a few leading psychiatric humanists of the older generation, such as Karl Bonhoeffer. These men became known as opponents of medical killing and, in varying degree, of the Nazi regime in general. In 1939, the politically suspect Bonhoeffer was replaced in the prestigious psychiatric position of the chair of Berlin University and Charité Hospital by Max de Crinis, Party and SS member. Bonhoeffer then became more active in helping his two sons and his son-in-law, all of whom were eventually killed by the regime for their opposition to it. He involved himself specifically in the struggle against medical killing by helping his son Dietrich, later a celebrated Protestant martyr, in the latter's contacts with church groups seeking authoritative psychiatric grounds for refusing to turn over their patients to the project.[4]

The unusual degree of respect accorded Bonhoeffer in the profession, together with his well-known opposition to medical killing, provided at least indirect professional and psychiatric support for other psychiatrists' efforts at resistance, however partial.[5]*

A psychiatrist for whom Bonhoeffer's influence was said to be crucial was Professor Hans Gerhard Creutzfeldt of Kiel. One of just two members of the medical faculty who did not join the Nazi Party, Creutzfeldt was somewhat protected by his academic dean, who discreetly let him know how far he could go in his anti-Nazi stance. Creutzfeldt went farther than most, and is said to have managed to protect most or all of the patients in his institution from the project. One psychiatrist told me that Creutzfeldt was known to have attacked "euthanasia" during his lectures, declaring, "They are murderers!" and was able to get away with it because the Nazis thought him very eccentric or even "a little mad."†Close relatives I interviewed doubted that he would have been able to say such things directly. In any case, he was perceived as being capable of uttering that truth.

"Certain Medical Objections": Gottfried Ewald

Just one psychiatrist, Professor Gottfried Ewald of Göttingen, openly opposed the medical-killing project. (But see the footnote on page 87 and pages 88–89.) Ewald had sufficient standing with the regime to be invited to become a leader in the medical killing project, sufficient personal and professional humanitarianism to refuse for reasons of principle, and sufficient courage to distribute his extensive critique of the program to high medical authorities.

At a planning meeting called by Werner Heyde, on 15 August 1940, to enlist prominent psychiatrists, Ewald refused to participate in the project and was asked to leave. He remembered Heyde presiding at a "long table," explaining that "the 'euthanizing' must continue" because, even though hospital beds were no longer urgently needed by the military, the institutions still had to be "freed" of patients, "since one does not know what is going to happen." It would be the task of the assembled psychiatric leaders to become "experts" or "senior experts," which meant rendering judgments on whether patients were to be "euthanized" (euthansiert). Heyde reported that there were plans to expand the program to senile and tubercular patients, and that Hitler was about to sign a law (whose text could be seen in the next room) that would provide "judicial security."[7]‡

*It must be said that Bonhoeffer originally favored sterilization and, moreover, did not take a strong stand against the Nazification of German universities, as he later had the candor to admit ("Unfortunately, neither I nor any of the other professors had the courage to get up and walk out in protest against the insulting attitude adopted by the Minister [for education and cultural affairs, Bernhard Rust] towards the academic profession").[6] He did, however, struggle to maintain an atmosphere of decency and balanced professional work in his department.

†Creutzfeldt later played a central role in exposing Werner Heyde and bringing him to trial (see page 119).

‡This text—if there actually was one—could have been the draft for such a law which, as we know, was never implemented.

Ewald felt so immediately preoccupied with formulating his objections that he could not recall what else Heyde said. When given an opportunity to speak, Ewald stated, "On principle I would not lend my hand to exterminate in this way patients entrusted to me." He pointed out that schizophrenics, the largest patient group concerned, were not as "empty and hopeless" as claimed, and could well benefit from new forms of therapy just then being developed. After giving additional arguments and making clear his refusal to become an expert, he was joined by two other psychiatrists. But those two reversed themselves, Ewald testified, when Paul Nitsche, Heyde's next in command and a man with considerable professional standing, spoke passionately of having personally lived through the tragedy of coping with a mentally ill brother-in-law and urged the group not to oppose the extermination of the mentally ill.* As Ewald said nothing more and clearly had not changed his position, Heyde "dismissed" him, in a firm but "very polite and collegial fashion," even expressing "respect for my point of view."[8]

Immediately after the meeting, Ewald made notes of what had happened at it, and these became the basis for a memorandum he sent to the dean of his faculty at the University of Göttingen, as well as to Heyde, Conti, a regional official in Hanover, and the psychotherapist Dr. Matthias Göring with a request that he pass it along to his cousin Hermann, the powerful air marshal.† Written essentially from a Nazi framework, the memorandum began by raising questions, not about the rights of patients, but about whether so "far-reaching" an action would be sufficiently beneficial to the *Volk* to justify it. Ewald conceded that, if a people were absolutely besieged, and "needed every grain (of food) for its healthy members, then . . . those unfortunate sick members would be the first to give their life in favor of the healthy population." But without that extremity, doctors should not "interfere with fate." .

*One of those two doctors, Arthur Kuhn (of Reichenau), disputed this and testified that he met the other man, a Dr. Meusberger (of Klagenfurt), at the train station, having left early while the rest of the group stayed late to drink and celebrate; but their overall roles remain obscure. Neither Kuhn nor Meusberger appears on lists of experts in Nazi documents. (I am grateful to Ernst Klee for a personal communication [November 1985] on this matter.)

†Matthias Göring was a psychiatrist and Adlerian psychotherapist who, largely because of his family connections, was made director of what came to be known as the Göring Institute in Berlin. Although an ardent Nazi who kept in constant touch with his eminent cousin and did not hesitate to exploit his name, Matthias Göring was generally perceived as being relatively benign (he was known within the institute as "Papi") and managed to maintain under one professional roof, with certain restrictions, Adlerian, Jungian, and Freudian psychotherapists and psychoanalysts, as well as those who were strongly pro-Nazi, anti-Nazi, or somewhere in between. Because he and his institute enabled psychotherapy to survive as a profession in Nazi Germany, and because he offered some protection to individual psychotherapists, he has been somewhat romanticized. Although he never achieved his goal of a "new German psychotherapy," he did press German psychotherapy into service to the regime and maintained active links with the military and the SS. The Göring Institute is a fascinating story on many levels, but I believe that Göring is best understood as a prototypical "decent Nazi"—a genre I shall have much more to say about later; and that he and his institute served the primary function of *Gleichschaltung* for German psychoanalysis, psychotherapy, and a small portion of psychiatry (the minority of the discipline concerned with a psychotherapeutic approach).[9]

He went on to argue that all people, not just the sick, should be willing to put their own lives and those of close family members "at the disposal of the State," especially during wartime, since "the *goal* for which we strive . . . [is] the greatest that we know . . . freedom, greatness and happiness of the people." He acknowledged the "higher medical and general goal" of ending life unworthy of life as compared with nursing it, but wanted to limit that concept to such situations as that in which a doctor would hasten the death of a terminal cancer patient who longed for it "for healthy [*gesund*] reasons." In that sense, Ewald sought to return to the true meaning of euthanasia. And he stressed the *"biological bond of blood"* that exists "even between a mother and her idiotic child—*and demands respect.*" Should a family, because of the economic burden created by such a child, consent to its elimination, the state would do better to offer aid to the family, "in order . . . not to differentiate between our countrymen who are in a better or worse economic position."[10]

Only then did Ewald raise "certain medical objections." He asked with italicized emphasis: *"Do we really know that all the patients who fall under this law are incurable?"* Here, focusing on schizophrenia, he pointed out that it contains no clearly recognized histopathology (tissue change) and that new therapies have resulted in "astonishing" recoveries. Going on to explore the psychological consequences for relatives and the general population, he noted that many will be "tortured" by self-blame, whether or not they actually gave consent; that there will be terrible conflict and reproaches within families; and that fear and distrust will be rampant, especially toward doctors, "because one knows that admission to a mental clinic or institution can lead to death." Not only would medical care for the entire population suffer, but the medical profession would lose its general standing, and people would associate it with everything that is "sinister, monstrous, and terrible." He boldly invoked the finality of killing: "One can live and even enjoy life without Fallopian tubes or a vas deferens (although most have suffered bitterly under the sterilization procedure), but death puts an end to everything."[11]

Ewald was at his most eloquent in affirming the integrity of the medical profession—but again within a Nazi context:

> Physicianship is built on the urge to *help* another, and comfort and not harm him. The psychiatrist in particular has learned to promote a higher good . . . the good of all. . . . Every sensible doctor will also approve euthanasia. Who, however, aspiring to become a doctor, will want to be put in the position of eliminating hopeless cases against the wish of their relatives, and, *without the most compelling need,* taking upon oneself the odium of killing? . . . I can certainly kill any time if it is a matter of saving the *Volk;* . . . I would also . . . approve the elimination of serious criminals and common vermin. But I cannot choose a profession whose daily business it is to eliminate a sick person because of his sickness after he or his relatives have come to me, trusting and looking for help.

And Ewald stressed that he spoke from many years of close professional observation, as a man who has had the opportunity "to really look into the psyche of his patients and of the people" to a much greater extent than "the best theorist . . . [or] statistician" concerned with hereditary research.[12]*

Ewald had been initially sympathetic to the Nazis, according to his widow, whom I interviewed in a nursing home: "He said his *Heil* Hitler enthusiastically like everyone else." Nazi Party documents confirmed this attitude, describing him, in 1939, as politically "reliable" and as having a "positive political attitude toward the Third Reich."[13] Yet Ewald's persistent attempts to gain Party membership during the 1930s were repeatedly refused for what were always described as merely "formal" reasons. Those formal reasons turned out to be related to Ewald's First World War injury, which had led to amputation of one of his forearms. As a "militarily disabled one-armed person" (as one investigation put it),[14] he was prevented from serving actively in the SA or an equivalent organization; he joined the SA Reserve so as to engage in their military maneuvers despite his handicap, as he had earlier those of the since-dissolved *völkisch Freikorps* "Oberland" which he joined in 1923. In being approved for renewal of his Göttingen professorship, Ewald was described in 1939 by a local Nazi personnel officer as "completely sympathetic to the aspirations of the NSDAP [the National Socialist German Workers', or Nazi, Party]."[15]

The Party documents further explained that an exception to formal requirements could be made for certain outstanding people considered "particularly desirable and regarded as a particular prize for the work of the Party," but that Ewald did not meet this criterion. The possible implication is that his professional standing, though certainly solid, was not outstanding; or that his Nazi identification, though strong, was not absolute. The latter "shortcoming" is suggested by his having placed (in late 1938, when he was director of the Göttingen State Hospital and after these judgments had been made) a Jewish patient eligible for work rehabilitation with a German farm family—an incident that outraged Party officials.[16]†

Yet he had what his widow called a "kind of connection" with Hermann Göring through having treated, and kept in the Ewald home, one of the

---

*Ewald received replies to the letter from his dean, Dr. Stich (cautious agreement and return of documents), from Conti (friendly disagreement), and from the state official, but apparently none from Heyde or Matthias Göring.

†The local Nazi leader in Mengershausen reported to the district leader in Göttingen that this Jewish patient had been observed at church festivals dancing with "German girls." This official then wrote to Ewald: "The understanding of the Third Reich of agrarian estate does not allow under any circumstances the presence of Jews on German farm land." Moreover this Jew's appearance in public had caused offense. Ewald returned the patient to the state hospital immediately, after explaining that he had been pressured by the government of Hanover to put as many patients as possible in home care because it reduced the burden to the state. Also, farmers were short of help and competed for such patients. However, no more Jews would be sent to farms.[17]

Prussian minister-president's subordinates so that the man's illness would not become known; Ewald had even gone to Berlin to report to Göring on the progress of the patient's therapy. This connection was undoubtedly a factor in Ewald's later decision to ask Matthias Göring to forward his critical memo on "euthanasia" to Hermann. Indeed, Ewald's way of articulating these views and making them known to high medical officials indicates some trust in the regime and some expectation that it would take seriously his moral scruples. The tone of his covering letters to Heyde and Conti is that of a friendly colleague discussing a serious matter. To Heyde, Ewald said, "I was sorry that I had to disappoint you"; and to Conti, he declared himself "gladly at your disposal for a personal consultation at any time, should this appear convenient to you." But, in these letters, he also spoke of his "medical conscience" and "inner need" to do what he did.[18] And he was not without fear of reprisal.

After his return to Göttingen from the meeting with Heyde in Berlin, Ewald said, according to his widow, "Please be sensible about things, but be prepared for the possibility that, any day from now on, I might be sent to a concentration camp." Also, he did not consult with colleagues about Nazi medical killing because, his widow believed, it was forbidden to talk about the subject to others, and he in any case "thought it would be of no use." She did, however, remember that later, sometime in 1944, he talked actively with psychiatric colleagues about joining in an effort to declare Hitler mad.*

Ewald's behavior became even more complex immediately after the German surrender. His wife told how he burned most of his psychiatric files because they "contained material against many people—they would lose their capacity to earn a living and could be sent to prison." Further questioning gave me the impression that the files contained correspondence exhibiting various degrees of support for Nazi positions, from *pro forma* expressions to strong enthusiasm, and could have been embarrassing not only to colleagues but to Ewald himself.

Ewald's widow also reported that he had "hidden" a considerable number of psychiatrists in his hospital, people who had been implicated in the "euthanasia" program. He enabled them to work there with minimal visibility (it is not clear whether they changed their names or took other measures to avoid being found), and at one time had "fifty-one guest doctors." She presented this as part of her husband's humanitarian impulse, his conviction that "it would not help anybody if these men

---

*There is some confusion concerning this remembered event. In 1938, at the time of the Czechoslovakian crisis, a group of conspirators, including Hans von Dohnanyi, who was Karl Bonhoeffer's son-in-law, considered capturing Hitler and trying him in a People's Court for endangering Germany's safety by courting war. Dohnanyi and another man had produced a report of Hitler's various illnesses which they showed to Bonhoeffer in the hope that he, or a panel he headed, would certify Hitler insane. A later attempt to question Hitler's sanity involved intrigue among high-level Nazis during the last year of the war. There is no written evidence of Ewald's participation in either of these attempts, but he could have been involved in still another, unrecorded effort by psychiatrists to declare Hitler mentally ill.[19]

suffered more, they had suffered enough already"; and she associated this activity with the same "simple sense of duty" he felt in his personal resistance to the medical killing project.

During the early postwar period, Dr. Ewald also gave willing testimony at "euthanasia" trials. He seemed to want to reassert his opposition to the project, but at the same time to offer personal help to psychiatrists who had been implicated. It may be that in certain ways he did not consider himself different from them. He had been a strong supporter of the regime, and his principled stand against its major "psychiatric" project was an attempt to reform it from within, even perhaps to preserve some of what he had come to admire in it. He could well have been left with a measure of guilt for this disaffection from his nation's representatives, and more specifically guilt toward his colleagues for stepping out of their group in a way that cast aspersions on them. After all, he was strongly identified with most of his colleagues professionally and politically, and probably went further than most in cooperating with the regime prior to his stand against medical killing. This guilt and identification contributed to his protection of his colleagues after the war. However one judges that behavior, the sensitivity to guilt it reflects could well have been related to the act of conscience that distinguished him. Also undoubtedly crucial was his injury, his status as a handicapped person, which made him more sympathetic than others to the potential victims of medical killing, a little more wary of the concept of "life unworthy of life." (Significantly, Dr. Kuhn, who seems also, at Heyde's Berlin meeting, to have refused full participation, had an amputated leg.)[20]

Ewald could not summon Bonhoeffer's deep-seated humanism and liberalism nor his professional stature. But I suspect that—and here Ewald resembles both Bonhoeffer and Creutzfeldt—earlier religious exposure affected this secular son of a Protestant minister.[21] Whatever the extent of such influences, and whatever one's prior relationship to the Nazi movement, there remains the inner integrity that permits one at a given moment to say no. A deeply concerned German physician who went over the entire Ewald story with me concluded rather sadly, "It seems that a hero is not really a hero." That may be so: Ewald was considerably less than an anti-Nazi hero. And yet perhaps he was a hero after all. He did perform, as a psychiatrist within a discipline that essentially complied with the regime, a direct, courageous, personal, and professional act of opposition to medical killing.*

*Of course, other secular psychiatrists took stands, in one way or another, against direct medical killing. They included Kurt Schneider (to be distinguished in every way from Carl Schneider [see pages 122–23]), Ernst Kretschmer, and Professor Karl Kleist, an internist with some psychiatric experience, who was described by an interviewed doctor as having mentioned in a lecture his refusal to join a "euthanasia" commission (see page 39). One young psychiatrist, Theo Lang, also approached Matthias Göring and asked him to sign a declaration against the extermination of mental patients. Göring declined;[22] he resisted efforts to gain his support on at least two further occasions (see page 91). The resistance of psychiatrists from religious institutions is discussed later in this chapter. Nor is this list in any sense complete.

Psychiatrists in Religious Institutions

Resistive psychiatrists and church leaders probably influenced each other more than has been generally recognized, but still in sporadic and limited fashion. Psychiatrists working within church institutions, however, could at times become part of more sustained and shared forms of resistance. At Schussenried, a Protestant psychiatric institution, the chief physician, a Dr. Götz, had a "violent quarrel" with the expert on the "euthanasia" physicians' commission because he "consistently evaluated [the work capacity] of the patients much too low." Dr. Götz remembered a previous situation "in which patients had been sent to their deaths"; now he felt that the visitor "put responsibility on [him for selecting patients for death], which was impossible for him to bear." He had been ordered to cooperate in the matter by the Württemberg minister of the interior, and was therefore aware that "he had not followed an order from the office of his superior and . . . that some day he would have to account for this."[23] That sense of potential guilt for patients' deaths could be a powerful fulcrum for resistance, especially in men with a strong Christian conscience.

Dr. Rudolph Boeckh, chief psychiatrist at the Evangelical Lutheran institution at Neuendettelsau (the site of the invasion of medical students and typists [see page 67]) was blunt in declaring "the commission's method of operation prejudiced and contrary to all medical practice." He added, "Since the final purpose of these reports on patients is known to the public, a heavy responsibility is imposed on me as the chief doctor, . . . even if several commissions are brought in prior to the final decision."[24]

In both cases, we see a tendency to protest the criteria and methods of operation rather than the overall project itself (a much more difficult and probably more dangerous undertaking): thus, Dr. Boeckh, for example, demanded the questionnaires be returned so that he could fill them out adequately.[25] That kind of compromise—pressing to save as many patients as possible while surrendering those one felt unable to save— was frequent.

Perhaps the most notable psychiatric resistance from within a church setting came from Dr. Karsten Jasperson, chief physician at the psychiatric institution at Bethel (separate from the associated institution for epileptics). As a Nazi Party member since 1931, Jasperson could go so far as to institute criminal proceedings against police groups associated with murder arrangements; refuse to fill out questionnaires, claiming that to do so was "aiding and abetting murder" according to existing criminal law; try to win support for that position from senior academic physicians, including his own Professor Rüdin (with whom he had little success) and Professor August Bostroem of Leipzig (who was responsive and apparently went on to make contact with Ewald). Jasperson's resistance could be expressed, as he put it, "precisely as a National Socialist doctor [for whom] these measures go directly and decisively against every conception of a physician's profession." He expressed these views to Martin Bormann, with whom he had a long-standing tie, and spoke of his concern that the absence of legal basis for the killings would impair "the ethical concepts of our *Volk.*" Bormann defended the program by contrasting the Christian view of wishing to keep alive "even those creatures least worthy of life" with the National Socialist position that keeping such people alive was "completely against nature."[26]

The People's Resistance

What eventually persuaded Nazi leaders to cancel the project officially was not psychiatric resistance but rather general resistance among the German people, articulated and heightened by a few courageous Protestant and Catholic religious leaders. Family members of patients wrote letters to institution heads (as excerpted in the epigraph to this chapter) expressing confusion and pain but also at times accurate knowledge and anger: references to "strange talk" about the fate of patients, questions about their dying "so fast," and resentment about relatives not being permitted a proper burial and not having a "chance to say goodbye."[27]

The unrest could reach high places. A provincial probate judge wrote to Franz Gürtner, the minister of justice, stating that he (the judge) had received formal charges from the guardians of patients and the personnel of institutions from which patients had been taken to their deaths at Hartheim. He went on to say to his judicial colleague, "Man commits an act of . . . extraordinary arrogance when he takes it upon himself to put an end to a human life because, with his limited understanding, he can no longer grasp the entire meaning of that life." In the same letter he also declared, "Everyone knows as well as I do" that "the murder of the mentally ill is as well known a daily reality as, say, the concentration camps."[28]

And Else von Löwis, a leader in the Nazi women's organization and a woman of the highest social standing who mixed regularly with regime leaders, wrote to a friend, the wife of the presiding judge of the Party Chancellery Court and a close friend of Himmler, of her horror at the regime's attempt to deceive the people in killing mental patients ("When the farmers of Württemberg see the cars go by, they too know what is going on—just as when they see the smoke pouring from the crematory chimneys day and night"); and at the policy of killing mental patients indiscriminately, including some only slightly ill or those sane for long periods of time, rather than only those "without the slightest glimmer of human consciousness" (which, she thought, would be accepted by the people if there were a proper law). She admitted that until then she had had "steadfast confidence in our Führer," but now she could feel "the ground . . . give way beneath our feet," though "people are still clinging to the hope that the Führer does not yet know of these things." The judge forwarded the letter to Himmler, who informed him "confidentially" that there was such a program, "on the authority of the Führer," being carried out by "medical experts . . . conscious of their responsibilities"; and that, if the project had become well known, "the manner of operating [was] at fault."[29]

Indeed, angry crowd reactions came close at times to public demonstrations against the killing of mental patients. One report to the SS Security Service from Absberg on 1 March 1941 states that "the removal of people from the Ottilien Home has caused a great deal of unpleasantness," tells of a priest offering communion to patients forced into a bus before large crowds of Catholic townspeople, complains of the visibility of the whole operation, describes how deeply troubled people were, and adds that "among those upset and crying are Party members."[30] This was one of the few issues on which sentiment against a regime policy was so openly and bitterly expressed.

Resistance from the Churches

Much of Protestant religious resistance centered on mental institutions; two leaders were pastors who served as nonmedical administrators of such institutions. These were Paul-Gerhard Braune, director of the Hoffnungstal Institution in Berlin and vice president of the central board of the Home Mission; and the Reverend Fritz von Bodelschwingh, director of the legendary Bethel Institution, mainly for epileptics, at Bielefeld. Both were active leaders of the Confessional Church, as opposed to "German Christians" who had allied themselves to the National Socialist regime. Both pastors also belonged to the group within the Confessional Church who believed that "where an institution was threatened by the killing, one should fight for the lives of the patients [against] those who were to take them away to have them killed"—rather than speaking out from the pulpit about the evil of the "euthanasia" project and its violation of God's commandments. The latter course, they feared, might harm the cause of actual patients.[31]

Bodelschwingh's institution at Bethel, initiated by his father, was renowned for creating a dedicated and harmonious Christian community. In that atmosphere Bodelschwingh could command the loyalty of his psychiatric physicians—including Jasperson—to join him in resistance to questionnaires, in expressing objections to Nazi officials, and in various maneuvers to keep patients from being drawn into the killing machinery.* Bodelschwingh also visited Matthias Göring in May 1940 to ask for help, and was told by Professor Göring "not to undertake anything [in the way of opposition], but only to do this when we have definite evidence" (though there surely was already evidence). Early in the next year, Bodelschwingh asked Professor Göring to deliver a letter addressed to the latter's cousin Hermann, pleading that his epileptic patients not be subjected to "economic planning" measures. Although Hermann Göring did see fit to answer, he claimed that Bodelschwingh's assertions were "in part inexact and in large measure false," and added that he would have Karl Brandt clarify things further. Bodelschwingh, in fact, negotiated endlessly with high Nazi officials and developed a close and friendly relationship with Brandt (see pages 115–16), partially cooperating while managing to stall the process despite a visit from a doctors' commission. Bodelschwingh succeeded in protecting most of his patients.[33]

Braune, described as a man of formidable "Prussian military bearing," had opposed the sterilization program[34]† and had taken the initiative in approaching Bodelschwingh concerning opposition to medical killing. Braune then worked closely with Bodelschwingh on gathering and exchanging information and paying visits together to high officials. In one, along with the surgeon Ferdinand Sauerbruch, they confronted Minister of Justice Gürtner, in the latter's apartment, with facts that apparently surprised him and caused him to be "genuinely horrified."[36]‡ Braune also produced a truly remarkable document, which combined passionate protest with detailed and systematic evidence, and was submitted to an official at the Chancellery and addressed to Adolf Hitler.

The document begins with general observations made in "various parts of the Reich" which "preclude any doubt that this is a large-scale plan to exterminate . . . thousands of 'human beings unworthy of life.' " These measures, he insists, "gravely undermine the moral foundations of the whole *Volk*" and were "intolerable." He then presents a chronology of directives, institutional experiences, questionnaire details, and methods of deception—even making statistical estimates of the number of people killed on the basis of the numbers on the urns of ashes received by families. He considers these events "shocking" and "simply unworthy" of therapeutic institutions.[37]

---

*Bodelschwingh was originally a supporter of the regime and even an advocate of eugenics, who spoke of his "deep reverence" for research in that area and accepted the sterilization program. But in his Christian view he looked upon the physically and mentally impaired as "God's admonition to man and reminders . . . of the connection between guilt and atonement."[32] He brought that Christian fervor to his protection of patients entrusted to him.

†Even he seemed to waiver a bit on sterilization. He apparently detested the wandering beggars he encountered as business manager of the German Hostel Association, and advocated that they be removed from society into work camps and even undergo "medical measures that would make these people no longer dangerous to the *Volk*."[35]

‡After that meeting, Gürtner asked the Chancellery chief Lammers whether the program should not either be stopped or else made legal.

He speaks also of the systematic creation of confusion: of patients "so completely mixed up in huge institutions [that] no one knows the other's fate." He tells how people "pine away in loneliness and die in total desolation" and offers as evidence the death of a jurist and son of a high government official.[38] In this way, Braune goes back and forth between carefully observed details and ringing ethical assertions.

He concludes, "We are dealing here with a conscious, systematic process of eliminating all those who are mentally ill or otherwise incapable of functioning in a community"—a process that "severely undermines the faith placed in . . . physicians and [health] authorities." He notes Germany's superior history in regard to providing well-run institutions and well-trained personnel with "unselfish readiness to serve," and asks whether these constructive inclinations will be forced "to die out slowly in our people?" He asks also how far the extermination of "life unworthy of life" can go, having already been extended to people who were "lucid and responsible"; and who the next target will be. Then he touches a particularly raw nerve: "What will happen to the soldiers who contract incurable afflictions while fighting for their fatherland?" He adds, "Such questions have already arisen among them."[39]

He then returns to moral questions concerning the sanctity of human life, and how violation of that sanctity "without legal basis" endangers "the ethics of the people as a whole. Whom if not the helpless should the law protect?" He points out that, after careful calculation, even if one hundred thousand people were to be killed (the actual estimate of the number who were eventually killed in the project),[40] it would be of no significant help to the economic well-being of the rest of the population. Braune concludes with a ringing declaration of the dimension of the danger and an intense plea for relief:

> We are confronted here with an emergency that deeply shocks everyone who knows about it, that destroys the inner peace of many families, and that above all threatens to grow into a danger whose consequences cannot even be predicted at this point. May the responsible authorities make sure that these disastrous measures are abolished, and that the entire problem is first examined from a legal and medical, from the ethical and political point of view, before the fate of thousands and tens of thousands is decided. *Videant consules, ne quid detrimenti res publica capiat!* ("Let the consuls see to it that the state suffers no harm!")[41]

Of all recorded expressions of resistance to Nazi medical killing, the Braune memorandum is unique in combining insistent documentation, compassionate identification with victims, concern for healing and healers, focus on the moral integrity of an entire people as well as on the broad ethical principle of the sanctity of life, exposure of the regime's vulnerability to general fear of "euthanasia" among the military, and passionate personal protest grounded in a spiritual tradition.

The Nazi leaders must have recognized the power of his statement, since Lammers, Chief of the Reich Chancellery, was said to have informed Hitler of it, then told Braune that the program could not be stopped. And about one month later, Braune was arrested under a warrant signed by Heydrich charging him with having "sabotaged measures of the regime and the Party in an irresponsible manner." Braune was held at the Gestapo jail on Prinz Albrecht Strasse for about ten weeks and then released (probably through Bodelschwingh's intervention) on the promise that he would undertake no further actions against policies of the government or the Party.[42]

While Bodelschwingh and Braune expressed their resistance essentially through official channels, certain local ministers spoke out directly from their churches, and could be sent to a concentration camp as a result. Ernst Wilm did so from a Westphalian village, and was denounced and sent to Dachau where he spent three years.[43]

The most ringing Catholic protest against "euthanasia" was the famous sermon of Clemens Count von Galen, then bishop of Münster.* It was given on 3 August 1941, just four Sundays after the highly significant pastoral letter of German bishops had been read from every Catholic pulpit in the country; the letter reaffirmed "obligations of conscience" at opposing the taking of "innocent" life, "even if it were to cost us our [own] lives."[44] The first part of Galen's sermon explored the Biblical theme of how "Jesus, the Son of God, wept," how even God wept "because of stupidity, injustice . . . and because of the disaster which came about as a result." Then, after declaring, "It is a terrible, unjust and catastrophic thing when man opposes his will to the will of God," Galen quoted the pastoral letter of 6 July and made clear that the "catastrophic thing" he had in mind was the killing of innocent mental patients and "a doctrine which authorizes the violent death of invalids and elderly people."[45]

He further declared that he himself had "filed formal charges" with police and legal authorities in Münster over deportations from a nearby institution. He went on in words that every farmer and laborer could understand:

> It is said of these patients: They are like an old machine which no longer runs, like an old horse which is hopelessly paralyzed, like a cow which no longer gives milk.
>
> What do we do with a machine of this kind? We put it in the junkyard. What do we do with a paralyzed horse? No, I do not wish to push the

*The Catholic Church as a whole was traditionally less identified with the German state than were the Protestant churches. Although Catholics were a majority in some areas of Germany, German Catholics still bore traces of "outsider" status.

comparison to the end. . . . We are not talking here about a machine, a horse, nor a cow. . . . No, we are talking about men and women, our compatriots, our brothers and sisters. Poor unproductive people if you wish, but does this mean that they have lost their right to live?

He pointed out that, should such a principle be maintained, "then think of the horrible state we shall all be in when we are weak and sick!" The danger extended not only to "invalids" who, when healthy, had been hard and productive workers and "brave soldiers, when they come back seriously wounded," but "none of us here will be certain of his life."[46]

And after a couple of poignant examples of specific people killed, the bishop concluded, as he had begun, with Biblical imagery, this time not of Jesus weeping but of "divine justice"—ultimate punishment—for those "making a blasphemy of our faith" by persecuting clergy and "sending innocent people to their death." He asked that such people (who could only be the Nazi authorities) be ostracized and left to their divine retribution:

> We wish to withdraw ourselves and our faithful from their influence, so that we may not be contaminated by their thinking and their ungodly behavior, so that we may not participate and share with them in the punishment which a just God should and will pronounce upon all those who—like ungrateful Jerusalem*—do not wish what God wishes![47]

With the authority of his office, a Catholic bishop invoked the wrath of God on those who were killing the innocent. This powerful, populist sermon was immediately reproduced and distributed throughout Germany—indeed, it was dropped among German troops by British Royal Air Force flyers. Galen's sermon probably had a greater impact than any other one statement in consolidating anti-"euthanasia" sentiment; hence, Bormann's judgment that the bishop deserved the death penalty.[48]†

Perhaps still more threatening to Nazi leaders was the protest of Werner Mölders, a Catholic *Luftwaffe* pilot and famous war hero who had

---

*Galen's image of "ungrateful Jerusalem" contains a troubling irony in its apparent reference to the Jews (as having violated God's wishes in rejecting Jesus). The image could well refer more broadly to any tendency to stray from God's wishes throughout Judeo-Christian experience; it nonetheless suggests the kind of sentiment within German-Christian doctrine and expression that enabled that clergy to virtually ignore Nazi persecution of Jews.

†Bormann was responding to a Nazi propaganda leader who suggested Galen be hanged. However, Bormann added that "under the circumstances of war the Führer will hardly order this measure." The propagandist responded the same day with a report of a conversation with Josef Goebbels, who had no answer on how to combat Galen; the propaganda chief feared that, if something were done to the bishop, the population of Münster could be "written off" for the duration, and that "one could easily add to that all of Westphalia." A memorandum within the Propaganda Ministry on 12 August warned that taking measures against Galen would create a martyr, and other bishops and priests would take up the charges. Father Bernard Lichtenberg, however, unique in his condemnation of Nazi persecution of Jews, was taken into custody and badly beaten; he died in transit to Dachau.[49]

received Nazi Germany's highest military decoration from Hitler himself. In a letter to superior officers, Mölders expressed his chagrin over the "euthanasia" program and threatened to return his decoration.[50]

Perhaps we could not have expected from the medical or the psychiatric profession as impassioned an ethical condemnation as Bishop Galen's. But we could have hoped for a statement as comprehensive and morally clear as Pastor Braune's or a commitment to patients as dedicated and tenacious as Pastor Bodelschwingh's. Dr. Ewald's actions and memorandum come closest. But he was constrained—other physicians more so—by Nazi affiliations, by the German tradition of psychiatric and medical subservience to governmental authority, and, more broadly, by ethical gaps in twentieth-century medical professionalism. I say this not to render the churches as a whole heroic: most Protestant and Catholic leaders either went along with the Nazis or did nothing. Rather my point is that the Nazi attempt at medical mystification of killing was given the lie not primarily by psychiatrists or other physicians, many of whom were directly involved in carrying out the program, but by a few church leaders, who gave voice to the grief and rage of victimized families with ethical passions stemming from their own religious traditions.

Nazi leaders faced the prospect of either having to imprison prominent, highly admired clergymen and other protesters—a course with consequences in terms of adverse public reaction they greatly feared—or else end the program. The latter was essentially the recommendation of Himmler, who noted that the secret was no longer a secret, though added, "If operation T4 had been entrusted to the SS, things would have happened differently," because "when the Führer entrusts us with a job, we know how to deal with it correctly, without causing useless uproar among the people."[51] Hitler apparently gave Brandt a verbal order on or about 24 August 1941 to end or at least to "stall" operation T4.[52]* But the killing of mental patients did not end: mass murder was just beginning.

---

*Dr. Friedrich Mennecke (see pages 139–42) told a postwar German court an anecdote that he thought explained the end of the program on which he had served as expert. One day, Hitler was traveling between Munich and Berlin on a special train when it suddenly stopped at a station. Looking out the window to see what the problem was, he saw a crowd watching the loading of a group of retarded patients into a train. Seeing Hitler at the window, the crowd became threatening.[53] Whether true or apocryphal, the story says something about perceptions of degree of opposition.

Although the "halt" was accompanied by a "whispering campaign" to the effect that Hitler had on his own initiative stopped a program about which he had previously known nothing,[54] many of the protests I have discussed came after 24 August and in reference to a program that the protesters clearly thought had not stopped. The halt was not only partial but apparently allowed for the possibility of resumption.

Chapter 4

"Wild Euthanasia": The Doctors Take Over

> For quite a number of doctors . . . Hitler not only had the power of a commander in chief in a political sense, but was also the highest ranking physician.
> —VICTOR VON WEIZSÄCKER

What was discontinued was only the visible dimension of the project: the large-scale gassing of patients. T4 officially ceased as a program, but that turned out to be still another deception. Widespread killing continued in a second phase, sometimes referred to in Nazi documents as "wild euthanasia" because doctors—encouraged, if not directed, by the regime—could now act on their own initiative concerning who would live or die.[1]

While the regime ordered most of the gas chambers dismantled (to be reassembled, as it turned out, in the East), it did nothing to stop the ideological and institutional momentum of medical killing. The regime's clear message, in fact, was that the killings were to go on, but more quietly. And more quiet killing meant more isolated, individual procedures. Doctors acted on their personal and ideological inclinations, along with their sense of the regime's pulse. That pulse emanated no longer from the Chancellery, which bowed out along with T4 itself, but from the Reich Interior Ministry and its national medical subdivision. There were changes in geographical location, but the regime continued to make transportation arrangements, required that patients' deaths be recorded centrally, and in some cases maintained T4 experts in a partially supervisory role. Patients were now killed not by gas but by starvation and drugs, the latter method in particular rendering the killing still more "medical."

The children's program was not included under the T4 "halt." Killing methods did not have to be changed: drugs and starvation, and not gas, had been employed from the beginning. The killing of children had been considerably less visible, taking place as it did on wards in smaller facilities without the telltale evidence of noxious smoke and odors that stemmed from large-scale gassing. The program had been based more on presumed eugenic and scientific grounds than on direct economic ones (the children did not work and ate less) and had not created the degree of public controversy that adult killing did. If anything, the reporting methods for ostensible abnormalities became more systematic. Research efforts, mostly post-mortem studies, also became more systematic, as sometimes happened in adult "wild euthanasia." Not only did the regime remain closely involved, but the greater part of the killing of children took place after the official ending of the "euthanasia" project. What did become more "wild" was the method of deciding which children should be killed. Now even the pretense of review boards of "expert opinion" was abandoned: any child considered in some way impaired, and sent through the administrative system to any of the "special pediatric units" of the original project, was still fair game. Beyond that, institutional doctors could proceed according to their own inclinations.

Adult "wild euthanasia" involved more radical changes for psychiatrists. No longer operators of gas chambers, they returned to the familiar terrain of syringes, oral medications, and dietary prescriptions for achieving the same end. From the regime's medical bureaucracy came the continuing message that mental patients were "useless eaters," burdens on the state and its war effort, "life unworthy of life." Permission to kill was clear enough, even if a little indirect. As one psychiatrist later testified, "In conversation with other participants in the program I learned that there would be no fuss if some physician or other in an institution stood ready to kill a patient by injection or overdose, if he was convinced that the patient's extinction was desirable." And there was a partial merger of child and adult "euthanasia" programs as the age limit of the children's program was raised to sixteen years: "to some extent this expansion was to offer a substitute for the cancelled program."[2] There were, in fact, documented cases of patients of about that age who had managed to survive the official end of the adult "euthanasia" program only to be fatally reclassified as a child.[3]*

That same psychiatrist added, "Such things would . . . happen without

*In late 1944, the directors of several Reich Committe children's facilities were told at a Berlin meeting to include adults. No reason was given, but they were told to omit the usual procedures because they "would take too long." The institutions' doctors were given the power of selection. Dr. Hildegard Wesse of the Uchtspringe facility recalled, when on trial, that she realized this was an extraordinary order, but thought that "those in Berlin" must be acting under pressure of war. Uchtspringe then had twenty-five hundred patients, with new transports arriving from the East daily. Dr. Walter Schmidt, head of a small children's section at Eichberg, recalled a "few so-called special authorizations [Sonderermächtigungen]": that is, severely malformed adults who arrived with Reich Committee documentation, often including a family request for killing.[4]

any method or procedure."[5] That anarchic situation prevailed at hospitals that had been emptied of mental patients by the original killing. The general disorganization was such that few became hospitals for soldiers or war injured—the original stated intent; and in the case of other emptied hospitals, used for schools and offices of various kinds, there were conflicting claims of possession by different groups. The general impression was that whatever facilities were gained by eliminating mental patients contributed relatively little to the Reich and its war effort. The regime was apparently more skillful and systematic in setting up conditions for killing than it was in utilizing the buildings that were emptied. Moreover, the dismantling of the killing centers was far from complete, and many "euthanasia" personnel expected gassing to resume when the war was over. The chambers at Bernburg, Sonnenstein, and Hartheim remained ready for operation when so ordered.[6]

"Special Diet"

Starvation as a method of killing was a logical extension of the frequent imagery of mental patients as "useless eaters." As a passive means of death, it was one more element of general neglect. In many places, mentally ill patients had already been fed insufficiently; and the idea of not nourishing them was "in the air." Moreover, the establishment of a new central accounting office clearly decreased the money available to the institutions.[7] (The decrease in heating in winter had similar causes and effects.) Dr. Pfannmüller was responding radically to such a mood when he instituted his method of starving children to death at Eglfing-Haar. In 1943, he would establish two *Hungerhäuser* ("starvation houses") for an older population.

On 17 November 1942, the Bavarian Interior Ministry held a conference with directors from mental hospitals throughout that area. The state commissioner for health, Walter Schultze, asked the directors to provide a "special diet" *(Sonderkost)* for hopelessly ill patients. Because several doctors were hesitant about this idea, it was suggested that a ministerial proclamation to that effect would be useful. Not at all hesitant was Dr. Pfannmüller, who "dramatically . . . told how he had once grabbed a slice of bread from a nurse who had wanted to give it to a patient." (Pfannmüller had been involved in the decision to hold the 1942 conference.) Also involved was the director of the Kaufbeuren Asylum, Dr. Valentin Faltlhauser, who had directed the child "euthanasia" program there and had also served as a T4 expert since 1940. Faltlhauser passed around the Kaufbeuren menu: "totally fat-free," it consisted of potatoes, yellow turnips and cabbage (usually green, occasionally red) cooked in water. "The effect," he claimed, "should be a slow death, which should ensue in about three months."[8]

The directive followed on 30 November, supported, it was claimed, by orders from Berlin. "In view of the war-related food situation and the health of the working asylum-inmates," it was no longer justified to feed everyone equally, "whether they contribute productive work or are in therapy or whether, on the other hand, they are merely being cared for . . . without accomplishing any useful work worth mentioning." The henceforth privileged patients were to be those performing useful work or in therapy, children capable of education, war casualties and those with senile diseases. Directors were ordered to institute such a program "without delay."[9]

It should be said that the number of patients included in this program was a fraction of the total hospital population. Their deaths would have made little difference to the state of nourishment of the German population, which, in any event, was much less affected than it had been by the First World War and its blockades. Yet in the Eglfing institution, for example, the Second World War mortality from starvation-related causes was twice that of the earlier war. Moreover, the exceptions, notably war veterans and the elderly, reflected those areas where popular disapproval was greatest.[10]

Pfannmüller and his colleagues had *carte blanche* on whom to choose for starvation. There were no forms or questionnaires. Indeed, this "pseudo-nourishment," in the words of Gerhard Schmidt, who took over as director at Eglfing at war's end, was a "method of killing . . . that in the classic sense is no killing, no one-time action with a recognizable cause or conclusion."[11] Pfannmüller often chose patients who had been considered insufficiently ill to be sent to the gassing centers. The motto at Eglfing was: "We give them no fat, then they go on their own."[12] The diet basically duplicated the Kaufbeuren model, with the addition of a slice of bread a day. When this proved ineffective at times—and, indeed, the kitchen staff sometimes added fat or meat to the soups against orders—rations were cut.[13]

When Dr. Schmidt took over the directorship at Eglfing-Haar at the end of the war, he encountered (as he told me) a total of ninety-four survivors on the two wards and a scene he would never forget: "Huge, dark halls . . . silent. No noise. Nothing. . . . The people showed no sign of life. A few stood. They said nothing. Like half-corpses."*

Doctors treating these surviving patients found that they experienced hallucinations of ghosts coming at night and eating their food; feelings of guilt over having done something bad for which they were now being punished; and dreams and fantasies of food of every kind in limitless amounts. The slow starvation method led many patients to believe they were getting the same wartime rations as everyone else, and few if any seemed to understand they had been singled out for starvation. On the basis of records, it was estimated that 444 Eglfing patients had died directly or indirectly from malnutrition, often from pneumonia, tuberculosis, or some other infection.[14]

*That image was the beginning of Schmidt's study of Nazi medical killing, a study that can be said to serve as the personal survivor mission of an anti-Nazi physician.

"Medication"

Killing by drugs gave more leeway to physicians. Their methods included injections of morphine; morphine plus scopolamine; or tablets, usually either veronal or luminal. Killing by drugs of already-weak patients was the preferred method at the killing centers now divested of their gas chambers. The proper dosage for gradual killing had been tested by Dr. Nitsche. Now, more literally, "the syringe was in the hand of the physician" or, as it happened, of an assistant or a nurse. There had been occasional killings by injection even during the height of T4: for instance, when a killing doctor at Hadamar refused to send a pregnant woman to the gas chamber, though she had been duly selected for that fate, the matter was resolved by a nurse who gave her a lethal injection.[15]

The year after the disassembling of the gas chamber (which had killed ten thousand patients in less than a year of operation),* a new physician named Adolf Wahlmann became medical director at Hadamar, an institution he had headed before the First World War and again in the mid-1930s. Wahlmann had joined the Nazi Party in 1933, but had been in some difficulty with the Party for what it perceived to be his greater commitment to a church choir he led.[17] Called out of retirement at the age of sixty-six to help with mental-hospital work before being transferred to Hadamar, he claimed at his later Frankfurt trial to have had no knowledge of the killing prior to his arrival. Whatever the truth of that claim, when Wahlmann arrived the chief administrator was then in the process of implementing a killing procedure, in which the chief doctor was expected to give orders to the head male nurse to kill male patients, and the head female nurse to do the same to female patients. When informed of that procedure by the administrator, Wahlmann refused to do so indiscriminately, insisting upon going about things more methodically—that is, medically. He developed his own "professional" system: he observed patients arriving on transports, made daily rounds, and studied medical records. He then held morning conferences where these observations were considered along with patients' records, and then would decide who was to be killed and what dose of what drug was to be used. Death certificates were also signed at these conferences, and plausible causes of death were determined for those already killed. The orders to kill were passed along by the head male and female nurses, present at the conferences, to the ward nurses, who carried them out. The "medication" (usually between six and twenty tablets of luminal, triomal, or a

---

*The ten thousandth victim at Hadamar had been celebrated as a milestone, as reported by an employee. Invited by a T4 doctor named Berner, the employees gathered that evening. Each was given a bottle of beer, and they adjourned to the basement. "There on a stretcher lay a naked male corpse with a huge hydrocephalic head. . . . I am certain that it was a real dead person and not a paper corpse. The dead person was put by the cremation personnel on a sort of trough and shoved into the cremation oven. Hereupon [the administrator] Märkle, who had made himself look like a sort of minister, held a burial sermon." Another witness reported that the celebration, which included music, degenerated further into a drunken procession through the institution grounds.[16]

related preparation) was usually given at night; those patients not dead the next morning were given lethal morphine-scopolamine injections. Over time, the method became routine, with greater reliance on injections and greater self-reliance on the part of nurses who increasingly came to decide upon necessary dosages of barbiturates or injected morphine-scopolamine for patients whose names were placed on the special "list."[18]*

As he involved himself in the process, Dr. Wahlmann discouraged one chief nurse from questioning it. And with the arrival, in 1944, of Polish and Russian workers mostly diagnosed categorically as "tubercular," the killing procedure became automatic. *The only examination performed on them by Wahlmann or any other doctor was done, after they had received their lethal drugs, for the purpose of confirming their death.* At his trial, Wahlmann justified that situation by explaining that the Russians and the Poles had been "sent to us by specialists who stated they were incurably diseased and were to receive the euthanasia on the same day"; and said that he was "not a [T.B.] specialist."[20] To gain the patients' cooperation for the injection, according to a former male nurse, "We told them that it was for treatment of their lung disease."[21]† The records of these laborers were then brought to Wahlmann's morning conferences, where his task was to decide upon a false but plausible cause of death in order "to write in the end to those case histories," as he later put it.[23]

In his legal testimony, he stressed medical principles concerning such things as the criteria used to determine the killing dosage of injections: "That is very different [for different people]. If I have a very strong person, then I have to use more. If I have a person who is used to morphine, then I have to use very much. If I have a very weak person, then I need very little." He could not remember the exact origin of the injections—whether "I ordered [initiated] it at that time or whether it was generally done then"; but he did stress that "injection is a completely painless method, and the term *euthanasia* comes from the Greek *eu,* which means beautiful."[24]

Killing with drugs, then, was the most "medical" form of all. There could be "conferences" where doctors discussed "therapy," the ordering of "medication," and further "clinical" decisions depending upon the effect of that medication. With the onset of "wild euthanasia," the doctor could share his syringe with a nurse, but he took on greater authority than

---

*Several nurses and nonprofessional employees, who sometimes also gave out the tablets, experienced anxiety about what they were doing, but most seemed to remain at their jobs and to consider themselves to be following orders. One employee experienced what was described as a "nervous breakdown" and was given six weeks' leave but then reassigned to the undressing room (which had so disturbed her in the first place) with the explanation that this was to "harden" her; she remained there a while and then succeeded in resigning by claiming to be pregnant.[19]

†At one of the trials, the chief female nurse, when asked whether she considered the Russians and Poles to have been murdered, answered, "Murder? How do you want me to understand murder? They died from injections." But pressed further whether in her opinion that was murder, she answered, "Yes."[22]

ever in deciding when and in what way the syringe or other medication would be used. "Wild euthanasia" can be understood as a continuation in still more medicalized form of the project of "euthanasia" killing. Simple medical technology—drugs, injections, diets—filled the murder vacuum as the regime's continuing desire to destroy "bad" genes was effected by the interaction of Nazi medical bureaucracy and individual Nazi doctors. The process continued until—in some places even beyond —the demise of the Nazi regime: there are stories of Allied troops liberating surviving patients at gunpoint.[25]

Chapter 5

Participants

Determined . . . to intervene therapeutically to attain healing and health for *everyone,* full of the desire to put themselves primarily at the service of the community, and full of impotent rage over the therapeutic inaccessibility of so many mental patients, psychopaths and habitual criminals (that is, the Jews!), they [the psychiatrists] actually moved from the individual to the "national body" [*Volkskörper*], to pervert "treatment" [*Behandlung*] metaphorically: to make extermination [*Sonderbehandlung*] the perfection of healing.

—KLAUS DÖRNER

At the Killing Center

A Psychiatrist Who Stayed: Horst D.

Dr. Horst D. worked at a killing center for about a year and was, at the time of our meetings, involved in an elaborate, unresolved legal procedure. A bearded vigorous man in his early sixties, I found him tense, cautious, and limited in his capacity to express feelings—wishing very much to explain himself and at the same time conflicted about his own explanation.

He thought he had been assigned to the T4 program because of a recommendation made to Heyde by a friend from student days with whom he (Dr. D.) had shared a semester of psychiatric work. His early enthusiasm for the Nazis together with his military experience and medical *in*experience were also undoubtedly factors in the assignment. Like others, he had been pressed into military service before completing his medical thesis,[1] and then was frustrated because he had virtually nothing to do and "there was no medicine at all." At that point, in mid-1940, "I was told I should come to Berlin and present myself at the Chancellery of the Führer," having "absolutely no idea what it meant, what it was all about." Upon reporting there, this very young and inexperienced doctor had an impressive encounter:

> Two professors of psychiatry met me. One was Heyde and the other was Nitsche. Both were wearing civilian clothes . . . and they talked about euthanasia. They talked about this problem, from the viewpoint of the work of Hoche and Binding [see pages 46–48]. . . . It was a very intensive conference and presentation of the necessity . . . of all this, and they convinced me.

Dr. D. was so impressed by Heyde and Nitsche's tone of quiet "persuasion," and by the "completely . . . extraordinary" situation of sitting down together with men of that professional standing, that he could turn over to them the responsibility for what he himself was being asked to do: "Whenever someone [of that standing] takes up that sort of thing, that means he's taking on a good deal of responsibility. I thought he [Heyde] would be well aware of what he was doing and of the responsibility involved."

The briefing included a discussion of the concepts of Hoche and Binding (brought up by the two professors) which, though not specifically familiar to Dr. D., were not inconsistent with the stress on organic and hereditary influences he had been exposed to during his psychiatric work as a medical student. Generally speaking, the encounter evoked his long-standing impulse toward obedience—an impulse inculcated during his rural childhood, especially by his civil-servant father. And when Dr. D. inquired of Heyde and Nitsche whether he could discuss the matter with an older respected friend, he was told quite sharply that "the entire matter was top secret."

He gained the impression that the project offered him better medical opportunities than the military situation he was then in:

> I found myself in a horrible dilemma. On the one hand there was the military idleness—with the likelihood that all of a sudden I would find myself in a medical situation I could not handle at all. That was horrible. . . . On the other hand, I did not think it would be just a killing institution. I thought I would have an opportunity to go on with my medical training—with patients—and that only certain patients would be selected, and then not just killed but given a mercy death. . . . Anyway, what was decisive then was the wish to work medically and not just as a soldier.

Or at least he could, partly and temporarily, convince himself of that —until he arrived at the actual killing center: "It was a great disappointment to see that there were no patients. . . . I imagined an institution with mental patients, and then some single rooms—well, what shall I say—

where special treatment would be performed. . . . But the patients came and were sent to the gas chamber right away."

Conflict developed in connection with the patients to be killed. While he described many of them as having been in a "hopeless condition" and as "living in a different world," he also acknowledged that "sometimes one could establish some kind of contact"; and he conceded, hesitantly, that at moments "it might have happened" that he felt sympathy for them as well. That sympathy, and the resulting guilt, was reflected in dreams and images then and now in which "I still see before me . . . one group of people . . . [and] I thought I should have saved them, that I should have helped them." He confused such dreams with actual memories of "a group of people who had come from far away, and I don't know who judged them." Having told me that, he paused and added, with quiet agitation, "This is getting dangerous," because "saying that, from the standpoint of lawyers, means that I have guilt feelings"—that he could be accused of having been aware at the time of wrongly killing people, rather than having acted out of genuine medical conviction: "What I just said could mean the death penalty to me legally."

Further contributing to his uneasiness and guilt were his doubts "about the way it was carried out":

Well, . . . there were so many, so many to take care of at once, not just the number, . . . but it was not one at a time. . . . I had imagined it would be done as an individual procedure, . . . one by one. Well, . . . it was done as a mass affair. . . . I think in human terms it is different whether you take care of someone who has to go this way as an individual . . . or whether you do it in groups with so many.

The killing method, that is, did not permit him to sustain the illusion that he was doing medical work: "*I* was the one who had to do it!" and "Who would like such a job?"

Concerning his activities as a killing-center physician, Dr. D. told of looking over patients and their charts in order to decide upon a "fictive cause of death" and to "supervise" the entire process. When I asked him whether it was his task as a doctor to press the lever to release the gas, he became upset and angrily demanded, "What does this have to do with psychological matters?"—implying that I was behaving like a lawyer or a prosecutor and could even have some connection with his trial. When he calmed down, he answered, equivocally, that doctors had to "determine whether the gas had had its effect" so that "the technical personnel could stop the gas." While he neither denied nor confirmed that he himself was the one who had released the gas, he left me with the impression that he was—a conclusion I drew not only from his response at the time but from the known activities of doctors at killing centers.

Dr. D. adapted to his work by means of two psychological maneuvers

—transfer of responsibility and the pursuit of science. He consciously renounced responsibility: "I told [Heyde] I could not take on any responsibility at all because I knew I was not qualified medically," and "Heyde said, 'All right, you will not have responsibility,' " emphasizing that professors and specialists would make careful evaluations and "the committee would make the final decision." *His* responsibility, Dr. D. was told, was to "render this . . . very valuable service to the colleague in charge" of the killing center. It was a matter of loyalty and sacrifice, for, as he came to feel, "the soldiers at the front also had to do things they did not like." The claim of his responsibility lay not with the patients but with his superior, his country, his race.

And responsibility became inseparable from his relationship to the *authority* of the regime: "The whole system radiated that authority. Like it or not, I was part of it. . . . I had no choice. I was in this web—this network of authority. . . . If you talk to people [in general terms about possibly leaving], they would say, you have to stay wherever you are, . . . where you are needed. Don't disturb the organization."

The opportunity for his second mode of adaptation occurred with the appearance of a leading German neuropathologist at the killing center to obtain brains for dissection. Dr. D. "took this as . . . an opportunity" to approach the visitor about the possibility of establishing "a pathology department" at the killing center, and of spending a few weeks in the professor's department "in order to get a better sense of things and be better prepared for this task." He saw this as a chance to spend time away from the killing center, as he sought to do whenever possible. But he also immersed himself in the task, studied medical histories of patients "and tried to find those whose brains might eventually be of interest," in accordance with the professor's research concerns. D. was even given a nurse assistant to help him in what he came to see as "preparatory work . . . that made further scientific work possible." Inevitably he came to see himself as serving science, and his duty as "saving those things that still could possibly be of value scientifically . . . for psychiatry in general . . . [so that] studying these brains would get us closer to understanding diseases, and of course curing those diseases." He was quite proud to add, "The Berlin Institute gave recognition to this . . . work."

Horst D. had, in other words, found a way to connect the killing work with *medical* research and to feel that he was doing his duty as defined both by his immediate group and by "science." Or to put things another way, a new sense of serving medicine and science enabled him, psychologically, to go on with the killing.

He welcomed the official cessation of the program, after which he was reassigned to the military for the remaining years of the war. In 1945, he went into medical practice, took "special pleasure in giving life," and described how "I brought children into the world in the middle of the night." Serving life helped ease a residual sense of guilt that he experienced only indirectly. He would feel "a little awkward" when with people, especially those he cared about, wondering "what those people would think if they knew what I have been doing." When eventually brought to trial, he felt the experience, painful as it was, to be "a kind of relief" because the matter was confronted: "I had nothing to hide any more. I could face everyone." He hoped that "I could really leave it behind me then"; but the trial dragged on, despite his original acquittal, because the state appealed that acquittal.

In addition to his regular medical practice, Dr. D. developed an interest in contemporary psychiatry, contrasting its "tremendous possibilities" for helping people with its "dead end" in the past, when "everybody shared the common conviction that these lives [of mental patients] were already ended—that these people were in Hoche's words, 'empty shells.' " He stressed that it is the responsibility of today's psychiatric leaders "to point out the human being in the patient, so that one feels obligated to help him and does not regard him as something one can shove away [*abschieben*]." Emphasizing how in the past "the professor for me was the highest," he declared bitterly that "it never would have occurred to me that a professor, in no matter what field, would expect a student or a young colleague to do something that would step over the boundaries of human ethics."

Concerning "euthanasia," or any program resembling that conducted by the Nazis during the war, he was unequivocal: "I would not agree to such a program today. . . . Who would do the work that had been expected of me? . . . Who would want to take the responsibility for the decisions?"

Horst D.'s experience epitomizes the tendency of Nazi doctors to experience conflicts about killing but to find ways to subdue those conflicts in adaptation to a murderous environment. His subsequent attitude, despite an occasional glimmer of self-examination, fell far short of genuine moral confrontation.

A Psychiatrist Who Left: Wolfgang R.

Another doctor who had worked at a killing center, Wolfgang R., experienced psychological circumstances closely resembling those of Dr. D. but with a significantly different outcome: R. managed to stop doing the work after about one month.

Tall and thin and ingratiating in manner, R., during our interview, was talkative but aware that, despite being generally outgoing, "whenever I talk about the subject . . . the words don't come easily."

His early enthusiasm for the Nazis—and especially for the military— even, as he described it, exceeded Dr. D.'s. Indeed, R. thought himself "predestined" for the military because of the strong military tradition of his area, and was among the first group of students to join the new *Wehrmacht* (the armed forces of which Hitler was supreme commander): "I valued the *Wehrmacht* in a very special way." He used words like "idealistic" and "free" to describe what he and other young people felt while participating in the Nazi youth movement, volunteering for resettlement work with ethnic Germans from Eastern Europe, and living out the "beautiful time" of Nazi student days. He did, however, recall a moment of pain when a popular Jewish teacher in his *Gymnasium,* or secondary school, was treated brutally and removed during *Kristallnacht,* the night of 9 to 10 November 1938 when throughout Germany, Jewish homes and shops were looted, burned, and destroyed, and many Jews were killed or imprisoned. Dr. R. said of his teacher then: "His facial expression was . . . deeply saddened . . . something I will never forget."

Like Dr. D., Dr. R. had been thrust into the military before completing his medical work, and was pleased to find there a physician mentor to whom he became very close. After a period of combat (in which he thrived) and then a lull (in which he had little to do), Dr. R. was called in and told that he was being assigned to an "indispensable" civilian position at the Führer's Chancellery. Excited by the prospect and congratulated by everyone, "I took off my beautiful uniform" and reported to Berlin. But instead of being briefed by Heyde or another psychiatric leader of the project, he was sent directly to the killing center where he was to work, and briefed by the chief doctor there, a nonpsychiatric medical professor and ardent Nazi. The latter impressed on R. the program's legality and priority as a direct Führer order, its application only to completely withdrawn mental patients who had been well screened by authoritative professors, its necessity during wartime to conserve food, and even its theological justification by a particular Catholic priest who had stated that "euthanasia" was morally justifiable in certain cases. Dr. R. had attended some of Heyde's lectures at medical school, and the fact that the professor's name was actively invoked "added to the reassurance" he felt.

That emphasis on acceptance of moral justification, one must keep in mind, is consistent with Dr. R.'s legal defense, as is his memory of not being shocked by the killing because he had been more or less persuaded of its propriety. Another factor might have been that, as a military doctor, he was "used to seeing death." What clearly did shock him was that "someone who didn't have the slightest inkling of psychiatry" would be sent to the killing center. He was bitterly disappointed: "I had imagined that I would be able to do medical work under the guidance of experienced doctors" and instead was "pulled out of the *Wehrmacht*" and "put in a place just wrong for me."

He went to the chief doctor and told him that, lacking any background or interest whatsoever in psychiatry, he was incapable of doing the work: the job "is not right for me." R. even managed to meet with Heyde and Brack at the Chancellery, told them the same thing, and was immediately offered a change in assignment "without . . . any difficulty whatsoever."

He was evasive about details of what he did at the killing center. While admitting that he checked patients against their charts to prepare plausible causes of death, he insisted that he was "excluded" from the actual

killing process because of his early efforts to leave—though he was implicated in the deaths of many patients.

Despite—partly because of—his vehement insistence ("I never had the
feeling of deserting—no, not at all"), I suspect that this ardent Nazi, who
loved the military and believed in obedience, experienced considerable
guilt at leaving. In discussing those feelings, he stressed that he "used this
period to try to learn as much as [he] could about psychiatry," though
he knew that "it may sound macabre." Here Dr. R. resembles Dr. D. in
seeking to minimize guilt by focusing upon medical-scientific experience,
though the guilt in D.'s case has to do not only with the activity at the
killing center but with his wish to "desert" his position there.

In leaving, R. was in no way in bad repute with the regime. He was for
a while given the task of tracing genealogies of prospective SS officers in
order to determine whether their family trees had been poisoned by
Jewishness or hereditary disease.*

But later, during the postwar years, he became increasingly resentful of
Nazi medical leaders who had deceived him. He spoke of their manipulations as "perfidious" and of the whole process as "all a very tricky thought-
out business." And during this trial, when one of the program's psychiatric
leaders testified about marking "Yes" or "No" on questionnaires, R. felt
himself become enraged and wanted to shout at the man, "You had people
killed without even seeing them!" R., in fact, attributed a subsequent
illness to those feelings: "I was so angry I had a heart attack." In that anger,
and in his description of the matter to me, he was expressing the deep
resentment of the dependent person toward authorities who had failed
and misused him, as well as a continuing effort to view them, and not
himself, as responsible for what he did. For he still had inner questions
about whether he could have left the program even earlier; and when
asked what advice he would give to young doctors to prevent them from
becoming vulnerable to that kind of project in the future, he immediately
answered, "I would advise them to leave—not to stay in such programs!"
Don't stay even for a minute, he seemed to be saying, lest you become part
of the killing. And even more strongly: "Today I would rather let myself be
shot than participate in such an action."

His attitude had been influenced by the question constantly asked by
his children: "Why didn't you leave [sooner]?" His answer, sadly put to
me and undoubtedly to them as well, was, "We simply didn't ask questions at the time." He stressed with approval the difference between his
and his contemporaries' unquestioning belief in Hitler and the new generation's insistence on questioning everything.

Finally, he expressed residual guilt in two additional ways. He said,

---

*In most cases, the policy was to transfer recalcitrant doctors from the program quickly
(or, as in the case of Ewald, to cease to enlist them for it) and to find more cooperative
replacements. If reluctance or refusal were expressed discreetly—that is, as a matter of
individual inability rather than of disapproval or condemnation of the program—there was
unlikely to be any punishment or loss of rank or standing.[2]

"Something that still weighs on my mind [is that the 'euthanasia' project] was experience in preparation for the mass killing later on [because he knew that] during this process, *Desinfektoren* were shown [how to kill] and these people later on worked in concentration camps in the East."

He also raised to himself a disturbing question—"the problem I cannot solve." That question was, "How would I have reacted . . . if I had psychiatric training and had done psychiatric work at the *Wehrmacht*—and were then sent to this place . . . if I had been the right man on the right spot?" He strongly implied that he might well have stayed, because "at that time Hitler was still for us the Führer. . . . Hitler couldn't have made a mistake."

Yet Wolfgang R. managed to leave, and we must ask why he was able to do at least that and Dr. D. was not. We cannot say with certainty, but the question Dr. R. asked himself suggests two probable factors: his greater sensitivity to guilt and his intense focus on technical issues. Concerning the latter, we shall see again and again that a plea of technical-professional limitation was the best way for a doctor (or anyone else) to avoid taking part in a Nazi project. But Dr. R. appeared to mean it: his uneasiness at being thrust into a killing situation would not have been sufficient *inner* justification for refusing an important assignment coming from the Führer, but his sense of actual technical (psychiatric) limitation could both add to that uneasiness and serve as that justification. There was an additional factor, an ironic one, that might have been the most important of all: Dr. D's intense idealization of the regime—his extraordinary attachment to both the Nazis and the German military. This idealization could turn to profound disillusion when confronted with the Nazi killing project, and especially when asked, as an "unprepared" doctor, to participate in it.

The Rank and File

In respect to the T4 programs, several ordinary psychiatrists I interviewed described various combinations of knowledge and confusion, and of cooperation along with gestures of resistance.

Dr. Günther E., who had worked in a few of the state hospitals where most German psychiatrists were then employed, represented one kind of response from the psychiatric rank and file. I encountered him as an old man living in rural retirement, at first friendly and responsive but increasingly uncomfortable over the course of the interview as the atmosphere of the Nazi era emerged.

Never an ardent Nazi but friendly toward the regime at the time, he had considered the sterilization program "a useful thing" because he agreed with the regime's contention that "the state should be associated with healthy inheritance." His only reservation was that the program had become too politicized.

He seemed similarly sympathetic to "euthanasia," which he stressed "was a medical term," but became critical of it when it seemed more "a political action." He told how confused he and his colleagues were as patients "were taken from us. . . . I didn't know where to"—until he learned from relatives that those patients "died soon" in specific institutions. Upon learning the truth, "I was shocked, . . . frightened to think it happened in an orderly state." He and his colleagues sought to find ways of saving people (by not diagnosing schizophrenia, by transferring them to private institutions less vulnerable to the killing project, or by sending them home) but mostly cooperated in ways they thought they had to. Psychiatrists varied between being "oppositional" or "indifferent." The latter seemed in the majority and "accepted [the project]. And since it was a state policy they did not wish to oppose it." Much depended upon the stance of hospital directors and of local medical-administrative authorities, some of whom were "radical Nazis" and pressed for maximum compliance while others sought to minimize the number of patients taken.

Dr. E. went on to explain that he and other psychiatrists came to distinguish between "dishonest" opinions from those experts who acted out of "sheer political motivation," on the one hand; and, on the other, "honest" judgments from those experts, much fewer in number, who based their opinions on genuine medical considerations. As he talked, it became clear to me that a focus on this distinction had enabled him and his colleagues to avoid moral truths concerning the "euthanasia" project: to avoid recognizing that what they viewed as "honest medical opinions" about schizophrenic or mentally deficient patients became the basis for mass murder of these patients. Yet his visible pain as he discussed these matters suggested that he could not avoid that recognition, and probably had not even then.

After we had been talking for a little less than two hours, he made it clear he did not want to say more: "I am nearly eighty years old, and . . . I don't want to have anything more to do with that era. . . . I don't want to think about it any more."

His story is that of the middle-aged psychiatric functionary in a state system as a dependent, essentially obedient civil servant. While the medical killing project was too radical for such a person, he could not risk or even imagine genuine resistance, and his compromise was to combine compliance with an effort to cling to professional psychiatric standards. The result was bitterness over his own moral corruption and disillusionment toward a regime he had served. Dr. E.'s personal experience epitomizes the dilemma that haunts all of German psychiatry: a murderous episode in the recent past whose memory can be neither confronted and absorbed nor wished away.

Psychiatrists in academic centers tended to be slightly more removed from the process than those in state hospitals. As one of the former put it to me: "We had to send them patients . . . but it [the killing] was done *there.*"* Yet in academic centers no less than state hospitals, psychiatrists made constant compromises, sending some patients and saving others, and at times even—according to the principle expressed to me by one such psychiatrist—"taking part in the selections [for the project] in order to prevent worse things from happening."

There was a generational factor, as a psychiatrist who took active part in the program made clear to me: "The younger ones [among whom he identified himself] were more in favor of it"; and it was only from among "one of the older ones [that a psychiatrist would occasionally] raise . . . his voice in warning . . . [and] point out to us that you can't do that, where do you want to draw the line?" Younger psychiatrists tended to identify themselves more with both the regime and the war effort, and might come to believe (as the same man went on to explain), "If the enemy is killing our healthy youth, than this ['euthanasia'] is not such a crime." Moreover, the term "unworthy life" was bandied about in discussions among psychiatric colleagues no less than in official documents, so that psychiatrists found themselves accepting it in varying degree, feeling that at least in certain cases "perhaps they [those running the program] are right after all," because "back then we were not unequivocally or clearly opposed." For, as he further explained, "in a dictatorship . . . the authoritarian regime takes responsibility away from [the individual]" so that rather than struggling over whether to act in one way or another, one feels, "I *must* act this way, . . . not get into a conflict situation, . . . which may be wrong . . . but . . . does have its advantages."

For the psychiatric rank and file, then, participation in direct medical killing was a way of going along with a regime one tended to be either in sympathy with or at least not opposed to. Whether one plunged into the project enthusiastically, made numerical compromises (gave up some patients to the killing process in order to save a few others from it), or focused on professionalism, one ended in some measure divesting oneself of responsibility for one's actions.

Concerning the specific mentality of psychiatrists, there are two aspects of their ideology I have only touched upon, having to do with their perception of psychiatric patients, psychiatric illness, and psychiatric hierarchy. First, many German psychiatrists (and psychiatrists working elsewhere in similar traditions) were committed to the idea of schizophrenia as an organic, incurable disease, whose natural course was deterioration. Indeed, for many, professional pride depended on that view. Any effort to penetrate the psyche of a schizophrenic patient as a means of understanding and a form of treatment was viewed by these psychiatrists as

*Killing centers were created from state hospitals, from large church-run institutions that had been expropriated by the state or, in one case (Brandenburg), from a prison.

"unscientific" and therefore a professional and personal threat. A distinguished German psychiatrist I discussed these matters with characterized that mentality as "the doctrine of the absence of empathy."* To be sure, this mentality in itself does not inevitably lead to killing in the name of "euthanasia"; there were psychiatrists who expressed empathy for their patients and yet became leaders in the "euthanasia" project: Carl Schneider, with his compassionate work-therapy program, is a case in point. Yet the general principle characterizes the psychiatric atmosphere within which medical killing could be readily embraced.†

If, at the heart of one's professional identity, one becomes easily susceptible to the idea that mental patients—and possibly other groups as well—lack ordinary human qualities, and hence to the idea of eliminating that group in favor of the ostensible health of all others, one might also be more amenable to embracing a new "therapy" that shows itself to be in accord with one's organic-genetic perceptions. In that way (as described in the epigraph to this chapter), many psychiatrists could harmonize with, even epitomize, the larger Nazi vision of curing by killing.

The second influential factor in German psychiatry was the traditional relationship of the profession to the state. Individual German psychiatrists had always identified themselves as servants of the state, rather than as independent practitioners. Mental institutions especially were part of the administrative structure of the state, and the same could even be said of university medical departments. The long-standing arrangement, when internalized and buttressed by German cultural stress on authority and obedience, made it difficult for individual psychiatrists to consider— or even imagine—defying the state when summoned to participate in virtually any kind of project.

---

*Walter Ritter von Baeyer, personal communication.
†One may carry the argument still further. During the period from the First World War (and before) to the Nazi epoch, there had been fierce battles in German psychiatry concerning the emerging school of psychoanalysis. While Freud had doubts about the efficacy of psychoanalytic treatment for schizophrenia, psychoanalysis in general stood for the principle of empathy: the psychoanalyst or psychiatrist is to enter the mind of the patient, to try to feel as the patient feels. Most German psychiatrists strongly opposed psychoanalysis. Among the most vehement of all was Alfred Hoche, the coiner of the concept of "life unworthy of life." At a medical congress, Hoche went so far as to read a paper on psychoanalysis called "A Psychical Epidemic among Doctors."[3] Psychiatrists like Hoche clearly felt their identity as physicians and scientists to be threatened by the spread of psychoanalysis. That sense of threat could well have intensified their commitment to their own credo—that of the doctrine of the absence of empathy. That credo contributed to the development of violent somatic treatment procedures (whatever their efficacy), such as insulin and metrazol shock therapy, electroshock therapy, and lobotomy. Under duress, those who held to the doctrine of the absence of empathy might have been more ready than otherwise to collaborate in killing their own patients.

Medical Leaders

The "Decent Nazi": Karl Brandt

Of the leaders of the "euthanasia" program, Karl Brandt (1904–48) must come first, as the Führer's choice to initiate the program—that is, as the Führer's conduit for it—and its ultimate medical authority, even if he came to have relatively little to do with its day-by-day operation. More than any other Nazi doctor, Brandt epitomizes the élite, highly educated, and dedicated healer joining actively in the medical killing.

Brandt came from a distinguished medical family in Alsace, trained under Ferdinand Sauerbruch, Germany's leading surgeon, and was himself, in his twenties, already emerging as a gifted surgeon and authority on head and spinal injuries.[4] He was also a fervent nationalist who embraced the Nazi movement as "the avenger, the party of hope," as part of what a friend and fellow medical student called Brandt's "fantastic dream" of Germany regaining the Alsace area he had been forced to leave in order to be a German national. Yet the same Karl Brandt had been strongly drawn to Albert Schweitzer, a fellow Alsatian, and was said to have been prevented from joining him in medical missionary work in Africa only by French requirements (Lambarene was in French-controlled Africa) of military service and citizenship. According to Brandt's old friend, "Schweitzer and Hitler were the two most influential figures in Brandt's life. They were his two models, his two mirrors."[5]

Brandt joined the Nazi Party and the Nationalist Socialist German Physicians' League in 1932; was introduced to Hitler that same year by his fiancé, a German swimming champion; and by 1934, at the age of twenty-nine, had become Hitler's personal "escort doctor." Within the inner medical circle surrounding Hitler, Brandt was the scientific figure and reliable traditional physician—as opposed to Theodor Morell, the Führer's personal physician since 1939, who was considered (accurately) a quack and a charlatan (see page 132).[6] While Morell retained his hold on Hitler, it was Brandt who developed what some called an "adopted son" relationship with Hitler similar to that of Albert Speer, Hitler's personal architect and later minister for armament and war production.[7] Both young men were tall and elegant, came from academic-professional families, and were well educated and steeped in German cultural and intellectual tradition—qualities that Hitler himself lacked but was drawn to and exploited.

Other Nazi doctors also held Brandt in unusually high regard, both professionally and personally. They spoke of him as decent, straightforward, and reliable. One doctor who knew him quite well described him as "a highly ethical person, . . . one of the most idealistic physicians I have ever met during my career." Albert Speer,* also a good friend of Brandt's, described him to me as a person who was widely appreciated and "very conscientious about his life—whatever he was doing." Speer was puzzled when he learned after the war of his friend's involvement in "euthanasia," and said that Brandt's integrity was such that "he must have believed in it."

Perhaps Brandt's most glowing testimony was that given a visiting writer in 1973 by the father of the child whose case Hitler used to initiate the entire killing project (see pages 50–51):

> It was right here. Karl Brandt was standing there near the window. He was tall and impressive. He seemed to fill up the whole room. . . . He explained to me that the Führer had personally sent him, and that my son's case interested the Führer very, very much. The Führer wanted to explore the problem of people who had no future—whose life was worthless. . . . From then on, we wouldn't have to suffer from this terrible misfortune, because the Führer had granted us the mercy killing of our son. Later, we could have other children, handsome and healthy, of whom the Reich could be proud. . . . Germany had to be built and every bit of energy would be required. That's what Herr Brandt explained to me. He was a proud man—intelligent, very convincing. He was like a savior to us—the man who could deliver us from a heavy burden. We thanked him and told him how very grateful we were.[9]

Brandt's near-mythic aura of elegance and purity made him the perfect advocate of "euthanasia" and the ideal delegate of the Führer. This aura even somewhat captivated the man most associated with protecting his patients *against* the medical killing project, the Reverend Fritz von Bodelschwingh (see pages 90–91). On a BBC radio broadcast during the summer of 1945, Bodelschwingh was said to have commented, "You must not picture Professor Brandt as a criminal, but rather as an idealist." Brandt had apparently been instrumental in sparing Bodelschwingh's patients.[10] After Bodelschwingh's death, his successor represented his views in an affidavit on behalf of Brandt to save him from the death penalty in Nuremberg. Bodelschwingh had been impressed by Brandt's willingness to listen to opposing views, and felt that he had greater restraint than others in the project in limiting its scope to "completely

---

*I use Speer's name because, during our interviews, he gave me explicit permission to do so. He and Brandt were not only close friends but acted to save each other's lives. In 1944, Brandt called in his own doctor allies to save an already ill Speer from an attempt at medical murder initiated by Himmler, who was disturbed by Speer's influence with Hitler. At the war's end, Speer tried to mobilize support to keep Brandt alive when Hitler sentenced him to death for "betrayal": for having arranged to send his wife and child to the American zone rather than having them perish in the mass suicide of loyal Nazis that Hitler intended.[8]

extinguished life" and was motivated "not by brutality, but by a certain idealism . . . inherent in his conception of life."[11]

Yet there were other sides to Brandt. François Bayle, a French psychologist who interviewed him repeatedly at the time of the Nuremberg Trial, described him as "a rich personality, vigorous . . . [but] undisciplined . . . pugnacious and childlike . . . made vulnerable by his ambition . . . [and] pride"; possessing "vivid intelligence . . . [but] little logical clearness, and much imagination which can be easily influenced and disordered"—"his character . . . equally easily influenced."[12] Bayle's stress on this combination of intense ambition and vulnerability to influence is consistent with Brandt's extraordinary attachment to Hitler and the latter's continuous hold on him.

There was also a strongly dissenting opinion from a Nazi doctor at the fringe of the Hitler circle, who described Brandt to me as dazzled by Hitler, deeply attracted to "the feeling of possessing power," but "a complete failure" in almost everything he did, including his attempt to have a network of military hospitals built in various parts of Germany. This doctor also felt that Brandt was criminally guilty, as judged at Nuremberg, for his responsibility not only for "euthanasia" but for various lethal medical experiments done in camps. This susceptibility to power is revealed as well in Speer's recollection of his friend Brandt's remaining for years at a relatively low SS rank until "suddenly he was jumping much more [in rank] than the others, . . . suddenly he was . . . a high SS man."

While Brandt was not viewed as strongly anti-Semitic, a story was told by a Dr. Hirsch of Tel Aviv of how a fellow medical student in Munich in 1925 once asked to see his notebook and returned it to him with a drawing of a gallows and a hanged man with the inscription: "The end of Hirsch: 19—?" The fellow student's name turned out to be Brandt.[13]

At Nuremberg, Brandt could well have expressed a genuine conviction concerning the value of "euthanasia" for incurable patients. But from what is known about Brandt's role in the "test demonstration" at Brandenburg comparing the killing effects of carbon monoxide gas and morphine injections, he surely became brutalized and numbed in equating that process with "major advances in medical history." A doctor who worked as Brandt's assistant told me that some of the psychiatrists went much further than Brandt thought they should have gone in "condemning . . . many people to death who should not have been," and that Brandt was angry when he found this out and wanted the practice stopped immediately. His attitude here was similar to his willingness to allow certain groups of patients to be saved, while in no real sense altering the basic killing project. Rather, he was the kind of Nazi who wanted such projects carried out as "fairly" and "humanely" as possible.

Of the greatest importance is the fact that Brandt never in any way disowned the German state, the Nazi regime, or Hitler himself. No wonder that the presiding judge could say that "there is an invisible figure sitting in the dock," and "that figure is Hitler."[14] Though Hitler turned on him viciously, Brandt never questioned their relationship or even his Führer's humanity in initiating "euthanasia," never broke away from the magnetic attraction Hitler held for him. Hence, Brandt could be sincere when he declared, in June 1948 before being hanged, "I have always fought in good conscience for my personal convictions and done so uprightly, frankly and openly."[15]

Brandt is, more than any other doctor, the prototype of what I shall call the "decent Nazi." Such a doctor was usually from an aristocratic or professional, often medical family whose general cultivation and pre-Nazi ethical concerns seemed strikingly at odds with the depth of his Nazi commitment. That commitment included a fierce involvement in the theme of collective revitalization; Brandt in particular embraced Hitler personally not only as a father but as a prophet and savior. In these doctors, a romantic-visionary inclination could combine with an embrace, even worship, of scientific-medical rationality. Brandt's religious-romantic involvement in the Nazi project contributed to his extensive numbing toward mass killing and to his extraordinary capacity to continue to see virtue in the total Nazi program. He could reinforce a sense of personal virtue by a measure of decency in immediate relationships and by opposition to the more "crude Nazis" around him. His powerful sense of himself as a physician, as a *healer,* was central to the process.

The "decent Nazi" did much of the work of the regime and was indispensable to Nazi mass murder.

The Medical "Old Fighter": Werner Heyde

Werner Heyde (1902–61) was of a very different stamp—the medical equivalent of the "old Nazi" or "old fighter," who became an SS "hit man" before taking over the "euthanasia" project. Even for doctors close to the regime, as one of them told me, Heyde had a "bad reputation . . . a real Nazi who had no inhibitions."

Neither his family background (he was the son of a textile manufacturer in Lausitz) nor his early academic showing (he was said to be "always first in his class") give any special clue to what he was to become. Two years older than Brandt, he was able to enlist in the military at the age of sixteen, during the last months of the First World War.

At the age of eighteen, he participated in the Kapp Putsch,* and then in a long series of organizations and events connected with radical nationalism and National Socialism.

Heyde was said to have attended Hoche's psychiatric lectures as a medical student during the early 1920s, and developed into a competent but unremarkable psychiatrist, described to me by another doctor as "an

---

*This putsch was an attempt by right-wing paramilitary and military organizations to overthrow the Weimar Republic in March 1920. It failed after four days, in large measure because of united and decisive opposition on the left.

ordinary person . . . [whom one] would never have thought . . . capable of doing such things." Originally a ward physician and eventually a clinical "chief doctor" (*Oberarzt*) in a psychiatric hospital, he enhanced his career by his standing as a Nazi (he joined the Party on 1 May 1933), and he became a full professor at Würzburg in 1939. In 1935, he became leader of the Würzburg Office of Racial Politics.

His SS career could be said to have begun as early as 1933 when he formed a close relationship to Theodor Eicke, who was first his patient and, in June of that year, became commandant of Dachau before being appointed overall inspector of concentration camps. Eicke, who became the architect of much of the concentration-camp system and mentor for many camp commandants, did much to institutionalize systematic physical and psychological brutality. It is not impossible that Heyde contributed to some of these conceptions (see page 153).

Heyde had joined the Party on Eicke's urging. Through this connection and then through that with Ernst Robert von Grawitz, the notorious SS chief physician, Heyde joined that organization in 1936, was immediately made captain, and in 1941, 1943, and 1945, he was promoted to major, lieutenant colonel, and colonel. Among his SS assignments were the creation of a neuropsychiatric division and supervising "psychiatric-neurologic and heredity research" on concentration-camp prisoners. This latter assignment was deemed "particularly urgent" because of its potential for "scientific applications." Heyde was also a consulting neuropsychiatric expert for the Gestapo in Berlin. This last assignment involved secret activities of which Heyde wrote in his Nazi *vita*, "naturally I can only hint," and which probably included advice on torture methods to induce prisoners to provide information as well as psychiatric evaluations useful to the Gestapo.[16]*

Heyde was a central figure, and the embodiment of medical legitimation, in the "euthanasia" mass-murder program. He played a large role in the planning of the entire structure of deception and overall killing procedures and, until replaced by Nitsche, was the main "chief expert" on ultimate decisions about who was to be killed. At the same time, as

---

*Walter Schellenberg, the head of the German Foreign Intelligence Service, paraphrased a report Heyde wrote on Georg Elser, the carpenter-electrician who nearly succeeded in assassinating Hitler in 1939, describing it as the "best analysis" made at the time, and revealing to us how far psychiatric corruption could go:

[Heyde] said that the assassin was a typical warped fanatic who went his own way alone. He [Elser] had psychotic compulsions, related especially to technical matters, which sprang from an urge to achieve something really noteworthy. This was due to an abnormal need for recognition and acknowledgement which was reinforced by thirst for vengeance for the alleged injustice which had been done to his brother [who had been arrested as a communist sympathizer and sent to a concentration camp]. In killing the leader of the Third Reich he would satisfy all these compulsions because he would become famous himself, and he would have felt morally justified by freeing Germany from a great evil. Such urges, combined with the desire to suffer and sacrifice oneself, were typical of religious and sectarian fanaticism. Upon checking back, similar psychotic disorders were found to have occurred in Elser's family.[17]

we have seen, he could be impressively reasonable, professional, and professorial in "guiding" other doctors, especially younger ones, in their participation. This activist psychiatrist-organizer and administrator of direct medical killing extended his participation in killing to the camps in the 14f13 program (see chapter 6).

After the war, Heyde escaped from custody; he obtained false papers and worked at a number of jobs. Finally he obtained a position as a sports physician in a school near Kiel, where—under the pseudonym of Dr. Sawada—he began to give expert medical legal opinions in various cases including psychiatric ones. As he earned a lot of money and lived flamboyantly, his true name and identity began to be known to leading political and judicial figures in the area, as well as to psychiatrists and other physicians. He was finally exposed by Professor Creutzfeldt, who recognized Heyde's hand in what the elderly anti-Nazi considered an objectionable forensic opinion, and one that countered his own; when Creutzfeldt wavered, his two physician sons pressed him to see the matter through. The court prepared an impressively detailed pre-trial dossier; but, in 1961, Heyde was found dead in his cell from cyanide pills before the trial could begin. The episode resembled earlier SS suicides at the end of the war, and there remains widespread suspicion that Heyde was helped, perhaps even pressured, to kill himself by people with ties to the SS, possibly including other doctors, who had infiltrated the guards and did not want the trial to be held.[18]

Heyde was a relatively ordinary psychiatrist whose passionate involvement with German nationalism and the Nazi vision of change led to near-absolute willingness to subsume professional principles to the Party, the SS, the Gestapo, the overall Nazi project. It may be that men like him held to the visionary Nazi principle of killing in the name of healing, while at the same time they had some awareness of being involved in filth and killing. But by means of psychological mechanisms I shall explore throughout this study, he was able to minimize that awareness and to continue to feel justified in in what he was doing. He also undoubtedly had psychopathic and sadistic tendencies, but these need not have been exceptionally prominent until called forth by his involvement with the Nazis. His career reveals to us how far certain doctors could go, propelled by ideology and by institutional arrangements, in abnegating a prior professional self and applying their medical skills to killing.

The Brutalized Physician: Hermann Pfannmüller

Hermann Pfannmüller (1886–1961)—who, like Heyde, joined the Party in May 1933—is another example of the corrupted, Nazified psychiatrist. It was this senior psychiatrist who, in his late fifties and director of an institution, held up by the legs a starving, nearly dead three-year-old child and declared, laughing: "This is the most simple method" (see pages 61–62). It is tempting to declare him a "psychiatric thug" and let it go at that.

Gerhard Schmidt, the anti-Nazi psychiatrist who took over Pfannmüller's institution at the end of the war, wrote a book on what he found there and elsewhere concerning the "euthanasia" project. Schmidt stressed Pfannmüller's deep commitment to the ideology of "life unworthy of life" and to a Nazi worldview that demanded the elimination of, as Pfannmüller put it, "the pitiful patient" who exhibited only "the semblance of a human existence."[19] And during talks I had with Dr. Schmidt, he described Pfannmüller, whom he met for the first time after the war, as "a simple man [who] was strongly convinced that [the "euthanasia" program] was urgently necessary," and belonged to the group who "thought they could make humanity healthier in this way." Schmidt also said that Pfannmüller had a reputation for being "very soft—a soft depressive type," who ordinarily "could not hurt a fly." It is likely that Pfannmüller was both a genuine ideologue and an extreme example of the depressed person who overcomes his own anxiety and death imagery by harming others. But when he had reached the point of starving to death infants, children, and adults, it is likely that there was operating within him a strong psychological brew of omnipotence and sadism. At the same time, he could have continued to see himself as for the most part idealistic and even decent. He later testified that he differed with Heyde in wishing to consider as "capable of work" even those adult patients who could perform only the simplest tasks. That testimony was undoubtedly self-serving but could also reflect his effort to see himself, even at the time, as a progressive and humane professional. In 1948, a Munich court declared him medically unfit for trial. The next year he was sentenced to six years' imprisonment.[20]

Pfannmüller remains the epitome of the brutalized physician-turned-killer. Contributing to his motivation is a mixture of ideological (biomedical as well as political) and bureaucratic passion, careerist ambition within the Nazi hierarchy, and tendencies toward depression and powerlessness which could be overcome by means of omnipotent and sadistic behavior.

The Double Life: Max de Crinis

Professor Max de Crinis (1889–1945), probably "the most outspoken and influential Nazi within the German psychiatric establishment,"[21] was striking in the double life he attempted to lead. Appointed in 1939 to succeed Karl Bonhoeffer to the psychiatric chair at Berlin and Charité Hospital, he was a psychiatric consultant at the highest level of the regime. As mentioned earlier, he was thought to have provided Hitler with the wording for the original "euthanasia" decree, and was certainly active in all aspects of the planning of that program and yet never identified as one of its leaders.

An Austrian, de Crinis had been active in anti-communist and *Freikorps* (see pages 126–27) activities since late 1918, joined the Nazi Party in 1931, and fled to Germany in 1934 following the failed putsch against the Dollfuss regime, in which he may have been involved. By 1936, he was active not only in the SS but in the SD; later it was officially understood that he should publicly camouflage these affiliations.* Similarly, while attending an early organizational meeting of the "euthanasia" program in 1939, de Crinis was said to have "demonstrated a positive attitude" toward all that was worked out, but was permitted to decline to serve as an expert "for personal reasons." He was, however, active in the SS Race and Settlement Office and, in 1941, became medical director of the Ministry of Education. He also took part in at least one bizarre intelligence mission to Holland as the impersonator of a military officer involved in a plot against Hitler.[22]

At his university and hospital in Berlin, de Crinis was reputed to have been "charming" and professorial in style. While his close Nazi connections were well known, he went to great pains to keep secret his "euthanasia" involvement, even to the point of appearing to be an opponent of medical killing. For instance, there was an incident, related to me by a doctor I interviewed, of a severely hydrocephalic child being brought to de Crinis for examination by him and his assistant. But when the question arose whether the child should be transferred into a channel leading to "euthanasia," de Crinis spoke sharply in the negative: "He has to go somewhere else." (After examining Hitler and diagnosing his Parkinson's disease, de Crinis also became involved in high-level, medically centered intrigue with Schellenberg, Himmler, and Conti concerning an armistice in the West.[23])

Word eventually got around the university and hospital about de Crinis's activities, and it is said that Bonhoeffer confronted him on some of these matters. Yet de Crinis did protect Charité patients from medical killing. And he actively pursued scientific work on the somatic basis for psychiatric disorders and for the emotions in general. De Crinis was a spokesman for the psychiatric establishment in attacking psychogenic assumptions and resisting nonmedical psychotherapy. Indeed, psychotherapy as such was suspect as a "Jewish" pursuit.

Aside from any reasons de Crinis may have had to hide the extent of his "euthanasia" and SS involvements, his pattern reveals a manifest "doubling" process (see chapters 19 and 20). It is possible that de Crinis, to a significant degree, inwardly maintained his sense of being a proper academic psychiatrist—an "older self" that coexisted somewhat autonomously with his Nazified "euthanasia" and SS-intelligence self. This latter self, constructed from Nazi ideological fervor and grandiosity, enabled him to carry out his important role in direct medical killing. De Crinis killed himself on 1 May 1945 in the prescribed Nazi manner by swallowing cyanide.[24] A historian of the Charité Hospital claimed in 1963 that,

---

*There is evidence of an official policy of "euthanasia" physicians obscuring their SS connections, but de Crinis seemed to carry this out to an extreme degree.

in its proud 250 years of existence, no other physician had been guilty of crimes approaching the magnitude of de Crinis's.[25]

Psychiatric Idealist: Carl Schneider

Carl Schneider (1891–1946), also an Austrian, exemplifies the moral descent of a distinguished academic psychiatrist into the Nazi worldview and a key role in the "euthanasia" killing project. Most striking about Schneider is the impressive record of empathy and rehabilitation measures for patients that he brought to his commitment to direct medical killing.

A woman psychologist I talked to who had worked for Schneider stressed his idealism, his and others' sense that a "euthanasia" project could end the horror—the "hidden crime . . . the black side of medicine" —of profoundly regressed, isolated, backward psychiatric patients. She thought Schneider unusually sensitive to psychological symptoms, and "not a bad man."

He was later described by a younger colleague as an "excellent psychiatrist . . . very sensitive . . . very impressive to younger psychiatrists." Schneider "detested force and cold routine," permitted psychiatrists to have lunch with patients, and disseminated principles of empathy, especially toward epileptic patients, he had learned from having spent some time at the Bethel Institution where he—a pastor's son—had been chief physician until 1933.[26]*

Schneider left Bethel to become director of the University Clinic at Heidelberg. He had joined the Party in 1932; and after the Nazis assumed power, associates observed his transformation from "a modest scholar with an umbrella and briefcase, occupied with the most subtle kind of investigation of schizophrenia," to a man who, as "a leader of German psychiatry, took on the mission of preaching National Socialism and offering his own enlightened program of work therapy as a National-Socialist approach par excellence."[27] Ironically, precisely that program of work therapy by Carl Schneider was referred to by Professor Ewald (see pages 83–85) as an extremely hopeful development in the treatment of schizophrenia, a development that argued strongly against subjecting schizophrenic patients to "euthanasia" killing, and against such killing in general.

His former associate, Walter Ritter von Baeyer, thought of him as "an ambivalent man." And Schneider himself, when discussing many patients, would put forward "two possible ways to help"—one of them work therapy, and the other sterilization and medical killing. Von Baeyer also felt that Schneider was the kind of "sensitive and weak person" who could be readily transformed by National Socialist convictions into "a very

---

*Despite his position at Bethel, Schneider had been involved in Nazi intrigues against Bodelschwingh for control of the Protestant church.

aggressive person" with new energy and confidence. He could have enormous impact upon younger psychiatrists because they "would first identify with this sensitive man, and then with his more aggressive side as they joined him in National-Socialist ideology."[28]

That new confidence could take the form of grandiosity—plans, never realized, for a vast research institute that would focus on hereditary influences in "idiocy"—and, more than that, would create a new "biological anthropology," which would "finally put an end to the old ideas about mankind." Schneider did succeed in obtaining large sums of money for a research institute where he initiated some of this work, using mainly brains obtained from the "euthanasia" project.[29]

Schneider's path of corruption was his psychiatric idealism. But, once on that path, he felt beckoned as well by immortalizing professional power. Whatever conflicts he experienced, he could connect his unusual empathy for psychiatric patients with the Nazi biomedical vision and its humane claim to end suffering and strengthen the race. A previously sensitive man's deep immersion in Nazi ideology in general enabled him to function as both empathic psychiatrist and medical executioner.

The Ultimate Healer-Turned-Killer: Irmfried Eberl

Finally, there is Irmfried Eberl (1910–48), unique among doctors in that he went from being head of major T4 gassing facilities to become, at age thirty-two, commandant—not chief doctor but overall commander —of a death camp.

Another Austrian, Eberl belonged to the younger generation of highly politicized early Nazi doctors, having joined the Party at the age of twenty-one. At the time of the test demonstration at Brandenburg in 1940, he was one of the first to be shown how the poison-gas killing technology worked. He made use of that knowledge extensively as head of that killing center and, when it closed down, as head of Bernburg. And, in addition to serving in the inner circle of psychiatric experts, he was given special authority to enter various psychiatric institutions and investigate their attitudes toward, and willingness to work energetically in, the "euthanasia" killing project.[30]

Eberl served as a special deputy to Heyde in supervising the all-important area of false causes of death, with the task of establishing consistency in the various killing centers and policies that could convincingly maintain the subterfuge.[31]* Eberl was actively involved organ-

---

*In this role, Eberl wrote a long, carefully argued letter to Dr. Rudolf Lonauer, director at Hartheim, objecting that one of his assistants had cited lung tuberculosis as a cause of death, because that disease was not likely to be suddenly fatal; moreover, tuberculosis necessitated such mandatory legal-epidemiological procedures as isolation and the closing of wards or institutions. The letter concluded with a remarkable paragraph:

In summary, I should like to state that because of all the cited reasons, the frequent diagnosis "lung tuberculosis" as practiced by you (about 40 to 50 percent of all cases that we have received come under this diagnosis) is not unobjectionable, and I ask you

izing special transports of Jewish patients to his killing institution at Brandenburg; a pocket diary of his denoted the various Jewish transports with the letter "J," together with the number of people and the names of the towns in which institutions sending transports to Brandenburg were located.[33]

Eberl's enthusiasm for "euthanasia" killing was expressed in his intense advocacy of the law that would openly legitimate the project as well as mercy killing on request. He pointed out that, whatever the existing reservations on the part of doctors, "the number of ideologically unacceptable medical officers will indeed shrink from year to year, since the new generation presumably will be ideologically correct to an overwhelming extent."[34]

Eberl was appointed commandant of Treblinka at the camp's opening in July 1942. An engineer from T4 had helped construct the gassing apparatus; and the personnel, as in the other death camps in Poland, came heavily from SS men earlier involved with "euthanasia." Ukrainian guards with dogs were a new feature. The fact that Eberl was the only physician known to have headed a death camp suggests that the Nazis had good reason to feel that he was indistinguishable from a nonphysician in his attitude toward killing Jews. It could also mean that the Nazis were at the time considering wider use of doctors as commandants of death camps, thereby extending the principle of medicalized killing.

If Eberl was a test case, he failed. An SS inspection visit to Treblinka a few weeks after the arrival of the first transport exposed a chaotic situation. Decaying corpses were piled up as new trains arrived, giving incoming Jews an all too clear idea of what awaited them, and making them difficult to handle; trains could not keep their schedule as one was held up behind another. Eberl was dismissed in short order. He had not been able to cope with the new dimension of murder, although his inefficiency in no way slowed down the process. At the peak in late August, trains were bringing in 10,000 to 12,000 Jews a day; by the end of that month, some 215,000 had been killed. (In comparison, as a T4 doctor, Eberl had killed "only" 18,000 patients in a little over a year and a half.[35])

During his brief tenure, Eberl was said to have worn his white physician's coat when walking about the camp. Whether or not he actually did, he became, for a brief period, the ultimate healer-turned-killer—even if he did not quite make the grade. Whatever his prior psychological propensity for omnipotence, sadism, and violence, he apparently experienced the kind of total immersion into Nazi ideology that would

---

in the interest of successful cooperation to refrain from using this diagnosis in such great numbers, especially if there have been no previous symptoms. I also must reject the advice of your office chief because, as a nonphysician, he is in no position to judge the facts properly, and I agree with him when he says that this question is a purely medical one and therefore is only to be decided by doctors.[32]

His consistent principle was that one needs a careful *medical* lie.

permit killing any individual or group in any way at any time to further the vision of purifying and curing the Aryan race.

Biological Romanticism: Johann S.

While Johann S. was not much involved in the "euthanasia" project, he lived out the full history and ideology of Nazi medical leaders. During about twenty hours of conversation over three full days, I found this canny, energetic, and fanatical old man, living in prosperous rural surroundings, to be the most unregenerate Nazi among all the doctors I interviewed. His life uniquely reflects the special Nazi blend of violent nationalism and visionary biology.

Soon after we sat down for the first time, he referred to a recent television program about a plan for a physicians' academy bridging the split between pre-clinical theory and clinical work, and declared that he had been working on such a plan during the Third Reich, at which time "doctors formed a tightly knit, completely self-contained medical organization" that integrated all health organizations and private institutions into "a complete medical sector." That set the tone of the interviews: nostalgia for the beautiful Nazi medical experience and justification for its failure, with no faltering in his embrace of the original vision. Indeed, he had spent virtually his entire medical life—as a medical "old Nazi," and a medical official in the upper reaches of the regime—pursuing and implementing that vision.

Johann S. described himself the "son of a doctor"—his medical family traceable back to the early seventeenth century and having ties to ordinary people (as veterinarians and blacksmiths) before emerging as part of the progressive rural élite (both grandfathers were National Liberal members of the Reichstag). As a child, he was involved with all forms of animal life; and when I asked him what subject interested him most, he answered emphatically, "Always, in life, in biology." When a little older, he began to read Bölsche and Haeckel. Ernst Haeckel, a towering figure in German biology and an early Darwinian, was also a racist, a believer in a mystical *Volk*, and a strong advocate of eugenics who "can be claimed as a direct ancestor" of the Nazi "euthanasia" project.[36] Wilhelm Bölsche was a literary critic who became a disciple and biographer of Haeckel and was known to have provided Hitler with "direct access to major ideas of Haeckelian social Darwinism" (see pages 441–42).[37]

When S. was eleven, his father moved his medical practice from the country to a large city—a move his son came to associate with a loss of idealized rural communal life, or *Gemeinschaftsleben* ("We would always have a friend dropping in to share what was on our table. . . . Our coachman would sit with us, . . . live with us") and the discovery of the "dreadful isolation of people" in the city ("People die in the same house, and the other person doesn't even notice it at all"). He went so far as to say, "The fact that I became a politician* can be traced back to this [dislocation]," by which he meant that a vision of rediscovering that ideal community became the *leitmotif* of his political struggles.

Overcoming War and "Betrayal"

In his early adolescence at the outbreak of the First World War, he remembers the "very powerful sensation" of the mobilization order and the euphoria of the general population at that moment and later at the announcement, in the marketplace, of each German victory. His entire family was directly involved: his father as an army doctor; his older brother training to become an officer; his mother, a leader in support activities; even his grandfather, a veterinarian with a cavalry regiment; and S. himself, a boy who was drawn to the military and hung around with officers quartered in his home. But before long victories and celebrations were replaced by defeats and by food shortages and hunger. Worst of all was the telegram announcing that his father had been wounded. The sight of his father "standing in front of me at the railroad station, . . . his arm in a bandage, . . . wearing a uniform together with . . . house slippers" was so overwhelming that it seemed like a *déjà vu* experience: he was convinced that he had encountered that exact scene in a dream the night before the telegram arrived. (It turned out that his father had been hit by a bullet from a German plane; but rather than acknowledge that absurdity, S. tried to make it a form of distinction by equating his father with Prince Wilhelm of Hesse, who was also hit by a German bullet, and in his case killed.) Though his father survived, S. recalled a series of subsequent events, almost equally disturbing, including the final defeat and returning troops shouting anti-military and anti-monarchical slogans, forming soldiers' councils, and tearing off the rank insignia from the uniforms of their officers (which caused S. to be especially "shaken"). To make matters complete, his older brother was wounded during the last days of battle, and "then the government collapsed."

In fact, the family never quite left the war. The older brother became one of the founders of a *Freikorps* unit (these "free corps" were voluntary paramilitary units composed mostly of demobilized soldiers); and S. himself, then age seventeen, joined to serve under his brother. He was eager to get into the military: "I belong to the age group that was not drafted for the war in 1918." While the formation of these units was initially encouraged by a weak government to help it keep the peace and suppress the threatened Communist revolution, members of the *Freikorps* came to see themselves as "cemented by their blood" to one another, struggling

*Since the word "politician" *(Politiker)* generally had a derogatory connotation for a person of Dr. S.'s rural background, his use of it here could suggest a certain inadvertent self-condemnation.

to keep the war going and to reverse its outcome, as destined to restore the glory of Germany.[38] Here S. entered directly into the romance of combat and death; he recalled proudly his unit's boldness in making use of patchwork equipment to defeat Communist troops, his brother's miraculous escape from execution by the Communists, and his living out the *Freikorps* principles (described by one participant) of "war and adventure, excitement and destruction." For the young S. the *Freikorps* was a profoundly formative experience; and for a leading historian of the phenomenon, "the real importance of the movement lies in . . . that brutality of spirit and in that exaltation of power which the men of the Free Corps bequeathed to the Third Reich."[39]

S. thought that the First World War experience "made a people of us," and that Germany had not been "militarily . . . defeated" but undermined by "strikes in the munitions plants." This was a version of the widely accepted right-wing "stab in the back" *(Dolchstoss)* theory of the First World War: Germany had been not defeated but betrayed—by leftists, Communists, non-Germans, and, above all, Jews. Over the course of his university and medical studies, S. took on the contours of an intellectual of the radical right, both élite and populist, scornful of the Weimar Republic ("We said, 'This mess has to be replaced by something completely different' "); reading Spengler and responding to his (in the words of a recent commentator) "celebration . . . of a national and racial soul that contrasts with a rootless international finance . . . locat[ed] . . . in the alien body of the soul of the Jews."[40] S. was also "greatly influenced" in his "historical views" by Houston Stuart Chamberlain, the Englishman who, early in the twentieth century, became a naturalized German citizen and married Richard Wagner's daughter Eva. Chamberlain wrote in German and his racist theory of history presents members of the Germanic (Nordic) race "as saviors of mankind" in a death struggle that "would decide whether the base Jewish spirit would triumph over the Aryan soul and drag the world down with it."[41] S. was part of a new nationalism, stressing the "community of blood" and the mystical transcendence of the "front experience" of combat in the First World War (in Ernst Jünger's words, "The last war, our war, the greatest and most powerful event of this era . . . [because] in it the genius of war permeated the spirit of progress . . . [and] the growing transformation of life into energy)."[42]*

During his student days, Johann S. followed a family tradition in becoming active in the national *Burschenschaften,* or student corporations, which he associated with deep Germanic roots and with *völkisch* princi-

---

*Jünger was the leading literary representative of the "front generation" and its "inner experience" of the trenches during the First World War. As a talented novelist and essayist, he "probably undermined the Weimar Republic more effectively than any other single author and helped foster a mental climate in which Nazism could flourish." He resisted joining the Party, however, and, after military experience in the Second World War, produced diaries "disdainful of the Nazi spirit to which he had once made no trifling contribution."[43]

ples: "Many of the first National Socialist physicians were *Burschenschaft* members."* Also connected with the *Burschenschaften* was a professor he admired who combined extreme eccentricity, ostensible clinical and therapeutic brilliance bordering on magic, the triumph of intuition over cold reason and the machine, and even the physician's prevailing over royalty (in one story, S.'s idol made a recalcitrant emperor pay an exorbitant fee for medical services). These themes would be consistent with Nazi medicine and, above all, with its and the regime's *Führer* principle.

S.'s family's struggle with Germany's extreme postwar inflation, his later medical practice with his father as "a worker's doctor and poor people's doctor," and his general preoccupation with community all inclined him toward a socialism of the right, sometimes termed "Prussian socialism," based on what Jünger called the *Gestalt* of the German worker-soldier.[44] That inclination played an important part in S.'s enlistment, at the end of 1930, in the SA, as did both his experience in the *Freikorps* (of which he considered the Storm Troopers "a continuation") and, in fact, his whole previous political formation. In addition, there was his romantic self-image: he described witnessing "a small troop wearing brown shirts and carrying the swastika flag† . . . singing the 'Horst Wessel' song‡ . . . real young workers . . . surrounded by jeering communists, . . . but they just marched right along," causing him to feel, "I should be ashamed of myself. These boys risked their lives and I don't do anything."

He plunged into their "completely militarized" marches, organized medical services for them, and saw himself, as did the SA leaders, as part of a revolutionary army that was responsible for Hitler's victory by reclaiming the streets from the "Reds." Above all, the *experience* was powerful: he felt himself in communal relationship with "the real workers. . . . This was one of Hitler's greatest achievements. . . . We came to live with these young workers in close community"; and finally, "we of the younger generation" had access to the "front experience," which S. had previously known only from his brother's renditions. Specifically denying the SA's terror tactics, S.'s nostalgia bordered on rapture as he described the beauty of the marches, the nobility of his group in "marching boldly past streets . . . filled with Reds," and he declared, "This was among the most beautiful times of my life." In addition, he considered his fellow

---

*The *Burschenschaften* emerged during the early nineteenth century as student groups committed to German national unity (in opposition to Napoleonic-French military, political, and cultural influence), on the one hand; and to political liberalization (in opposition to Prussian-authoritarian repression), on the other. Originally disdainful of the traditional student corps and their focus on dueling and drinking, the *Burschenschaft* movement itself eventually took a conservative direction and came to emphasize these same activities, while holding to a fierce nationalism.

†The swastika flag was the emblem first of the Nazi Party and later of Nazi Germany. Devised by Hitler, the flag had a red background in the middle of which was a black hooked cross (the swastika [meaning, in Sanskrit, well-being or good luck], an ancient symbol in many cultures) within a white circle.

‡The Horst Wessel song was composed by a young SA leader who was killed in a Berlin brawl in 1930. His death was systematically manipulated by Goebbels in a way that transformed into an ascetic martyr a man who had literally been a pimp.

doctors to be developing within the SA something on the order of a revolutionary medicine and, indeed, of a biologized state: "And they were all doctors like me, who tried to think biologically, [of] biology as the foundation of medical thought. . . . We didn't want politics—we were critical of politics—but [were concerned] with the way human beings really are—not just an idea or philosophy."

National Socialism as Applied Biology

The nation would now be run according to what Johann S. and his cohorts considered biological truth, "the way human beings really are." That is why he had a genuine "eureka" experience—a sense of "That's exactly it!"—when he heard Rudolf Hess declare National Socialism to be "nothing but applied biology" (see page 31). Dr. S. felt himself merged with not only Hess (he told me, with some excitement, "I was standing no more than ten meters from him at the time!") but with the Führer himself: "Hess knew exactly what Hitler thought. . . . He was the only one closely involved with him all the time." S. quickly joined the Party and devoted himself to the realization of that biological claim.

He pointed out proudly that these early SA doctors formed the nucleus of the National Socialist German Physicians' League *(Nationalsozialistischer Deutscher Ärztebund),* the doctors who, as he put it, "were the first intellectuals to have complete confidence . . . in National Socialism to march in the streets"—in effect, to put their bodies on the line.

Now S.'s hero was Gerhard Wagner, who had served in the First World War, the *Freikorps,* and the SA and was a founder and the head of the Nazi Doctors' League. Described accurately by one observer as "a notorious public advocate of the anti-Jewish racial laws,"[45] Wagner was to Johann S. "a fantastic person—an all-around doctor from a medical family, [who] had a personal influence on Hitler." Wagner was a protégé of Rudolf Hess, and Dr. S. understood both of these leaders to favor something on the order of permanent revolution and to view the National Socialists "as a movement rather than a party, constantly growing and changing according to the 'health' requirements of the people's body [*Volkskörper*]": "Just as a body may succumb to illness, the *Volkskörper* could do the same."

S. worked closely with Wagner in the Nazification of German medicine, the two men sharing Hess's *Volk* mysticism, advocacy of lay practitioners, a Nazi version of holistic medicine that would "put in the foreground . . . questions of the psyche that had been neglected" (see pages 40–41), a broad medical outreach to all institutions (holding to medical authority so that "employees of a factory knew that their boss could not give orders to the doctors"), and "a new medical *Weltanschauung.*" This worldview replaced two false doctrines—that of Christianity, which understood human beings "only in a spiritual sense"; and that of the French Revolution, which claimed that "all human beings are equal"—both of which, according to S., "came into conflict with biological experience, . . . with the laws of life."

During those heady years from 1934 to 1939, S. became a missionary for this biomedical vision, making hundreds of speeches to doctors' groups, Party meetings, and general audiences. He combined his mystical concept of "biological socialism" with Nazi leadership principles, especially concerning the hegemony of physicians as the authentic, practicing biologists in matters of race and population, judgments about the needs of the people, and much else. As for anti-Semitic attitudes and actions, he insisted that "the racial question . . . [and] resentment of the Jewish race . . . had nothing to do with medieval anti-Semitism . . . but only [with] the aim of self-fulfillment, *völkisch* self-fulfillment." That is, it was all a matter of scientific biology and of community. Again S. declared nostalgically, "It was a beautiful time for me."

Everything changed in 1939, the year Gerhard Wagner died and the war began. While S. took the Nazi view of the war (as being forced upon his country by Poles mistreating ethnic Germans), he felt that it interrupted his biological mission and, indeed, that it "ended the whole National Socialist movement." He saw the medical aspect of the movement, under Conti, Wagner's successor, increasingly bureaucratized within the Interior Ministry, with lawyers taking over and Party-based visionaries like himself having less to say. Even before then, S. had been critical of this legalistic trend as manifested in the Nuremberg racial laws and the sterilization program. Rather than its courts and elaborate legal machinery, S. wanted it run completely by doctors, who alone would decide which people had dangerous hereditary traits, and who could alter policies according to changing medical knowledge.

Another villain in the piece was the SS leader, Himmler, whom S. characterized as "a mere animal breeder . . . [who] thought he was competent in racial questions," and who never represented the real view of the National Socialist Party and was the reason for much unfair criticism of it. S. arranged to be reassigned out of Berlin in order to escape the "grotesque" bureaucratic situation.

Concerning "euthanasia," he was sympathetic to the concept, emphasizing what a "blessing" it was for regressed mental patients to be "released." But he was extremely critical of the actual project, considering it a product of "Himmler's circle," and its timing a bureaucratic disaster. He also objected to the Nazi state—the representative of the whole community, or *Gemeinschaft*—taking human life, and seemed to prefer here also that the matter be left *completely* to doctors. He believed that the "loudest protest" against "euthanasia" came from old Nazi doctors who were district medical officers; that Karl Brandt's execution at Nuremberg was "completely unjustified"; and that the responsible people were Brack, a "failed doctor" who sought only his own advancement, and Bouhler, also a nonphysician, who implicated Brandt at Nuremberg to save his own neck. But the whole subject embarrassed S.: from it, he

went into what became for him a characteristic end-of-the-interview dia-
tribe in which he blamed the atmosphere of brutality "brought about by
the Russian troops," the "declaration of war" by Chaim Weizmann, the
Zionist leader, against the Germans, and the "brutality of the air raids on
Germany."

In all this, S. presented himself not only as a biological idealist but as
a "reasonable Nazi" countering the excesses of others. He defended the
concept that "there are certain qualities of the Nordic race," and claimed
that this was "a scientific idea," and that "we wanted to call forth the
spiritual substance of the northern European, really European culture
[*Kultur,* in Nazi usage, could mean 'racial culture']": "Just have a look at
who's running your country . . . basically the Nordic race." But he would
grant that the German people were a mixture of races, and that "we saw
things too narrowly" in equating *Volk* with race. He attributed these
errors, however, to insufficient knowledge of genetics at the time—that
is, to a kind of innocence.

Clearly a fierce anti-Semite at least during the Nazi era, S., upon learning that I was Jewish, declared unctuously, "The Jewish question became
our tragedy and your tragedy." He explained that it was initiated "by the
flood [of Jews] from the East, and by Darwinian principles enabling Jews
to become especially able "through such a hard selection during these
two thousand years" to take so many medical positions that German
doctors were excluded from; but he added, "Nowadays we know that all
of us, Jews and Germans, belong to the same cultural community" and
must stand together against the "adverse cultural community," including
China and Russia but especially the expanding numbers of the people of
Islam, which "is where the danger comes from." Except for rearranging
his cast of characters, Dr. S. had not changed much. Racially, he practiced
what he preached, and had an enormous family: "I have always believed
that those who are fit should have as many children as possible, and those
who are unfit should have as few . . . as possible."

His attitude toward Hitler was generally worshipful: "He . . . was an
extraordinarily nice person, and took care of his men just like a father.
. . . he was a genius . . . brilliant . . . had an incredible memory," and was
not responsible for such excesses as "euthanasia" or the killing of Jews,
which were the work of men like Himmler maneuvering behind Hitler's
back. Moreover, "Hitler was not really anti-Semitic" but "of course
. . . got angry when the Jews started a war against him" (here Dr. S. was
referring to a 1941 book by Theodore N. Kaufman, entitled *Germany Must
Perish!*).* Yet S. could also say that it was very unfortunate that Hitler had

---

*Published in 1941, this book does indeed advocate "the extinction of the German
nation and the total eradication from the earth, of all her people"—an end to be accomplished, ironically enough, by a systematic, "main and thorough" program of "Eugenic
Sterilization." The rationale for such a program is the prevention of future wars, given the
existence from virtually the beginning of history of a German "war-soul" or "war-lust"
manifesting itself in one way or another.[46] The book was seized upon by Nazi propagandists
generally in terms not unlike Dr. S.'s.

been made into "a Godlike being"; that he was the kind of man who had to "talk himself free" of problems, and would contradict himself, and that people were too quick to rush to do what they thought he wanted; and that, like all geniuses, he was psychologically unstable and "what we doctors would call a psychopath." S. described telling Conti, before he himself went off to war, that "you cannot ask me to follow a Führer . . . who I am convinced is no longer sane." In the end, however, S. exonerated Hitler by attributing his mental difficulties to his medical mismanagement by Morell, the quack doctor, who constantly gave Hitler drugs and created what Dr. S. was convinced were addictions to both amphetamines and to intravenous glucose.* In this way, he invoked a medical explanation for the errors and excesses of Hitler himself and the Nazi regime.

Concerning the concentration camps, Dr. S. said that those physicians who worked there "had nothing to do with us"—that is, were not part of the physicians' groups he worked with or presided over. He insisted that he had heard nothing of the camps until after the war, that doctors' roles in experiments and selections were "disputed," that "the whole Himmler shop" responsible for it all was so secretive that it was hard to learn the truth; and finally that "the doctors in those institutions [camps] were the least National Socialist," and "if they had been genuinely National Socialist, they would have been at the front!"—which is where Dr. S. went.

In 1943, when he saw signs of Hitler's "deterioration" and other "big mistakes," he went to see Conti and berated him for his shortcomings, especially his failure to protect Hitler from Morell, and abruptly enlisted in an SA unit as a common soldier and left for the Russian front. S. was seeking a form of purification, following an important personal quest ("I wanted to experience war"), and, above all, sought the mystical "front experience" associated with the First World War. Referring again to his brother and father, he said, "All this left such an impression on me that, even though I was leaving seven children, I volunteered for . . . this war experience, . . . right there at the front." He was not disappointed. He wrote glowingly about his experience as both common soldier and military doctor, and added, "Humanly speaking and also from a physician's viewpoint, I would be lacking a great deal had I not lived this."

Johann S.'s life story illustrates the interaction of historical forces with individual-psychological tendencies. Concerning that interaction I would emphasize his intense belief in the immortal *Volk;* the mystique of war and

---

*Dr. S. gave a psychohistorical twist to the matter by saying that Hitler's distress at not being able to realize his dream of an alliance with England caused chronic stomach trouble, which Morell was called in to treat. There is little doubt that Morell was a charlatan, but there is dispute about whether he created amphetamine or other addiction in Hitler. One study concludes that "amphetamine toxicity is an extremely probable diagnosis"; but a still more recent study concludes that no such addiction existed.[47] Whatever Hitler's relationship to amphetamine, one should recognize the danger of invoking addiction as "the reason" for his or the Nazis' extreme behavior or negative historical direction.

its culmination and bitter frustration in the First World War; the over-whelming death immersion of that war and the degradation of defeat, remarkably reversed in the glorification of the "front experience" and the "stab in the back" explanation through which German resurgence becomes a survivor mission and debt to the dead who "are not really dead at all . . . [but] climb out of their graves and visit us at night in our dreams";[48] the violence of the collective redemptive-revitalizing impulse as expressed through militarized male bands (the *Freikorps* and the SA) with ambivalence that could become murderous toward their homoerotic tendencies;[49] the combination, within a single mystical constellation, of those elements of *völkisch* romanticism, the warrior ethos, and national revitalization with visionary biologism, Nordic-centered racism, and pas-sionate anti-Semitism; and a vision of physician-philosopher kings with mythical medical-alchemist powers (see pages 481–84) who both exem-plify and serve the *"Führer* principle" in bringing about immortalizing racial revitalization.

Dr. S.'s decision for purification in battle could well have been an effort to fend off perceptions of overall failure, wrongness, even evil, having to do with the entire Nazi project. (A somewhat parallel purifying impulse may have motivated Hitler in his effort to destroy all of Germany at the end of the war.) Whatever S.'s front experience served, he emerged from it regretting nothing. He knew the Nazis had been excessive in their killing of Jews, but purported to prove that the numbers were exag-gerated, that much of it was done not by Germans but by Ukrainians, and that "numbers don't count anyway," as he struggled (successfully) to hold on to his Nazi religion. His conclusion was not that National Social-ism was wrong or bad but that "the time was too short"; that for its purposes to be achieved, it "will take many generations"; and that Hitler, presumably like Moses, "opened the gate into a new century but did not cross the threshold" and essentially "was a man of the nineteenth cen-tury." And, finally, "National Socialism failed because we could not de-velop enough biological teaching—it was not possible to educate people sufficiently in biology"—so that "the tragedy of National Socialism was that it was never realized."

While Dr. S.'s swings between modes of logic and madness could be attributed to senility, they were characteristic of someone caught between an elaborate belief system with a certain internal coherence and that system's larger intellectual absurdity and moral madness. Crucial was the extensive sharing of the project, so that the most bizarre ideas and poli-cies "seemed normal to all concerned."[50] Johann S. demonstrates how Nazi doctors could combine certain logical structures with flamboyant and murderous expressions of that moral madness and continue to func-tion in the process.

Chapter 6

Bringing "Euthanasia" to the Camps: Action Special Treatment 14f13

> [I]t must be the duty of racial hygiene to be atten-
> tive to a more severe elimination of morally inferior
> human beings than is the case today.... We should
> literally replace all factors responsible for selection
> in a natural and free life.... In prehistoric times
> of humanity, selection for endurance, heroism, so-
> cial usefulness, etc. was made solely by *hostile* out-
> side factors. This role must be assumed by a human
> organization; otherwise, humanity will, for lack of
> selective factors, be annihilated by the degenera-
> tive phenomena that accompany domestication.
> —KONRAD LORENZ (1940)

It was probably inevitable that the T4 killing project would be extended
to the concentration camps, but the program under which that was done,
bearing the code name 14f13, has always been something of a mystery.
From the standpoint of this study, we may view this program as a key
means of linking the direct medical killing we have been discussing with
the medicalized killing in the concentration camps—that is, linking the
Nazi version of "euthanasia" with genocide.

The SS did not run T4, though it had close ties with the program. We
have seen how it provided the means for killing: the carbon monoxide gas
chamber, as developed by the SS officer Christian Wirth, as well as other
personnel and equipment necessary for transportation and for murder.
Equally important was the SS's tie to leading T4 psychiatrists and

Heyde's involvement since 1936 with the camps themselves as supervisor of "neurologic and hereditary control" of prisoners.

Early in 1941, T4 leader Bouhler agreed to let Himmler use T4 personnel and facilities to rid the camps of "excess" prisoners—notably those "most seriously ill," physically and mentally. Sometimes called "prisoner euthanasia" or (by prisoners) "Operation Invalid," the resultant program was officially "Operation [or Special Treatment] 14f13."* The designation came from the reference number for the operation in documents of the Concentration Camp Inspectorate.† That spring, "experienced psychiatrists" from T4 were sent to the camps, assured that their work in selecting out "asocial" elements had scientific importance. Their work, as in T4, was based on prior questionnaires. For this purpose, however, they were shorter, asking after a prisoner's name, race, and "health" (that is, whether incurable).‡ The short form was explained by the T4 doctors' lack of time, although camp commandants or camp doctors did the initial screening. To camouflage procedures, those selected were told that they were being sent to a "rest home." (In fact, people apparently volunteered until it was realized what was happening when personal effects, but no "rested" prisoners, returned.)[6]

As low as T4 standards were, those in 14f13 were worse. "Examinations" by T4 doctors were perfunctory or non-existent, and the questionnaires frequently contained no medical information at all, but only a list of an inmate's ostensible crimes and political deviations. Ordinary SS camp personnel could construe political beliefs or rude comments about the Führer as "mental deficiency" or "psychological aberration," and the visiting doctors' commission almost never objected to an SS request for "transfer" (to a killing facility). Whatever the travesty of medicine, inmates observed that "the doctors were dressed in white coats," although other prisoners apparently assumed that they were Gestapo in disguise.[7]

Toward Jews these white-coated doctors developed an approach that was to become a Nazi trademark—that of collective diagnosis. For Jews, neither "examination" nor health considerations were necessary. As one participating T4 psychiatrist recalled, "it sufficed to take the reasons for arrest (often very extensive!) from the documents and transfer them to the questionnaires."[8] This meant that the only thing to be considered was

*There is some evidence—Friedrich Mennecke's recollection in his testimony at Nuremberg[1]—that, as early as the summer of 1940, psychiatrists from T4 were sent to concentration camps to evaluate inmates, whose original questionnaires were filled out by camp doctors. One commentator sees in this early sequence an "experimental" phase in the expansion of medical killing.[2] But others question whether any such phase actually occurred.[3]

†Similarly, for example, natural deaths were 14f1; 14f2 was a suicide or accidental death; 14f3, shot while attempting to escape; 14fI, execution.[4]

‡This contradicts Nitsche's later testimony that "the combing out of the c[oncentration] c[amps] was done according to precisely the same viewpoint, by means of the same questionnaires, as those in the insane asylums." He claimed that, because of rumors of popular unrest over the placing of the mentally ill in camps, they were being returned to proper institutions.[5]

that they were Jews and could be presented *as a group*—a process, as we shall observe, close to that of selections in Auschwitz. That same psychiatrist had copied phrases from the SS files of Dachau and Ravensbrück on the backs of their photographs. On one: "Inflammatory Jew hostile to Germans; in camp lazy and insolent." Another: "Anti-German disposition. Symptoms: Well-known functionary of the KPD [German Communist Party], militant agitator." And still another: "Diagnosis: Fanatical German-hater and asocial psychopath. Principal symptoms: inveterate Communist, ineligible for military service."[9] As a postwar German psychiatrist stated, "It would be difficult to find a clearer documentation of the political manipulation of the psychiatric profession."[10]

One key to the nature of 14f13 lies in the term "special treatment" (*Sonderbehandlung*) as part of the program's name. "Special treatment," though it was to become a euphemism for killing in general, was used originally (from 1939) as a specific Gestapo concept and code term legitimating extralegal execution. Thus, Reinhard Heydrich issued decrees, on 3 and 20 September 1939, distinguishing cases that could be taken care of "in the accustomed manner and those which require[d] special treatment": the latter, because of their seriousness, danger, and "propaganda consequences deserve to be considered for elimination, ruthlessly and without respect of persons." The concept was consistent with Hitler's formally articulated claim (made in October 1939, soon after the outbreak of war) to "the right of deciding over life and death of all Germans, without regard for existing laws." T4 itself had been initiated under this claim, but 14f13 structured it specifically in connection with the principle of "special treatment." The term then was extended to a variety of cases in the work of the secret police, and to decrees by leaders of the Race and Resettlement Office concerning the handling of racially undesirable people. By the middle of 1941, the term was being used "matter-of-factly" in connection with extermination of Jews in the East, even to the creation of different verb forms such as a past tense, "specially treated" (*sonderbehandelt*). In June 1942, Himmler approved a "euthanasia" death for tubercular Polish workers by stating, "I have no objection to giving special treatment to the Polish nationals . . . who have been certified by authorized physicians to be incurable."[11]

The use of the term "special treatment" followed a sequence, then, of being applied first to allegedly dangerous criminals, then to medically determined "unworthy life" in the greater society (in the T4 program, where, however, the term was not widely used), and finally to still-medicalized "euthanasia" in the camps (via 14f13, where it was always used) of all groups considered by the regime to be undesirable (Jews, homosexuals, political opponents, ordinary criminals, "shiftless elements," Catholic critics, etc.) and now inclusively viewed as "unworthy life." The extension of the aura of "euthanasia" into the camps in this way widened indefinitely the potential radius of medicalized killing. And that form of extralegal but legitimated killing took on a special priority and absoluteness: the minutes of the 1 January 1940 SS conference on race-related immigration questions state that an individual judgment on "special treatment" was to be "incontestable, like that of a physician" (see also pages 430–33).[12]

Although the code name had originated from the office of the Inspectorate of Concentration Camps, orders and directives came only from T4 headquarters, and doctors reported from the camps back to that headquarters for appointments with Heyde or Nitsche and to drop off completed forms for processing; transfer lists were prepared there, so that inmates on the lists could be sent directly to one of the still-operative killing centers (such as Bernburg and Hartheim) where they were gassed in the same manner as patients in the T4 program. One variation from T4 procedure was that death notices were sent out from the camps rather than centrally, though with similarly contrived causes of death. (By early 1942, no notices were sent out.) The continued pseudo-medical "euthanasia" idiom was reflected also in Nazi documents in their reference to "prisoners' euthanasia" and in camp inmates' references to "invalid transports."[13]

Medical Bridge to Genocide

The 14f13 program went through several changes in focus over its period of operation. Its emphasis shifted almost immediately from the mentally ill (if that emphasis ever actually existed) to political prisoners, Jews, Poles, draft evaders or those deemed militarily unsuitable, those guilty of "racial" crimes, habitual criminals—until the mentally ill became hardly relevant. Yet in March 1942, an SS directive went out to camp commandants emphasizing that prisoners capable of work were *not* to be included under 14f13. (The decision to keep workers may have been somewhat affected by the fact that remaining T4 facilities were full.) And in April, as more camp inmates were being pressed into armaments work, commandants were even told that only the truly mentally ill were to be selected for "mustering out" (*Ausmusterung*). Even the bedridden could be given appropriate tasks. As we shall see in the discussion of Auschwitz, the camps were always involved in conflict between two factions, both of which could be found within the SS bureaucracy. One faction wanted maximum extermination; the other, exploitation of slave labor.[14]

According to Dr. Hans-Günther Seraphim, an expert witness at several postwar trials, "ruthless extermination" was more likely to have been pushed by the 14f13 physicians' committees, with their bureaucratic location in Hitler's Chancellery, than by the concentration camp administration.[15] This may well have been true through most of the program's history. In early 1944, however, 14f13 entered something of another phase as the war continued to take its human toll. The camp at Mauthausen near Linz, for example, had become severely overcrowded and suffered from increasingly unsanitary conditions. The assistance of the nearby T4 facility at Hartheim was thus requested. Since the need here was simply for space, there were no questionnaires or experts. Camp personnel made selections, and those killed included slave laborers from the East, Russian prisoners of war, Hungarian Jews, Jehovah's Witnesses, and above all *Muselmänner.* *

Hartheim also received shipments from Dachau and Ravensbrück. Even prisoners who might have worked were eliminated in this situation. Gold dental work was removed and sent to the T4 center. Apparently so many prisoners were designated for killing that gassing was resumed at Hartheim. The facilities there were finally dismantled in December 1944, at which time the turn-of-the-century Renaissance castle became a children's home, intended to camouflage what had happened there. At Hadamar, this was the point at which slave laborers from the East, diagnosed categorically as "tubercular," were being injected on SS orders (see pages 100–102).[17]

A close observer notes that 14f13 was initially aimed at exterminating those in the camps who had psychiatric disturbances; and that, given the crudeness of the deceptions employed, "it is difficult to understand why Himmler did not trust his own camp doctors to execute the selections, since with the criteria applied, any SS-sergeant could have acted with the same competence . . . [and] the expert professors could have put on their signatures in Berlin."[18] The answer, I believe, lies in the powerful Nazi impulse, sometimes conscious and at other times inchoate, to bring the greatest degree of medical legitimation to the widest range of killing.

The 14f13 project provided two crucial bridges between existing concepts and policies and unrestrained genocide. There was, first, the *ideological bridge* from the killing of those considered physiologically unworthy of life to the elimination, under the direction of doctors, of virtually anyone the regime considered undesirable or useless: that is, from direct medical to medicalized killing. The fraudulence of the process was clear enough even to those carrying it out—even one of the 14f13 doctors put quotations around the word "examination" when writing to his wife[19]— but the continuing medical idiom served ideological and psychological purposes for individual participants.

The second is the *institutional bridge* from the T4 project to the concentration camps (these had been established in 1933 [see chapter 7]). The camps themselves became connected with a principle of medical-eugenic killing. The sequence in managing the killing was from T4, to the central offices and inspectorate of the camps in general, to ever-enlarging greater initiative from individual doctors. In that way, camp doctors increasingly took over the function of "euthanasia," and that function merged with their participation in mass murder. This sequence was made clear in an investigative report by the SS judge Konrad Morgen on corruption in the

---

*"Musselman" or "Moslem" was camp jargon for the living corpses who were so named, according to Hermann Langbein, because "when one saw a group of them at a distance, one had the impression of praying Arabs."[16]

camps. Morgen distinguished between illegal and legal forms of killing in them. As legal, he mentioned "those cases where physicians, upon their personal decisions, relieve incurably ill patients from their suffering by administering a drug for mercy killing." And, in the next sentence, he added, "The same applies to those cases where physicians acted in a state of emergency, where they killed victims of epidemics and those who could be suspected to have been infected, and killed them painlessly, in order to prevent mass deaths."[20] Such murder could be easily juxtaposed with "mercy killing" in that both were perceived as medical functions. (In part II, we will observe how such a "preventive" approach to epidemics was systematically pursued as part of mass murder.)

With the exception of Auschwitz, all camps where 14f13 was operative (for example, Dachau, Sachsenhausen, Ravensbrück) were of the standard kind, within which prisoners were beaten, starved, subjected to slave labor, and often killed; but the overall function of the institution was not mass murder *per se.* By providing these ordinary camps with killing centers as well as with a corrupt selections process for facilitating mass murder, 14f13 transformed them into functional equivalents of extermination camps. The arrangement could be temporary, or sustained as in the case of Mauthausen and Hartheim. T4 doctors made extensive selections at Mauthausen during the early part of 14f13; subsequently, Mauthausen camp doctors did the selections for people to be killed at Hartheim. The connection continued until the center was dismantled, when the order came not from the SS but from Hitler's Chancellery, specifically from Viktor Brack, central administrator of the "euthanasia" program.[21]

Ultimately, then, 14f13 provided for virtually unlimited application of the "euthanasia" program—especially to Jews, but also to Gypsies, Russians, Poles, and other Germans. The Nazi message—for victims, for possible observers, and mostly for themselves—was: all our killing is medical, medically indicated, and carried out by doctors. The 14f13 project is thought to have killed more than twenty thousand people, but the concepts and policies it furthered contributed to the death of millions.

An Inside View of 14f13: Friedrich Mennecke

The series of letters Dr. Friedrich Mennecke wrote to his wife (herself a T4 laboratory assistant) from the various concentration camps he visited provide an inside view of 14f13; appropriately enough, these letters were often written on the back of printed "euthanasia" questionnaires.

Mennecke was an ardent Nazi, having joined both the Party and the SS in 1932 and served as a deputy Party leader in his area—somewhat unusual for a medical man, as was his background as the son of a bricklayer. He claimed, in Party correspondence, strong professional involvement in "hereditary biology" and sterilization. He had just three years of psychiatric experience at the state mental hospital at Eichberg before being made its director in 1939. A special unit was formed there for extensive killing of children. Just thirty-seven in 1941, he was one of the youngest of those central to the 14f13 program.[22] His letters suggest a variety of ways in which a physician could experience professional enthusiasm in connection with participation in murder.

There is the sense of special professional opportunity: "Our work here [at the Sachsenhausen camp] is very, very interesting. . . . I am collecting . . . large quantities of new experiences" (4 April 1941). Three days later: "I am putting particular value on these examinations for eventual future scientific utilization." There is pride in the assumption of increasing responsibility: "I spoke with Dr. Heyde on the phone and told him I could handle it all by myself, so no one else came today to help" (20 November 1941). There is professional busyness: "On 13 December [1941] we're again going to Berlin only to leave again on 14 December to Fürstenberg [Ravensbrück] where we will begin working on the 15th. We have to be finished with Ravensbrück by 21 December" (25 November 1941). There is the statistically based aura of efficiency: "Although today I had to begin working half an hour late, a record was broken. I managed to complete 230 forms, so that now a total of 1,192 are complete" (1 December 1941). And after finishing 80 additional forms by working "briskly" for less than two hours the next morning, he expressed a sense of triumph over his total of 320 forms, "which Dr. Müller [his 14f13 colleague] certainly could not do in 2 full days. Whoever works fast, saves time!" (2 December 1941).* And his professional zeal in conveying to a camp doctor and the commandant "my ideas about which inmates should come into consideration for registration," resulted—happily for him—in the decision that "the number is to be expanded by 60–70 [inmates]" (20 November 1941).

At the same time, his at least partial awareness of the fundamental fraudulence of the operation emerges in his frequent use of quotations around the word "examined," and in such comments as: "There are only 2,000 men, who will be finished very soon, because they are just looked at assembly-line style" (3 September 1941) and, "About the composition of the pat[ients at Ravensbrück], I would not like to write anything here in this letter" (20 November 1941). Clearly disillusionment set in, since he wrote to his wife on 19 November 1941 that, when asked by Heyde to continue to devote himself indefinitely to the work, "I very politely declined," and told Nitsche in a later discussion in early 1942, "that I wanted to go back to my institution [Eichberg]" (14 January 1942).†

---

*And, it should be noted, brings home more money. Serving as a T4 expert was piecework. The monthly payment for up to 500 questionnaires was 100 marks; up to 2,000, 200 marks; up to 3,500, 300 marks; over 3,500, 400 marks.[23]

†In testimony given in November 1946, Mennecke claimed that, from 1942 on, he became aware that "all these methods of the Nazi government were inhuman and cruel and completely undiscriminating and sinful"—indeed, that he had recognized some of these truths by 1940. While we should be skeptical, it is possible that he was fending off that kind of awareness even as he enthusiastically proceeded with his deadly work. He claimed that,

One of the ways Mennecke continued to function in the face of his awareness of that fraudulence was by condemning what he took to be excess within the project ("[Dr. Hans] Gorgass . . . is said to have behaved dreadfully while at Buchenwald, . . . he supposedly acted more like a butcher than a doctor, thereby damaging the reputation of our whole operation. We will now have to iron out these wrinkles" [25 November 1941]). By contrast, Mennecke implied a dignified professionalism for himself and a good medical reputation for the project.

Like many involved in medical murder, he condemned "Berlin"— meaning the project leaders—for pressing him too hard: "In Berlin (Jennerwein!)* the word is simply do 2,000 more—whether or not so many come under the basic guidelines does not seem to bother anyone!" (20 November 1941). And he developed the submissive bureaucrat's anger toward inefficiency from above—which, in this case, required him to return to certain camps a second time. But expressing sentiments like "Today Berlin's disorganization hit a high point" may have provided precisely the outlet for feelings that enabled him to carry on with the work. Even more important in sustaining him was the opportunity to hobnob with the same "Berlin" élite at luxury hotels, such as Munich's Bayerisches Hof: "We went to the train station at 7:00 P.M. to pick up Professor Nitsche (and Professor Heyde) as well as Frau Nitsche" (3 September 1941). "[Heyde] was very, very friendly. . . . [Professor Nitsche] was very, very cordial and asked about you." Mennecke was beside himself with pleasure when praised and treated collegially: "Heyde also spoke very highly of my work. . . . I discussed with him several interesting points pertaining to our work" (19 November 1941). That suggestion of paternal approval, of merging with authority, and of confirmed professional-medical standing helped Mennecke maintain his callousness: "A second batch of 1,200 Jews followed [a smaller group of non-Jews], but they did not have to be 'examined' " (25 November 1941).

That numbing becomes an important part of a "medical killing self" that more or less separates from the rest of the self in the process of doubling which I shall examine in connection with the Auschwitz doctors. Important to the process is the affirmation of his prior self through endearments to his wife: "Next time my *Mutti* ['Mommy'] is coming along. . . . Most affectionate kisses from your devoted *Vati* ['Daddy'] . . . dear little kisses from your always devoted Fritz-Pa." Pleasant social

---

during his earliest concentration-camp visits, prisoners were examined individually "to establish the presence of psychosis or psychiatric symptoms," and that it was still "a medical question."[24] The claim could be entirely false. But if even partly true, it would suggest the highly dubious medical dimension of the project even in its origins.

*Jennerwein was the code name for T4 chief administrator Brack. Since Brack was not a physician, Mennecke's resentment here may be partly directed at some perceived "non-medical" ignorance or unreasonableness. It is difficult to say what he meant by the "basic guidelines" being violated. It is likely that these had to do with ability to work, and that T4 officials were pressing for more and more nonworkers (or inmates judged inadequate workers) to be included in the net.

arrangements with 14f13 leaders and colleagues connected the two elements of self, as in a postcard sent from the famous popular scenic area, the Starnberger See, near Munich ("Since we first begin working tomorrow, we have taken a beautiful outing" [3 September 1941]) and signed by not only Mennecke himself but also Dr. Gerhard Wischer, head of the Waldheim institution in Saxony; Dr. Nitsche; Dr. Victor Ratka; Dr. Rudolf Lonauer, director at Hartheim; Erich Bauer, chauffeur; and, added separately, Dr. Theodor Steinmeyer. There is also a group photograph of these relaxed excursionists.[25]*

Also contributing to balancing his two selves was pride at being classified as "essential" to (and therefore not liable to military draft), and honored by, the regime. Mennecke was sentenced to death by a German court, but died in prison in 1947 of tuberculosis contracted during his "euthanasia" work.[26]

The Evolving Genocidal Mentality

Of the number of people killed in the T4 and the 14f13 projects, the following statistics are usually given: adult mental patients from institutions, 80,000 to 100,000; children in institutions, 5,000; special action against Jews in institutions, 1,000; concentration-camp inmates transported to killing centers (14f13), 20,000 (Klee estimated that at the end of 1941, some 93,521 "beds" had been emptied for other uses [70,000 patients gassed, plus over 20,000 dead through starvation and medication]—in other words approximately one-third of the places for the mentally ill.)[27] But these figures may well be too low; twice these numbers of people may have perished. The fact is that we do not know and shall probably never know. Elements of deception, imposed chaos, and the destruction of many records make anything like an accurate estimate impossible.

The same is true concerning the total number of people murdered at specific killing centers. Hartheim victims of both ordinary "euthanasia" and 14f13 are variously estimated from 20,000 (by Dr. Georg Renno, Lonauer's successor as director), to 400,000 (by Franz Ziereis, the former commandant of Mauthausen, on his deathbed); 30,000 is believed to be the best estimate.[28] While these figures may seem unimpressive when placed next to the millions killed in the Final Solution, they represent the murder of shockingly large numbers of people—all in places characterized as hospitals.

Mennecke described to his wife, on 12 January 1942, an obscure but

---

*Mennecke revealed similar patterns in thanking the director of an institution he had visited in order to press "euthanasia" selections: "We will think back with joy on the days we spent with you . . . and have the nicest remembrances of the individual wards."

central moment in the sequence from T4 to genocide. "The day before yesterday," he wrote, "a large team from our Operation left for the East under the leadership of Herr Brack to help save our wounded in the ice and snow." This mission was "top secret! Only those who could not be spared from carrying out our Operation's most urgent work have not come along." The team, consisting of twenty to thirty doctors, nurses, and office personnel, drawn particularly from Hadamar and Sonnenstein, apparently crossed the Russian border and went somewhere in the area of Minsk. On the face of it, there is no reason such an ostensibly humanitarian and patriotic mission should have been kept secret. The camouflage was apparently twofold. First, some observers believe that this team carried out "euthanasia" on German soldiers, whether severely wounded, particularly brain-damaged, or simply rendered psychologically unfit to fight.[29] Such killings would, of course, have been publicly taboo. Second, this project apparently related to the setting up of death camps in Poland, for which some of the mission personnel stayed in the East. Key figures were Christian Wirth (see pages 71–72), whose technical knowledge of T4 gas chambers was now to be used in the East (Belzec was then being built); and Dr. Irmfried Eberl, who would soon become commandant at Treblinka.[30]*

Another doctor from the mission, Horst Schumann, would soon complete his trajectory from the Grafeneck and Sonnenstein killing centers to Auschwitz (see pages 278–84).

The previous summer Dr. Ernst von Grawitz had recommended the use of gas chambers to Himmler as the best way to go about mass killing. The carbon monoxide method developed for "euthanasia" was subsequently used in all death camps, with the exception of Auschwitz.

All of these developments were expressions of an evolving genocidal mentality. The Nazis were moving toward violently carrying out Lorenz's vision (quoted in the epigraph to this chapter) of replacing the evolutionary forces of selection.[31] For, as Raul Hilberg and others have emphasized (and as I shall discuss in part III), Nazi genocide seems not to have been the end result of a clear, long-standing plan but rather to have evolved from shared imagery in the minds of Nazi leaders.[32] A crucial period for the evolution of this genocidal mentality was early 1941, when restraints were increasingly abandoned and bold action was first countenanced, then demanded. This was the period of preparation for the invasion of the Soviet Union, of activation of the *Einsatzgruppen*, of the extension of the T4 program to 14f13, and of the conversion of the biomedical vision into the Final Solution. The actual invasion of the Soviet Union in June had extreme importance. It enormously strained all German resources, including those necessary to maintain large numbers of Soviet prisoners. The invasion also brought about the increasing con-

*Many of those originally sent to the East were returned to Germany before being assigned to the death camps.

centration in ghettos of very large numbers of Jews, with attendant problems of not only starvation but epidemics that could spread to German personnel—and came after the rejection of various large-scale plans for Jewish immigration, including the Madagascar Plan. These problems, within the framework of the Nazis' biomedical vision and war mentality, could be solved by ever-expanding "euthanasia"—by a policy of "dispensing of existence" as literal and total as any in human history.

PART II

AUSCHWITZ:
THE RACIAL CURE

Introduction to Part II

Had the Nazis named their "euthanasia" institutions according to their concepts, they might well have referred to the "Hartheim [or Grafeneck] Center for Therapeutic Genetic Killing" and, correspondingly, to the "Auschwitz Center for Therapeutic Racial Killing."

It was a Nazi doctor, Heinz Thilo, who gave Auschwitz a much more appropriate name—*anus mundi*, "anus of the world"—a term meant to characterize what another Nazi doctor, Johann Paul Kremer, described as "the most horrible of all horrors": "the particularly unpleasant . . . action of gassing emaciated women."[1]

An astute Polish psychiatrist has suggested that the term *anus mundi* accurately reflects the Nazi vision of "the necessity to sweep clean the world," a vision "of the Germanic superman, . . . of a world where there would be no place for sick people, cripples, psychologically immoral people, contaminated by Jewish, Gypsy or other blood."[2] All these, he is saying, were for the Nazis biomedical waste material. In Auschwitz, that especially meant Jews.

While Auschwitz genocide came to encompass Gypsies, Poles, and Russians, only Jews underwent systematic selections.* For the primary function of Auschwitz, once it had been reconstituted, was the murder of every single Jew the Nazis could (in Himmler's words) lay their hands on anywhere.

The SS doctor did no direct medical work. His primary function was to carry out Auschwitz's institutional program of medicalized genocide.[3] Consider the SS doctor's activities in Auschwitz. He performed initial large-scale selections of arriving Jewish prisoners at the Birkenau camp (chapter 8). These selections were usually conducted according to formula: old and debilitated people, children, and women with children all selected for the gas chamber; while relatively intact young adults were permitted to survive, at least temporarily. The victim's experience, with which we begin, gives the truest picture.

After the selection, the presiding doctor was driven in an SS vehicle, usually marked with a red cross, together with a medical technician (one

---

*Poles and others underwent limited selections, conducted within the camp, early in Auschwitz history. And the Gypsy camp was selected *en masse* for death in 1944 (see pages 185–86). But institutionalized selections for the gas chambers involved only Jews.

of a special group of "disinfectors," or *Desinfektoren,* from within the *Sanitätsdienstgrade* or SDG) and the gas pellets, to a gas chamber adjoining one of the crematoria. As *Führer,* or "leader," of the team, the doctor had supervisory responsibility for the correct carrying out of the killing process, though the medical technician actually inserted the gas pellets, and the entire sequence became so routine that little intervention was required. The doctor also had the task of declaring those inside the gas chamber dead and sometimes looked through a peephole to observe them. This, too, became routine, a matter of permitting twenty minutes or so to pass before the doors of the gas chamber could be opened and the bodies removed.

SS doctors also carried out two additional forms of selections (chapter 9). In one, Jewish inmates were lined up on very short notice at various places in the camp and their ranks thinned in order to allow room for presumably healthier replacements from new transports. The other type of selections took place directly in the medical blocks in a caricature of triage. Rather than simply permitting those closest to death to die —in order to use limited medical resources to treat those who might be saved—as in traditional medical triage (the meaning given the term as originally used by the French military), the Nazis combined triage with murder by sending to the gas chamber those judged to be significantly ill or debilitated, or who required more than two or three weeks for recovery.

Medical triage-murder became a standard SS policy, influenced both by the vision of the Final Solution and by I. G. Farben's economic arrangements. But an additional factor also of great importance was the residual influence of the 14f13 "euthanasia" action in the camps. In other words, the principle of killing the weak, the sick, and the generally undesirable had been established in medical circles, extended specifically to concentration camps, and then institutionalized (still within medical circles) in Auschwitz, and Auschwitz alone, on a phenomenal scale. That 14f13 influence involved both the mentality and the legality of a medical form of a triage murder, so much so that the Frankfurt court could view medical-triage killings as probably derived from 14f13 policies. In other words, the Nazi versions of "euthanasia" and the Final Solution converged on Auschwitz medical blocks, thereby rendering them an important agency of the Auschwitz ecology of murder.[4]

SS doctors also conducted murderous forms of "epidemiology": prisoners with a contagious disease, usually typhus but also scarlet fever or other conditions, would be sent to the gas chambers, sometimes together with the rest of the patients on that medical block (many of whom might have been free of the contagious disease) so that the empty block could then be completely "disinfected." (Nazi doctors played a similar role in Jewish ghettos in Poland, where they contributed to oppressive policies in the name of controlling epidemics, especially typhus.)[5]

SS doctors ordered and supervised, and sometimes themselves carried out, direct killing of debilitated patients by means of phenol injections into the bloodstream or heart given on the medical blocks (chapter 14). These injections were most extensive during the early years of Auschwitz (1941–43) prior to the full development of the gas chambers. They were usually performed by medical technicians or brutalized prisoners, who served as surrogates for the doctors. SS doctors had similar responsibility for another group of phenol injections ordered by the Auschwitz Political Department (actually the Gestapo) for what were known as "hidden executions": the killing of such people as Polish political prisoners or occasionally German military or other personnel condemned to death for various reasons. Doctors also attended other executions of political prisoners—usually by shooting—in order to declare the victim officially dead.

In connection with all of these killings, doctors signed false death certificates, attributing each death of an Auschwitz inmate or an outsider brought there to be killed to a specific illness (cardiac, respiratory, infectious, or whatever). Those Jews selected for death at the ramp, never having entered the camp, required no death certificates.

SS dentists, who worked closely with doctors and also performed selections, were in charge of supervising prisoner work *Kommandos* in pulling out gold teeth and fillings of dead Jews after they had been gassed.

SS doctors (according to Höss) were supposed to perform abortions on "alien" (*fremdvölkisch*) women found to be pregnant. Whether or not that category was meant to include Jewish women (as opposed to their being in a separate category of their own), abortions were performed on them in secret by Jewish prisoner doctors when it was learned that a diagnosis of pregnancy in Jewish women meant immediate gassing.

In the case of official corporal punishment (for instance, whipping), SS doctors were required both to sign forms attesting to the physical capacity of an inmate to absorb such punishment, as well as to be present while it was administered.

SS doctors also consulted actively on determining how best to keep selections running smoothly—making recommendations, for example, about whether women and children should be separated or allowed to proceed along the line together. They also advised on policies concerning numbers of people permitted to remain alive, weighing the benefits to the Nazi regime of the work function against the increased health problems created by permitting relatively debilitated people to live.

Doctors' technical knowledge was also called upon with regard to the burning of bodies, a great problem in Auschwitz during the summer of 1944, when the arrival of enormous numbers of Hungarian Jews overstrained the facilities of the crematoria, so that bodies had to be burned in the open.

Selections, the quintessential Auschwitz ritual, epitomized and maintained the healing-killing paradox. The first selections performed by the arriving SS doctor were his ritual of initiation, his transition from ordinary life to the Auschwitz universe, and the early calling forth of his Auschwitz self.

In terms of actual professional requirements, there was absolutely no need for doctors to be the ones conducting selections: anyone could have sorted out weak and moribund prisoners. But if one views Auschwitz, as Nazi ideologues did, as a public health venture, doctors alone became eligible to select. In doing so, the doctor plunged into what can be called the *healing-killing paradox.*

For him especially, killing became the prerequisite for healing. He could arrange for medical care only so far as the slaughterhouse was kept at full function. And his healing area (the medical block) was simultaneously a clearinghouse for further killing. He became an advocate of killing on two fundamental levels: that of the ecology of the camp (selecting larger numbers at the ramp and on the medical block when the camp was overcrowded, hygienic conditions were threatened, and the quantity of sick or weak inmates strained medical facilities and lessened work efficiency [see pages 180–81]); and in connection with the larger biomedical vision (curing the Nordic race by ridding it of its dangerous Jewish infection), whatever the degree of intensity or amorphousness of his involvement in that vision. The healing-killing paradox was what Dr. Ernst B. called the "schizophrenic situation." But that situation was an enduring institutional arrangement, the basis for social equilibrium in Auschwitz (see pages 210–13).

But prisoners could not be permitted to kill themselves; suicide violated the logic of the healing-killing paradox. Indeed, overt suicide, such as running into the electric fence, was considered a serious violation of discipline and often exhaustively investigated. (Suicides by Treblinka prisoners were described by one commentator as the "first affirmation of freedom" contributing to significant prisoner rebellion in that camp.[6]) More gradual submission to death as in the case of the *Muselmänner,* could be tolerated or even encouraged because it did not seem to challenge Nazi life-death control. The healing-killing paradox, if it was to be internalized by the Auschwitz self, required exclusive control of life and death on the part of Nazi perpetrators.

The key word in the healing-killing reversal is *Sonderbehandlung,* or "special treatment," carried over from Nazi practice and from the 14f13 project in particular (see pages 136–37). We have seen how this euphemism for killing insinuated something on the order of medical therapy, along with a standing that was "more legal than legal." (In general bureaucratic usage, "special" [the prefix] was the opposite of "regular": special trains and regular trains, special courts and regular courts, etc. Special procedures were deemed necessary because of special conditions. The word not only detoxified killing and aided in its routinization but, at the same time, infused that killing with a near-mystical priority for the "Auschwitz self" in carrying it out. Killing assumed a certain feeling of necessity and appropriateness, enhanced by the medical, as well as the military, aura surrounding it.

Sonderbehandlung was part of the mystical imperative to kill all Jews; and once Auschwitz took on that imperative, any Jewish arrival or prisoner could be experienced by the Nazi doctor's Auschwitz self as designated for death, and, psychologically speaking, as already dead. Killing someone already dead need not be experienced as murder. And since Jews, long the Nazis' designated victim, were more generally perceived as carriers of death, or bearers of the death taint, they became "doubly dead." Just as one could not kill people already dead, one could do them no harm however one mutilated their bodies in medical experimentation. The human experiments performed by Nazi doctors (chapter 15), while tangential to questions of ecology, were fully consistent with the regime's larger biomedical vision.

For their regulation of the Auschwitz ecology, SS doctors needed the actual medical work of prisoner doctors, who in turn needed SS doctors to make that work possible—to keep others alive and stay alive themselves. What resulted were profound conflicts within prisoner doctors concerning their relationship to the Auschwitz ecology and to their SS masters as they (the prisoner doctors) struggled to remain free of selections (chapter 11) and to retain a genuinely healing function (chapter 12). There were antagonisms among these prisoner doctors along with a few examples of close identification with Nazi medical policies (chapter 13). But it was the SS doctors who pulled the strings, who, while not without their own significant inner conflict, managed to adapt sufficiently to the Auschwitz system to maintain its medicalized killing (chapter 10). Their adaptation involved the process I call "doubling," which permitted them to select for the gas chamber without seeing themselves as killers.

At the end of part II, I examine in greater detail the behavior and psychological experience of three individual SS doctors: one who managed to avoid doing selections and to help many inmates despite his Nazi contradictions (chapter 16); another, the notorious Mengele, who found full self-expression in Auschwitz (chapter 17); and the chief doctor (chapter 18), who sought to "reform" the Auschwitz system in ways that might benefit prisoners, even as he set up the full machinery of medicalized killing.

Chapter 7

The Auschwitz Institution

> Sure, there are peoples who have hated each other
> for centuries. But that one kills people so sys-
> tematically, with the help of physicians, only be-
> cause they belong to another race, that is new in the
> world.
> —Brother of chief SS Auschwitz doctor

Auschwitz can be understood only in relation to its three historical identi-
ties: as a Nazi concentration camp, or *Konzentrationslager;* as a work camp,
or *Arbeitslager,* with a special connection to I. G. Farben Industries; and
as an annihilation camp, or *Vernichtungslager.*

Auschwitz as Concentration Camp

Concentration camps were instituted almost from the moment the Nazis
seized power. Dachau, the first, was created by Himmler on 20 March
1933, as a place where Communists, Social Democrats, and other alleged
political enemies were to be "concentrated" and held. These political
prisoners had been arrested in considerable numbers following the emergency "protective custody" decree of 28 February, which was implemented immediately after the Reichstag fire.* Dachau, after a brief phase
of quixotic brutality by the SS administration, became the model for the
concentration camp. Now Himmler established the camps as "legally
independent administrative units outside the penal code and the ordinary
processes of law."[2]

Under Theodor Eicke—first as commandant of Dachau after mid-1934,
and as inspector of concentration camps and SS brigadier general in

---

*This fire occurred on 27 February. Although there is some historical debate whether
the Nazis arranged it as a provocation, they clearly used it as an occasion to round up
political opponents and to begin consolidation of their dictatorship.[1]

charge of the Death's Head Units*—quixotic brutality was replaced by a policy of impersonal, systematic terror. Earlier, because of his own violent acts, Eicke had been imprisoned on orders from Himmler and then transferred briefly to the Würzburg University Psychiatric Clinic where, as we have noted, he was Heyde's patient; it was upon his release that Eicke was assigned by Himmler to run Dachau. Whatever happened between psychiatrist and patient, this sequence suggests that very early Heyde contributed significantly both professionally and medically to concentration-camp policies. In any case, those policies under Eicke grew into what Rudolf Höss, who trained at Dachau for his post as commandant of Auschwitz, later called a "cult of severity" and a "Dachau spirit" according to which *all* inmates were enemies of the state; and camp guards were to be trained in cruelty and to dispense it with pitilessness (or "hardness"), detachment, and incorruptibility.[3] In fact, corruption was endemic to such a system.

During the middle and late 1930s, categories of camp inmates were extended to include people considered "habitual criminals"; "antisocial elements" (beggars, vagabonds, Gypsies, vagrants, "workshy" individuals, idlers, prostitutes, grumblers, habitual drunkards, hooligans, traffic offenders, and so-called psychopaths and mental cases); homosexuals; Jehovah's Witnesses (whose organization was outlawed because of its absolute pacifism); and—especially from the time of *Kristallnacht* (9–10 November 1938)—Jews. A system of identification was instituted, according to which each prisoner had a rectangular piece of material sewn onto his or her uniform, upon which was imprinted a colored triangle: red for political prisoners, purple for Jehovah's Witnesses, black for asocials (for example, prostitutes), green for criminals, and pink for homosexuals. Jews wore a triangle (usually red), under which an added yellow triangle was sewn on to form a hexagram (Star of David). Late in 1944 this "Jewish Star" was abolished and replaced by a horizontal yellow bar above the classification triangle.[4]

The legal and social theory of the camps, as articulated in 1936, had a distinctly biological and therapeutic hue. Werner Best, Himmler's legal authority, identified the "political principle of totalitarianism" with the "ideological principle of the organically indivisible national community," and declared that "any attempt to gain recognition for or even to uphold different political ideas will be ruthlessly dealt with, as the symptom of an illness which threatens the healthy unity of the indivisible national organism, regardless of the subjective wishes of its supporters."[5]† Thus, the disease-cure imagery was extended to the concentration camps—a still larger reversal of healing and killing. That reversal dominated the

---

*The Death's Head Units (*Totenkopfverbände*) were created by Himmler at Dachau under Eicke's command and became the general concentration-camp guards. They took their name from their skull-and-crossbones insignia.

†At issue was the Prussian law on the State Secret Police of February 1936, which removed the Gestapo, particularly its use of protective custody, from judicial restraint.

camp hospital blocks virtually from their beginnings. More often than not, "to become sick in a concentration camp meant to be doomed," as Eugen Kogon put it. SS doctors or corpsmen would frequently contribute to that fate by means of lethal injections. At Buchenwald, for instance, an SS doctor "finished off a whole row of prisoners with injections of sodium evipan" and then "strolled from the operating room, a cigarette in his hand, merrily whistling 'The End of a Perfect Day.' "[6]

Kogon, who had been prisoner secretary to the chief doctor in Buchenwald, described the power held by prisoner functionaries on the hospital blocks; how prisoners brought there as patients, if considered dangerous (because they were brutal to other prisoners who informed on them or because they belonged to a rival political faction) could be either medically neglected by prisoners in charge or even killed by them by means of lethal injections. In most camps, ordinary criminals were at first in charge of hospital blocks, and under them abuses were greatest; conditions improved considerably when political prisoners wrested power from the criminals, and when prisoner doctors were permitted to do medical work. But long before, SS doctors and corpsmen had used camp medical blocks for killing; in Dachau, there were "convalescent" blocks in which the sick and debilitated were simply left to die.[7]* And we know of the use of the medical blocks to collect ostensibly incurable or otherwise undesirable inmates for "euthanasia" killing.

But the medical block could also become what Kogon called "a rescue station for countless prisoners." More than anywhere else in the camp, prisoners could be hidden, numbers could be switched, and patients slated for killing could be warned and discharged. Another effective device was to hide prisoners on contagious wards where SS personnel rarely strayed: Kogon states that on three occasions he himself hid on the tuberculosis ward in order to avoid transfer to Auschwitz to be killed.[9] There could also be genuine convalescent blocks and other medical arrangements that helped one to survive, such as "convalescent slips" enabling one to spend several days under relatively favorable conditions.

The SS doctors assigned to the early concentration camps tended to be medically undistinguished, strong in their Nazi ties, and personally self-aggrandizing. "Generally speaking, they were more adept at feathering their own nests than at healing, and usually their skill lay in killing rather than in saving."[10] Experiments on prisoners were also done mainly in these traditional camps, though for the most part not on an extensively organized basis until the early 1940s. More characteristic of Nazi doctors was their regular participation in "triage" killing of the weak and the sick as well as of prisoners designated by others for destruction. Camp doc-

---

*This license to kill did not always extend to healthy prisoners, at least in the early stage of the camps. In June 1933, the Munich Prosecutor's Office implicated a camp doctor at Dachau together with Eicke's predecessor in an inmate's murder.[8] Such legal scrupulosity in the camps must have been rare.

tors did at times conduct something on the order of a sick call for inmates, but usually only grudgingly or even brutally.

The doctors' manner tended to be military: from the start, their medical function was subsumed to requirements of the camps and the legitimation of brutality and killing. For instance, doctors signed forms attesting to prisoners' capacity to withstand corporal punishment or to undergo transfer to another camp. While the doctors also had the actual medical function of controlling and preventing epidemics, their concern tended to be solely with the health of SS personnel.

Auschwitz was created, in June 1940, on the model of the traditional concentration camp, and was apparently intended then mainly for Polish prisoners and as a quarantine and transit camp from which prisoners were sent to camps in Germany. The medical arrangements at Auschwitz were originally the same as those in traditional concentration camps.

Auschwitz as Work Camp

In concentration camps, work was always required of prisoners, was generally part of a systematic program of terror and humiliation, and was often a means of gradual but intentional killing—of Poles as well as Jews. From 1937, the work force in camps became sufficiently organized to be considered an important national source of forced labor, and increasing arrests were motivated by the need for such labor. As with T4 inmates, prisoners came to be judged as worthy of life only to the extent that their ability to work contributed to the power of the Third Reich—which made them, as has been pointed out, "less than slaves."[11]

But underneath that pragmatism was the Nazis' worship of work, and their mythology that prisoners could earn their freedom by means of work. This mythology was especially promulgated by Eicke, who probably was responsible—without irony—for the notorious *Arbeit macht frei* ("Work brings freedom") sign first put up at Dachau and then at the entrance to Auschwitz.*

From at least late 1941, the work function began to take on central importance in the camps and that led eventually to relative improvement in conditions for prisoners concerning such things as confinement arrangements and food, and in some cases monetary awards, cigarettes, and access to camp brothels. The focus on work coincided with the camps' becoming subordinated, in March 1941, to the SS Economic and Administrative Department (*Wirtschaftsverwaltungshauptamt,* or WVHA)

---

*In Höss's words, "It was Eicke's firm intention that no matter what category, those prisoners whose steady and zealous work marked them out from the other should in due course be released, regardless of what the Gestapo and the Criminal Police Office might think to the contrary. Indeed this occasionally happened, until the war put an end to all such good intentions."[12]

which, headed by Oswald Pohl, was concerned with economic issues in the use of inmates. In contrast, the Central Security Department of the Reich (*Reichssicherheitshauptamt,* or RSHA), as the political and police unit, was preoccupied with the brutal detention of prisoners and the mass murder of Jews (see pages 174–75).[13]

Auschwitz was to become a major source of slave labor serving an enormous I. G. Farben enterprise for the manufacture of synthetic oil and rubber. Indeed the factory site was chosen in early 1941 largely because of its accessibility to the camp and to resources of coal and water. The overall operation became known as I. G. Auschwitz. Auschwitz inmates were working on the construction of that factory, known as I. G. Buna,* even before the establishment of the subsidiary camp at Birkenau where most of the killing was done. During 1942, I. G. Farben set up its own outer camp at Monowitz, still part of the overall Auschwitz constellation. This facility was meant to increase Farben's control over labor, to lower expenses, and to reduce the loss of time and energy in marching to the work site. In the Monowitz economy, Farben was responsible for food, housing, and medical care; the SS, for security and punishment. There was always close liaison between camp authorities and I. G. Farben officials in the brutal exploitation of inmates, who generally worked from three or four in the morning until evening darkness on close to a starvation diet (see pages 187–88). But whatever measures they took either to abuse the prisoners further or slightly improve their lot, work efficiency was always poor.[14]†

From early 1943, other big firms joined I. G. Farben in exploiting Auschwitz labor. These included Krupp, which moved a bombed-out fuse plant to Auschwitz; the Hermann Göring Works (coal mines); Siemens-Schuckert (electrical parts); and the *Jägerstab* (Pursuit Planes Staff) from the Speer ministry, whose attempts in 1944 to recruit inmates for the construction of underground aircraft factories were hampered by the increasing shortage of prisoners capable of working. These and other firms drew mostly upon inmates of Monowitz (known as Auschwitz III) and set up a network of satellite camps for miles around.[15]

Höss has made the point that, because of the official policy of keeping significant numbers of prisoners alive in order to work, "Auschwitz became a Jewish camp . . . a collecting place for Jews, exceeding in scale anything previously known."[16] But in actuality, since most Jews were killed on arrival, they probably did not begin to constitute a majority of camp inmates until 1944, and even then remained dominated in the prisoner hierarchy by smaller groups of Germans (political prisoners and ordinary criminals) and Poles.

The work function required not only large-scale selections to deter-

---

*Buna, a synthetic rubber developed by I. G. Farben, was made experimentally first from coal and later from oil.

†In initial discussions between the SS and Farben, it was estimated that efficiency of no more than 75 percent (compared with German workers) could be expected from slave laborers; in practice, they were less than one-third as efficient.

mine which prisoners would be killed immediately and which permitted to work and thus live a while longer,* but also a functioning medical block where prisoners could be treated by prisoner doctors. Indeed, Auschwitz, more than any other camp, reflected the inner Nazi struggle between pragmatic strengthening (through forced labor on war work) and visionary murder. But however elaborate the work arrangements became, they remained secondary to the camp's killing function.

Auschwitz as Annihilation Camp

The annihilation camp emerged in late 1941 and early 1942. There were six such camps in Poland: Chelmno (Kulmhof), Belzec, Sobibór, Treblinka, Majdanek, and Auschwitz. The first four devoted themselves exclusively to the killing function, though sometimes only Chelmno and Belzec are viewed as "pure killing camps," since minor industrial activity with forced labor was conducted at Treblinka and at least planned at Sobibór. But only Auschwitz and Majdanek combined a significant amount of forced labor with the systematic killing function. The four exclusively death camps were run by SS police units, not by the economic and administrative division of the SS that ran Auschwitz. And unlike Auschwitz, much of their killing equipment and personnel (with the added exception of Chelmno) came directly from the "euthanasia" program, including the carbon monoxide gas chambers and the killing-center staff. A great deal of the early installation and function of their killing apparatus was in fact supervised by Christian Wirth, who had done the same for the T4 killing centers (see page 71).[18]

Auschwitz marked a radical escalation in both the vision and the technology of mass murder. The biological image was intricately involved in the Auschwitz vision as revealed by Höss's recollection of Himmler's description of the purpose of the camp:

Jews are the eternal enemies of the German people and must be exterminated. All Jews within our grasp are to be destroyed without exception, now, during the war. If we do not succeed in destroying the biological substance of the Jews, the Jews will some day destroy the German people.[19]

As Höss recalled, he had been "suddenly summoned" by Himmler in the summer of 1941 and told, "The Führer has ordered that the Jewish question be solved once and for all and that we, the SS, are to implement that order." Himmler explained that existing extermination centers in the East could not carry out "the large actions which are anticipated."

*The life expectancy of Jewish workers at the Farben works was three or four months; in the outlying mines, about one month.[17]

Auschwitz had been "earmarked" for the task because its location was favorable for communications and transportation as well as isolation and camouflage. Himmler impressed upon Höss the gravity of the undertaking, the "difficult and onerous work," requiring "complete devotion notwithstanding the difficulties that may arise." Höss was to "treat this order as absolutely secret."[20]

Auschwitz took on a special status as the primary institution for carrying out the soon-to-be clarified policy of mass murder of the Jews. The task required Höss to explore—together with Adolf Eichmann, who held the Jewish desk at the RSHA—"the ways and means of effecting the extermination."[21]

Despite earlier remarks by Hitler regarding annihilation of Jews, the Nazis considered a variety of plans for expulsion, voluntary immigration, resettlement in Madagascar, etc. Only after these plans had been abandoned—found unfeasible for various reasons, including the reluctance of other nations to accept large numbers of Jews—was the definite decision made to implement the "Final Solution." In 1938, there were still 350,000 or so Jews in Germany (reduced from 515,000), and the Nazis' invasions and annexations kept acquiring more Jews. In March 1941, Keitel signed an order for the operation of Himmler's killing units in Russia, once that invasion took place. Then, on 31 July, after the invasion, Göring signed an order for Heydrich authorizing him to make "all necessary preparation" in respect to organizational and financial matters for the "complete solution of the Jewish question in the German sphere of influence in Europe."[22] Other agencies had been ordered to cooperate as needed.

The power of organizing deportations was now given Eichmann, the RSHA expert on Jewish affairs. Höss's remembered interview with Himmler may have followed this order. On 21 November, Heydrich ordered various state secretaries and SS chiefs to a meeting to discuss the Final Solution. The resulting so-called Wannsee Conference, after the RSHA address, was held on 20 January 1942. The Führer's authority was cited for a discussion of evacuation to the East, where the survivors of their labor utilization would be "treated accordingly" (entsprechend behandelt). While there was some discussion of side issues, such as mixed marriages and old Jews and war veterans—who, it was said, would go to the model camps at Theresienstadt—the point of the conference was clear, if largely unspoken. As Hilberg puts it, "Gradually, the news of the 'Final Solution' seeped into the ranks of the bureaucracy. . . . How much a man knew depended on his proximity to the destructive operations and on his insight into the nature of the destruction process."[23]

During early 1942, the details of the killing procedure were not yet clear, and were not solved until spring with the establishment of gas-chamber camps in Poland. The resulting time lag between the beginning of deportations and the construction of killing facilities led to overcrowding in some eastern ghettos and to bureaucratic myths of Jewish "migration." Höss's recollections make clear how much this "solution" was influenced by individual initiative once it was known what the Führer, in fact, wanted.[24]

Finding a "Suitable" Method

The severe psychological obstacles experienced by the *Einsatzgruppen* troops in carrying out face-to-face killing were known to Nazi leaders. As Rudolf Höss later recalled:

> I had heard Eichmann's description of Jews being mown down by the *Einsatzkommandos* armed with machine guns and machine pistols. Many gruesome scenes are said to have taken place, people running away after being shot, the finishing off of the wounded and particularly of the women and children. Many members of the *Einsatzkommandos*, unable to endure wading through blood any longer, had committed suicide. Some had even gone mad. Most of the members of these *Kommandos* had to rely on alcohol when carrying out their horrible work.[25]*

In the fall of 1941, one of the leading *Einsatzgruppen* generals, Erich von dem Bach-Zelewski, stunned Himmler by declaring to him, after they had witnessed the killing of about one hundred Jews: "Look at the eyes of the men in this *Kommando*, how deeply shaken they are! These men are finished [*fertig*] for the rest of their lives. What kind of followers are we training here? Either neurotics or savages!"[27] And Bach-Zelewski himself was to feel the effects: hospitalized with severe stomach and intestinal ailments, he experienced, according to Dr. Ernst Robert von Grawitz, chief SS doctor, "psychic exhaustion" and "hallucinations connected with the shootings of Jews" he instigated and "grievous other experiences in the East" (see also footnote on page 437).[28]

As a consequence, as Höss explained, only gas was seriously considered, "since it would have been absolutely impossible by shooting to dispose of the large numbers of people that were expected, and it would have placed too heavy a burden on the SS men who had to carry it out, especially because of the women and children among the victims."[29] Inevitably, they turned to earlier Nazi experience with gassing, and Eichmann familiarized Höss with the "euthanasia" project's use of carbon monoxide gas released through showerheads. But the method was inadequate for large numbers of people because of the great amount of gas and the many installations with gas chambers that would be required. Mobile gassing units used in the East had similar limitations. Hence, "Eichmann decided to try and find a gas which was in ready supply and which would not entail special installations for its use." As late as November 1941, Eichmann and Höss had not yet discovered a suitable gas, though the

---

*Himmler is said to have become ill while watching a mass shooting, after which he ordered "more humane" killing.[26]

camp commandant had chosen an isolated Auschwitz site for the killing
—a former peasant farmstead, which was made into the gas chamber
Bunker I. They had not yet thought of burning the corpses, and the site's
meadows allowed long pits for burials.[30]

On one of Höss's trips away from Auschwitz in August 1941, his deputy, SS Captain Karl Fritzch, "on his own initiative" conducted successful
experiments with Zyklon-B (the German trade name for hydrogen cyanide or prussic acid) on Russian prisoners of war on Block 11, the punishment block. Zyklon-B "was constantly used in Auschwitz for the destruction of vermin, and there was consequently always a supply of these tins
of gas on hand."[31] Höss joined in on repetitions of the experiment on his
return, observing the killing while wearing a gas mask, and noting that
death came very quickly; although he later claimed, "During this first
experience of gassing people, I did not fully realize what was happening,
perhaps because I was too impressed by the whole procedure."[*]

During Eichmann's next visit to Auschwitz, he and Höss decided on the
gas "for the mass extermination operation." After two provisional sites,
operations shifted in the spring of 1942 to bunkers I and II in the area
initially chosen by Eichmann and Höss. The victims included Jews from
Upper Silesia (territory lost to Poland at Versailles) as well as Russian
POWs. Now Höss began to take pride in the new method. Visiting the
extermination camps at Chelmno[†] and Treblinka, he observed that their
use of carbon monoxide was inferior: the exhaust gas produced by truck
engines was not always sufficient, so that a number of victims "were only
rendered unconscious and had to be finished off by shooting." Even after
the war, while in Polish incarceration Höss remained proud of the efficiency of "his" gas: "Experience had shown that the preparation of prussic acid called Cyclon B caused death with far greater speed and certainty,

---

[*]There is some evidence that Höss and his deputy cannot claim exclusive "discovery"
of Zyklon-B as an agent for killing large numbers of human beings. According to testimony
at his trial (by a British Military Tribunal in Hamburg beginning 1 March 1956), Dr. Bruno
Tesch, owner of the firm TESTA (acronym for Tesch and Stabenow) which distributed the
gas to Auschwitz, himself conducted experiments bearing on its feasibility not only as a
pesticide but as a means of killing efficiently large numbers of human beings. There is
another report of an Auschwitz SS man named Breitwieser, who apparently assisted in the
early Auschwitz experiments and was said to comment, upon noting how efficient Zyklon-B
was for delousing: "Now we have the means for the extermination of prisoners." Yehuda
Bauer and Erich Kulka believe that this intense focus on the use of Zyklon-B for killing is
partial evidence for an even greater centrality of Auschwitz in the Nazi projections of the
Final Solution than has previously been recognized. The victimization of some sick inmates
in those early Auschwitz experiments with Zyklon-B also suggests the Auschwitz focus from
the beginning on its murderous reversal of healing and killing. It is likely that, with the
existing experience of Zyklon-B for delousing and the known need for an efficient agent
to kill human beings, the idea of using that agent occurred more or less simultaneously both
to the "theorists" at firms making and distributing the gas on the one hand, and to the
Auschwitz "practitioners" on the other.[32]

[†]Höss had gone to Chelmno partly to investigate methods of cremation used there. In
the summer of 1942, Himmler ordered that mass graves be opened and corpses burned,
and the ashes disposed of "in such a way that it would be impossible at some future time
to calculate the number of corpses burned."[33]

especially if the rooms were kept dry and gastight and closely packed with people, and provided they were fitted with as large a number of intake vents as possible."[34]

Mass killing of Jews began either in late 1941 or early 1942. The Auschwitz administration had procured Zyklon-B indirectly from the manufacturer, DEGESCH, an acronym for German Corporation for Pest Control. DEGESCH, largely controlled by I. G. Farben, distributed the gas through two other firms—in Auschwitz's territory, through TESTA.[35] In 1942, its distribution within the SS became centrally regulated by the SS Hygienic Institute in Berlin under Dr. Joachim Mrugowsky. Given its extensive prior use against rodent and insect spreaders of disease, we might say that Zyklon-B was always considered a form of medical equipment. Yet it was placed under stricter medical supervision only as the prime chemical of extermination, and was even stored in the Auschwitz pharmacy for a period of time.*

Another change took place as well. In the past, Zyklon-B had by law been combined with a small amount of an irritant gas designed to warn of the presence of the dangerous substance when premises had not been sufficiently ventilated after fumigation. Sometime in 1943, the gas began to be distributed to Auschwitz without the irritant, and bore the warning: "Attention! No irritant!" Removing the irritant clearly expedited the killing process, but that step also, however, posed greater danger for those handling this lethal gas. Special training had always been required for that purpose. The group handling the gas had originally been drawn from personnel associated with the manufacturer, but the responsibility was transferred to a special group of "disinfectors" from among the SS medical corpsmen. These *Desinfektoren* became a noncommissioned élite, and part of the duty of the doctor on the Auschwitz ramp was to take necessary measures to protect them from exposure to Zyklon-B and to be prepared to treat them should such exposure occur. We can say, then, that Zyklon-B became a dangerous "killing medicine," to be handled only by medical personnel.[36]†

---

*One doctor I interviewed, who held a senior advisory position within Nazi civilian and military structures, told me of serving as chairman of a high-level committee on allocating scarce medical equipment to civilian and medical groups, including the SS. After the war, he claimed to be horrified and chagrined to learn what the SS had used Zyklon-B for. The story tends to confirm the medical status of the gas. Concerning the doctor's claim of ignorance, I would say that he had demonstrated in a variety of ways an extreme capacity for invoking the psychological defenses of denial and numbing, of the will not to know. In his case, those defense mechanisms would have to have been extreme—one suspects that in at least part of his mind, he knew—given the increasingly large amounts of gas the SS required for Auschwitz: for example, for fumigation, camps got delivery about every six months; Auschwitz got one every six weeks.

†The manufacturer opposed the removal of the irritant because its patent had been on this irritant addition, rather than on the gas itself. Involved in this change was Kurt Gerstein, then chief disinfection officer in the SS, who worked under Mrugowsky in Berlin. Gerstein had an engineering background as well as a certain amount of medical training. Few figures have been as confusing to historians and biographers, given his intense SS involvement at

From 1943, there were shortages in Zyklon-B because Allied air raids interfered with production. At times it even became necessary for camp officials to pick the gas up by truck at the production factory near Dessau, about 300 miles to the northwest. Höss later (in testimony) estimated that Auschwitz used a total of 1,900 kilograms of its killing medicine.[38] From the beginning, he consulted Auschwitz doctors on the effects of the gas:

> I had always thought that the victims would experience a terrible choking sensation. But the bodies, without exception, showed no signs of convulsion. *The doctors explained to me* that the prussic acid had a paralyzing effect on the lungs, but its action was so quick and strong that death came before the convulsions could set in, and in this its effects differed from those produced by carbon monoxide or by a general oxygen deficiency.[39] [Italics added]

The explanation falsely implied painless killing. But this general medical effectiveness was reassuring to Höss, as he no longer had to experience the horrors of face-to-face killing: "I always shuddered at the prospect of carrying out exterminations by shooting. . . . I was therefore relieved to think that we were to be spared all these blood baths, and that the victims too would be spared suffering until the last moment came."[40]

But his greatest relief—and the most important personal "therapy" the gas provided him—was its contribution to the solution of the technical and bureaucratic problem assigned him: "I must even admit that this gassing set my mind at rest, for the mass extermination of the Jews was to start soon and at that time neither Eichmann nor I was certain how these mass killings were to be carried out. . . . Now we had the gas, and we had established a procedure."[41] That "procedure" was the "assembly line" basis for killing—the phrase, appropriately enough, of an Auschwitz camp doctor.[42]

---

the center of mass murder, along with his fanatical SS demeanor; yet also his Protestant evangelical anti-Nazi connections and desperate efforts (including a dangerous conversation with a Swedish diplomat) to inform the outside world about the Final Solution. Gerstein later claimed—and was believed by one biographer—that he had proposed that the irritant be discontinued on the grounds that, without it, death was more humane, and that by rendering the gas undetectable, he could find a pretext for destroying consignments with the claim of dangerous leakage. Most observers—notably Rolf Hochhuth in his 1964 play *The Deputy*—have emphasized Gerstein's extraordinary acts of resistance; others, such as Hilberg, are primarily impressed with his role in the mass murder process. There is a sense in which both groups are correct: I believe Gerstein to have been the most extreme example of the doubling process encountered in this study.[37]

Chapter 8

Selections on the Ramp

> They were all doctors.
>
> —Auschwitz survivor

The Victims' Experience

To Jews arriving at the ramp, nothing medical seemed to be occurring —though much of their experience there was orchestrated by Nazi doctors. It was a terrifying scene of vast confusion, in many ways an extension of a journey of persecution that had begun when they were driven from their homes, and continued through the days or weeks of the slow, cruel, dehumanizing train journey to the camp in brutally overcrowded railroad boxcars. Arriving Jews usually saw the SS doctor standing on the ramp as just another SS officer with absolute power over them. Many had little sense that a selection process of any kind was taking place.

The experience of Marianne F., who arrived at Auschwitz from Czechoslovakia in early 1943 as a seventeen-year-old girl, is typical. First, the bizarre reception:

> We arrived at night. . . . Because you arrived at night, you saw miles of lights—and the fire from the . . . crematoria. And then screaming and the whistles and the "Out, out!" [now she shouted] *"Raus! raus! raus! raus!"* [colloquial German for "Out!"], and the uniformed men and the SS with the dogs, and the striped prisoners—we, of course, at that time didn't know who they were—and they said, "Throw everything out. Line up—immediately!"

And then the confusing, rapid-fire selections:

> They separated you and then lined up everybody in fives, . . . and there were two men standing. . . . On one side, was the doctor, one was Mengele, . . . and on the other side was the . . . *Arbeitsführer,* which was

the . . . man in charge of the work *Kommando.* And it was, . . . "You go, you go by truck. You walk, you go by truck." . . . A pattern pretty soon developed that you could see—under fourteen about and over thirty-five were assigned to the trucks. And not until we actually marched into the camps did you know exactly where the trucks had gone, . . . and this was done, I mean, very fast, very efficient.

Next was a ritual reception by old inmates:

[We went] directly on foot to the camp, . . . and . . . the minute you came into the camp, . . . [there was] a so-called welcome committee of prisoners that would watch you until you could be processed into the sauna [shower]. Those were prisoners—Slovakian girls who had already been there since about one year before. . . . The only thing they were interested in first of all was to get everything they could get before the SS would get it from us—jewelry or watches, what have you—because they already were in the inner circle knowing how to manipulate and organize for food and things. And secondly, to *immediately* tell us what was waiting for you and what has happened—somehow [they thought]: *"We've* been [here] so long, *you* might as well know."

That knowledge, attained within hours or even minutes, called forth and maintained the extreme numbing that characterized all life in the camp:

And then of course immediately you realized what the unbelievable smell was . . . that you have been smelling. . . . Somehow or other they . . . were already so inured. . . . You come to the point that if you were in there long enough, you had absolutely *no* emotions left—and all you were concerned [with] was survival.

But most did not survive. The terrible knowledge imposed on this Czechoslovakian girl was recorded by Dr. Otto Wolken, an Austrian-Jewish prisoner physician, who observed closely what went on in the camp, especially the behavior of SS doctors:

Over time, five crematoria were built in which the gas chambers were also located. People from all nations, of both sexes, of all ages were gassed. . . . Gassings of unthinkable dimensions took place at the arrival of prisoner transports from France, Belgium, Italy, Hungary, Greece, Czechoslovakia, and Germany, as well as from the Polish camps and from Norway. When the transport trains came in, the arrivals had to pass before the camp doctor . . . on duty. He pointed his thumb either to the right or to the left. Left meant death by gas. From a transport consisting of about 1,500 people, about 1,200 to 1,300 went to the gas chambers. Very seldom was the percentage greater of those who were permitted to live. At these selections Mengele and [Dr. Heinz] Thilo made their selections while whistling a melody. Those elected for the gas chambers had to undress in front of the gas chambers and were then chased into them with whip lashes, then the doors were closed and the gassing took place. After about eight minutes (death occurred after about four minutes) the chambers were opened and a special *Kommando* for this purpose had to take the corpses for cremation to the furnaces, which were burning day and night. There were not enough ovens at the time of the Hungarian transports [beginning in late May 1944] so that large trenches had to be dug to burn the corpses. Here the wood was sprayed with petroleum. Into these trenches the corpses were thrown. Often living children and adults were thrown into the burning trenches. These poor ones died a terrible death by burning. The necessary oil and fats for the burning were obtained partly from the corpses of the gassed in order to save petroleum.[1]

For those entering the camp, as Marianne F. went on to describe, there were a series of initiatory humiliations: undressing completely in front of SS men when entering the shower or "sauna"; having all of one's bodily hair shaved ("I grant you, good for . . . preventing all the lice, which of course were there, but psychologically, . . . it was unbelievably degrading . . ."); the issuing of minimal, ill-fitting clothing, mostly old Russian prisoners' uniforms; and the tattooing ("I remember when . . . that thing [the number tattooed on each prisoner's forearm] was put on, . . . it got infected and everything, and I suppose swollen and what have you—I never felt any pain—you were really numb").

She spoke of the psychological effectiveness of the whole process:

> [There was] this fiendish insight that whoever organized . . . it had. And the fact that if you do something that is totally unbelievable and . . . you are incapable of believing, you don't believe it. And the things that went on in Auschwitz . . . the gas chambers—nobody would have believed that. And then the houses that the crematoria had—you know, brick houses, windows, curtains, white picket fences around the front. And people never thought of anything—regardless of chimneys smoking. They could not believe it. . . . There was a touch of diabolic genius.

Wolken stated, similarly, that, although told about Auschwitz before being taken there by a Pole who had been to the camp, he and his friends "did not want to believe him. . . . We said that he must not have been there and that he is telling us fairy tales."[2]

Nazi doctors and others involved in the reception process varied greatly in their tone. Another survivor, whose work gave him the run of the camp, explained that "they [the Nazis] were psychologically very [well] prepared for every situation," so that at times "the doctor was very friendly to the people, . . . asking, 'How are you?' and, 'What occupation [do] you have?' " When an arriving inmate mentioned illness, looked weak, or was too young or too old, the same doctor made the decision to send him or her to the gas chambers. This survivor went on to tell of an incident (described to him by members of the *Sonderkommando*)* when a doctor appeared in the room outside the gas chamber where prisoners had to undress, noted a broken glass on the floor from shattered eyeglasses, and told the people there, "Please be careful that you . . . [don't] injure your[self]." The survivor's conclusion: "So they [the Nazis] were, tó the last moment, . . . using [the] hoax."

He went on to list the series of steps in SS doctors' involvement in the killing: first, the chief doctor's assignments to his subordinates concerning duty schedules and immediate selections policies; second, the individual doctor's service on the ramp, performing selections "in a very noble [seemingly kind] manner"; third, the doctor riding in the ambulance or Red Cross car to the crematoria; fourth, the doctor ordering "how many [pellets] of gas should be thrown in . . . these holes from the ceilings, according to the number of people, and who should do it. . . . There were three or four *Desinfektoren*"; fifth, "He observed through the hole how the people are dying"; sixth, "When the people were dead, . . . he gave the order to ventilate, . . . to open the gas chamber, and he came . . . with a gas mask into the chamber"; seventh, "He signed a [form] that the people are dead . . . and how long it took"; and eighth, "he . . . observed . . . the teeth . . . extraction [from] the corpses." This was the survivor who concluded that "the killing program was led by doctors—from the beginning to the end."

Other survivors conveyed their sense of bizarre unreality ("Living skeletons in striped uniforms, their skulls shaven, . . . like silent shadows, climbing onto the trains, . . . strange 'porters' [who] took out our luggage") and the depth of their confusion ("Wild men in striped suits. . . . Half Yiddish, half German; leave everything; clubs descending, blows").[3]

One could be so numbed as to be catatonic, as a Jewish woman doctor, Gerda N., arriving in late June 1944, described:

> We were in such a confusion, . . . in such a shock. . . . They shaved off our hair and we got such terrible clothes. . . . They took everything away. Our luggage, everything, . . . and I came to a camp which was called Mexico. . . . There was nothing in it, . . . even no water. . . . I think one thousand [people] in one barrack. . . . We got our first meal

*The *Sonderkommando* consisted of Jewish inmates assigned to dispose of corpses of Jewish victims. *Sonderkommando,* literally "special command," could refer generally to groups performing extraordinary tasks, including SS murder teams in the East.

the next day. . . . I must say I was in a . . . stupor. . . . I couldn't move. I just sat and couldn't move. . . . I really didn't move at all the first few days, maybe a week or ten days. . . .

"You cannot realize it" was the way another prisoner doctor put it— meaning that one could not take in or absorb the experience.

From late 1942 or early 1943, those who arrived as doctors were not only permitted to live but were made a special category of prisoner. They were usually singled out at the ramp, though some were admitted to the camp (rather than being dispatched to the gas chamber) on the basis of their relative youth and strength, and only there identified as doctors. The process could be haphazard. Some older doctors were sent to the gas without ever having been admitted to the camp. At the other extreme, a survivor doctor stated that, upon arriving at Auschwitz with a transport for which he had medical responsibility,

> the doors were pushed open and we were told to hurry out onto a platform. There was a high-ranking SS medical officer near us and I told him in my best German that Nora [this survivor's fiancée] and I were the nurse and doctor in charge of the transport. He seemed friendly and told us where to stand, and not to let anybody move us. He treated us as colleagues. He even told me to hold onto the books I had in my hand, to contact him later in the camp, and added that I would be well taken care of.[4]

One suspects that even the relief at being treated so well was accompanied by an underlying terror which this doctor partly suppressed.

Moreover, to be identified and favored as a doctor could intensify pain and self-condemnation concerning the fate of family members. One prisoner doctor stated simply that when the SS doctor doing the selections identified him as a physician, "he directed me to the right and my mother to the left." Another doctor, who arrived in Auschwitz in September 1943 from a transit camp in Holland, conveyed to me the primal feeling of both the strength of his urge to survive and his guilt that he alone of all his family survived because he was a doctor:

> We were . . . my wife, my child, and her parents. We came out of the train. There was a German. He said women to the one side and men to the other side. And then I—what really happened I don't know exactly. . . . But at the moment I was standing with my father-in-law. He was about, over seventy. He was an old man. And I was thinking, "Maybe I can help him." And when I was standing there, then I heard someone saying, "Doctors [in English], *austreten* ['Come out of the ranks']." And I went out and they put me to the other little group of younger people. . . . You see, if I should not have heard this outcry [call for doctors], I should not have been here. Luck is such an important

thing. I heard it. And I went out. I was not thinking . . . that it was
something special. I was thinking maybe . . . it means something.
. . . But I would stress the fact that I owe my life to be[ing] a doctor.
That I owe to my parents [who had little money and sacrificed to give
me an education]. I have never thanked them for this. . . . That's also
a feeling of guilt, you see. . . . But . . . [from] the gas chamber, they
saved my life.

    One hour later someone told us that the rest of our transport was
gassed. There you get a shock. What is normal? If you hear, *Gott behüte*
["God forbid"] that there should be a phone call that your wife and
your children are gone, what's the normal reaction? . . . And so I heard
my wife, my child, my parents, my parents-in-law, my sister—they were
killed. And still I want to live. And you can say [it's] Freud's *Selbsterhal-
tungstrieb,* or *Lebenstrieb* ["instinct of self-preservation," or "life instinct"], or how you call it, but it is impossible to understand. It's so
difficult to accept. That there is not a moment in life that you can say
no. This is the end. . . . You hear your whole family is gassed. And one
hour later they were calling again, "Doctors, *antreten* ['line up']" and
I went.

Some arriving doctors, having heard that the Nazis tended to kill the
intelligentsia and wanted only people capable of physical labor, were
reluctant to reveal that they were physicians—as one described upon
arrival in Auschwitz in November 1943:

    So I hear that they are asking . . . age and profession. And I heard
    that all who say some physical profession or physical work, they are
    going not with the elderly people and not to the trucks. So when I came
    . . . there, . . . I stand with the military way of standing, and I say my
    age and that I am [a] concrete worker. . . . And when we arrived at the
    camp, then the clerks, who were prisoners too . . . took . . . different
    details: name and then profession. And then one of them, a Jew, said
    "If there are some doctors among them, don't be afraid. Say that you
    are doctors because doctors are now needed." It's no more extermina-
    tion of doctors. Because before there was total extermination of doc-
    tors, and not only doctors . . . but—how do you call it?— . . . intelli-
    gentsia, . . . people who study to be professionals. . . . And [only] then
    I said . . . that I am a medical doctor.

As many survivors told me, at the time of selections "they called out
for doctors and twins." But being permitted to live as a doctor meant that
one witnessed others' deaths. Thus one prisoner doctor, Henri Q., who
arrived in July 1942 when selections had not yet been formally instituted
but conditions in the camp were at their most brutal, told how within a
month 90 percent of the eight hundred people on his transport were

dead, and "at the time of the liberation, fourteen of us [fewer than 2 percent] were still alive."

Twins, too, were separated out, since Mengele was collecting twins for study. At selections there were shouted orders: *"Zwillinge raus!"* ("Twins, out!") and *"Zwillinge heraustreten!"* ("Twins, step forward!"). One woman who arrived in her teens with her twin sister and their mother heard that call, to which her mother responded; indeed the next day an experienced prisoner told them, "It's because you're a twin that you have a chance to stay alive."

There were tragic efforts to protect family members that had the reverse effect and left surviving inmates with especially painful feelings of guilt. A woman who arrived at the age of seventeen told how she was placed in a group with her little sister, four years younger than she. Seeing that the child was confused, "I practically pushed her" toward the line with their mother and grandmother, telling the SS people, "Her mother is over there." Unknown to her, that line was going to the gas chamber: "This is what I have to live with."

A similarly painful story was told by Dr. Abraham C., a radiologist, who arrived with his wife on a cold night and gave her his parka to wear and his scarf to put over her head. Because, he recalled, "she looked like a little old lady," she was ordered to the line that went to the gas chamber. "So in a way it was because of the precautions I took for her that she was put on the wrong side because otherwise—she was young, active, and should have been among the thirty or forty young women who went to the camp alive."

The Sequence of Killing

These incidents stemmed directly from manipulations and deceptions promulgated by Nazi doctors. The truth they were concealing was to be found in the gas chambers and crematoria and has been described by a Polish Jew who spent most of his ten months in Auschwitz from March 1944 working as a member of the *Sonderkommando*. Such direct testimony is rare because members of that *Kommando* were usually killed after a certain time in order to eliminate witnesses, a fate this man escaped from only because of the liberation of the camp by the Russian army.* He tells how camp policy shifted from early brutality to "another method that made their work easier by telling the new arrivals that they had to take a shower to be clean after the long trip." Now it became the task of the Jews in the *Sonderkommando* to "calm the people [arrivals headed for the gas chamber]." These Jews engaged in this deception because they "were

*Members of the *Sonderkommando* could be permitted to survive because of their technical skills, or because of the general confusion during the last months of the camp.

in a slaughterhouse from which there was no escape and everybody clung to his own life," and also because "it was better to save the victims from . . . tortures" (the previous policy of exposing Jews to beatings, vicious dogs, and fiendish shouting); thus, "by taking over the task of the SS men, they rendered a last service to the death candidates."

This same witness went on to say that when *Sonderkommando* Jews did tell arrivals that they were going to be gassed, "they became insane, so that we later preferred to keep quiet."[5]

He then described the sequence of the killing:

> After the arrivals were taken to the location next to the crematorium, they had to undress entirely because they were told they would have a shower. Then they were chased—often with beatings—by the SS into the so-called bath, which in reality was a gas chamber. This was a hermetically sealed room about 80 square meters large and about 2.25 meters high. There were two doors—one was the entrance, the other one served to take out the corpses. Through two little windows which were located right under the ceiling the Zyklon-B gas was thrown into the room by an SS man. The death agony of the people lasted about fifteen minutes*. . . .
>
> Our task consisted of taking corpses on a stretcher to the ovens and to throw them into them. Every ten minutes four corpses were thrown in. When there were enough ashes gathered in the oven, we had to take them out (about once a week), pulverize them, and load them on the trucks. The ashes were then taken to the river Wisla and thrown in.[6]

An SS judge investigating "corruption" in Auschwitz noted that the crematoria did not attract much attention:

> A large door led to the so-called undressing rooms. There were numbered seats and even wardrobe tickets. Arrows on the wall pointed to the shower rooms. The lettering was in six or seven languages. Everything was shiny as a mirror in this huge crematorium. Nothing pointed to the fact that only a night before thousands of people were gassed and burnt there. Nothing was left of them, not even a tiny piece of dust on the oven armatures.[7]

The *Sonderkommando* worker explained further that, when relatively few people were to be killed, and "it didn't pay to gas them," an *Unterscharführer* (or sergeant) named Georgi "had the duty . . . of shooting the people personally." Victims would be "brought out by two of us" to Georgi, who then "shot him or her from the back with a shot in the neck." And later, when bodies were burned in open trenches because the crema-

---

*Most probably died a little more rapidly.

toria could not handle the number of arrivals, Georgi "became braver and more brutal" and at times had victims brought "by the *Sonderkommando* to the burning trench, [where] they were ordered to lie down, and [he] shot them one after another."[8]

The mass killing was done systematically, with elaborate organization:

There were five crematoria where about 800 prisoners worked. The crematoria consisted of four rooms especially built for them, as well as a converted room that had been a farmhouse before. In each crematorium about 180 prisoners worked. . . .

In each oven about 800 corpses could be burned within 24 hours. That was not sufficient. Further mass graves were dug, which were about 2 meters deep, 10 meters long, and 5 meters wide, to burn humans. . . .

When the four crematoria were no longer sufficient to exterminate the growing transports, . . . we had to throw the corpses into burning trenches. There the Germans found out that, to save benzine, human fat could be poured on the corpses and drained into a lower trench. We poured the human fat from pails on the people so they would burn faster. Here we worked from May 1944 to October 1944. We worked 12 to 16 hours daily; four SS men were next to each crematorium and were helped by 180 prisoners. The fire burned continuously—day and night.

No wonder that "the horrible screaming of these people I still hear in my mind to this day and I cannot get rid of it."[9]

Hilberg has pointed out that the four Birkenau crematoria could burn a maximum of about 4,400 bodies a day. But in May and June, Hungarian Jews alone were being gassed at nearly 10,000 a day, so that the added trenches were required for burning bodies. When those trenches had to be dug, the four Jewish *Sonderkommando* units contained a force of between fifteen hundred to two thousand men, and by August 1944, over twenty thousand corpses were burned on certain days.[10]

The doctors were central to the elaborate medical subterfuge, as Dr. Henri Q. stressed:

The [Nazi] doctors' . . . collusion in deception . . . was a real staging; . . . a Red Cross truck to reassure people, and in that truck was the prussic acid that was to kill them. There was a Red Cross ambulance when transports arrived. Those details were meant to appease people. When one sees an ambulance, one thinks there is medical care. It was a deliberate psychological manipulation to keep people from reacting. . . .

There were trucks where sick and old people, children and pregnant women were told to get on. People believed that the Germans were civilized and sent trucks for the sick, the old, the children and the women. They actually thought the Germans were not that bad. But the healthy went to the camp and the trucks to the gas. People chased the trucks [saying they had] diabetes or a heart condition. They should have gone into the camp but they thought the trucks were better.

Even Dr. Q. and fellow prisoner physicians could be deceived: "It took us a while to realize that the doctors . . . took part in it all."

SS Doctors: Professional Arrangements

Selections were conducted, from within a medical hierarchy, by camp physicians *(Lagerärzte)* under the direct authority of the Auschwitz chief doctor, or garrison physician *(Standortarzt)*. The latter—who was Eduard Wirths (see chapter 18) for most of the period we are concerned with— operated within two separate chains of command. He was subordinate to the chief concentration-camp physician of the SS Economic and Administrative Department, or WVHA. This position was held from 1942 by Enno Lolling, who was stationed in Berlin but came frequently to Auschwitz and other camps. At the same time, Wirths was also subject to the authority of the camp commandant, with whom he dealt regularly on a day-to-day basis.*

Other doctors had different duties and different chains of command and were not expected to perform selections. These included the troop physicians *(Truppenärzte)* who took care of SS personnel; doctors who were sent to Auschwitz specifically to do experiments on inmates (notably Carl Clauberg and Horst Schumann) and tended to have more direct ties with Himmler; and doctors who belonged to the local camp Hygienic Institute, located outside the main camp and part of a chain of command separate from either that of the camp doctors or the camp commandant. The Hygienic Institute was officially concerned with questions of epidemiology and bacteriology and was installed in Auschwitz after an extensive typhus epidemic in 1942.

"Medical activity in Auschwitz consisted only of selecting people for the gas chamber" was the way that Dr. Ernst B., who had been there, expressed the matter to me. (I discuss Dr. B. at length in chapter 16.) Certainly what was called "ramp duty" was a central function of Auschwitz camp doctors. Generally about seven SS doctors shared that duty, and their performing selections was considered a matter of military jurisdiction: within the military-institutional structure, selections were a medical task only they were considered competent to perform.

The principle—established from above—that only doctors should se-

_____

*This double chain of authority was characteristic of Nazi bureaucracy—often involving the hierarchy of both one's immediate institution and the Party itself or an affiliate structure.

lect was adamantly defended by Wirths. Indeed, he himself insisted upon setting an example: not only did he himself select, when he as chief would not have had to, but he put off other obligations that might have prevented him from carrying out ramp duty for which he was scheduled.[11] His attitude was close to that of Höss, the camp commandant, who felt compelled to be present at times during not only selections but the entire sequence of killing: "I had to show them all that I did not merely issue the orders and make the regulations but was also prepared myself to be present at whatever task I had assigned to my subordinates." Significantly, he claimed that doctors had this expectation of him as well, that he felt it necessary "to look through the peephole of the gas chambers and watch the process of death itself, because the doctors wanted me to see it."[12]

The SS doctor Ernst B. thought that having a *physician* conduct selections "made it perfect"—by which he meant, "If somebody from some other place comes and says we don't have enough people or we have too many, . . . then it can be claimed that the doctors have done it [the selections]—that it has been done with precise medical judgment." That "perfection" involved the appearance of appropriate medical activity—Auschwitz's "as if" situation—and that policy of doctors' doing selections was (according to Höss) largely laid down by the chief SS doctor, *Reichsarzt* SS Ernst Robert von Grawitz.[13]

Wirths was understood to have had additional reasons for insisting upon the medical control of selections, reasons having to do with constant friction between his office and the commandant or military command in general. As Ernst B. put it: "As far as the head doctor was concerned, everything that the military was doing was foolish and wrong, and if he gave away his responsibility to them—in this case, the selections —then his influence on the military was reduced. He had to support his power any way he could, and avoid relinquishing his hold on various levels." Dr. B. was implying that Wirths considered himself, as a physician, more humane but was at the same time involved in a classical bureaucratic struggle. And for the same reason, Dr. B. believed that the chief doctor preferred that he, rather than his medical subordinates, should retain control over selections in order to maintain his general influence: "In every bureaucracy everyone tried to enlarge his 'writing table' [*Schreibtisch*]."

In holding to the principle of medical efficiency for the entire operation, Wirths oversaw the selections process, including its personal arrangements, and thereby maintained the efficiency of Auschwitz killing. (I shall examine his behavior and his conflicts in chapter 18.)

Performing selections was constantly compared to being in combat. The message from Himmler, from the camp commandant, and from the medical hierarchy was that this difficult assignment had to be understood as wartime duty. Selections were often compared more directly to medical triage in war. Thus Dr. B. could quote his friend Mengele as having repeatedly said that "the selections during the war with his own people in connection with emergency care—who got care and who didn't—that these were much more problematic" than selections in Auschwitz.

Duty arrangements for selections were simple enough.* The chief doctor (Wirths) provided the names of physicians—and later of pharmacists and dentists—under his jurisdiction to the ranking noncommissioned officer of the medical unit (usually a top sergeant [SS-*Stabsscharführer*] or a technical sergeant [*Oberscharführer*]) and ordered him to make up a duty roster for ramp service. The rosters included the doctor with primary responsibility for the selections on a particular day as well as a back-up doctor. The latter was supposed to be present, but was by no means always there, especially toward the last phases of the gassings in 1944. Rosters had to be signed by Wirths and posted one week in advance. Similar rosters were prepared for the ramp duty of medical corpsmen, including *Desinfektoren* who were the only ones permitted to handle the gas.

When the commandant's office was notified of the arrival of a transport, it immediately informed the SS medical division. That office in turn notified the physician on duty as well as the highest-ranking noncommissioned *Desinfektor* and the responsible people in the motor pool, from which the ambulance or other vehicle (usually bearing the Red Cross sign) was sent. This careful set of internal arrangements ensured that the selections, *from the standpoint of SS doctors and personnel,* were conducted in an orderly and proper fashion—that is, according to regulations.† That controlled orderliness extended to the functioning of the Jewish *Sonderkommando* in the crematoria, who were coordinated closely with this medical structure.

Each selection was greatly influenced by instructions from above concerning the relative number of arriving Jews to be killed or permitted to survive. In general terms, policy was set in Berlin by higher SS officials, including Himmler himself. But decisions were also greatly influenced by Auschwitz deliberations between the chief physician and the commandant. Overall, there was a basic conflict between the police arm of the SS, which considered itself responsible for the annihilation of all Jews; and the economic arm of the organization, which responded to the increasingly desperate wartime need for productive slave labor. Wirths and other doctors saw themselves as essentially in the second group because, in addition to performing selections, their task included maintaining the health of these slave laborers, at least to the degree of enabling them to work. But SS doctors could take the opposite view as well, claiming that overcrowding and extremely poor hygienic conditions could lead to devastating epidemics. They would therefore insist that fewer arrivals be admitted to the camp; that, in effect, a greater percentage of them be

---

*These were discussed by a former inmate who had worked closely with Wirths, and by Dr. B.

†The term frequently used to describe this is *ordnungsgemässer Ablauf* ("proper course").

killed. Wirths and Höss constantly consulted about such matters, and there was known to be considerable disagreement and tension between the two men. Wirths constantly sought better medical facilities, while Höss was preoccupied with facilities for maximum efficiency in mass murder. According to Dr. B., they conferred on many things, including especially those that could "go wrong."

One of the things that could go wrong was for officers other than physicians to conduct selections illegally: either because they represented the Reich Security (police) position (Eichmann) and wanted to see all Jews killed, or because they represented the views of the economic and administrative division and wanted to keep as many Jews as possible alive for work. Höss claimed that medical authority supported his own police position of maximum killing:

> The *Reichsarzt* SS [Grawitz] . . . held the view that only those Jews who were completely fit and able to work should be selected for employment. The weak and the old and those who were only relatively robust would very soon become incapable of work, which would cause a further deterioration in the general standard of health, and an unnecessary increase in the hospital accommodation, requiring further medical personnel and medicines, and all for no purpose since they would in the end have to be killed. . . .
>
> I myself held the view that only really strong and healthy Jews ought to be selected for employment.[14]

The conflict within the SS was never fully resolved. In a way, it did not have to be. Advocates of maximum murder could take satisfaction in the killing of overwhelming numbers of arriving Jews; selections provided the slave-labor advocates with their slaves. And doctors' recommendations were met by both tendencies: the extensive killing prevented overcrowding; and the selections, by providing stronger inmates, eased the doctors' task of maintaining the health of the inmate population.

They could in fact come to see their physician's task, as Dr. B. said, as rendering the killing "humane": "The discussion [among doctors] was about how the matter could be carried out humanely [*die Sache human durchgeführt*]. That was the problem of the physician. . . . The discussion about the possibility of humanity [in killing], . . . [of] humanitarian [methods in the face of] . . . the general overload of the apparatus—that was the problem."

"A Regular Job"

The selections became simply "a part of their life," as a prisoner doctor, Jacob R. commented to me. And Dr. B., too, noted that, whatever reservations SS doctors had at first, they soon viewed selections as "normal duty," as "a regular job." Indeed within the Auschwitz atmosphere, as another survivor testified, "to kill a man was nothing, not worth talking about": a doctor who was perfectly polite and decent most of the time "felt no compunction about sending people into the gas."[15]

From the late spring of 1944, when an enormous influx of Hungarian Jews placed a strain on the scheduling of doctors on the duty roster, the way of conducting selections changed. Now, as Dr. B. explained, mass arrangements had to be made. At a special meeting of medical officers, Wirths announced that dentists and pharmacists were to take regular turns along with doctors in performing the selections. And selections were done by "teams": "When the train arrived, there were announcements through a loudspeaker, such as " 'Mothers and children go left!' "

Although two doctors were present, neither any longer made decisions about individual arrivals. Rather, the doctor became "only a supervisor." It was still important that he be present because he had the responsibility of overseeing the behavior of noncommissioned officers, others on the selections team, and prisoners—all of whom took part in placing arriving men and women in lines according to their category. With thousands of people arriving every day—as many as ten thousand in one night—selections were done "only by groups. . . . One couldn't select individuals. . . . In the regulations it was stated that every individual must be judged capable of work—'camp-worthy'—or not on medical grounds. In practice, that was never carried out—because it was impossible. One . . . selected only according to categories." But the doctor was still central, Dr. B. emphasized: *"He stood there and led the thing."*

Doctors could become very engrossed in questions about the method or technique of selections:*

"The people who participated in [a particular] selection would discuss it for days. 'Which is better: to let mothers go with their children to the gas or to select the mothers later by separating them from their children?' . . . Those were the type of problems in Auschwitz—not ideological problems but purely technical problems. And wars were virtually waged over these issues."

Dr. B. explained how advice would be given to doctors and SS camp leaders by women criminal *capos* (prisoner functionaries) drawn from among actual German criminals; these *capos* found it much less difficult to handle arriving mothers whose children were still with them.

They engaged in elaborate exchanges about how many people should be killed and how many admitted to the camp, always from the standpoint of medical and hygienic considerations:

There were numerous discussions: Should one gas more or should one [gas fewer]? Where is the limit to be set? That is, if you take more old people into the camps, then there are more diseased people, and

---

*Contrastingly, they virtually never discussed the *nature* of selections (see pages 193–94).

that, for many reasons, is the worse problem if they are in the working camp . . . where there is only so much possibility [for keeping limited numbers of people alive]. . . . Then the camp leadership comes . . . and says, "You're sending us people we can't do anything with. They'll only croak." . . . You understand that about these purely technical issues there were heated and intense discussions.

Dr. B. told me that "the doctors really became active" in confronting the overriding technical problem of burning large numbers of corpses. With the crematoria unable to take care of the enormous new load, trenches were dug and piled high with corpses.

> One had to burn . . . great piles—enormous piles. Now that is a great problem, igniting piles of corpses. You can imagine—naked—nothing burns. How does one manage this? . . .
> They had been through the gas chambers and now thousands were lying there and had to be burned. How does one do that? One tested numerous methods—and here the doctors were drawn in to try to solve this problem and they helped find solutions.

Ernst B. himself became a bit excited as he explained in more detail the technical problem:

> The gas chambers were sufficient, you see, that was no problem. But the burning, right? The ovens broke down. And they [the corpses] had to be burned in a big heap. . . . The problem is really a large technical difficulty. There was not too much room, so first one thought one would have to take small piles. . . . Well, . . . that would have to be tried out. . . . And then everyone contributed his knowledge of physics, about what might possibly be done differently. If you do it with ditches around them, then the air comes up from below and wooden planks underneath and gasoline on top—or gasoline underneath and wood in between—these were the problems. Well, the solution was not to let the fire die. And maintain the cooperation between the gas chamber and the crematorium. When [the fire] reached a certain intensity, then it was just right—but then you could not get to it, so it was still too hot, etc. Those were the problems.

He went on to explain how different people did different things to help:

> And the actual work was of course done by the subordinate commanders [*Unterführer*], you understand, the NCOs [*Unteroffizier*]—people who were experienced in cleaning out [*wegräumen*], who . . . had to deal with these prosaic [*hausbackenen;* literally, "home-baked"] problems. There are technically talented people . . . physicians as well as

. . . NCOs and also company commanders and camp leaders. Some
were . . . how shall we say? . . . well, one cannot put it any other way
—interested in it. They pressed forward, or rather they engaged themselves. . . . They said, "What those others are doing is all rubbish!" Or
. . . some who had already been in other concentration camps where
one was experiencing these matters because, for instance, the crematoria had been out of operation or were small. . . . Physicians and other
people—all those who believed themselves to be experts—they engaged themselves there.

As Dr. B. summed up the matter: "The problem . . . was not the
selections but how one can burn the colossal quantities [of corpses] if the
ovens are not working. That's what was being talked about, and nothing
else."

The problem led to antagonisms among doctors and other SS leaders
("Why didn't *you* have an idea?"), and to disclaimers of responsibility
("That is not *our* job—*you* go ahead and do something"). Soon discussions of the nagging problem were no longer confined to small medical
or technical circles but were extended to casual off-duty moments, with
such comments as, "This fool, he did such and such—how can he do that
when—?" Dr. B. explained that the "best ideas" did not necessarily come
from doctors or other officers but came from "very simple people"
among SS personnel. And his message again and again was that the focus
was always pragmatic, on what *worked*—"not [on] moral or aesthetic or
any other such considerations . . . because that [area of feeling] was
already blocked off [*abgeblockt*]. . . . It was purely a technical matter." And,
with chilling consistency, on the subject of ethics: "No. 'Ethical' plays
absolutely no [part]—the word does not exist."*

B. then provided a simple but telling model:

> The whole pattern of things within the camp atmosphere . . . was just
> the way it is in a civilian community, with all the human squabbling, you
> understand. . . . It was like the planning of construction or something
> on that order, things you observe in any community. . . . Not only
> professional conflicts but also positions of power . . . were fought out
> just as in any civilian organization, but here it was all about the Ausch-
> witz crematorium and such things. . . . It is exactly the same. . . . Human
> beings living in communities have a task, . . . administering something
> somewhere, and . . . they always function in the same way—according
> to rules—for instance, Parkinson's Law.† . . . And it was exactly that way
> within the concentration camp—especially so because of the secrecy
> and because it [the camp] had such an exceptional position [*Sonderstell-*

---

*In the original German: *"Nein. Ethisch spielt überhaupt—das Wort gibt es nicht."*
†The semi-humorous principle—put forward in C. Northcote Parkinson's 1980 book,
Parkinson: A Law—that bureaucracy expands to fill up available space.

ung; here suggesting "special function"]. . . . And the extraordinary [nature] of those . . . actions [the killing], . . . that was not a matter of debate . . . but had been accepted. For instance, the problem of the crematorium and its capacity, etc.—that was equal to the ordinary problem of sewerage or the like elsewhere.

One was getting rid of the waste material of a routinized communal enterprise.

For the most part, doctors raised objections not to the project but to being themselves victimized by violations of what they considered fair play: "For instance, . . . one had to be on duty three nights in a row. . . . because another . . . was shirking and organized for himself an outer camp inspection [assignment] with which he made himself a better life."

Yet communal spirit could be mobilized: "If, for instance, doctors were off duty and another [doctor who was on duty] wasn't able to handle it, . . . they would have helped him, according to their [technical ability to give advice on how to get the crematoria going again]."

The use of a vehicle marked with a red cross seemed perfectly natural: "That was a military vehicle. What else should they have used? Gassing was the physicians' responsibility. Physicians had only cars marked with Red Cross markings. So what should [one expect them to use]?"

Ernst B.'s accurate description leaves out the sense of filth and evil retained by SS doctors at some level of awareness. Thus, in his diary (see page 147), Kremer commented, "In comparison . . . Dante's inferno is almost a comedy. It is not in vain that they call Auschwitz an extermination camp!"[16] True, this and his *anus mundi* comments came after his first and second selections; thereafter, Kremer's diary, detached even then, became still more so over the few months he was in Auschwitz. But Dr. B. himself, referring to ramp duty more than thirty-five years later, acknowledged, "There is no way to describe selections in Auschwitz."

Chapter 9

Selections in the Camp

A doctor was not a doctor. A doctor was the selection. That was what the doctor was—the selection.
—Auschwitz survivor

General Camp Selections

Selections could take place virtually anywhere in the camp, including of course the medical blocks. We may designate as "general camp selections" (or simply as "camp selections") those that took place anywhere but in the medical areas. General camp selections could take place on one or more blocks, or in front of the various blocks (sometimes at roll call), or at work *Kommandos* (often when setting out in early morning), or at any gathering place of the camp. They varied in size from tens to hundreds of people taken from a relatively small area of the camp, to thousands of people from a larger camp unit. Here, too, only Jews were selected.

Like all selections, these were part of the overall equilibrium between extermination and work productivity—part of what I have called the Auschwitz ecology. And they, too, were influenced by "hygienic" considerations within the camp—namely, the drain on "health" facilities and the danger of epidemic created by relatively large numbers of *Muselmänner*, or extremely emaciated prisoners. Although general policies were handed down from above, there was considerable room for variation and creative improvisation from below.

The fact that the basic Auschwitz policy of killing inmates unable to work began with an order (in May 1942) from Enno Lolling, chief physician of the concentration camps, suggests high-level *medical* participation in the implementation of the selections policy.[1] And we know of significant medical involvement in its formulation as well. In any case, that policy of killing ostensibly weak inmates was pursued so ruthlessly during the next eighteen months (the last half of 1942 and all of 1943) that frequent additional directives were issued warning that enough prisoners had to be kept alive to perform the necessary work.[2] Toward the end, the selections diminished considerably—except for the destruction of two entire camp units in mid-1944.

At times the orders for camp selections seemed to be sufficiently precise—at least sufficiently translated by command and medical authorities into precise numbers—that doctors performing the selections did so with rather exact requirements. More often there was considerable leeway so that it could be, as one knowledgeable survivor put it, "very, very arbitrary," and the individual selecting doctor could frequently "do as he liked."

Selections could be requested unofficially as well as officially. (The head of a subcamp, as the same survivor tells us, might approach an SS doctor with the complaint of *Überlag* ["overcrowding"].) In either case, there was likely to be a combination of pressure on the doctor to follow a general policy and considerable discretion on his part as to how to do that.

Dr. Otto Wolken, the prisoner doctor who kept records, told of a mass camp selection, held on "the last Sunday in August in 1943," in which four thousand Jews were sent to be gassed. He referred to a sequence of ramp selections; of individual killings by *capos,* encouraged by camp authorities; of prisoners admitted to the camp but unable to do the heavy work assigned to them—and when "these heroes lost their pleasure in doing this [killing], . . . the camp doctor appeared." His appearance was synonymous with the dreaded order of *"Blocksperre!"* ["Block sealed!"], which meant that no one could leave his or her block and curtains or blinds were drawn to prevent vision into or from the affected blocks:

> The camp doctor, accompanied by some SS, went from block to block. He received from the office the number of Jews in each single block. The Jews were taken from the blocks . . . and their numbers were checked at roll call. Then they had to strip completely, whether it was summer or winter. And now the doctor went along the rows of naked people, and all who appeared weak or frail, who had bandages, showed boils, or even scars or scabies were . . . sent along with those to be killed.[3]

Wolken went on to convey the systematic organization of the process from block to block, with those selected taken to a specially emptied block where they remained for a day or two, "packed like sardines," the near-starvation rations allocated for them largely intercepted by *capos* who traded food for alcohol and "had drinking orgies, which usually ended with severe mistreatment of the selected." It did not matter that some prisoners were killed in this way because "only the [total] number had to be correct, they didn't have to be alive." When transporting them at night in trucks to the gas chamber, SS men engaged in "rough jokes," again enhanced by alcohol, and in additional beatings and killings.[4]

This combination of efficiency, extreme randomness, and brutality and humiliation, was especially true of camp selections. Dr. Jacob R., a Czech-Jewish prisoner doctor, described how "sometimes the SS would take a whole *Kommando*—tell them to take down their trousers—and look to see if they had no buttocks or gluteal muscles [indicating near starvation and weakness]—and then send them to the gas chambers." Wolken told how the selecting doctor chose prisoners who "for some reason or another, didn't please him. . . . There was no medical examination," so that a friend of his "was sent to the gas chamber simply because of an old wound from an appendicitis operation." For, as he added, "the fact that such a doctor could in ten minutes inspect all the prisoners in a block, an average of 500 people, gives some idea of how selections were carried out."[5]

Marianne F. described the process as even more haphazard and unpredictable:

> This [the criteria for selection] frankly never [had] any rhyme nor reason—because when I had typhoid fever and I look like this [she made a grotesque face]—no hair and a skeleton [and I was not selected]. But people next to me, before me, and behind me, that had survived already—five, six months—and already looked halfway more normal—were taken. You did not know.

And she went on to describe how it felt to be exposed (as she was from January to May or June 1943) to twice-daily selections, upon leaving the camp for work in the morning and upon returning at night:

> The day—you got up at four o'clock, and it was pitch dark, I mean in winter . . . then you—roll call, and you stood, and stood, and stood . . . sometimes two hours or more—lines of five—until the roll call tallied. And that—to this day I don't know—I can't figure out how it was tallied. I mean how the numbers were supposed to tally, because *gobs* of people . . . died overnight, . . . the people that were beaten to death, . . . as they didn't want to crawl out [of their bunks to come out for the selection]. I mean, I never could figure out what their mathematics were. But it had to be very precise mathematics, because sometimes if the roll call didn't tally we stood till seven and to eight o'clock! And then, as soon as you were through with the roll call, you always marched out. . . . Orchestra on the left, [playing] rousing marches. On the right, the doctor and the *Arbeitsführer* [chief of work]—and selection.
>
> Sometimes it was Mengele only, sometimes it was [one of] the others [among the doctors] only, sometimes it was both. . . . They would just stand there at the gate—that was part of their duty. . . . You would come up to the gate and [there would be the order] "Stop!" And he [Mengele or the other doctor] would look down the row, . . . look at the faces.

"You!, you!, you!—out!" The ones from the back had to move forward so as to make the row five again. . . .

And the same reception committee as you walked back at six o'clock at night. . . . We were too damned pooped [after a full day of hard physical work] to do anything! . . . And then had to *trot* in, the whole time, and they selected you as you trotted into the gates. And believe me, I didn't feel like trotting. . . . We know that the doctor was part of it.

Selections were sometimes done on a sacred Jewish holiday or on a day of shared celebration, such as Christmas. This survivor, herself Jewish but promoted to work in a clerical group of mostly Polish non-Jews, told of "[sitting around] . . . the Christmas tree [in 1943] and singing Christmas carols, and . . . probably three or four trucks going right by there into the gas."

Prisoner doctors, though likely to be protected from late 1942 and early 1943, could, if perceived as weak or sick, be selected with other prisoners. But they were better able than others to study the selections process and find ways to survive it.

Prisoners resorted to every possible device to create the appearance of health, strength, and, above all, ability to work. Some stuffed rags under their clothes to look fatter (when not required to strip); others rubbed whatever substance they could find on their faces, or simply massaged their faces briskly, to overcome pallor and produce color; and everyone tried to make vigorous physical motions (trotting or running in place) quite beyond what they considered their capacity at the time. Marianne F. explained to me that, without understanding just why or how, "I kept a determined grin on my face . . . [and] was determined never to show fear," and took pains to get her teeth brushed and to wash her face—all part of the extraordinary effort called forth by certain prisoners to stay alive.

Some women tried to drape their clothes in ways that would hide pregnancy (which for Jewish women meant being sent to the gas), and some had secret abortions by Jewish prisoner doctors. One woman told how Mengele asked her suspiciously whether she were pregnant, and said, if she was, "I will send you to another place with better conditions"; she claimed to have answered, "From what?" and was spared.[6]

The message prisoners fought against was articulated by a Rumanian-Jewish survivor: "Everybody said to us: 'Because you're dirty you have to die' "—the word "dirty" standing for every impurity assigned to Jews that necessitated their annihilation.

And frequently prisoners, particularly doctors, attempted to save a few people by manipulating records and reports and especially camp numbers. Wolken told how he cooperated with a Jewish clerk in saving people who had already been selected: by assigning them the numbers of dead people, by removing the names of people when possible from the list of

those selected, and "once I even stole before the eyes of the camp doctor
. . . a pile of . . . reports from which the numbers for the gassing list were
supposed to be taken."[7] But mostly, like all selections, those in the camp
proceeded inexorably.

Selecting Entire Camps

On two occasions entire camp populations—the Czech family camp
and the Gypsy camp—were, in effect, selected for the gas chambers.
These were not selections in the usual sense: there was no doctor dividing
people into those who died and those who lived.* But there was in each
case a high-level order (from Berlin) for the annihilation of a specific
group of thousands of people which had previously been kept intact. The
events were perceived in the camp as large-scale selections.

It is likely that doctors were involved in these decisions, considering
the health problems posed by these family camps—particularly the Gypsy
camp, which was described by many as a quagmire of starvation and
disease to a degree exceptional even for Auschwitz. Certainly, when the
order did come from above, doctors were key figures in conducting the
mass killing.

Consider the following description by a former prisoner—then part of
the Sonderkommando and therefore a close witness of these events—of the
first of two mass annihilations of the Czech (Jewish) family camp, which
took place on 8 March 1944 and claimed (according to Wolken) 3,792
men, women, and children. The Nazis had utilized the Czechs—most of
whom arrived in September 1943 from the model ghetto at Theresienstadt—for extensive propaganda campaigns, including the careful creation of a documentary film radically falsifying camp arrangements—all
this associated with a rumor that the camp was under the protection of
the International Red Cross. But, in carrying out the killing, the SS
realized that inmates there had been in Auschwitz long enough to recognize what was happening, and therefore treated them with great and overt
brutality:

> [In the dressing room of the crematorium] people's blood-stained
> and battered heads and faces proved that there was scarcely anyone
> who had been able to dodge the truncheon blows in the yard. Their
> faces were ashen with fear and grief. . . . Only a few days ago had
> Lagerführer [Johann] Schwarzhuber promised them, on his word of
> honor as an SS leader, that they and their families would be going to
> Heydebreck [an I. G. Farben plant]. . . . Hope and illusions had van-
> ished. What was left was disappointment, despair, and anger.
>   They began to bid each other farewell. Husbands embraced their
> wives and children. Everybody was in tears. Mothers turned to their chil-

*But doctors could arrange to save a few people (see pages 232–33).

dren and caressed them tenderly. The little ones . . . wept with their mothers and held on to them. But, . . . when several SS leaders—among them *Lagerführer* Schwarzhuber and Dr. Mengele—appeared in the doorway of the changing room, those standing near flew into a rage. Suffering and sorrow gave way to unrestrained hatred for those men. . . .

After a while I heard the sound of piercing screams, banging against the door, and also moaning and wailing. People began to cough. Their coughing grew worse from minute to minute, a sign that the gas had started to act. Then the clamour began to subside and to change to a many-voiced dull rattle, drowned now and then by coughing. . . .

It seemed to me that today death came more swiftly than usual. Barely ten minutes had passed since the introduction of the gas crystals when there was quiet in the gas chamber.[8]

When this member of the *Sonderkommando* came down on the elevator from the crematorium with a few of his fellow-prisoner workers, he found the camp commander (head of the subcamp) and Mengele standing just outside the gas chamber:

The doctor was just switching on the light. Then he bent forward and peered through a peep-hole in the door to ascertain whether there was still any signs of life inside. After a while he ordered the *Kommandoführer* to switch on the fans which were to disperse the gas. When they had run for a few minutes, the door to [the] gas chamber, which was secured with a few horizontal bolts, was opened.[9]

SS doctors were similarly involved—again especially Mengele—in the killing of the four thousand inhabitants of the Gypsy camp on 1 August 1944 (see also page 375). Mengele was chief doctor of that camp, and so active was he in the annihilation process that many prisoners I spoke to assumed that he himself was responsible for it and had given the specific order. There is evidence that he actually opposed that annihilation; but once it was ordered, he applied extraordinary energy toward carrying it out (see page 323).

Prisoner doctors who had worked there at the time told me that Mengele seemed to be all over the camp at once that day, actively supervising arrangements for getting the Gypsies to the gas chamber. He had been close to some of the Gypsy children—bringing them food and candy, sometimes little toys, and taking them for brief outings. Whenever he appeared, they would greet him warmly with the cry, "*Onkel* ['Uncle'] Mengele!" But that day the children were frightened. Dr. Alexander O. described the scene and one child's plea to Mengele:

Mengele arrived at around eight o'clock or seven-thirty. It was daylight. He came, and then the children. . . . A Gypsy girl of eleven, twelve, . . . the oldest [child] of a whole family—maybe thirteen, with malnutrition sometimes they grow less. *"Onkel* Mengele [she calls], my little brother cries himself to death. We do not know where our mother is. He cries himself to death, *Onkel* Mengele!" Where did she go to complain? To Mengele—to the one she loves and knows she is loved by, because he loved them. His answer: *"Willst du die Schnauze halten!"* . . . He said it in a common, vulgar way . . . but . . . with a sort of tenderness: . . . "Why don't you shut your little trap!"

Others told how Mengele combed the blocks, tracking down Gypsy children who had hidden, and how he himself transported a group of those children in a car to the gas chamber—drawing upon their trust for him and speaking tenderly and reassuringly to them until the end.

With the adults it was a little different. Dr. Alexander O. remembered their protesting that they had "fought for Germany." Another prisoner physician, recalling a *Blocksperre,* said, "Whenever I see a picture of Dracula, I think of Mengele running through the *Zigeuner* [Gypsy] camp—just like Dracula. . . . We could hear the terrible crying from the beating and torturing as they put the Gypsies on those cars. . . . [On nearby blocks] they were crying and shouting, 'We are worried that Mengele and his assistants will come and burn us.' "

Medical-Block Selections: The Triage of Killing

Nazi doctors were best observed—and perhaps most revealingly—when selecting on the medical blocks. In those selections, the SS doctor performed his healing-killing reversal within a medical context. They were therefore a key to medicalized killing and a special truth of Auschwitz. Selections on a medical block were a murderous caricature of triage: the doctor sorted out the sick and the weak to be fed to the killing machinery.

A leading Polish prisoner physician, Wladyslaw Fejkiel, described the "main purpose" of the Auschwitz "health service" as serving *"as a link in the mass extermination campaign."* "Outpatient centers" were a "place for selections"; and hospital areas, " 'waiting rooms' before death." Auschwitz hospitals, in his view, also provided medical legitimation: "If somebody learned about the existence in the camp of the[se] . . . institutions, it was impossible for him to believe that the inmates were subjected to starvation, terror, or mass murder." There was also the function of isolating the sick, especially those with contagious diseases, in order to "prevent possible epidemics, which could affect the SS personnel and the civilian slave labour, employed by the German industry, attached to the camp." The additional function of the medical blocks became the provision of some actual treatment for those slave laborers, the prisoners who worked in the camp. But, during the early phase of Auschwitz, there was virtually no such treatment available, and limited medical practice of any kind. Moreover, as Dr. Fejkiel went on to explain, the average diet in Auschwitz permitted a prisoner to remain alive no more than three months, after which time symptoms of emaciation and "hunger disease" set in; and the early hospital blocks served as places "where the people suffering from the hunger disease could spend the time from the beginning of the sickness until their death."[10] In that sense, the medical blocks became a particularly direct means of maintaining the murderous ecology of the camp.

In terms of general Auschwitz function, medical blocks remained a contradiction. In the face of camp conditions and the near-starvation diet, they could not contribute significantly to the health of the work force; and enough Jews arrived constantly to replace weaker members of that force. The medical blocks probably existed because of prior concentration-camp practice, concern about epidemics, the professional and psychological inclinations of Nazi doctors, and above all the broad Nazi impulse toward medical legitimation of killing.

With the arrival of Eduard Wirths as chief SS physician in September 1942, and the increasing official emphasis on the working capacity of large numbers of prisoners, medical facilities were considerably expanded and improved. Prisoner doctors were permitted to do real medical work; responsible political prisoners (many of them German Communists) replaced the often brutal criminal prisoners in important medically related positions; and SS doctors, for the most part, lent their support to these developments. Yet at precisely the same time, the mass murder of Jews was also expanded to reach its most extreme proportions, and SS doctors were major coordinating figures. They "did everything the command wished": that is, "cooperated closely . . . in the annihilation of the prisoners, and simultaneously did everything to make believe that they administered the proper medical treatment and in such a way they helped to conceal various crimes." Their falsifications included certification of the food rations as sufficient for life as well as the subsequent death certificates (required for prisoners admitted to the camp).[11]

I. G. Farben contributed a significant economic dimension to Auschwitz murder-triage. In March 1941, it agreed to pay the SS three *Reichsmarks* a day for each unskilled concentration-camp inmate and four *Reichsmarks* for skilled inmates. The price set for children was one and one-half *Reichsmarks.* I. G. Farben representatives sometimes complained about SS brutality to prisoners insofar as it impeded their work (though also sympathizing with the SS position that "only brute force has any effect on these people," and "it is impossible to get any work done without corporal punishment"); but perhaps the main complaint was that "transports from Berlin [meaning Berlin authority] continued to have so many women and children as well as old Jews" (that is, not enough able-bodied male workers). And by September 1942, I. G. Farben was running its own concentration camp at Monowitz.[12]

This I. G. Farben–SS collaboration departed from "the conventional

economics of slavery" (where the slave is "capital equipment to be maintained and serviced for optimum use" with gradual "depreciation" over
a full lifespan) and instead

> reduced slave labor to a consumable raw material, a human ore from
> which the mineral of life was systematically extracted. When no usable
> energy remained, the living dross was shipped to the gassing chambers
> and cremation furnaces of the extermination center at Birkenau, where
> the SS recycled it into the German war economy—gold teeth for the
> *Reichsbank,* hair for mattresses. . . . Even the moans of the doomed
> became a work incentive, exhorting the remaining inmates to greater
> effort.[13]

The whole process was consistent with the official Nazi policy—applicable to all "asocial elements" (including Auschwitz inmates)—of *Vernichtung durch Arbeit* ("destruction through work") which in practice meant
literally working people to death.[14]

Although I. G. Farben was forced to expand its hospital facilities in
Monowitz, it established a rule that no more than 5 percent of the inmates
could be kept in those facilities at any one time. And within that 5 percent,
patients had to be able (in the estimate of doctors) to return to work
within fourteen days—or else be sent to the gas (I. G. Farben records
used the euphemism *nach Birkenau,* or "to Birkenau"). The two-week
criterion carried considerable weight because I. G. Farben was able to
establish a policy of ceasing payments to the SS for a particular prisoner
after that period. The arrangement functioned as a kind of "health insurance" that I. G. Farben provided to the institution that, so to speak,
owned the slave laborers.[15]

In coming to these agreements and carrying them out, I. G. Farben
officials mixed with their counterparts in the SS in such pastimes as
hunting and ceremonial dinners and the like: for instance, "on December
20 [1941], representatives of the I. G. took part in a Christmas party of the
Waffen S.S. which was very festive and ended up alcoholically gay."[16] It is
likely that SS doctors were involved in some of these fraternal activities.

In late 1942, the Lolling order that all prisoners unable to work were
to be killed was extended to include sick prisoners who could not be
expected to recover within four weeks. In practice, however, the period
of illness permitted was usually no more than two or three weeks. And
the number of prisoners in the hospital (in the Auschwitz main camp and
Birkenau, as opposed to Monowitz where I. G. Farben set a still more
stringent policy) was not to exceed 7 percent of the camp population in
the summer and 10 percent in winter.[17] *

---

*Sometimes the figure is given as 6 percent. It seems to have been somewhere in the
range of 5 percent to 7 percent and there were constant efforts on the part of prisoner
doctors to circumvent the rule by surreptitiously keeping in hospitals more than the permissible percentage of inmates.

The medical block was not only the locale for selections but also the place where records of killing were kept. A Polish woman survivor who had done clerical work on a medical block, told how "we had files . . . a record of every person's death—when the death machine was operating full blast. We knew everything." This woman's medical block kept a file on all female inmates of the camp, and inmates responsible for it "were ordered to cross out . . . those women [designated for the crematoria] as 'transferred.' " In other words, the medical block was the final common pathway for Auschwitz death control, and the book in which all was written.

It was also an autonomous unit within the camp, technically subject only to the authority of the camp doctor and his SDG assistants, and not even to command authority.

But the authority of the SS doctor could be quickly murderous, as Dr. Robert Levy described in a later article: "On January 21, 1944, in my surgical block, because of the irrevocable decision of SS physician Thilo, I lost in a few instants 96 of my 100 patients."[18]

At the Frankfurt Auschwitz trial of 1963–64, the sequence of a selection on the medical block was accurately summarized:

> Between 8:00 and 9:00 A.M. the SS camp doctor [Friedrich Entress] appeared . . . [and] went to the doctor's room in Block 21. . . . After his correspondence was taken care of, he went with [Josef] Klehr [a notorious SDG noncommissioned officer, implicated in murder on many levels (see pages 265–67)] to the outpatient room in Block 28. There he had new sick patients brought to him. . . . The prisoner doctor stated his diagnosis. The camp doctor just looked at the sick person quickly and with a glance at the index card given him by the prisoner doctor or nurse, saw whether the person was Jewish or not. Then he decided immediately what was to happen to the prisoner; either to keep him in the hospital or send him back to the barracks, or for *"Sonderbehandlung"* ("special handling") which meant killing by phenol. Only Jewish prisoners were given *"Sonderbehandlung"* and especially those who looked weak (*Muselmänner*) or had a sick condition that made it unlikely they would be able to return to work soon. . . . Sometimes Dr. Entress put the cards of the "examined" prisoners in various piles. Everyone in the know [SS assistants, prisoner doctor, etc.] . . . understood which pile contained the cards of the prisoners destined for *Sonderbehandlung*. . . . Many [of the prisoners selected] suspected nothing. . . . Others had an idea that they would be killed because despite strictest secrecy, it leaked through the camp that prisoners were murdered in Block 20 with phenol injections given by Klehr. That's why many Jewish prisoners only reported sick in extreme emergency.[19]

Some commentators differentiated between "small selections" and "large selections" on the hospital blocks. In the smaller kind, as just described, the SS doctor would take a quick look around the hospital blocks, or have a number of patients brought to him, and select a few of the weaker ones for phenol injections. With the larger selections, all prisoner patients would be brought, usually naked, before the camp doctor who, with a glance, decided which among them could remain and which were to be killed. These large selections could involve two hundred or three hundred prisoners; and within a day or two of the selection, the prisoners were loaded into trucks and taken to the gas chambers.

There were especially large medical-block selections in connection with typhus epidemics or fear of an epidemic. The most notorious of these took place on 29 August 1942. Typhus had been spreading rapidly through the main camp, affecting SS personnel as well as prisoners, and necessitating that a special wooden barracks be set up specifically for typhus patients. The decision to "liquidate" those typhus patients apparently came from Berlin, and Entress selected seven hundred or eight hundred people, including typhus patients, those suspected of having the disease, and those convalescing. Prisoner doctors and nurses were originally supposed to be included but were saved apparently by means of some form of negotiation.[20]

Dr. Jan W., a leading Polish prisoner physician, pointed to the SS doctor as the one who acted on the principle that "a person can live only if he works—unless he works, . . . he must die"; and who, together with his assistants, "had in fact the task of speeding up . . . [that] death."

"Skeletons Marching"

Prisoner doctors could observe what those medical-block selections were really like. The highly respected Lucie Adelsberger, who worked on the overcrowded Jewish block* of the women's hospital in Birkenau, reported a hospital scene:

> The sick lie on straw sacks, all jumbled together, one on top of the other, and cannot stretch their sore limbs nor rest their backs. The beds bulge with filth and excrement, and the dead and the decomposing press with their stiffened bodies against the living who, confined as they are, cannot move away. Every illness in the camp is represented here: tuberculosis, diarrhea, rashes induced by crawling vermin, hunger edema where the wasted skeleton has filled itself with water to replace the vanished cell tissue, people with bloodshot weals caused by lashes of the whip, people with mangled limbs, frozen feet, wounds from the electric wire, or who have been shot at for trifles by a trigger-happy SS.

*Regulations required that Jewish inmates be treated by Jewish doctors, and "Aryan" inmates by non-Jewish doctors. How scrupulously this segregation was maintained varied with Nazi doctors, but seemed to be held to more strictly in the women's hospital in Birkenau than elsewhere.

They are all in torment, groaning, hungry, thirsty, shivering from cold under their meager coverings and yet fighting for their pitiful lives.[21]

The French-trained prisoner doctor, Alexander O., described an equivalent situation on the men's side:

> We had mostly Jews to take care of, . . . the "'convalescence' ward" on the second floor of Block 20. The room was called the "diarrhea room," and there we would get patients who for the most part had edemas of the lower limbs which we would call "general weakness." Almost all of them had ulcers, ulcers that did not heal because of the edema in the legs. So all these patients, classified as ill, were simply waiting their turn to go to the gas.

Dr. O. went on to tell how, when a selection was expected soon after his arrival on that ward, he had been confused by his prisoner colleague's insistence that he urge inmates to get down off their bunks, even beat them if necessary: this, it turned out, was the only way to save their lives. After the two doctors had managed to get all but a few of the patients down, the selection began:

> They announced, *"Achtung, Lagerarzt!* ['Attention, camp doctor!']." A young man, nicely built, thin, tall, an SS officer, came in, followed by a noncommissioned officer. These were called . . . let us say medical staff, with a caduceus. . . . All, in turn—naked—go before the doctor, running past him, chest out, in a very military fashion. . . . Whoever has not seen this military bearing in a skeleton does not know what degradation and contempt are. . . . If a skeleton walks stooped over, slowly, slowly, that is a skeleton presenting a normal appearance, one might say even a decent appearance. But to see this procession of skeletons marching at a military pace, chest out, shoulders thrown back, and coming to a stop abruptly—well, it is something saddening, debasing, beyond description. A skeleton marching that way—the edema [fluid] in the scrotum swinging, the completely emaciated scrotum swinging —that is something one cannot forget.

In order to avoid being deceived by prisoner doctors' attempts to save lives, the more fanatical and vicious SS doctors, such as Friedrich Entress, created what became known, according to a survivor and nonmedical scientist, as the "negative selection": "That is, he picked the healthiest-looking in order to uncover the ones hidden by block personnel—to uncover deceptions of one kind or another. The SS never discovered a foolproof way of preventing these deceptions. Entress did not do it often —but he did do it. He was the only man I knew of who did that negative selection."

Even when the selection was only partial, as was more usual, large numbers of patients could be doomed, as Dr. Adelsberger described:

At about ten the *Lagerarzt* [camp doctor] appears on a visit. *"Achtung!"* Jewish block with 683 patients! The *Lagerarzt* has a long time for the block today and looks at each of the patients separately. Those who can walk have to file past him. Those who don't march smartly enough, those with swollen feet or with superficial sores, those who can't get out of bed, all these have their numbers noted. After barely an hour, more than 400 numbers have been written down. When the *Lagerarzt* leaves the block there is a paralyzing silence. More than 400 know that in a few hours time they will be transferred to another block where perhaps many hundreds more are waiting . . . a block isolated from the rest of the camp where only the corpse bearers have entry, for the death that awaits in the gas chamber has already stamped its irrevocable seal.[22]

Chapter 10

Socialization to Killing

> They [the SS doctors] did their work just as some-
> one who goes to an office goes about his work.
> They were gentlemen who came and went, who
> supervised and were relaxed, sometimes smiling,
> sometimes joking, but never unhappy. They were
> witty if they felt like it. Personally I did not get the
> impression that they were much affected by what
> was going on—nor shocked. It went on for years.
> It was not just one day.
>
> —Auschwitz prisoner doctor

Virtually all Nazi doctors in Auschwitz complied in conducting selections,
although they varied in how they did so and in their attitudes toward what
they were doing. These attitudes ranged from enthusiasm to ambivalence
to reluctance and temporary refusal, and in at least one case, to successful
resistance or at least avoidance.

For most SS doctors, selections were a job—somewhat unpleasant and
often exhausting, and an occasion for heavy drinking, as Dr. Karl K.
explained:

> The selections were mostly an ordeal [*Strapaze,* suggesting exertion,
> fatigue, physical strain, drudgery]. Namely, to stand all night. And it
> wasn't just standing all night—but the next day was completely ruined
> because one got drunk every time. . . . By the last half of the night he
> is already half high, and at the end he is drunk. . . .
> [The drinking] was during the selection. . . . A certain number of
> bottles were provided for each selection and everybody drank and
> toasted the others. . . . One could not stay out of it [the drinking]. And
> the result was—when it was getting to be two, three o'clock, and one
> started getting very tired, then one just drank more.*

---

*SS doctors in their own way shared in the sense of entitlement described by Konrad
Morgen (see pages 138–39) when visiting an SS guard room that, far from spartan, con-

Moreover, for some of the long-standing SS doctors, the selections process was an improvement over earlier camp conditions:

> There were old-timers who had experienced much worse things than selections earlier on—personally beating someone to death and such things. . . . [The duty] was disliked, unpleasant. Yet the real old-timers who were around at the introduction of these selections, who experienced the time when people just expired in the camps and the prisoners beat one another to death or beat to death those who were dying or were suspected of having typhus.* . . . For them the selections were practically—one can't quite say relief—but in any case a situation that had improved. It got better—things were systematized.

Newcomers who had not experienced those earlier brutal camp conditions "suffered initially" at the selections, but "then it got to be routine —like all other routines in Auschwitz." SS doctors rarely made selections a topic of conversation: "If they did, it might be to complain. . . . Someone might feel cheated if he had to stand one more night more often [than the others], or if he were not relieved [from duty when he was supposed to be] or the like."

Adaptation: From Outsider to Insider

A survivor and leading chronicler of Auschwitz, Hermann Langbein, classified Nazi doctors as falling into three categories: zealots who participated eagerly in the extermination process and even did "extra work" on behalf of killing; those who went about the process more or less methodically and did no more and no less than they felt they had to do; and those who participated in the extermination process only reluctantly.[2] Langbein referred mainly to selections within the camp, which could be observed closely by prisoner physicians and certain other inmates (he himself observed a great deal as Wirths's secretary). But those differing attitudes applied to ramp selections as well—both in the drinking patterns just described and in overall ramp "styles."

For instance, another survivor contrasted the style of Dr. Franz Lucas, generally acknowledged to be a reluctant participant, with that of Josef

---

tained couches with SS men "with glassy eyes" lying about and being served "like pashas" by beautiful Jewish female prisoners. The SS person (probably an officer) escorting Morgen, upon seeing how appalled the judge seemed, "only shrugged his shoulders and said: 'The men have had a tough night behind them, they had to get several transports out of the way.' "[1] The escort too believed in that entitlement.

*Dr. K., though mostly accurate about Auschwitz details, tended at times, as here, to stress the brutalized behavior of prisioners while minimizing that of SS men.

Mengele: Lucas was "an easygoing, fatherly man who carefully and with slow movements selected on the ramp," while Mengele "did it with graceful and quick movements." Mengele's exuberant style reflected a set of ideological and characterological qualities we shall examine in chapter 17. Lucas's more cautious style was that of a man who, according to prisoner doctors, "was always decent toward the patients and . . . treated us well," and "was a human being . . . [who] gave me back my faith in the German man," and whose relative softness toward prisoners put him in repeated conflict with other SS doctors and officers. Yet despite all this, he, too, did selections.

While those differences were real and meant a great deal to prisoner physicians and other inmates, Dr. Ernst B. has claimed that they were not nearly as great as they appeared. He himself had been revered by a number of survivors as a rarity, a humane SS doctor. But he thought that more critical and fearful attitudes toward other doctors had to do with their "typical SS" authoritarian demeanor, and went so far as to suggest that it was little more than a question of bedside manner. Discussing himself and his Auschwitz medical superior (mostly feared and avoided by inmates), Dr. B. drew the analogy of two doctors who enter a community with the same professional qualifications; and even though they both use the same medications, "in the opinion of . . . people, one is a good doctor and the other is not," the source of the difference in their reputations being only "their personal relationships with patients, . . . little personal things."

Needless to say, "little personal things" could have staggering importance in Auschwitz; and Dr. B., for psychological reasons of his own, minimized important actual differences between himself and fellow SS doctors (for instance, he alone managed to avoid performing selections [see chapter 16]). He acknowledged that doctors differed in their approach to selections, but there was truth to his point that all SS doctors were greatly influenced by what he called "practical" (meaning pragmatic) issues: their shared relationship to an institution and to its selections demands, as regulated by higher medical and command authorities. And as greater numbers of transports arrived, selections were going on much of the time; as Dr. B. put it, "There was no way of avoiding [viewing] them if one had work to do in the camp."

Under increasing pressure to select, most SS doctors underwent what he viewed as an extraordinary individual-psychological shift from revulsion to acceptance: *"In the beginning it was almost impossible. Afterward it became almost routine. That's the only way to put it."*

This shift involved a *socialization* to Auschwitz, including the important transition from outsider to insider.

Alcohol was crucial to this transition. Drinking together, often quite heavily, evenings in the officers' club, doctors "spoke very freely" and "expressed the most intimate objections." Some would "condemn the

whole thing" and insist that "this is a filthy business [*Schweinerei*]!" Dr.
B. described these outbursts as so insistent as to be "like a mania
[*Sucht*], . . . a sickness . . . over Auschwitz and . . . the gassings."

Such inebriated protest brought about no repercussions—indeed, may
even have been encouraged—and was unrelated to commitment or action. Consequently, "whether one condemned it or not was not really so
much the issue." The issue, as Ernst B. defined it, was that "Auschwitz
was an existing fact. One couldn't . . . really be against it, you see, one
had to go along with it whether it was good or bad." That is, mass killing
was the unyielding *fact of life* to which everyone was expected to adapt.

Whenever an SS doctor arrived at Auschwitz, the process was repeated
as questions raised by the newcomer were answered by his more experienced drinking companions:

> He would ask, "How can these things be done here?" Then there was
> something like a general answer . . . which clarified everything. What
> is better for him [the prisoner]—whether he croaks [*verreckt*] in shit or
> goes to heaven in [a cloud of] gas? And that settled the whole matter
> for the initiates [*Eingeweihten*].

This ostensibly humane argument, Dr. B. was saying, was itself an
assertion of Auschwitz reality as the baseline for all else. His language of
initiation is appropriate in that selections were the specific "ordeal" the
initiate had to undergo in order to emerge as a functioning Auschwitz
"adult." And by exposing and combating doubts, the drinking sessions
helped suppress moral aspects of the prior self in favor of a new Auschwitz self.

Doubts could include the fundamental matter of a physician engaging
in killing: "One would say, 'Selecting is not the province of the doctor,
because it is a completely nonmedical activity.' . . . I must refuse to select
because my only purpose is to sustain life." That, too, always evoked "an
answer . . . to which nobody was able to object: 'What do you do in war,
. . . in battle, don't you have to select there as well?' Since not all can be
treated and not all can be transported, this [need to select] is the problem
of every military doctor."

However absurd the comparison by any logical standards, in that setting it could seem credible. For, as Dr. B. added, "Whether you believe
something or not always depends on the situation." And the "essential
psychological situation" of Auschwitz doctors, in his view, was resignation to its killing structure: "I'm here. I cannot get out. If prisoners come,
that is a natural phenomenon [*Naturereignis*]. And I have to do [make] the
best of it." (This last sentence was spoken in English.)

Beyond mere resignation, SS doctors moved psychologically into that
perceived Auschwitz reality. Through the drinking sessions, their resistance was "talked out" *(ausdiskutiert)*, so that after about fourteen days the
newcomer "no longer spoke of these things," and since "everyone [knew]

everyone else's point of view . . . there [was] no longer any discussion [of it]." And at that point one became an "insider."

Dr. B. summed up, with considerable feeling, the extremity—and mystery—of this transition process:

> When you see a selection for the first time—I'm not talking only about myself, I'm talking about even the most hardened SS people, . . . you see, . . . how children and women are selected. Then you are so shocked . . . that it just cannot be described. And after a few weeks one can be accustomed to it [*kann man es gewöhnen*; also suggests becoming inured]. And that [process, change] cannot be explained to anybody. But it is the same phenomenon that takes place right now in terrorists, in relation to close terrorist groups. . . . And one can . . . only experience [it to know it]. The expert can record it, but he cannot enter into it [*nachempfinden*; "know it from the inside"]. . . . But I think I can give you a kind of impression of it. When you have gone into a slaughterhouse where animals are being slaughtered, . . . the smell is also a part of it [*es gehört auch der Geruch*; literally, "the smell is what is required (for your reaction)"], . . . not just the fact that they [the cattle] fall over [dead] and so forth. A steak will probably not taste good to us afterward. And when you do that [stay in the situation] every day for two weeks, then your steak again tastes as good as before.

The slaughterhouse example is all too apt, but Dr. B. was struggling to convey both an explanation and his retrospective awe and anxiety at the fact of such a psychological transition.

But, as he also explained, doctors inwardly *wanted* to make that transition because of the great urge to become an insider. For in so extraordinary a situation, he implied, personal isolation would be intolerable, and one would become desperate to "establish contact somehow" with others. Newcomers would seek out men with whom they could identify—because of relatively similar backgrounds and outlooks. For instance, a young doctor who had just joined the SS would seek out men in that category rather than medical "old fighters" who had been in the concentration-camp system for years. There would be shared regional attitudes (such as Bavarian antagonism to Prussians) or educational and class affinities. Sometimes experienced Auschwitz doctors were assigned as mentors to arriving neophytes (in ways I shall discuss), which suggests that the authorities were aware of the pattern of conflict during the early transition experience.

Pressure and Mentorship

At the same time there was constant pressure from above toward maximum involvement in selections, particularly from the spring of 1944 when dentists and pharmacists were also ordered to take their turns on the ramp. One of those dentists later testified that his plea to Wirths that he did not feel capable of performing selections, and wished to leave the camp, was met with a cool declaration that "according to a 'Führer order,' service in a concentration camp was considered front-line duty, and that any refusal was considered a desertion" (see pages 393–94).[3]

Pressure and mentorship could combine, as in the case of Franz Lucas who, known to have a certain reluctance to select, was taken to the ramp by Wirths and Mengele and more or less shown how to go about things. Lucas apparently tried several ploys, including feigned illness, to avoid selecting; and even after complying, his kindness and medical help to prisoners led to a dressing down and an eventual transfer.[4]

In general the evidence suggests that Wirths preferred persuasion to threat; but that a doctor could, if sufficiently determined, avoid performing selections without repercussions—though only if he expressed his reluctance as inability rather than defiance. There were a few accounts of noncommissioned officers who broke down in response to ramp duty. While Wirths in one case was reputed to have "raged and screamed" and insisted that, during the fifth year of the war, one could not afford "sympathy with such sentimentalities," such men were generally given different duties. Official attitudes varied; and Wirths is even said to have responded to an SS doctor's reluctance to select with the comment: "Finally, a person with character."

Whether he said exactly that, he fiercely retained his prerogatives regarding medical control of selections. Dr. B. reported, for instance, that during the crisis of the Hungarian transports, when a camp commander learned that there were too few doctors to perform all of the selections required, and offered to assign some of his own people, Wirths replied firmly, "No, that is *my* responsibility. I don't want anyone else doing it."

After describing selections as having so permeated Auschwitz routine as to become "like the weather," Dr. B. immediately added, "like a snowstorm" so that "when it is there one is unable to think about it," thereby suggesting that selections were not a calm but an agitated fact of life.

The socialization of SS doctors to Auschwitz killing was enhanced by the camp's isolation from the world outside. The connecting medical figure with outside authority was Enno Lolling, who came frequently to the camp from his Berlin office and was essentially incompetent and a heavy drinker. Ernst B. had the impression that Lolling's superiors preferred not to know too many details about the camps, and that there was a general policy of "screening them off" from regular SS units. Camp doctors perpetuated the isolation by their reluctance, in Dr. B's phrase, to let others "see their cards." The result was, as he put it with only partial exaggeration, that "a concentration camp [became] a totally self-contained entity, absolutely isolated from everything—especially Auschwitz."

Doctors assigned there, then, had limited contact with anything but Auschwitz reality. They became preoccupied with adapting themselves to that reality, and moral revulsion could be converted into feelings of discomfort, unhappiness, anxiety, and despair. Subjective struggles could replace moral questions. They became concerned not with the evil of the environment but with how to come to some terms with the place.

They then became creatures of what Dr. B. described as the all-important Auschwitz milieu or atmosphere: "In that atmosphere everything is seen differently from the way it would be viewed now." On the basis of all the pressures and adaptive inclinations I have described, "after a few weeks in that milieu, one thinks: 'Yes.' "

The selections machine did not function impeccably. There could be not only too many transports for the facilities but poor organization in handling transports, too little room in camp quarantine where new inmates were kept, and occasionally an insufficient supply of gas. Among the troops, efficiency could be impaired by drinking too much, and the same was true of doctors. Doctors indeed drank heavily, though, according to Dr. B., only one was a recognizable alcoholic, and even he "had sufficient discipline not to get drunk when he was on duty doing selections." One could say that whatever the technical problems or human frailties, Auschwitz could mobilize a collective determination to keep the gassing process going.

Psychological Distance

Participation in selections was also enhanced by a sense that they did not come first in the hierarchy of horrors. Dr. B., for instance, stressed that "other things were much worse"—such as scenes of starving children in the Gypsy camp," where 80 percent of the inmates in general were starving to death while a few could be "living very well." He stressed the difficulty of "having this in front of you every day, continuously," and how "it took a long time to be able to live with that."

There, as in other situations, what mattered was what one could see, what confronted one's senses: "The killing was mostly excluded [from conversation], . . . [since] it was not what was directly visible. But very visible were the so-called *Muselmänner*. [Also] visible were the ones who were starving . . . to death. . . . That was a bigger problem. . . . One was more oppressed by that."

By not quite seeing it, doctors could distance themselves from the very killing they were actively supervising. The same purpose was served by drawing upon their having witnessed what they claimed were worse horrors—in camps for Russian prisoners of war and in other concentration camps—which enabled them to conclude that "they've got it a lot better here." As Dr. B. went on to explain: "What made Auschwitz especially notorious were the gassing installations. Right? And those were now somehow or other a bit further off, and one could only actually sense them by means of smell." But, as he earlier implied, one gets used to a smell.

Furthermore, there were more "fundamentally controversial" activities about which SS men had greater qualms. Among these, Dr. B. mentioned Gestapo methods for extracting confessions, about which "one had very great reservations." With doctors buffered from the killing, selections could be accepted as an established activity and seem less onerous than special brutal tasks (such as medical collusion in torture to produce confessions) and immediate confrontation with inmates dying of starvation. But one may turn that point around and say that the selections were so onerous, so associated with extraordinary evil, that Nazi doctors called forth every possible mechanism to *avoid taking in psychologically what they were doing*—every form of psychic numbing and derealization (see pages 442–47). Hence Dr. B., who witnessed many selections without performing them, could say that "what remains are a few personal impressions, and these impressions are in themselves not even the really cruel events. If one tried to describe a selection now, that would be almost impossible . . . because it is a technical process. . . . I can describe many isolated images; . . . they are still there, but one must drag them out of one's memory." This difficulty of recall suggests that Nazi doctors never quite felt—that is, emotionally experienced—their original act in performing the selections.

Doctors were further enabled to do selections by the shared sense that Auschwitz was morally separate from the rest of the world, that it was, as Dr. B. put it, "extraterritorial."* He referred not to Auschwitz's geographical isolation, but to its existence as a special enclave of bizarre evil, which rendered it exempt from ordinary rules of behavior. He also stressed its extreme contradictions as contributing to its function.

For instance, he spoke of an aura of élite and highly detached military professionalism on the one hand, and of all-pervasive corruption on the other. That military professionalism, derived from both the SS and the earlier Prussian tradition, required ramrod posture, demeanor, and integrity and a form of self-control that would have made it "inconceivable . . . to speak about [inner or intimate] feelings." The underlying corruption was in the nature of shared open secrets involving *all* and, to a degree, contributing to cohesion:

> Every single SS man had so many possibilities for being corrupt in some way that almost everyone did something—had "dirt on his walking stick" [*Dreck am Stecken*]. And everyone knew about everyone else's improper activity, which is why nothing ever came of it—because everyone knew about everyone else. That's why the SS troop *Kommando* always held together so well—at least externally.

By "dirt" he meant such things as keeping gold and other valuables taken from Jews before they were killed instead of turning it over to the

---

*The word means outside territorial boundaries and, in a modern historical sense, has special reference to areas in which citizens of a dominant Western country were exempt from the legal jurisdiction of a weaker country (either colonized or in some way threatened or controlled) where they resided.

state, or making exchanges or other deals with prisoners through which Nazi personnel, including doctors, obtained gold or money from them. He went on to point out that, moreover, Auschwitz rules were such that "the very moment [an SS physician] fraternized, he was . . . committing a crime." In the vicious circle of contradiction and illegality that developed, whatever means one took to curb illegal practices could usually be accomplished only by further illegalities: to curb excessive trading of food or hoarding of gold on the part of corrupt SS men or *capos* required that special arrangements (essentially forms of bribery) be made with others in authority. And since anything was possible in that atmosphere, it was difficult to separate fact from mere rumor or from what Dr. B. called "latrine talk." As he declared, "Even in the case of Rudolf Höss, certainly the most incorruptible and most correct camp commandant that ever existed, . . . there was this rumor, . . . much talked about, . . . that he had an affair with a Jewish woman."*

The food situation was a perpetual source of corruption. With near-starvation rations further siphoned off at various points, the ordinary prisoner could not survive on the amount of food made available to him or her. Everyone therefore "organized," as the Auschwitz term had it: arranged a way to get enough food to stay alive and help friends do the same. Corruption in that sense was life preserving—but, as Dr. B. put it, "All those who survived Auschwitz lived from food that was taken away from the others." What he did not say was that the SS policy, as carried out by camp medical and command authorities, imposed this fundamental life-death corruption. They used the situation for reward-and-punishment control over prisoners and frequently for additional trading that filled their own pockets.

The ultimate corruption was the existence of the mass killing, around which the camp essentially revolved. Since that killing process depended upon extensive prisoner involvement, it could be maintained most effectively when camp conditions were relatively good. In other words, whatever Nazi doctors contributed to the health of inmates—and they did improve camp hygiene, expand medical facilities, and support prisoner doctors—was in the service of not just the work force but the murder machine. That was the real "dirt" on all of their "walking sticks."

Yet many Nazi doctors kept pressing for better medical conditions—searching everywhere for useful equipment, accumulating it in their barracks, seeking to have better operating rooms—but always faced what Dr. B. called the "barrier," the threat of starvation, so that the medical structures they built were part of a "fiction." Even if enough food could be "organized" to keep patients alive for a while, "the primary founda-

---

*Characteristically, the rumor was partly true (he did have an affair with a prisoner, Eleonore Hodys) and partly false (she was not Jewish)—and, in this latter aspect, more scandalous than the truth. But there was much more to question about Höss's alleged incorruptibility: he in fact tried to murder Hodys when she became pregnant.[5]

tion was lacking because they were starving to death." And, we may add, because the same patients helped one day would be sent to the gas chambers another day, or else utilized to keep the killing structure functioning. This is what Dr. B. called the "schizophrenic situation," by which he meant ostensible efforts to heal and help in the midst of the fundamental Auschwitz mission of mass killing.

Nazi doctors, Dr. B. tells us, "lived like lords," because "everything that amounted to actual work was done by the inmates." This "good life" gave them additional incentive to participate in selections, especially since the alternative, should they have strongly requested a transfer, would probably have been the Russian front, where their lives would have been in extreme danger.

That "good life" included elegant demeanor, especially from the standpoint of inmates ("SS doctors were extremely well dressed, . . . distant gentlemen, who did not touch an inmate," according to prisoner doctor Henri Q.), and an encompassing presence in the camp ("They managed the situation . . . at the infirmary . . . selections, . . . at the station . . . the crematoria. . . . They were everywhere").

These legitimaters not only of "medical" triage-murder but of medic*alized* Auschwitz killing were aided in their function by their sense that all Jews were already condemned. What Dr. Magda V. said of Mengele applies more generally to SS doctors: "It didn't matter to him [whether he selected someone or not]. because he thought that sooner or later they're going [to the gas chamber]. . . . For him I think we . . . were just dead anyhow." Another survivor similarly called the whole process "only a play": that is a staged drama in which "we were all there to be killed. The question was only who was to be killed first."

For the SS doctor, efficiency in selections became equated with quarantine arrangements and the improvement of actual medical units, all in the service of keeping enough inmates able to work and the camp free of epidemics. Within that context, the SS doctor inevitably came to perceive his professional function to be in neither the killing nor the healing alone, but in achieving the necessary balance. That *healing-killing balance*, according to the SS doctor Ernst B., was "the problem" for Auschwitz doctors. From that standpoint, as he further explained, the principle of "clearing out" a block when there was extensive diarrhea—sending everyone on it to the gas chambers—could be viewed as "pseudo ethical" and "pseudo idealistic." Dr. B. meant that such a policy in that environment could be perceived by the doctors themselves as ethical and idealistic in that they carried out their task to perfection on behalf of the higher goal of camp balance.

Detoxifying language contributed to this self-deception. As Dr. Jacob R. explained, SS doctors were surely cruel in sending people to the gas chambers but "never admitted it": "They called it going on a transport back to camp." Another prisoner doctor suggested how far this kind of euphemism contributed to a pervasive atmosphere of denial:

> I couldn't ask [Dr. Fritz] Klein, "Don't send this man to the gas
> chamber," because I didn't know that he went to the gas chamber. You
> see, that was a secret. Everybody knows the secret, but it was a secret.
> If I said to him, "Herr Doktor Klein, why should you send this man to
> the gas chambers?," I suppose that he would say, "Gas chamber? What
> do you mean?"

Partly out of boredom, but for important psychological reasons as well,
all Nazi doctors took up what Dr. B. called "hobbies." These hobbies
might include approximation of actual medical work or research; or collaboration with more experienced prisoner doctors in various medical
enterprises including surgery and both clinical and laboratory studies. In
these the Nazi doctor, in relationship to the prisoner doctor, was both
student and arbiter of life and death. Certainly the avid construction of
ambitious hospital units was still another hobby. And the reason these
were all hobbies is that, as Dr. B. put it, "We could do [them] at the pace
of a hobby or with the attitude of a hobby." Or, to put matters more
simply, such was the nature of Auschwitz that everything not concerned
with killing—and to a lesser degree, with work production—was no more
than a hobby.

All such hobbies come down to a particular purpose, as Dr. B. tellingly
put it: "And there one could seek out, lay out, a task. And in it also achieve
success. And in that way sweep the problem [of Auschwitz killing] under
the table." Building medical facilities, then, served the psychological
purpose of avoiding awareness of one's own killing and of others' dying.
In that milieu, as Dr. B. said, "a hospital is a *contradictio in objecto* [objective
contradiction]. . . . The doctors escape into . . . illusion."

Also crucial to SS doctors were a series of personal alliances. Each
doctor sought to have good relationships with the members of the SS
team he worked with on the ramp. In a different way, the SS doctor could
also experience various kinds of psychological satisfaction from his contacts with prisoner doctors (to be discussed later) and develop what Ernst
B. called "small cells of personal communication," giving rise in turn to
"many, many small islands of humanity." However precarious, these
"islands of humanity" enabled SS doctors to feel that they could "really
do [people] a lot of good" and helped them block out the Auschwitz
mainland of murderous *in*humanity.

Ideology and the "Jewish Problem"

Crucial to the capacity to perform selections was a doctor's relationship
to Nazi ideology. Important here was the basic early attraction on the part
of most of these doctors to the Nazi promise of German resurgence—a
tie that could sustain them through reservations and discomfort: "We

looked at it [Auschwitz] as a totally messed-up thing. [But] you could not change it, you see. That's like in a democracy, where you may find many things wanting, but you cannot change it. Or rather you stick with it nonetheless. Because [you] think democracy is better." The strong implication is that Nazism *even with Auschwitz* was the best of all possible worlds.

However ironic, these medical participants in mass murder were held to the regime behind the murder by the principles of what Dr. B. called "coherent community" (*zusammenhängende Gemeinschaft*, which also means "community that hangs together") and "common effort" (*allgemeine Anstrengung*, which implies intensity and exertion) in discussing his and others' sense of the Nazi movement's commitment to overcoming staggering national problems. Hence he could speak of "a faith" [*Glaube*] and, more than that, of a "practiced faith" joined to a community [*Gemeinschaft*]; in all this, "the bridge . . . is the ideology." And that "bridge" could connect the Nazi doctors to an immediate sense of community and communal purpose in their Auschwitz work.

Anti-Jewishness was an active ingredient in that ideology. While there was individual variation, Dr. B. claimed that "all physicians were absolutely convinced that 'the Jews were our misfortune' "—the phrase first uttered by Heinrich von Treitschke, the nineteenth-century politician-historian who contributed to the sense that "there was something virtuous about being anti-Semitic" (see pages 35–36).[6] When I mentioned the phrase "gangrenous appendix" an SS doctor had applied to Jews (see pages 15–16), Dr. B. quickly answered that the Nazi doctors' overall feeling was: "Whether you want to call it an appendix or [not], it must be extirpated [*ausgerottet*, meaning also 'exterminated,' 'destroyed,' or 'eradicated']." He went so far as to say that even the policy of killing all Jews was readily justified by this "theoretical and ideological" stance, so that "of course they supported it."

On other occasions, B. spoke differently, stressing that Auschwitz Nazi doctors were not for the most part ideologically minded. But he was consistent in stressing their sense of a "Jewish problem" and their tendency to speak in what he called the usual propaganda phrases: "That all cultures have realized that the Jews . . . must be kept outside of the regular [*normal*] culture. . . . That German culture cannot grow [*ausbreiten*; also 'spread,' 'unfold,' 'open out'] if it is being infiltrated 'Jewishly,' or something along that line."

But to perform selections, the Nazi doctor had to make the psychic shift from ideology to actual mass murder (as Karl K. explained):

> There was no one in Germany or in the whole world who had not heard Hitler's and Streicher's proclamation that the Jews had to be exterminated [*vernichtet*]. . . . Everybody heard that. And everybody "heard past it" [*vorbeigehort*; "didn't take it in"]. Because nobody believed that such a reality would come into practice. . . . And suddenly one is confronted with the fact that what one used to, my God!, take

for propaganda verbiage [*Propagandageschwätz*] is now totally, completely, wholly [*ganz, ganz, ganz*] matter-of-fact [*trocken*; literally, "dry"] and strategically concrete, that it is being realized [*verwirklicht*] with 100-percent strategy. That above all shook one. That one did not foresee [but] . . . you knew it, and all of a sudden you are standing in front of it. Did you *really* know it?

The passage is clear enough on the doctor's shocking confrontation with the literal enactment of victimizing imagery. But I believe it also suggests the widespread German psychological resistance to taking in the dark side of Nazi actuality, whatever the extensive evidence of its existence—a form of psychological resistance still present today in Nazi doctors despite, and because of, their exposure to the darkest Nazi reality of all.

Doctors could call forth an absolutized Nazi version of good and evil as both justification for what they were seeing and doing and further avoidance of its psychological actuality (as Ernst B. explained):

Precisely because they were convinced of the justness, . . . or of the . . . National-Socialist "world blessing" [*Weltbeglückung*] and that the Jews are the root evil [*Grundübel*] of the world—precisely because they were so convinced of it did they believe, or were strengthened—[in that belief], that the Jews, even existentially, had to be absolutely exterminated [*die Juden eben existentiell, also absolut vernichtet werden müssen*].

And although "not everybody approved of the gassing" and "many theories were discussed," one had to admit that gassing was an improvement over the inefficiency of previous methods:

The main argument for the gassing was that when one tried to create ghettos, . . . they never lasted longer than one or two generations. And then the ghetto—let us say—would become porous [*undicht geworden*; "would become leaky"]. That was the main argument for the gassing. Against the gassing there were a number of different kinds of the most nonsensical speculations . . . forced sterilization and so on. . . . Lots of theorizing went on.

Now there was a more successful approach to the "Jewish problem" and, as Dr. B. added, "a means of confirmation" of that success.

In talking about these matters, he never directly answered one question I repeatedly asked him: whether doctors disagreed with one another about the necessity to kill all Jews, or agreed about that and disagreed only about the means. I believe that the ambiguity has psychological significance beyond this evasion. From what Dr. B. and other observers have conveyed, it is probably accurate to say that most Nazi doctors in Auschwitz believed that something they perceived as "Jewishness" had to be eliminated, whether that meant sending all Jews to Madagascar, forcing most Jews to leave Germany while permitting a small well-established minority to remain and undergo complete assimilation, or murdering every last one of them. By clinging to this ambiguity, Nazi doctors had an additional means of avoiding the psychological reality of the decision for mass murder and its implementation. And by viewing the whole matter as a problem that needed to be "solved," by whatever means, that pragmatic goal could become the only focus. The very term *Endlösung,* or "Final Solution," served both psychological purposes: it stood for mass murder without sounding or feeling like it; and it kept the focus primarily on problem solving. So given a minimum agreement on the necessity of solving the "Jewish problem," doctors and other Nazis could come to accept, even to prefer, the mass-murder project, because it alone promised a *genuine* solution, a clearing up of the matter once and for all, and a *final* solution.

But there were different combinations of ideology and attitude. Even older career doctors—for instance, Hans Wilhelm König—could be in accord with SS principles but retain a measure of humanity so that (as Dr. Jacob R. stated) "As long as a person is allowed to be alive, he could be treated as a person." It was König who was friendly with a woman prisoner artist (pages 232–33); and Dr. R. told how König had, on the forced march out of Auschwitz, saved his life by helping him up when he found it difficult to continue and was in danger of being shot.

Friedrich Entress, in contrast, was consistently perceived as brutal. According to Dr. R., "he was only interested in the system and had no interest in patients, and Jewish doctors were non-persons." Polish prisoners had their own special reasons to be terrified of Entress (see pages 262–63).

But, for Dr. Lottie M., "the fanatic was Klein." It was he who insisted upon maintaining separation between the Aryan and the Jewish medical blocks, who considered the Jews a "gangrenous appendix" to be removed, and was at one with the selections process. "He felt that the right thing to do was to kill these people, . . . [that] it was right to do so," Dr. M. stated, still with a certain degree of incredulity. More generally, Nazi doctors, as a Czech doctor, Erich G., observed, would "treat Jewish people as having a human form but not a human quality" and as "potential polluters of the German race"—which was why a Nazi doctor "became a killer instead of a healer," a phenomenon "I saw daily."

Careerist concerns became bound up with ideology in ways that reinforced one another. From the standpoint of career, the Auschwitz assignment was of mixed value. Its advantage lay in the likelihood of official recognition, including promotion and future advantages, for performing difficult duty, all the more so for a doctor identified as efficient and zealous in his work. But in terms of useful medical experience, always important for one's career, Auschwitz offered very little. Dr. Lottie M. observed that Nazi doctors wished to be always professionally "on top of what is going on," so that if they would say, "No, no, that wasn't good," they would mean that something "wasn't good because their career was interrupted."

Nazi doctors did not recall being especially aware in Auschwitz of their Hippocratic oath, and were, not surprisingly, uncomfortable in discussing it with me. A number of them, in fact, told me directly that the oath of loyalty to Hitler they took as SS military officers was much more real to them than was a vague ritual performed at medical school graduation (see also page 435). The latter oath had enormous power, as I learned from a doctor who, though long anti-Nazi, refused to listen to the BBC toward the end of the war because of his oath to Hitler. (An oath for Germans especially can be experienced as an absolute commitment to an immortalizing principle, an association of self with a transcendent morality). Dr. Lottie M., however, felt that the Hippocratic oath was always in some sense present for German doctors, in contention with more immediate loyalties and with the oath to Hitler. And this woman prisoner doctor thought the Hippocratic oath, however dim in awareness, an important factor in certain situations, as when Nazi doctors insisted upon better conditions for prisoners or when, for instance, König insisted that "pregnant women cannot be kept in a camp."* With all their participation in murder, the residual influence of a healing self once bound to the Hippocratic oath rendered the SS doctor, according to a prominent non-Jewish prisoner and resistance leader, "the weakest link in the SS chain." But his oath to Hitler maintained the link nonetheless.

Making the System Work

Dr. B stressed the absoluteness of the situation, the need to decide immediately that "you've got to go [here]—and you will go *there!*—with utterly no room for additional discussion."And that absoluteness was consistent with membership in a ramrod SS military élite. As Dr. B. also pointed out, "The SS doctor was from the start different from other military physicians" in that only he among them carried a pistol, and there was the sense that "if the need arises, he becomes a soldier like anyone else." Moreover, through Himmler's messages, that special status was particularly associated with serving in the camps: "Himmler always made clear to us that this task of concentration-camp personnel was especially significant [*wichtig*; 'weighty, essential, vital'], . . . a matter of the highest level, . . . high and elevated, . . . so somehow in this way [conflict or expressions of revulsion] were cut off [*abgeschnitten*]." Dr. B.

---

*König meant that pregnant non-Jewish women should be released.

believed that doctors were "certainly" affected by Himmler's message because it heightened the sense on the part of SS officers and personnel that working in a camp made them a special élite, and the doctors' further sense of being an élite within that élite.

That special recognition received for participating in murder helped shift doctors' conflicts to intra-organizational ones—questions of personal loyalty to either the chief doctor or the camp commandant, and general issues of one's "sense of duty as a civil servant," or at least its military equivalent. For these and other reasons, Ernst B. could say that he saw no direct expressions of revulsion toward selections, though he "always wondered" why that was so. A partial answer is that a combination of ideology and cynical detachment became a much more comfortable psychological stance—here described by the prisoner nonmedical scientist who observed a few Nazi doctors closely and read some of their records:

> They considered themselves performing *Therapia Magna Auschwitz-ciense.* They would even use the initials T.M. At first it was mockingly and ironically, but gradually they began to use them simply to mean the gas chambers. So that whenever you see the initials T.M., that's what it means. The phrase was invented by Schumann who fancied himself an academic intellectual among the intelligentsia of Auschwitz doctors. By that phrase they meant, for instance, saving people from typhus epidemics. They were doing them a favor. And there was also a sense of humane method in what they were doing. . . . A second part of the concept of *Therapia Magna* was doing things for science—learning things for science, etc.

In connection with those few doctors who resisted selections, Dr. B. groped unsuccessfully for their reasons. He concluded only that, after one has "witnessed the whole procedure from the beginning . . . then you can only in a clearly intuitive way [*nur rein gefühlsmässig*] say, 'This is impossible!' I don't have any explanation for it." (Just one SS doctor so far as we know—Dr. B. himself—succeeded in refusing and holding to it, though with the help of a special relationship to chain of command; and one other SS doctor—Hans Delmotte—tried to, for a while.)

The very contradictions and complexities concerning healing and killing that caused Dr. B. to speak of a schizophrenic situation also militated against resistance at the time—and against comprehension later on. On trying to explain Auschwitz by writing about it, Dr. B. said, "For me, it's impossible because . . . if you start at one point, then the [endless] problems [of nuance and explanation] come and because nothing is concrete, you see."

What did become clear was the power of the Auschwitz environment, as one SS doctor recalled years later: "One could react like a normal human being in Auschwitz only for the first few hours. Once one had spent some time there, it was impossible to react normally. In that setup everyone was sullied." And SS doctors, as a survivor added, were "doing what the society wants you to do."

Dr. Henri Q., noting angrily that doctors "who are to care for the sick" instead "participated in such a massacre without resisting," pointed out that only one SS doctor (and there is actually some doubt about him) asked to be sent to the Russian front instead. Dr. Q. contrasted that record with consistent resistance by prisoner doctors who risked their lives changing lists and protecting people from selections in various ways. And he observed closely the relationship between routinization and extreme moral blunting—the "relaxed" manner of "gentlemen who came and went" described in the epigraph to this chapter. And the prisoner doctor Magda V. pointed out (as did the SS doctor Ernst B.) that, whatever the difference in the Nazi doctors' attitudes toward selections, they did them as "part of their job"—with such compliance that "I think those bastards knew what they came for."

But Dr. V. nonetheless noticed that doctors could behave differently from one another. One factor was fear. Of Dr. König, she said that he took more people from the medical blocks in selections than he need have taken "because he was scared," and added, "[Among SS doctors] there [weren't] . . . many brave men there. . . . We didn't get the cream of . . . humanity."

The doctors were affected as well by the impending German defeat. Some became considerably more pleasant and helpful, looking for the support from liberated prisoners they knew they would soon need. But some had a reverse reaction, selecting people to die all the more energetically; as Dr. Lottie M. observed, "it seemed to them more necessary to believe that they [were] right. . . . Somehow you felt them say, 'We are still right.' " Individual psychological attitudes toward women and men could also be important in ways to be discussed. Dr. M. told me, for instance, that Rohde was relatively considerate to women prisoner doctors—and, in fact, was especially active in arranging release from the camp of pregnant non-Jewish women inmates (made possible by later Auschwitz rules)—but was at the same time "an awful man toward the men."

Another element was their education and general knowledge. The Polish doctor Tadeusz S. stressed that they were "not educated doctors," "did not understand either human beings or medicine," and sometimes resembled medical students whose basic ignorance enabled them to think of "fantastic experiments," all the more so when combined with Nazi ideology. This ignorance was greatest in older SS doctors who had been early Nazis, the medical version of the "old fighters." But Dr. S. was referring to the overall Nazi impairment of the profession and to medical versions of the Nazi pseudo intellectual: the half-educated visionary, highly ideologized, intellectually undisciplined and fundamentally anti-intellectual, insecure and radically arrogant.

Also affecting their behavior were powerful blocks to empathy and compassion for patients. Several Nazi doctors stressed the absence of any principle of empathy in their medical education; and although the emergence of doctors with minimal empathy is a worldwide phenomenon, it is probably fair to say that it has been especially true of German medicine independent of the Nazis. The Nazis of course accentuated the pattern in cultivating medical versions of their principle of hardness, which reached an extreme of brutalized cynicism in the comment of a Nazi physician to the SDG *Desinfektor* inserting the gas: "Now go on and give the Jews their feed."[7]

The Schizophrenic Situation: Doubling

The SS doctor was deeply involved in the stark contradictions of the "schizophrenic situation" that Ernst B. considered to be the key to understanding Auschwitz; I see it also as a further expression of "extraterritoriality"—of the sense that what happened there did not count. The heart of that schizophrenia for doctors lay in the idea of doing constructive medical work within a "slaughterhouse." A related dimension of the schizophrenia, as B. explained, was the "split situation" between the idealism of a world-bettering great German state along with the specific Nazi "world blessing"—and what he called (still reluctant to speak directly of mass murder) "the other situation, the one working with those . . . methods there."

Dr. Magda V. was impressed by the difference in behavior of some doctors when performing selections: "It was . . . a different person, . . . doing different things. I'm telling you, . . . they were schizoid." She was trying to say that they seemed to be two different people. Rohde, for instance, when doing selections, would "be uneasy, . . . probably . . . louder or, you know, rougher certainly." Tadeusz S. recalled Rohde's firing a shot into the air from his pistol on one occasion when "he saw people going to the gas chamber after he had sent them there," out of "a combination of anger, being drunk, and anxiety—a problem of conscience." Nonetheless Rohde "was doing exactly the same things [selections] as the others."

There were gradations depending upon a doctor's attitude toward selections: Rohde, according to Dr. V., "hated it" and drank heavily; König "was extremely disciplined, . . . considered it a duty"; Mengele "was detached, . . . like he would exterminate vermin"; and Klein "enjoyed it, the bastard." Tadeusz S. characterized Horst Fischer and Friedrich Entress, as "the worst murderers, . . . [who] had faces like priests . . . but were very cold." But the inner division present in most was evidenced by the fact that they tended to leave quickly after the selections and turn things over to the underlings (as if, as Dr. V. put it, "they [themselves] didn't . . . do anything"): that is, as a means of distancing themselves from what they had actually done.

Dr. Peter D. commented on this inner division in Dr. Horst Fischer (who had supported D.'s work in otolaryngology): "[His] manner was human . . . when he was alone with me; [yet concerning selections, he] never had a regret for what he did." Dr. D. "wondered how he could . . . go on doing that [selections]."

Another way Nazi doctors coped with Auschwitz was to lead a double life that both reflected and enhanced their psychological doubling. Thus, they spent most of their time in the camp (except for occasional professional or pleasure trips to nearby areas) but went on leave for a few days every other month or so to spend time, usually in Germany, with their wives and children. They remained extremely aware of the separateness of the two worlds. One's wife, children, and parents came to stand for purity, as opposed to an inner sense of Auschwitz filth. Ernst B., for instance, managed to get home every two or three months for about a week's time but spoke strongly against the idea of his wife ever visiting him at Auschwitz: "I could never have subjected my wife to a closer look at things. . . . I can't even express myself properly, [but] the thought of her coming there would have caused [me] great [inner] resistance. One simply gave it no consideration whatsoever."*

Dr. B. observed that each SS doctor could call forth two radically different psychological constellations within the self: one based on "values generally accepted" and the education and background of a "normal person"; the other based on "this [Nazi-Auschwitz] ideology with values quite different from those generally accepted." The first tendency might be present on one day, the second on the next, and it was hard to know which to expect on a given occasion or whether there would be a mixture of both.

Only a form of schism or doubling can explain the polarities of cruelty and decency in the same SS doctor. Klein is perhaps the best illustration here. This cruel and fanatical racist was seen by Dr. Magda V. as profoundly hypocritical and simply a "bad man," and by another prisoner physician, Olga Lengyel, as "one of the fervent zealots" who ran the Nazi annihilation project. Yet this latter doctor also spoke of him as a person capable of kindness, as when he brought her medicine for her patients and protected her from cruel SS personnel (see pages 226–27); he was, Lengyel said, "the only German in Auschwitz who never shouted."[8]

---

*There were exceptions: Höss's family lived with him in Auschwitz as did the wives or families of other commandants; and among doctors, Wirths's family lived there some of the time, and the wives or families of a few others periodically or more briefly. Even in those cases, however, the men seemed to maintain the separation between the world of Auschwitz killing and their family life nearby (see also page 319).

SS officers also had social and sexual opportunities involving German women, mostly civilians, who did clerical work at nearby command areas or in some cases in the camp itself.

Another prisoner also had a surprisingly positive experience with Klein: when walking in the camp, this man took the highly unusual and dangerous step of approaching the SS doctor directly in order to ask him to have his (the prisoner's) wife, a nurse, transferred from an attic working place, where a great deal of sawdust caused her to cough incessantly, back to a medical block where she had worked in the past. Instead of saying, "Away with this fellow!" as everyone thought he would, Klein complied. This survivor commented, "These things are so intermingled —murdering and extermination on the one hand, and the very small details where something could work out quite the other way." He further reflected:

> When I tell this . . . after thirty-five years, I think, How could it be possible? . . . That one could influence this god and make a man who . . . exterminated thousands of people . . . to have interest in one prisoner girl, and save her. . . . There are things that happen in human nature . . . that an experienced analyst even cannot understand. . . . This split, . . . it can be very delicate. . . . Maybe with these small [positive] things—with Klein, there [was] something of . . . medical tradition in them. But, in general, I believe they were no longer doctors. They were SS officers. In these things, the group spirit is one thousand times mightier than the individual spirit.

This survivor was saying that Klein functioned primarily in relation to the collective SS ethos, or what I call the "Auschwitz self"; but that he had available a humane dimension of self that could emerge at certain moments.

The existence of that humane element of self may, in fact, have contributed to Klein's and other Nazi doctors' cruelties. For instance, when SS doctors asked pregnant women to step forward so that they could receive a double food ration—only to send those who did to the gas chamber the following day—it is possible that a brief sense of potential "medical activity" (improving the diet of pregnant women) contributed to the doctors' psychological capacity to carry out this hideous hoax.

In my interviews with Dr. Lottie M., she raised several questions she asked me to explore with Nazi doctors: How far did they look upon all of Auschwitz as "an experiment [on] how much a person can stand"? How much were they able to recognize "the irrationalism of . . . the racial theory"? At what point had "they started to be afraid of the end"? But what she was most curious about was "this question of split loyalty"—of conflicting oaths, contradictions between murderous cruelty and momentary kindness which SS doctors seemed to manifest continuously during their time in Auschwitz.

For the schism tended not to be resolved. Its persistence was part of the overall psychological equilibrium that enabled the SS doctor to do his deadly work. He became integrated into a large, brutal, highly functional system. Thus Dr. Henri Q. could wisely urge me to concentrate upon Nazi doctors' relation to this system rather than upon a single, infamous individual such as Mengele: "What impressed us was the fact that Auschwitz was a collective effort. It was not just a single person, but many. And the disturbing thing was that it was not something passionate [irrational]. It was something calm—there was nothing emotional about Auschwitz."

Dr. Jacob R., in discussing Nazi doctors' continuing function, stressed "this question of power—of having uncontrolled power over somebody." And in regard to the evil use of that power, Dr. Tadeusz S. quoted Dr. Fischer as having told him, "We [Nazis] have gone so far now that we have no way out." There are two possible implications here: the moral principle that the evil could not be undone; and the psychological principle that, having maintained a death factory for a period of time, one felt impelled to continue its function. The psychological point is that atrocity begets atrocity: continuing to kill becomes psychologically necessary in order to justify the killing and to view it as other than it is.

That dynamic of living with the schism and the numbness was revealed also in what Dr. S. took to be later attitudes of Nazi doctors: "Oh, they still live all over the world. They have no moral problem. They are only unhappy that they lost the war."

These last few remarks by prisoner doctors suggest that the collective process of medicalized killing was, psychologically and technically, self-perpetuating; and that Nazi doctors found a way to engage in the process —the schism of which I speak—with sufficient detachment to minimize psychological discomfort and responsibility, then and over time.

Chapter 11

Prisoner Doctors: The Agony of Selections

> They dealt with me nearly like a human being—but
> all the while there was the reality of the camps.
> —Auschwitz prisoner doctor

For prisoner doctors to remain healers was profoundly heroic and equally paradoxical: heroic in their combating the overwhelming Auschwitz current of murder; paradoxical in having to depend upon those who had abandoned healing for killing—the Nazi doctors. And before prisoner doctors could be healers in Auschwitz, they had to succeed in the very difficult task of surviving, mentally as well as physically.

Only from late 1942 were significant numbers of prisoner doctors permitted to work on hospital blocks, often at first as an orderly or a nurse rather than a doctor. Earlier, there had been near total neglect of the sick: a handful of prisoner doctors (mostly Polish; and in the women's camp German and then Czech-Jewish as well) had virtually nothing in the way of medicine or treatment to offer the overwhelming numbers of moribund patients. Patients were further victimized by SS men and prisoner *capos* who were medically ignorant, often sadistic, and inclined to try their hand at medical procedures (a notorious former locksmith, for example, boasted of having performed many amputations).

Terror and Privilege

From late 1942 or early 1943, Jews who arrived as doctors were not only permitted to live but were made a privileged category of prisoner. But they, nevertheless, retained an underlying terror from what they had experienced in the camp. And we have seen how favored treatment as a doctor could be accompanied by pain and guilt concerning murdered family members (see pages 167–69).

Until called on to practice in this way as doctors, many prisoners had been as subject to murder, brutality of various kinds, and extreme humiliation as any other inmates, sometimes even more so. Dr. Alexander O. described to me how, when he was at first put together with about twelve other doctors in a *Kommando* assigned to demolition work, he came upon a large ditch that had served as a toilet and was filled with fecal matter: "As doctors it was our special privilege to empty this enormous ditch, to demolish the toilet shack and clean up, but to do so camp style—that is, not with pumping tools but with our hands." Others, while ostensibly serving as prisoner-block physicians were assigned, as one of their main functions, "to transport cadavers—there were ten, twenty, thirty of them each morning in front of each barracks—to the cadaver depot."[1]

The improvement brought about by the new chief physician, Eduard Wirths, included the utilization of political prisoners who in some cases had experience of medical work in Dachau and other camps, but also a more professional SS medical contingent: the SDG corpsmen and among them the *Desinfektoren* who had been trained for both healing and killing. As an aid to combatting epidemics, the Hygienic Institute (see pages 304–5) was also brought to Auschwitz at about that time, and was to provide employment for knowledgeable prisoner physicians—"many famous professors from Prague and from Budapest and from everywhere," as the SS doctor Ernst B. put it.

But the greater number of prisoner physicians had to work on hospital blocks where, under the control of SS doctors, they were more vulnerable to being drawn into selections.

Some came to the medical blocks first as patients and learned quickly about medical selections, sometimes by going through them. Even when sent to work on these medical blocks, they were technically registered as patients, so that I. G. Farben could avoid paying for them as workers. And the first exposure to a medical block, when checking in as a patient, could take on the characteristics of a prisoner-doctor initiation rite. The Czech doctor Jacob R. told me, "I saw from the collecting room of the patients, the loading of the corpses in the cellar of the hospital—the way they were handled like logs. [It was] my first impression of what Auschwitz really was."

A working assignment as a doctor, especially for a Jewish inmate, could literally elevate one from the dregs of Auschwitz to a situation of special privilege. Dr. Michael Z., who spent two months on a *Kommando* carrying dirt back and forth in his jacket ("Always running and all the time there were *capos* who beat up on us"), was transferred to a new block, which "was reserved for the *Prominenz* ["celebrities"], for the V.I.P.'s, for the *capos,* for the block chiefs." When Dr. Z. became ill with typhus, he was protected from selections for a while by a colleague; and even when that failed and he was "put on a truck to the gas chamber," he was rescued by a Polish block chief "whom I had taken care of in the past."

Moreover, one could finally take *active* steps for one's own survival or that of others; and sometimes for getting oneself transferred to a better or less dangerous situation, one could make use of influence, have special access to food on the medical blocks, or even arrange that certain records be altered.

But a prisoner doctor quickly came to see the series of falsifications that underlay the medical structure. These included elaborate falsification of the cause of death, not only for prisoners selected for phenol injections or the gas chambers, but even for special executions ordered by the Political Department and carried out in medical blocks by means of phenol injections. In the latter, there could be arrangements resembling those of the "euthanasia" project, as Dr. Jan W. made clear: "Telegrams, . . . official forms, statements to the family—the exact time of death in hours and minutes, though the victim died four days earlier, . . . the cause of death . . . this or that—pneumonia, for instance." However appalled by the world of SS doctors, prisoner doctors had no choice but to adapt to it.

For Dr. Henri Q., what Nazi doctors did was "an abomination" of medicine by "men who were trained to heal, help, relieve suffering and prolong life, and there they did just the opposite." A prisoner doctor, aware of how little he or she could do, could feel (as Dr. Gerda N. put it) like "a prisoner in a camp [who] had a [medical] degree but really didn't do [the] work of a physician." Prisoner doctors had to connect with, even as they struggled to attenuate, the Auschwitz medical reversal of healing and killing.

Whatever their privileged state, prisoner doctors were constantly reminded of Auschwitz truths and of the extreme danger just underneath any apparent security. Dr. Q., for instance, remembered one Sunday morning:

> We had seen parades of deported women [women inmates] for three hours. They were coming from the crematoria to the station. Each woman was pushing a child's baby stroller. . . . And those were the strollers that their children had been taken to the gas chambers in. They were taking them back to the station for the Germans to send to Germany to be used there. We understood, . . . but even we refused to believe this concrete image.*

SS doctors applied considerable pressure to involve prisoner doctors in the overall Auschwitz system because they needed the latter's coopera-

---

*It is not clear from this description how much the mothers understood about the deaths of their children, or whether the mothers themselves were destined for the gas chamber in accordance with the policy of killing mothers with children, or whether the incident occurred at a time when mothers were permitted to survive.

tion on many counts. For one thing, since only prisoner doctors were in direct touch with sick patients, especially typhus cases, their cooperation was necessary to control epidemics in the camp. As Ernst B. explained, before mid-1942 if several cases of typhus broke out in a particular area of the camp, "it was shut off. . . . All inmates were gassed (whether or not they showed signs of typhus). . . . Then it was disinfected, and one hoped it would work." But Dr. B. knew that prisoner doctors used "every available means to hinder the SS doctor in recognizing . . . an epidemic" and hid typhus cases or falsified diagnoses.

SS doctors sometimes more or less recruited prisoner doctors they thought would be useful to them. For instance, Dr. Magda V., although very young and medically inexperienced when arriving in Auschwitz in early 1942, was skillful with her hands, impressed an SS doctor who saw her perform an emergency tracheotomy, and was almost immediately made head woman prisoner doctor, a position of authority she retained during her entire stay in Auschwitz.

Similarly, Dr. Peter D., an accomplished otolaryngologist working in a small, outlying camp, saved the life of a fellow prisoner by diagnosing his condition as acute mastoiditis with extradural abscess (external to the brain membrane, the dura mater) and operated on him with carpenter's tools, the only instruments available. This was, in Auschwitz, a dangerously illegal act. Nonetheless, when the SS doctor in charge of the camp, Horst Fischer, found out about it, he quickly had Dr. D. transferred to a large hospital at Monowitz and given a special ward of fifteen beds for work on ear, nose, and throat cases, as well as appropriate surgical instruments.

These prisoner doctors were recruited, first of all, because the SS doctor needed to maintain actual medical work in the camp. In addition, many of the prisoner doctors knew the German language; and their knowledge was useful for certain kinds of reports and records, often false ones, which could be more important than actual medical treatment. Their recruitment could even depend on neatness. One prisoner doctor, for example, was tested by the SS doctor Bruno Weber, head of the Hygienic Institute, for his capacity to prepare an accurate, well-turned-out graph on the basis of numbers derived from work in the laboratory. This prisoner doctor was inspired to something close to perfection by the memory of "a young Frenchman" who had been similarly tested and whose graph was "a little fuzzy and had a few smudges from erasures" —resulting in his rejection. A few months later he was a *Muselmann*. [2]

But the most remarkable recruiting procedure of all was that of Dr. Wanda J., whose ability as a surgical gynecologist and hospital organizer was recognized while she was a prisoner at a different camp, and led to a visit from Dr. Enno Lolling, overall head of concentration-camp medical services. Lolling explained to her that she was to be transferred to Auschwitz under an unprecedented arrangement in which her hair would not have to be shaved and she would not have a number tattooed on her arm (in fact, she was given an Aryan rather than a Jewish number). It turned out that Dr. J. was needed to provide actual medical care for the women on the notorious Block 10, where various experiments were done.

Since the real medical work of Auschwitz—treatment of sick inmates—was inseparable from selections, when SS doctors involved prisoner doctors in the first they brought them at least to the periphery of the second. In so doing, the SS doctors sought to avoid recognition of their own guilt by bringing prisoner doctors as close as possible to the dirtiest of all medical work. To the extent that they could succeed in tainting those they ruled over, they felt themselves to be less tainted. In that way they could blur, at least for themselves, distinctions between victimizer and victim, between physician jailer and physician prisoner.

When discussing these matters, Dr. B. would revert to this view, emphasizing again his conviction, quoted earlier, that "all those who survived Auschwitz lived from the food that was taken away from the others."

Thus, the ultimate adaptation of prisoner doctors involved a *quid pro quo*—that is, "something for something." The "something" given by the SS via the SS doctors to prisoner doctors was, first of all, survival. And not only one's own survival but the capacity to contribute to the survival of others. Prisoner doctors were very clear about the relation of their medical status to staying alive: "If I were not in the hospital [as a doctor], I'd be dead too"; or, "For me to be a doctor has been life saving"; or, "We survived because of our profession."

One prisoner doctor tells of the concrete ways in which this was true:

> Bread was . . . the main currency, the symbol of power and status. . . . I realized that, as a doctor-nurse, I was sort of upper middle class in the camp society: the better fed I looked, the more authority I seemed to have. As a member of the [medical] staff, I received a double ration of soup and occasionally some extra bread. It was important to husband one's energy. I managed, following the example of my veteran co-nurse, to sneak a little after-lunch nap in a corner.[3]

One way prisoner doctors overcame this potential guilt toward other prisoners was by helping them.

The "something" gained by SS doctors from prisoner doctors involved the work of the camp, work that took them to the edge of selections—as another prisoner doctor put the matter self-laceratingly when he declared, "We did the work. They gave us something extra—extra food. . . . But [they said], 'You must help us. You must do the work.' They are shrewd. They know a lot about human psychology."

There were further paradoxes about what prisoner doctors did. Many of those who worked closely with SS doctors, and appeared to be actively collaborating in selections, were actually using their position to save as many people as possible. And those who expressed themselves vehemently, then and later, against any cooperation with SS doctors tended to have made their own adaptation, their own *quid pro quo* which had to include a measure of such cooperation.

The ultimate healing-killing paradox within which prisoner doctors lived was their recognition, at some level of consciousness, that as their capacity for healing increased (with the general improvement of medical and living conditions in Auschwitz), the gas chambers and crematoria were achieving their maximum function. Dr. Jacob R. had that paradox in mind when he contrasted (in the epigraph to this chapter) his own relatively favorable treatment ("nearly like a human being") with "the reality of the camp." Although he himself, according to later testimony, helped many fellow inmates medically and spiritually, he nonetheless expressed the moral dilemma of prisoner doctors. At one point, he said, "We could keep our values—basic values—our *medical* values," but another time: "The whole set of values [for prisoner doctors] was completely changed. One really didn't know what was right or wrong." To different degrees and in varying ways, both of his observations were true.

Dr. Ernst B. gave the SS doctor's point of view on how the latter needed help from the prisoner doctor even to perform "good" selections (that is, kill the weak and retain the relatively strong for working): "He [the SS doctor] personally treated absolutely no one. . . . How should he know on his own that he is selecting correctly? He can't. So he is dependent upon the chief of the prisoner physicians."

An SS doctor who "wanted to do it the easy way," Dr. B. further explained, would say to that ranking prisoner physician, "I need a list of one hundred people tomorrow." A reluctant prisoner physician would be encouraged by the SS doctor to pass along the requirement to a prisoner colleague, or the SS doctor might himself approach a different prisoner doctor he knew to be more compliant. If he thought he had received a "good list" so that . . . he could say, . . . when they were marching past, "Those are really the worst," he would continue to go about things that way. But if he considered himself to have received a "bad list," he would either turn to a different prisoner doctor or take the attitude, "Next time I'll do it myself."

Another kind of SS doctor—whom Dr. B. described as "the self-confident, responsible, ideologically absolute SS-firm type"—would check the patients' records, have them appear before him, and take over the entire process himself. But even that kind of SS doctor was likely to draw prisoner doctors into the process in some degree by asking them about the physical status of patients. In practice, SS doctors might go about matters a little more indirectly, seeking as much cooperation as possible from prisoner doctors in locating the weaker patients and making decisions. Prisoner doctors could find indirect ways of resisting some of these pressures, and avoid the dangerous position of becoming a specific target for an SS doctor's anger. A man with a sensitive conscience, Dr. Jacob R.

was so troubled that he wondered, "Should one continue to work and help the situation [facilitate the selections in that way] . . . or should one quit [get oneself transferred to a work *Kommando*] and know that another person . . . [would be] worse?"

Inmates, especially Jewish inmates, came to know how dangerous the medical block was. A Czech woman survivor, for instance, remembered with gratitude the first piece of advice she received in Auschwitz—"Stay out of the hospital"—and spoke of two forms of suicide in the camp: "To go to the [electric] fence or to go voluntarily to the hospital." In contrast, for an inmate to be assigned to *work* in the hospital was ideal: light, indoor work instead of the life-destroying outside work details, more available food, and a place of potential influence. Prisoners working there sought both to help people and to consolidate their own position.

But when medical facilities became severely overburdened, these privileged inmates could come to feel the whole situation as completely untenable, and some prisoner doctors (as Ernst B. explained to me) "were of the opinion that if a selection is done right, it is better for those involved [selected] than if they starved to death in the camp." While recognizing again the self-serving aspect of such a statement from an SS doctor, the dedicated prisoner physician Lottie M. confirmed the general principle:

> You saw them arrive. . . . The line went next to our camp, our sick [block], . . . and I said [to myself], "Oh, will they come into the camp or will they go to the gas chamber? If they come to the camp, how awful. No beds, no sheets, no food, nothing. It will be more and more." You see? And we couldn't stand it. We always said, "Oh if we are [able to stay at] the number we are now, . . . it's tolerable. But one more is already too much for us." So [at] the same time you hope that they won't come [t]here, though you know that if they don't, . . . there was no alternative besides the gas chamber. . . . And I say that is the big problem [in relation to later] . . . guilt feelings.

She was saying this as a woman of considerable candor and integrity making a personal confession. The fact that prisoner doctors could experience this ambivalence served to increase SS doctors' acceptance of their own deeper schism.

Dr. Magda V. conveyed the dedicated prisoner doctor's mixture of helplessness and reluctant acquiescence in overall triage:

> I asked the other girls [prisoner doctors] who were there. . . . You know, we said, how many are dying? All right—so, roughly we knew what we can show them [the SS doctors]. The rest, . . . we just tell them, look healthy . . . or stand up or do something or, you know, pull yourself together. They [the people close to death] will die anyhow. There was no chance of saving them, no chance. . . . If you selected . . . them, all right, so they were dead a day earlier or two hours earlier.

That degree of cooperation could save the lives of at least the relatively healthy patients.

Dilemmas

But the problem then was, as Dr. Jacob R. put it, "becoming part of the system—this was the most troubling thing." Dedicated to trying to help people, he told me with characteristic sadness and honesty of "the practice which haunts me all the time—which I have never spoken about . . . the practice of selections of . . . prisoners . . . unable to work." He went on to describe how certain patients would be very weak and show no improvement after days of hospitalization: "So sooner or later they would be [recognized as] unable to work—and we were unable to help. So they went off . . . to the gas chambers—controlled [selected] by the SS doctors. And we had to decide who he [the SS doctor] would see."

The dilemma for prisoner doctors was how much to become a part of the system (in Dr. R.'s words); how much to cooperate in selections. When requested or ordered by SS doctors to make lists of patients, prisoner doctors would often consult with one another to try to come to a common position—usually a compromise in which they would agree to limited cooperation (listing obviously emaciated patients) while struggling to save those they could.

They also had disagreements with each other, which, according to Dr. Lottie M., could be difficult to discuss candidly because of resulting feelings of pain, conflict, and anger toward one another. Thus, prisoner doctors were pressed by their Nazi medical rulers into a moral dilemma which, however resolved, had to result in a sense of guilt: one could save lives only by contributing to Auschwitz selection policies; one could avoid that involvement only by refusing to exercise one's capacity to save lives.

Pressures from Nazi doctors could cause prisoner doctors' behavior toward one another to swing from solidarity to silence to contention. So convoluted could matters become that one prisoner doctor's not helping out with a selection could be experienced by another as a form of betrayal. Dr. Gerda N., for instance, told me how she and a colleague served under their Jewish doctor friend and superior, who generally protected her two younger colleagues. They, in turn, would cooperate with her when she conveyed to them Mengele's orders for identifying sick patients: "We . . . tried to select the ones which were likely to die in a day or two." But on one occasion, she herself was particularly agitated and told them, "You have until tonight to give me . . . twenty-five people who have to be selected," because Mengele had demanded this. "And if you don't do it, he said he will shoot us." At that point, Dr. N. and her friend "broke down" and "decided to stop it [their cooperation]," and hid themselves until well past the deadline. Dr. N. was not clear exactly why they did this, but it had to do with a mixture of fear and resentment of her superior ("[She had all the] advantages [of status and authority]. She should do it [the selections] herself") and with frustration once more at being given this "responsibility" while her own medical side was cruelly destroyed ("We were not doctors at all. . . . We had no rights, . . . no drugs, . . . nothing. . . . We were like puppets"). When the superior finally located her two subordinates, Dr. N. said, "She was very angry . . . [at] how we let her do this thing alone, and [she said]: 'Do you think [it] is collegial to do such a thing?' "

Prisoner doctors used their connections with SS doctors to attempt every possible ploy to save people from selections. One prisoner doctor conveyed their combination of ingenious dedication ("We managed to conceal essential records and told patients to go to the bathroom") and something close to futility ("In this way, even if we could not do very much, they perhaps had a chance or at least could die a more or less natural death").

Friendly relations could also be cultivated with certain SDG noncommissioned officers, some of whom had been medical and theological students. A prisoner doctor described one who was considered especially decent and would say quietly, "It is likely that they will come [for selections] tomorrow." Others could be bribed so that requests that they help arrange for numbers to be changed in life-saving ways would be accompanied by envelopes with money.

Dr. Henri Q. stressed the importance of humor, telling of a middle-aged French-Jewish dentist who kept "making jokes, laughing, and telling us stories": "I told myself he was completely crazy." He would say such things to Dr. Q. as "Dear Marquis, at five o'clock we are to have tea together," making Q. wonder whether the dentist "did not realize what was going on here." But, in retrospect, he helped the prisoner doctors "by telling his stories"—that is, by creating a consistent debunking alternative, however unreal, to the terrible actuality.

One cannot overemphasize the sea of death in which prisoner doctors lived. In addition to constant selections, there were, especially during the early days, punitive roll calls on medical blocks in which everyone, no matter how sick, was forced outside to the front of the block, either to stand at attention or, if unable to do so, to lie on the ground. Even in cold weather they were dressed only in underwear and were sometimes doused with cold water, resulting in many deaths. One had to carry on as though life could be continued: "Strange how everybody knew and did not know the everpresent proximity of death."[4] Together with the daily routine was constant talk (and evidence) of "going up the chimney." Even as they committed themselves to the struggle to live, prisoner doctors could believe, as did Gerda N., "that the death sentence was given to all of us . . . [whether for] . . . today or tomorrow."

Threats and pressures from SS doctors could make that death sentence feel imminent. A prisoner doctor told how the SS doctor Fritz Klein kept demanding more information about sick patients in order to send larger numbers of them to the gas chamber, and so then added in his characteristically pained tones: "It's not honest in life to ask from a man such things. Maybe you have to be a holy man to say no. I'm not optimistic about my own behavior, you see. And still I am not a bad man. Really not. But life asks me, 'You or me?' and I say, 'Me.' "

Apart from selections, prisoner doctors had to engage in a certain amount of triage (in their case the actual medical kind) of their own. For instance, when Jan W., a young Polish doctor, could obtain a limited amount of invaluable typhus vaccine from his underground contacts, he did not simply dispense it on a "first come, first serve" basis. He avoided giving it to inmates whom he considered "too weak to recover" or who were in general elderly and infirm (precisely the people one would give the vaccine to under ordinary circumstances), and instead chose "people who were young and who would be helped by the vaccine." Moreover, Dr. W. favored his own "network of acquaintances," meaning Polish political prisoners like himself: "A friend from school in Krakow . . . is much closer to me than a Dutch Jew whom I saw for the first time in my life."

Another doctor, a Dutch Jew, had the same inclination toward favoring his own kind. He told of giving all twenty sulfa tablets he possessed to a man with erysipelas, and of thereby curing at least one person. But, this doctor added, "[He] was a Dutchman, of course. It was easier for me and for him. We could speak to each other and we understood each other. Should he have been a Pole, I don't know."

Aside from the question of one's own group, there was the constant moral and medical question of whether to spread the twenty or thirty tablets of sulfanilamide or other medication among ten people, and use up one's supply in a day without any effect; to two or three people, and perhaps give each a full day's dose but no more after that; or to one person, whom one could treat effectively over the several days necessary. As Dr. Erich G. put it: "This [was] the dilemma for doctors . . . every day."

There were at least three kinds of situation in which prisoner doctors felt it necessary to participate in killing. First, the killing on medical blocks of *capos* who murdered and beat other prisoners, as described by Dr. Fejkiel (pages 186–87). Such killing saved numerous lives—but was killing nonetheless: someone, usually a resistance leader or group, had to decide that a particular *capo* was "dangerous," and agree with others that he should be killed; and someone had to do the killing, usually a cooperative effort between a prisoner doctor and other inmates working on the medical block.*

Second, there were situations in which prisoner doctors felt certain patients had to be killed. Dr. Elie Cohen, in a book whose subtitle is "A

---

*There were resistance networks in Auschwitz, the most prominent of which was Communist-led. (See pages 388–90).

Confession," tells how, when he was in charge of a "lunatics' room," one of them escaped into the camp and caused a disturbance, leading the SS commandant to issue a warning that such things had better not happen again. Cohen's reaction, which he shared with a prisoner friend who worked with him, was that if they could not keep things quiet on the ward "we'll all be for the gas chamber." Since this mental patient was extremely difficult to control, the friend responded by questioning his "sacrificing 600 people for one lunatic!" The two men cooperated in the killing by injecting an overdose of insulin, and Cohen later wrote:

> On that occasion I . . . yes, I infringed the ethical rule that one is a doctor not to murder people, but to try to keep them alive, to try to cure them, help them. And . . . it's always the first step that counts. For a few weeks later, it happened again. But by that time I had far fewer moral scruples about going upstairs again and saying to V., . . . "Same old thing. We'll have to do it again."
> And we did too, and that man died as well.

There was no problem about reporting the matter:

> It was quite simple, of course, for you just filled in something on the deceased's cards. Pneumonia . . . anything you liked. For it was all a farce in that room. I kept a very neat chart for each patient, showing his temperature and even the medicines we were giving him. Or were *not* giving him rather, even though they were entered on his chart.[5]

Auschwitz could thus impose upon certain prisoner doctors some of the elements of the direct medical killing, or "euthanasia," program discussed in part I.

Cohen and other prisoner doctors struggled against the overall brutalization of an environment in which, as a former prisoner orderly told me, "the corrupting of all human and ethical standards took place so rapidly . . . that one had to be very stern to prevent the somewhat stronger prisoners hastening death of the weaker fellow prisoners." The extreme example was the behavior of hardened criminal psychopaths who joined with SS personnel in killing people on work *Kommandos*, after which prisoners would be sent out to bring back the corpses to fill in the necessary "rows of five" and obtain the proper count—sometimes taking place while the prisoner orchestra played the tune (mentioned earlier) of "That's How We Live Every Day" (*So leben wir alle Tage*).[6]

There was a third form of killing that certain prisoner doctors engaged in: abortions performed during various stages of pregnancy, and the killing of newborns after secret deliveries. These abortions and killing of newborns were done because women (especially Jewish women) discovered to be pregnant or to have given birth to an infant were killed by the SS. There have been many reports of these clandestine events. Dr. Gerda

N., for instance, told of a courageous prisoner physician whom she considered a "heroine of abortions."

On one occasion, Dr. N. herself was present when the Hungarian doctor induced labor in a woman who was not far from delivering.* As Dr. N. said, the Hungarian doctor's focus was to "save the life of the woman," and "she [the doctor] did it at the risk of her own life," depending upon the fact that "nobody talked—there was . . . a silent conspiracy." Dr. N. spoke of the psychological pain of everyone involved: "For the mother [it was] something terrible. But it was strange enough—the women in the end agreed. Some said no, I don't want it. They [would] rather die together with the children. But at the end they all agreed. Some of us said, 'Oh you can have another baby still [in the future], and so on.' "

There were other accounts of newborns left in the block to die and of others being strangled or suffocated in order to avoid detection. For Dr. N. stressed that, had the SS found out, they would have insisted that the Hungarian doctor and helpers—and not they (the Nazis) themselves—were "murderers."

Dr. Olga Lengyel has written poignantly about these matters in her book *Five Chimneys* (1947), where she describes the necessity, when infants were delivered on the medical block, to "make [them] pass for stillborn." She tells of sneaking a woman onto the block for a delivery: "[Afterward,] we pinched and closed the little tike's nostrils and when it opened its mouth to breathe we gave it a dose of a lethal product. An injection . . . would have left a trace." Of her own residual guilt, Dr. Lengyel says: "Yet I try in vain to make my conscience acquit me. I still see the infants issuing from their mothers. I can feel their warm little bodies as I held them. I marvel to what depths these Germans made us descend!" And who cannot be haunted by her terrible additional comment: "And so, the Germans succeeded in making murderers of even us."[7]

Dr. Cohen, in his "confession," commented more generally: "As a student, as a doctor, you . . . had such very different things in mind."[8]

---

*Dr. N. was not sure of the method employed ("I think she gave some [form of] injection") but saw her make use of a portable stand "like a little operating table" and "a little instrument . . . very primitive."

Chapter 12

Prisoner Doctors: Struggles to Heal

> One day I broke the syringe. I was terrified. It was a much worse crime to break a syringe than to kill a man. A syringe was worth more than a human life.
> —Auschwitz prisoner doctor

> Our pride—my pride—is to have been able to remain human there. . . . I believe we remained doctors in spirit in spite of everything.
> —Auschwitz prisoner doctor

"On a Certain Level Collegial"

Yet the prisoner doctors' impulse to heal persisted impressively. That impulse, in fact, bound them to SS doctors and created strange, contradictory, and yet important relationships between the two groups. As the SS doctor Ernst B. told me, Auschwitz regulations strictly forbade "fraternization" with prisoners; but, as he added, "the psychological fact is that men cannot live together without fraternization." Living together in this sense meant having to work together for at least some common goals.

Dr. B. also said that "the doctors wanted more hospital buildings; the others [SS Command] said fewer and more fueling of the fire [the killing]." Whatever the inconsistencies of SS doctors on that matter, the principle of more hospital facilities and more actual healing appealed to their sense of themselves as physicians even as it became consistent with official policy. And there were occasions when they allied themselves with prisoner doctors against representatives of command. For instance, Olga Lengyel told how Dr. Fritz Klein befriended her owing to their common Rumanian language and origin in Transylvania, and defended her against the threats of the notoriously cruel camp overseer Irma Grese. There was even a confrontation between the two SS officers when Klein called Dr. Lengyel out from a punishment roll call on a Sunday in order to bring her medications for patients, and succeeded in his purpose despite Grese's angry declaration: "Do not forget, Doctor, that I give the orders here!"[1] Yet Klein was the same Nazi medical ideologue who had compared killing Jews to getting rid of a gangrenous appendix (see pages 15–16).

There was one remarkable SS man—not a physician but an SDG non-commissioned officer named Wilhelm Flagge—who was associated by the prisoners *only* with healing. Flagge was always gentle and helpful with patients, constantly countering the influence of a cruel chief guard, Hanna Bormann (who would claim they were feigning illness in order to avoid work), by insisting on the autonomy of the medical division (as Dr. Lottie M. remembers): "You have no authority in here. It is my area. I say they stay." The fact that other SDG personnel inserted the gas and gave the phenol injections intensified inmates' gratitude toward Flagge.

In their degradation, prisoner doctors could be extraordinarily moved by the slightest expression of humanity emanating from their Nazi masters, and especially from Nazi doctors. Dr. Erich G. remembered with almost mythic intensity a brief encounter with a German doctor in the camp: "[He] shook hands with me. [He] was really human." And Dr. Gerda N. similarly spoke of a cherished memory of a "very young" German doctor whom she encountered after being evacuated from Auschwitz to another camp, and who asked to see the very sick children on her ward: "I suddenly saw in his eyes . . . tremendous pity. . . . He pitied those children who were there so sick without real treatment [and] he pitied me."

Medical teaching and learning patterns provided some of the most paradoxical aspects of these relationships, where the mentors were the prisoner slaves—Jewish, Polish, and German prisoner doctors—and the students were their jailer masters. For instance, when the SS doctor Horst Fischer, impressed with Dr. Peter D.'s surgical skills, decided to transfer him to the large Monowitz hospital and provide him with instruments and beds for his patients, the arrangements did not stop there. Dr. D. was required to let Fischer know whenever he planned to operate because Fischer insisted upon being there and in fact "scrubbing" (the term for the disinfection procedure one follows as part of a surgical team) and assisting in the operations. Dr. D. remembered Fischer as "a doctor who wanted to learn . . . [and] was interested . . . in everything [pertaining to the case]."*

Peter D. and other prisoner doctors told of Fischer's involvement in a situation of psychiatric learning as well. A Polish professor of psychiatry,

---

*But Dr. D. had to be careful with his assistant: once, when congratulating Fischer upon successfully completing his first mastoid operation under Peter D.'s supervision, the former replied angrily, "You make fun of me as if I were a mere student." And D. commented to me, "I have to say that, apart from his SS side, he was a real human being."

who had some knowledge of electroshock therapy, then quite new, demonstrated to Fischer an apparatus he had constructed with the help of the electrical section of the Monowitz subcamp. Fischer arranged for women considered to be in need of the therapy (because they were "mad" or emotionally disturbed in some way) to be brought to the professor for shock treatments. Again, Fischer was a conscientious student, attending most or all of the therapy sessions conducted by the professor, while the other prisoner doctors of the hospital attended only the first two (see pages 298–300.)

While collaborative efforts like these were unusual, the kind of medical bond they suggested was common enough. And however these bonds were tainted by the existence of selections, they meant a great deal to prisoner doctors and served a purpose for Nazi doctors as well.

There was sometimes even a suggestion that the bond was intensified by their having survived together the unpleasantness of the selections procedure. One prisoner doctor told of getting to know Dr. Klein, who performed selections every fortnight but "was very kind," and emphasized the bond they formed: "If you see a man every week and especially at the moments of the selections," you come to know him "very, very well." Dr. Magda V. clarified the matter: "It was something like what you read about the way victims of terrorists can feel about the people who took them prisoner." The bond, that is, is formed by extreme coercion and includes elements of a sense of shared fate, at least temporarily.*

The bond required the prisoner doctors to move into realms of numbing and derealization inhabited by the SS doctors. Dr. Magda V., for instance, demonstrated considerable skill both in medical areas and in handling pressures from Nazi doctors; but when I asked her about her knowledge of phenol injections (see chapter 14), she said that she was "so numb" that she did not "take in details. . . . Somebody said something, but it was . . . unreal." Similarly, about selections and other aspects of experience: "The whole thing was utterly unreal, . . . and I'm sure that I'm not the only one who had the feeling that you were in a kind of ivory tower and it [was] not happening."

Dr. Jacob R., who spoke of Nazi doctors as being at times "on a certain level collegial," also told me that, for him and other prisoner doctors, "it was impossible to live in Auschwitz without a sort of emotional anesthesia." Not until almost twenty years later, when called to testify at a trial taking place in England, did he overcome that anesthesia: "It was a terrible shock to be confronted with [Auschwitz victims], . . . their life stories, . . . the experimentations. . . . [At that time] my faculties were restored."

Dr. Erich G. spoke of a "psychic immune reaction," which was "like wearing an asbestos jacket, so that if there is a fire breaking out the fire

---

*She refers here to the kind of bond—known as the "Stockholm syndrome"—that has been observed to develop between hostage takers and hostages, in which the shared death encounter can be a central factor.

does not affect you." Moreover, "he who could not get this [psychic immune reaction] died." Nor could one, when confronted with selections, surrender the bond with Nazi doctors so necessary to one's own life and to one's capacity to save others.

While the bond was precarious in the extreme, and prisoner doctors never fully lost their image of all Auschwitz Nazis as murderers, there were some exceptionally positive relationships—for example, between a few prisoner doctors and two SS doctors in the Auschwitz Hygienic Institute, Ernst B. and Delmotte G. Several survivor doctors made clear to me that these two SS doctors were genuinely considerate to them, helped arrange illegal meetings with wives or family members in the camp, and could be trusted with personal confidences. But even in those unusual cases, prisoner doctors could hardly be completely relaxed.

Sometimes a Nazi doctor used such relationships for a kind of catharsis, for expressing (though hardly confronting) his feelings of guilt derived from participating in selections. Dr. Jan W., the Polish prisoner physician, described Werner Rohde (whom several inmates considered relatively decent) to be a "kind of German *Bosch,* * . . . more sociable [than other Nazi doctors]," and a man who treated prisoner doctors "more as fellow physicians." In addition,

> he [Rohde] sometimes even told of dreams that he had the previous night. I'll tell you about one of those dreams. He came in one day and told us, "What a dream I had last night. It was a terrible dream. I dreamt that [I saw] fried Jewish heads—Jewish heads on a frying pan." This was immediately after a selection in which a large number of people were gassed and burned.

Rohde's dream probably reflected a combination of guilt feelings, death anxiety, and a degree of sadism. Such a confession could be made only to Polish or possibly German prisoner doctors. But this apparent freedom did not mean that they could be casual in their response to the SS doctor's catharsis.

The ostensible collegueship with the SS doctor could be perceived as entrapment. One prisoner doctor told how Klein would sometimes address him as *"Herr Kollege"* or *"Herr Doktor Kollege,"* how "friendly" and "very kind" Klein was, and how Fischer, Klein, and Rohde "were quite normal to us" and "talked medicine with us." This man's point was that he and other prisoner doctors were manipulated and exploited in the relationship:

> They didn't lash us. No, not at all. There was no need for them to do it because we were very obedient. We were slaves. You always stood to attention [here he clicked his heels and brought himself to attention

---

Bosch was a First World War derogatory term for a German but here also suggests a rough-hewn, spontaneous person.

to demonstrate this military subservience]. . . . We did the work. . . . So you can control a whole country with a very few men. You put the right boys [in] the right place.

Dr. Peter D. put a more positive value on the relationship: Fischer became "a friend and colleague to such an extent that he would never take someone from my work to send to the camp [select for death]." Dr. Magda V. was struck by the use of such relationships to "kind of spread the responsibility" in a situation within which "everybody pushes the responsibility on someone else." But for SS doctors there was also the principle that Dr. B. has mentioned: their need to "escape into this illusion . . . that they were doing good professional medical work."

SS Doctors and Women Prisoner Doctors

SS doctors' relationships with women prisoner doctors were complex and could include elements of "chivalry" and at times even affection, but also deception and danger. Rohde in particular could, as Dr. Lottie M. put it, view the camp as a "war of German men against Jewish men, . . . [but he] somehow helped the women and protected them."[2] She and others reported that he "was very much in love with our Jewish chief doctor . . . [and] very impressed by her" in ways that enabled her to have considerable influence with him. Dr. M. described Dr. V. as a "good-looking and very intelligent woman"; and there were widespread rumors among inmates that she became Rohde's mistress. Some inmates attributed Magda V.'s seemingly privileged status to this alleged affair, and it was a factor in an attempt to bring charges against her in Czechoslovakia after the war. On the basis of having been observed working closely with SS doctors and going around with them, she was accused of complicity in selections—an accusation Dr. M. considered "simply crazy," because, as she pointed out, Dr. V. was really doing everything possible to save lives.

Lottie M. and Magda V., during separate interviews with me, expressed regret that Rohde was hanged immediately after the war as they considered him, respectively, "a better one" compared with other Nazi doctors, and "in his own way a thoroughly decent chap." Dr. V. somewhat exaggerated Rohde's virtue, maintaining the impression that "he refused to do selections and went to the Russian front" (which was not the case). She also said she chastised him for giving opinions, presumably negative, about Jews without having known any: "How can you talk about the Jews?" At the same time, she ridiculed accusations of both collaboration and sexual liaison with Rohde, stressing the Nazi principle of *Rassenschande* ("racial disgrace or crime") that would apply to sexual relations with a Jew: "I was only a *Häftling* [prisoner], for crying out loud!" and,

"You have to visualize the situation." It seemed clear to me that Dr. V. had been neither collaborator nor mistress. But in speaking of how Nazi doctors looked approvingly on her poise and linguistic and medical abilities and considered her to be "fair" and "doing a job in a good way," she revealed once more the potential taint in any relationship a prisoner doctor made with SS doctors. Another prisoner doctor may have characterized the bond most accurately when he spoke of Dr. V. as a "mother-confessor to Rohde."

Dr. Lottie M. owed her life to Rohde. When she became extremely ill with typhus, Rohde announced to the prisoner doctors who took care of her, "I don't want her to die," and saw to it that she received good care and nourishing food. He went so far as to bring her first a dress, and upon her further request a brassière, so that she could get out of bed. All this was not lost on the *capos* and SS personnel, who "felt that [she] was protected by him . . . and that they shouldn't interfere with that." His friendly attitude toward her began when he learned that she had done university and medical studies in the same place as he, and he responded with enthusiastic reminiscences and questions about professors, restaurants, and shops. Rohde apparently found Dr. M. to be bright and attractive as well, so that, as she put it, "I didn't feel close to him, but he did to me." She had no great respect for him, describing him as "silly, . . . a . . . good-looking sports type, . . . no bright ideas"; but she had still further reason to be grateful for him: "The funny thing was, he always tried to get me free." He felt that, as a non-Jewish German, she should be helped to leave Auschwitz, and with that in mind even arranged for her to talk with a new commander. When she came back from the meeting discouraged, explaining to Rohde that the new subcamp commander "seems to be a great anti-Semite [she had been imprisoned partly for helping Jews]," Rohde replied, "Well, we are *all* anti-Semites." Dr. M. told him she had not had that impression about him, to which he answered, "Well, in the camp the situation is different." He was saying—in still another manifestation of Auschwitz healing-killing schizophrenia—that the "informality" of the camp permitted one to be more relaxed with individual Jews (as he was with Dr. V.) even as one subjected them to mass murder as a group.

Rohde attempted to convey to Dr. M. his reluctance concerning selections and his need to drink in order to perform them. While protective toward favored prisoner doctors such as Lottie M. and Magda V., he seemed to want them to share the numbing he could induce in himself through drinking. Thus once when a block was sealed off for selections (*Blocksperre*), Rohde observed Dr. M. peeking out at the prisoners being dragged into lorries and taken away to be killed, and said with some agitation, "Why do you [try to] see it? Aren't you lucky that you needn't look at that? It's better not to look."

Dr. Klein—who, as Dr. Ella Lingens-Reiner told me, was a *"real"* anti-Semite—was delighted to discover that she was not Jewish and was Ger-

man. Because he would seek her out and "liked to talk with me," there
were also rumors among inmates of an affair between them. Actually Dr.
Lingens-Reiner felt that she had to be careful to placate him. But she was
sufficiently comfortable with him (as Dr. B. pointed out) to be able to
raise the question that led to his "gangrenous appendix" remark:

> Klein was there at a time when they were gassing . . . very much.
> . . . Then you saw the crematorium. You saw the black smoke and the
> fire—even the fire coming out of the huge chimneys. And I was stand-
> ing there and looking at it and Klein next to me. And then I said, "I
> wonder, Dr. Klein, that you can carry out this business. Are you never
> reminded of your Hippocratic oath?" And he said, "My Hippocratic
> oath tells me to cut a gangrenous appendix out of the human body. The
> Jews are the gangrenous appendix of mankind. That's why I cut them
> out."*

Actually Klein's romantic interest was focused on an attractive young
Polish doctor, with whom five women prisoner doctors shared a room.
While (in Dr. Lottie M.'s view) there was no physical relationship here
either, Klein got into the habit of appearing in the room early on Sunday
morning, while the women were still in bed, in order to "flirt" with the
attractive Polish doctor, mostly by describing his political views at some
length ("His . . . idea was that the Poles should unite with the Germans
and go against the Russians"). And Dr. M. went on to explain in a way
that said something about the basic nature of these relationships: "We
didn't want to die, you see, so we stayed in bed until he had finished his
flirt with this lady." Klein was transferred from the women's camp when
an SDG noncommissioned officer happened to walk in on one of his
Sunday-morning visits and, as Dr. M. put it, "made mention to the head
of the . . . camp that this Dr. Klein is on too good terms with prisoners."

Eva C., an artist who was in her late teens in Auschwitz and also very
attractive, tells of a relationship with another SS doctor, Hans Wilhelm
König, that saved not only her own life but her mother's as well. She
described, not without affection, her first impression of König as "a
nebisha [Yiddish for 'unimpressive' or 'nonentity'] SS man, looking like
Don Quixote, with his sleeves too short," and told how he began to
appear every day at the little office where she did her medical drawings,
and chat with her pleasantly about everything except "subjects concerning the camp—that was a no-no."

In early 1944, she heard (through a relationship she had with a male
prisoner who was the block senior) of the plan to gas the entire Czech-
Jewish family camp of which they were a part, and told the news to König
when he next appeared after a couple of weeks of absence. Shortly afterward, almost certainly at König's instigation, she was called before Men-

---

*This was her remembered version of the conversation also quoted in her book (see
pages 15–16).

gele so that her number could be taken to be included among those very few who were to be permitted to survive. Her insistence that she would not consider "staying alive alone" was interpreted to Mengele by another prisoner doctor present as meaning that she had a mother in the camp who was still young and strong and could work; and Mengele, after first protesting, gave in and took the mother's number as well. And, at the second and liquidating selection of the Czech family camp soon afterward, König not only arranged for mother and daughter to survive once more but, when the prisoners were forced to march naked before the SS doctors, much to Eva C.'s humiliation (all the more so because she knew them): "I [could] catch a glimpse of [König's] eyes looking straight in my eyes and no place else, and I was very grateful for that." She sensed that he was reassuring her that "things would be all right, that he was a friend": "I felt he cared."

But her evaluation of König's attitude was: "He made me a kind of pet, . . . and when there was a kind of skit when the lower SS people had a special party with the higher SS people—there were amusing skits—I heard about it—in which he was teased because of always bringing presents—cigarettes, food, and so on, to the 'beautiful artist.' " Her persistent ambivalence concerning the relationship emerged in what is for a survivor an ultimate question: "He saved me. But I sometimes wonder, if I had the chance to save his life, whether I would."

In these relationships, women prisoner doctors could uncover pockets of humanity in Nazi doctors and thereby save lives. At times they could do so by means of a calculated psychological attitude. Dr. Lottie M., for example, who had studied with the early psychoanalyst August Eichhorn, tried to apply to SS men, and even Nazi doctors, what Eichhorn had emphasized as the best attitudes with which to approach juvenile delinquents:

> Either say something very severe in content, and friendly in the way of saying it—or the opposite, you say [something] friendly but in a strict way. . . . So [Eichhorn] said, "If you have this little boy, you say, 'Well, Franky [in a stern tone], it's the last time that I'll help you out of this mess.' Or, you say [in a soft tone], 'Frank, you know that I like you— I think you are a nice and clever boy—but what you have now done is impossible and I have to punish you.' " . . . And I thought—well all of the SS people are like that, so the best way would be to treat them like that.

She combined those approaches with occasional surprise, candor, and even humor. (When an SS doctor overheard her referring to him in a derogatory way in French, which she had not thought he understood, and said threateningly to her, "Have you finished complaining about me?" she replied, "No, I have not finished but, if you wish, I will interrupt myself and stop," causing him to look astounded and to slam the door and leave the room.) She acknowledged, "You had to be in a certain position" to act so boldly (she was German and non-Jewish and also held a leading medical position); but she had learned to use such attitudes, she added, not only from Eichhorn but from Magda V., a Jewish woman prisoner doctor who was notably poised in her relationships with SS doctors.

Magda V. herself, in further discussing Rohde, made an observation about psychological influence: "I might have influenced Rohde without knowing [it]. . . . Maybe I inhibited Rohde. . . . It's very, very difficult to kill somebody whom you know for five years or . . . five days. . . . You develop a certain association." But she had to admit that saving lives was extremely difficult; "Everything was really very quick. . . . They were selected, and half an hour later, they were up in smoke."

Medical Values and Medical "As If"

SS doctors' deception and hypocrisy were pervasive. Dr. V. told how Klein "pretended to be nice" and was "everyone's picture of a family doctor, . . . smallish, roundish, . . . a nice family-type of doctor who was very concerned about you." And when a woman with a fifteen-year-old daughter once complained to him about their not receiving treatment from V. herself, Klein patted the child's head and told the mother, "My dear, not to worry. . . . You're going to hospital. I'm going to look after you." But V. "knew what it meant: the gas chamber for both." She further asked, "How can a doctor who's trained to save lives do this?"

The sequence she perceived, at whatever level of consciousness, was something like this: He and I are both physicians committed to healing; he not only violates our oath but does it while pretending to be a kindly healer; I must depend upon him in order to survive and remain a genuine healer, but to do so requires me to become enmeshed in what he is doing and to run the risk of becoming like him.

Here a key theme in the prisoner doctors' struggle was what Dr. Jacob R. called "keeping one's medical values" as a means of "keeping alive as a human being" and "resist[ing] accept[ance] of the values of the camp." One could combine a certain numbing with low-key activity, so that for this doctor, "it was . . . not important to be a leading personality" but preferable rather to focus on quietly helping patients and "to do what is possible under the general circumstances."

The difficulty was that they had to work within a medical structure that was both part of the killing and built on deceptions of the medical "as if" situation. As Dr. Henri Q. put it:

> In the hospital that the Germans have finally created for the inmates, . . . a temperature chart, an observation sheet is much more important

than a human life. It is not necessary to treat a patient well, but one has to mention on the observation form [medical chart] that he received all the medication required for his condition, so that the Germans can prove to the world afterward, black on white, that if he died, it was because he was weak and not as a sequel of the poor treatment he was subjected to.

Prisoner doctors were especially drawn into the illusion of medical authenticity in their connections with Nazi doctors, as Dr. M. has made clear in describing her working arrangements with Mengele:

> I act[ed] as if it were a normal hospital, though I kn[e]w it [was] not. But . . . when Mengele entered the block, I said, "May I show you this patient? . . . Could I take this one to the men's camp for [an] operation because we have no surgery but the men's camp ha[s]. . . ." I showed him ten of these patients. He said yes or no and went away. And it all had the forms of the normal head doctor's visit.

Lottie M. had a certain standing as a German non-Jew. Gerda N., a Jewish doctor, told me of her own pain concerning questions of "responsibility" and described as a "farce" her and other inmates' attempts at medical work. With virtually no medication ("We got ten aspirins a day for a block of thousands"), they were expected to treat patients with the most severe and debilitating symptoms. The resulting sense of helplessness was magnified and infused with guilt and frustration by expectations that could not be fulfilled: "What can a doctor do . . . with nothing in his hands? . . . There's even no water . . . but we still had to . . . do [things] as if we were responsible for something. . . . [To] be responsible for something you cannot take the responsibility [for], . . . it's sort of . . . schizophrenic, . . . very schizophrenic."

Like Dr. Ernst B., Dr. N. used the term "schizophrenic" to describe the reversals and confusions of healing and killing—of attempts at, and claims for, the former in the face of the latter. But she went further in revealing the terrible psychological consequences of those healing-killing paradoxes for a prisoner doctor clinging to a sense of medical responsibility. Without directly saying so, she suffered from the Nazi doctors' sinister extension of the idea of responsibility to encompass culpability and blame: they accused prisoner doctors of being "responsible" for patients' deaths as a way of exonerating themselves and other camp authorities. This pattern of "blaming the victim" (in this case the physician-healer-victim) was, as we shall see, psychologically important to Nazi doctors; but here we may note especially its potentially devastating psychological impact on prisoner doctors, even when they were consciously aware that the accusation was absurd.

A related contradiction was the experience of providing, with SS doctors' encouragement, extensive and ultimately successful treatment for patients, who were then murdered. Dr. Henri Q. told of cases involving "complex open fractures, complex reduction [bone-setting] apparatus, and osteosynthesis [operation for uniting the fractured ends of a bone]," in which treatment was elaborate and painstaking: "And when they would be cured, they were killed—because they were weak." And Dr. Jan W. described a similar pattern in which Friedrich Entress, notorious for his zeal in conducting selections, was taught a surgical procedure by a Polish prisoner doctor, which the SS doctor, in turn, performed on patients. But

> if the treatment had to last longer than a very brief convalescence, even after a successful operation, he [Entress] would consider the patient a burden on the hospital, affecting the rate of turnover in the hospital. So, even then, after the operation performed by this SS doctor who learned the art in this way, he could just as swiftly send the patient to the gas chamber or to an injection of phenol.

This schizophrenic contradiction between healing and killing remained until the end. As Jacob R. said:

> My last duty in Auschwitz [before he was transferred to Buna] . . . was typical of the attitude of negating reality—of the prisoners and of the SS too. The Russians were coming nearer and nearer. And [yet] we prepared a course of lectures for doctors in camp [telling them how] to be better prisoner doctors. That was September 1944. . . . We were ordered [to do it] by the SS doctors, very much against the idea [opposition] of the orderlies. It was a matter of power position.

It was also a matter of maintaining the Auschwitz "as if" medical situation, a deception in which prisoner doctors were required to be key figures. Dr. Erich G.'s observation that Nazi doctors "could not suppress all humanity" may have a double truth: they could not suppress *all* of their own humanity; much less could they suppress that of their prisoner-physician-slaves.

Remaining Healers

Mostly prisoner doctors struggled to work together in ways that could sustain life. Besides their "caucuses" on establishing policies toward selections, in different ways—as Dr. Gerda N. said in connection with her contacts with other women doctors—"they were just great, . . . as hungry, . . . thirsty, . . . [and] under the threat of being put to death as all the others were, but still they functioned [to help others]."

While their lives were sometimes saved by grateful patients, prisoner doctors were more likely to be saved by one another. Dr. Erich G. told of a colleague, now a lecturer in biology in Eastern Europe, who, when in Auschwitz, lost his motivation to live and would certainly have died except for two interventions on the part of prisoner colleagues. On one occasion, G. himself grabbed his friend after spotting him walking toward the electric fence; and on another, a third colleague took him from a group of people selected for the gas chamber (the depressed man had sought the selection), "gave him a slap in the face, . . . hauled [him] away, and he survived." That mutual expectation of support could carry over from Auschwitz to postwar life, as in the case of another colleague G. helped save after the latter's health had deteriorated so far he was almost a *Muselmann.* Years later, this man, then ill and working in the same medical department as G., came to him and said, "Please save my life the way you did in Auschwitz."

Another aspect of Auschwitz healing was the necessity for prisoner doctors to falsify diagnoses in order to prevent patients from being selected for death. Dr. Michael Z., for instance, told how, when working in the bacteriological laboratory of the Hygienic Institute, "I often gave false results because when there were cases of Koch bacilli, . . . tuberculosis, . . . [or] malaria, [if I did not report] negative results, . . . it was automatically the gas chamber. . . . [So] I took it upon myself, when I knew it was an inmate, to give a result that would not harm him." Again, Z. and other prisoner doctors took advantage of the SS doctors' ignorance and distaste for sick inmates. For example, prisoner doctors (when working on the hospital block) would diagnose actual typhus cases as flu, knowing that these patients were "dirty . . . and full of wounds, sores," and that the SS doctors would not come near them: "Then it was easy to tell them [the SS doctors] stories."

But at other times, saving lives depended upon struggling to establish the true diagnosis—as when SS doctors wrongly diagnosed typhus in people whose fever was actually due to pneumonia. Dr. Rudolf Vitec testified about one such situation, when he was unable to prevent these misdiagnosed patients from being sent to the gas chamber, and was himself transferred to a corpse-carrying detachment for remonstrating with SS doctors.[3]

Also necessary was for prisoner doctors to learn to refuse certain requests, as well as the proper way to refuse. Dr. Z. resisted the ultimate threat to his healing identity—the strong suggestion on the part of a prisoner functionary that he give lethal phenol injections. Dr. Z. insisted, "I do not know how, . . . and what I do not know how to do I cannot do." He had apparently sensed (correctly) that inability rather than opposition was the attitude that enabled one to resist without dire consequences.

In order to remain healers, prisoner doctors had to exploit SS doctors' antagonisms and rivalries. Dr. Wanda J. believed that she was able to put together good hospital facilities on notorious Block 10 (the experimental block) "because it was all mixed up" and "because they hate[d] each other. . . . [Wirths] hated Professor Clauberg. . . . Professor Clauberg hated him. He hated Höss. Höss hated him. And so it's a farce."

Dr. J. was given a special opportunity to exploit the situation when Höss's mistress was admitted to the medical block with tuberculosis of the hip following an earlier abortion for a four-month pregnancy (see page 201). Dr. J. immediately gave all this information to Wirths because "I was Wirths's woman" (she worked under his authority, and he went to some lengths to protect her), and because "the underground [of which she was a part] of the camp was living on hate between Höss and Wirths." She learned from Wirths's prisoner secretary, also in the underground, that Wirths had quickly called Berlin in order to make use of the information; and without knowing the consequences, she felt that it was "our good luck that they were fighting."

When a relatively friendly SS doctor like Rohde, as Dr. Jan W. put it, permitted "very little distance between him and prisoner doctors . . . and [a] spirit of professional people at work," prisoner doctors had to exploit that spirit and at the same time keep it limited in order to distance themselves from selections and remain healers. As Dr. Henri Q. explained, "We suffered and [acted] within the limits of the possible. . . . Doctors did provide some comfort, I believe. There was the comfort for the patient and the fact that he was not alone, that someone understood and was trying to help to do something for him—and that was already a lot. . . . We were a group, not just the [individual] doctors of our block." He could then conclude (as in the epigraph to this chapter) that he and his friends "remained doctors . . . in spite of everything."

Helping children could greatly contribute to the prisoner doctors' struggle to maintain a healing identity. Dr. Henri Q., for instance, told of the impact of a nine-year-old boy from a Jewish ghetto in Poland, who "made such a racket on the truck that was to take him to the gas chamber that the SS took him out" and permitted him to do errands for them. The doctor added proudly that the boy had been on his block and "is still alive and we see each other often . . . in Paris." He spoke even more intensely of a still younger Russian child ("a rare thing in the camp") whom he once took to the infirmary:

I walked in front of all the blocks, and you could feel all the men, over ten thousand men, who were looking at this child. I was very proud to walk with him, . . . as if I were walking with the president of the Republic. There is only one president and there was only one child.

Chapter 13

Prisoner Doctors: Collaboration with Nazi Doctors

> We would accept being mistreated by locksmiths, barbers, common criminals, etc. . . . but that a fifty-year-old [prisoner] physician could strike younger colleagues in the most brutal manner, and that he would send them to the gas chamber, that seemed to us a monstrosity.
>
> —Auschwitz prisoner doctor

A few prisoner doctors came to identify themselves sufficiently closely with Nazi doctors and camp authorities to be viewed as collaborators. Such collaboration could be related to the anti-Semitism of various national groups and to antagonisms between ordinary criminals and political prisoners, and among Jews themselves.

Long-standing Polish anti-Semitism loomed especially large. Dr. Jacob R., a Jew with much understanding for others, spoke of the "nationalistic and anti-Semitic" Polish doctors and the even worse prisoner orderlies, who "really abuse[d] Jews . . . in a way that caused people to suffer and to die." While some Jews had their own antagonisms to Poles, it was the latter who arrived first in Auschwitz and who were given inmate positions of relative authority, including medical authority. While the Poles suffered grievously, their intelligentsia being a particular target for direct and indirect Nazi killing, they were "Aryans" (although Slavs) and certainly not an anti-race like the Jews. Some Poles could make common cause with Nazi authorities in being (as one prisoner doctor put it) "so anti-Semitic they didn't care about Jews being gassed or getting [fatal] injections" because "they had the feeling they were some kind of superior being." Hence, many Polish prisoners engaged in the Auschwitz pattern of violence toward Jews—in the form of (sometimes lethal) physical beatings—and some Polish doctors got into the habit of slapping or imparting a few blows, with Jewish physicians among their victims. Jews in authority could also on occasion "slap one another"; but (as Dr. Erich G. put it) for "the Polish or the others to strike a Jew, it was no problem." Even when Polish colleagues behaved "in a very correct manner," (as a Czech woman survivor explained), they could be perceived by Jews as condescending: "We knew they were anti-Semitic."

The entire Auschwitz structure—its death sentence for Jews—contributed to deadly callousness toward Jews, as a Polish survivor who worked in a medical block described in partly defending Polish doctors:

> Consider the situation of a young [Polish] doctor or [advanced] medical student. He knows that 90 percent of Jews will be put to death sooner or later, and the same percentage of *Muselmänner* [in general]. He had to fill quotas. If he had refused, he wouldn't have helped anyone and would have died himself—and another person would be put immediately in his place to do what he refused to do. . . . People grow indifferent to certain things. Like the doctor who cuts up a dead body [does a post-mortem examination] develops a certain resistance.

This Auschwitz death taint greatly intensified the pre-existing antagonism of some Polish doctors toward all Jews, including patients; and there were frequent stories of the former's efforts to have Jewish doctors transferred from medical blocks to places in the camp likely to result in their death. While these attempts were generally successful, they were sometimes defeated by appeals to other prisoners with influence and, on at least one occasion, to Dr. Wirths himself.

Occasionally a Jewish doctor who had some authority, such as Magda V., could speak frankly to Polish colleagues: "Look, we are all equal here. . . . I can't have it [anti-Semitic attitudes] here. . . . We're all in the same boat." As she explained, "[They knew] that I would stick my neck out for the Poles the same way I would . . . for the Jews, and I told them that." And she emphasized that many Polish colleagues were "all right" and some even "fantastic" in their help to everyone. Other Jewish doctors told of their lives being saved by strong interventions on the part of Polish colleagues. But for the most part Jews, including Jewish doctors, had to be wary of Polish authority as well as of pervasive anti-Semitism in Polish doctors and functionaries, which contributed in a variety of ways to Jewish deaths.

Polish-Jewish struggles intertwined with profound conflicts between political prisoners and ordinary criminals. The latter brought about much suffering and death until the political prisoners gradually took over, their medical contingent spearheaded by a group of German Communists transferred from Dachau where they had been associated with Wirths, an effective contact they were able to maintain in Auschwitz. The struggle could become violent, including arrangements in medical areas (as Dr. Tadeusz S. described) "to send . . . to their deaths" criminal *capos* who killed and beat inmates. Over time, SS doctors tended to support the political prisoners, as they helped maintain better medical arrangements and better organization in general.

Jewish doctors had conflicts with one another: for example, more experienced women doctors resented Dr. V., who was given considerable authority upon her early arrival in Auschwitz despite having only recently completed her medical studies. Others understood (as Dr. Lottie M. explained) that "this is no normal medical performance . . . and she's a good organizer and [handled things] in a very clever way" useful to other prisoner doctors. There were other antagonisms between Jewish doctors of different nationalities, including feelings on the part of French doctors that they as a group should be in charge of a medical block, and resentment when a doctor from one group thought that a doctor from another was "threatening me with Mengele"—that is, attempting to use a relatively close relationship with an SS doctor to enhance his or her own position.

Doctors were susceptible to sudden humiliations concerning their Jewishness: Michael Z. was assigned to the Gypsy camp but "stayed [only] a very short while because a decree was issued stating that Jews did not have the right to take care of Gypsies." Furthermore, under certain circumstances (on particular blocks and during a relatively early Auschwitz phase), Jewish doctors could be in considerable danger from their own "élite" patients, Polish and German *capos* for whom they had to serve as orderlies. "They would sometimes give us our daily round of blows [as] . . . their way to acknowledge our care," Dr. Z. observed; and he wondered, "How many [Jewish] university professors, physicians did we see killed by their patients?"

Jewish doctors also faced resentment from ordinary Jewish prisoners, who complained about the superior or "faceless" attitude on the part of some Jewish doctors and their inclination to give curt orders rather than be considerate or even offer a smile ("They don't shoot people normally for a smile"). And one Jewish survivor told me how her infant, a twin, became ill. Hearing of a "famous professor" from Eastern Europe, she carried the sick infant across the camp but could not get the doctor to make an examination, and the child died ("I don't say he could have saved him, but he didn't even try. . . . He neglected his responsibility as a doctor").

Although privileged compared with other Jewish prisoners, Jewish doctors could share with them the sense of being in overwhelming danger at all times—and from virtually everyone. One prisoner doctor recognized that "there were good people" among the Poles, but his more general feeling was that "the Poles were anti-Semitic, all the Poles," and

he described hearing them say, upon the arrival of Jewish transports:
"For us Poles, Hitler has one good side—he is freeing us from Jews."
Although he knew there to be admirable people in the resistance "from
all over Europe," all the "non-Jewish prisoners were anti-Semitic, . . .
merely with different nuances."

Four Medical Collaborators

It was inevitable that at least a few prisoner doctors would cross the line
into what was perceived by other inmates to be active collaboration with
the SS. We will examine four of them—three Poles and a German Jew—
each identified with a particular form of collaboration: respectively, selections, experimental operations, physical violence, and "Jewish collaboration." These four patterns of collaboration tell us much about not only
the men themselves but the Nazi doctors who orchestrated the collaboration and the Auschwitz environment where it occurred.

All four of them were men, probably for several reasons: the greater
number of male prisoner doctors, the greater authority given them in
general, and perhaps the greater capacity of women doctors—as women
—to adapt flexibly to Auschwitz and, specifically, to SS doctors without
succumbing (or at least doing so less extremely and less frequently) to
the lure of a "power position" in the Auschwitz hierarchy.

Performing Selections: Adam T.

Adam T. was the only one of the four medical collaborators still alive.
I found him not in Poland but in Germany, where he had been living since
the end of the war, having even Germanized his last name. Dr. Jacob R.
echoed other prisoner doctors in describing him as "an opportunist
. . . and anti-Semite"—a judgment R. somewhat qualified by adding, "All
of us preferred to help ours [our own people]." Dr. Peter D. also considered Adam T. anti-Semitic as well as "overzealous," a man who "wanted
to be on the good side of the [SS] doctor because he had a better chance
[that way] as a Christian of getting out of the camp." But Dr. D. added,
"With me he was very nice." A non-Jewish former inmate able to observe
him closely placed Adam T. among those prisoner doctors "who selected
more people than even the SS doctors would have." And the nonmedical
scientist, also a close observer, summed the matter up: "Adam T. was a
rabid anti-Semitic Polish nationalist with an evil temper. He was quick to
rouse. He could swing from cruelty to kindness. He could go either way.
He was unpredictable."

Having been received by most survivors in tones of warm colleagueship
and sympathy with my work, I was struck by Adam T.'s discomfort about
meeting me ("Well, that all happened so long ago. I don't like to talk

about it. I'm quite old now.") and by his combination of wariness and defensiveness when we did meet. I encountered an elegantly dressed man who received me in a lavishly furnished home and referred quickly to his large clinic and his summer home on the Mediterranean.

But he also showed me the tattooed number on his arm and pointed out how low it was, meaning he had been at Auschwitz very early and very long—four full years. He told me that, when a member of a Polish resistance group, he had been arrested for listening to Allied broadcasts, had undergone six months of brutal treatment in a prison in Krakow ("You keep . . . expecting that at any moment they are going to shoot you"), was subjected to a severe beating at the hands of SS personnel upon his arrival in Auschwitz (from which he emerged with a broken arm), and soon afterward developed a serious case of typhus. As a patient on the medical block he observed "the way the SS did things" (giving phenol injections and removing the corpses to vehicles to carry them off); the day after his discharge, "the whole hospital was put in the gas chamber." Even if he stressed these things in order to exculpate himself, there was no doubt about his violent initiation not just to Auschwitz (though he also worked awhile as a laborer) but to the essence of Auschwitz "medicine."

He recalled with some feeling the terror of the early Auschwitz period: how large numbers of Polish prisoners died every day from various forms of brutality; and how this was in accordance with the overall Nazi project of destroying the Polish intelligentsia. Then he added in a way I thought odd, "For their strategy, maybe that was right"—odd because he seemed unusually empathic toward "their strategy."

His situation improved greatly when he was permitted to do medical work and then to run a large medical block at a major subcamp. There he described himself as beleaguered by political prisoners whom he referred to as "old German Communists," "Jewish Communists," and "German Jewish Communists" who, he claimed, constantly made trouble for him by intriguing against him. He insisted that some of those people were still doing so in attempts to accuse him falsely (he was referring not only to attitudes held about him but to talk of bringing him to trial).

Jacob R. gave what is undoubtedly an accurate picture of the situation Dr. T. referred to. A Jewish Communist prisoner, who was an influential functionary in the hospital, told Dr. R., when he arrived there, that T. was anti-Semitic and fascistic and had to be countered; while T. went much further at the time and confided to R. that it was necessary "to eliminate certain Communists" and that R. could have the functionary's job when the latter had been properly taken care of. Jacob R. had the impression that his troubled retreat from any such suggestion was viewed by Adam T. as "very dumb," that Dr. T. had taken on Auschwitz mores to an unusual degree, that "he considered himself like a god in the hospital" and embraced "his absolute power" without restraint. T. came to resemble Nazi doctors in performing surgery on Jewish prisoners "just to learn the operation," while insisting that an experienced surgeon assist him; otherwise, he had little concern for patients and treated Jews "as though they were nonexistent." For T., "the most important thing was that the system worked smoothly," and that he retained his power and privilege.

In talking to me about SS doctors, Adam T. at first dismissed them as "just big Nazis" with "no idea about medicine." But over the course of our interview, his references to them became increasingly sympathetic. He told how they helped him to replace nonmedical people with "real doctors," but how later one of them along with an SS noncommissioned officer were unfairly imprisoned. For in evoking SS doctors sympathetically, he was defending his own behavior. For example, he claimed that he would say to SS doctors during a selection that "certain people would be able to work after a couple of weeks," and they said, "Good, they can stay here." The SS doctor "always said yes" to such requests from Dr. T. Moreover, it was not the SS doctor but the camp commandant, T. insisted, who demanded the selections, and "the first proud killer was the Political Department [which had] nothing to do with the [SS] doctors." SS doctors, he claimed, "were very nice [and] talked quietly with us" and, rather than putting pressure on prisoner doctors to become involved in killing, took pride in improving medical facilities and medical statistics in their camps. In any case the "liquidation" was performed by nonmedical personnel, and "the doctors didn't do that much." Also, SS doctors were under pressure to comply: "The SS could kill SS too," and "I always say it's not so easy to be a hero."

In this way, Adam T. mixed kernels of truth, half-truth, and falsehood in presenting an apologia for SS doctors and for the prisoner doctor who cast his lot with them. The apologia included elements of blaming the victim: stressing the difficult "psychological situation" of Jews who had previously lived comfortably, but now developed "prison neurosis" and, finally despairing, committed suicide by plunging toward the wire, and being shot from the tower.

T. tried to present himself as a healer, as someone who "kept people alive" in this sea of death, and who worked closely with prisoner colleagues to improvise equipment and do what could be done for patients.

But he became tense when talking about selections; and in telling how patients were sent away when his hospital became overcrowded, he used a euphemism for the gas chambers I had not previously heard—"the central hospital." He referred to that euphemism in a way that tended to justify selections by equating them, as SS doctors were told to do, with combat medical triage. He talked about the extraordinary situation of the one occasion when the camp was bombed, and five hundred people were killed and one thousand injured:

> People came to our hospital. Some were very bad. The SS would say, "It is not possible you can make these people healthy. You must trans-

fer them to the central hospital." It was no problem for the SS. There was the same situation at the front. If a German soldier would have an open break [bone fracture]—a leg amputation—if it would heal in three or four weeks, he was sent to work in an office. But with soldiers they couldn't help—they had to die. They did it with their own soldiers. That was the war—a very hard situation.*

In addition to the exaggeration and probable falsehood contained in the account, it presents the Auschwitz authorities as a beleaguered group trying to do their best with "a very hard" wartime situation. Dr. T. could thus add the equally dubious contention that "usually if someone was sent to the gas chambers, he was *very* sick . . . [and would] have no chance to live in the camp."

Despite his general sympathy for SS doctors, Dr. T. condemned Wirths as largely "responsible for the whole catastrophic situation . . . [in which] they made this extermination from the medical point of view." His anger probably reflected both a residual fear of SS doctors ("In the evening they [could] send a piece of paper down to the office, which means [someone] will be killed the next day") and, more important, his recollection of Wirths's connection with the group of Communist political prisoners he, Adam T., considered to be his enemies. At one point, however, he softened notably in talking about Wirths and gave me the distinct impression that he was unconsciously associating the chief SS doctor with his own moral dilemma: "I ask myself, why did Wirths stay in Auschwitz? He could go away. He could say he wanted to go to the front. Of course the commandant may say, 'I have no one else. I need you.' "

Dr. T. made a point of his frequent contacts with Jews in the German city in which he lived. One prisoner doctor, in commenting on Dr. T.'s extensive contact with the Jewish community, said with gentle sarcasm, "I hear he has become a *Tzodik,* " using the Hebrew term for "saint." The turnabout, hardly convincing to Jewish survivors, was a part of T.'s postwar adaptation.

Another Jewish survivor, Isaac K., who had worked as a nonphysician in the same hospital, confirmed Adam T.'s clear anti-Semitism but acknowledged that he would occasionally help save a Jewish prisoner's life when requested, though in such cases he usually had to be bribed (with food, money, clothing, or whatever). K. condemned Dr. T. for performing selections—as he apparently did on occasions when the SS noncommissioned officer evaded the task—though adding that within the Auschwitz structure "somebody had to make the selections [because of] the overcrowding of the hospital." K. was saying that Dr. T. had gone beyond what a prisoner doctor was required to do even in Auschwitz. K. made a still more damning accusation: "We have proof that he collaborated

*Concerning "euthanasia" of German soldiers, see page 143.

with the . . . SS" in connection with reporting on the attempted escape of three Jewish prisoners, who were soon captured and, in keeping with prevailing Auschwitz practice, publicly hanged. K. went on to tell how Dr. T. had learned surgical techniques from Jewish doctors, but added that "he treated the doctors very nicely" and that he himself remained on a friendly basis with T.: "[He could be] very, very nice, . . . but I felt from the beginning I can't trust him."

K. was suggesting a pattern of doubling in Dr. T., which I have identified in Nazi doctors (and will discuss in detail later). Adam T.'s combination of right-wing Polish nationalism and anti-Semitism, along with his stance of omnipotence in response to his own overwhelming death anxiety, led to his developing an "Auschwitz self" very similar to that of an SS doctor. Dr. Jacob R. made the point to me that it was a case not so much of "identification with the aggressor" (in psychoanalytic terminology) as one of identification with the overall Auschwitz structure of authority, an identification Dr. T. could half maintain and half reverse during the postwar years. In Auschwitz, however, that form of adaptation enabled him to enter directly into the healing-killing reversal epitomized by selections.

Experimental Operations and "Libel": Wladislaw Dering

The second of three Polish prisoner doctors, Wladislaw Dering, performed cruel experimental operations on Jewish inmates, which became widely known through his being the plaintiff in an extraordinary libel trial that took place in London in 1964.[1]

Dering, who had been imprisoned because of his activities in the Polish underground, arrived very early in Auschwitz (15 August 1940) and underwent severe beatings by the Gestapo. In Auschwitz he first did hard physical labor and then became a nurse, before emerging as a leading Polish physician who "in the beginning had a good reputation" among prisoners.[2] During this early phase, he helped many people, especially fellow Poles, and was recognized by inmates and SS doctors as an unusually skillful surgeon.

In an important early incident, he was told by a German doctor to give a phenol injection. In the version he gave at his later trial, he claimed that, upon discovering the nature of the substance in the syringe, he refused to give the injection. A prisoner doctor testified afterward, however, that Dering actually gave the injection on an order from Dr. Entress but did not know what he was injecting. And when the prisoner died almost instantly, Dering was "shocked and declared that he would never again give any injections."[3] Whichever account is true (I am inclined to believe the latter version), Dering was undoubtedly stunned and terrified by the experience, which may nonetheless have served to take him over the threshold into atrocity.

In 1943 he was given unprecedented authority for a prisoner doctor when appointed by Wirths to be block elder at the infirmary, making him not only chief prisoner doctor but a leading *capo* as well. During this period, he was enlisted by Horst Schumann (with the aid of Wirths) to perform surgery in connection with sterilization experiments. Dering removed ovaries and testicles of about two hundred Jewish inmates after these organs had been subjected to radiation, to make them available for pathological examination to determine whether the radiation had been effective. He administered spinal anesthesia in a crude and painful manner (rather than following the usual procedure of first anesthetizing the track of the main injection), often while patients were forcibly restrained. Operations were done without sterile procedures for hands and instruments, were performed extremely rapidly, and were followed by hasty and rough suturing. The entire procedure took about ten minutes. (Dr. Wanda J. recalled Schumann telling her—when she, pleading lack of surgical facility, resisted his request to perform the same operations—"I'll show you a surgeon who'll do it in ten minutes each.")

Although Dr. J., who had known Dering from medical school days in Poland, knew that "he wasn't very . . . pro-Jewish," she was at first pleased to learn he was block elder in the infirmary because she thought, "He will help me." But he rebuffed her dietary request for very sick patients because, she thought, he believed that "we [Jews] are condemned to death."

Since she was asked to calm the young women Dering operated upon, she witnessed much that went on. She told me with some bitterness how during an operation she asked Dering in Polish, "Do you realize what you are doing?" to which he answered, "Of course. I have to remove the ovaries . . . because, you know, Schumann is here." She added that "he did ten girls in one day . . . one afternoon" under conditions that were simply "septic" (meaning infectious and non-antiseptic). In subsequently taking care of these women, she observed the extensive tissue destruction and infection resulting from the combination of deep X rays, crude surgery, and general Auschwitz conditions. She had to struggle not only to keep these patients alive but to find ways to protect them from official scrutiny since, as "bearers of secrets" (*Geheimnisträger*—secrets, in this case, of the surgical experiments), they were always in danger of being sent to the gas chambers.

Other prisoner doctors observed Dering's increasing brutalization. Dr. Jacob R. told how once, when making rounds together, Dering looked at a patient he had operated on, and remarked, "Sterilization magna"—an intentional *double entendre*, since the same term, "great sterilization," referred in medicine to the discovery of sterile procedures to prevent infection. Dering also made a tobacco pouch out of the scrotum of one of the testicles he had removed from Jewish prisoners, and sometimes displayed it to other inmates.[4]

Concerning Dering's anti-Semitism, Dr. R. reported that, on the same day of the rounds, Dering said to him, "You see that what is going on with the Jews is not very esthetic, but it's the only way, the only solution."

Dering was thought to have informed on other prisoners to the Political Department. He used his influence to have certain Jewish prisoners he did not like, including at least one physician and a nurse, sent to the gas chamber without even the formality of a selection.

Dering was rewarded for his efforts by being released from Auschwitz, and then went to work in the clinic of Carl Clauberg (the other Auschwitz doctor engaged in experimental sterilization) in Germany. Dr. Wanda J. saw Dering leave, carrying two suitcases and looking fit. As she said, "He was a kind of German anyhow—a *Volksdeutsch* [ethnic German]."*

After the war, Dering went back to Poland, soon fled to England out of fear of Polish legal proceedings, and was held for nineteen months in a British prison until it was finally decided not to extradite or deport him. He worked in Africa for ten years as a physician with the British Colonial Medical Service and then returned to London where he practiced under the National Health Service.[5]

His quiet medical life was startlingly interrupted in 1959 with the publication of the novel *Exodus* by the American Jewish writer Leon Uris. Uris spoke of Auschwitz's Block 10 where Nazi doctors "used women as guinea-pigs and Dr. Schumann sterilized by castration and X-ray and Clauberg removed ovaries and Dr. Dehring [*sic*] performed 17,000 'experiments' in surgery without anesthetic."[6] Feeling pressed to clear himself in the eyes of his son and his second wife (his first wife was said to have divorced him upon learning what he had done in Auschwitz), Dering initiated a libel suit against Uris and the British publisher and printer of the novel. An extraordinary trial ensued in which Nazi sterilization experiments and Dering's relationship to them were dramatically revealed by three leading women prisoner physicians, two of them Jewish, as well as by surviving victims of those operations, every single one of whom was brought to London as a witness. The women prisoner doctors played a large part in the legal proceedings, both in giving damning testimony and in contacting the women who had been operated on and arranging for not only them, but the surgical records from the Auschwitz Museum, to be brought to London. The latter, in keeping with the German penchant for orderly records, contained (according to one of these doctors) "the number of girls . . . that he [Dering] operated on . . . [what] he did to them, and the numbers of the boys—everything was in this book."

At the trial two former Polish prisoner doctors testified for Dering, mainly concerning his life-saving efforts on behalf of themselves and others during the early Auschwitz years. Another Polish male prisoner doctor testified against him. But the testimony of the three women doc-

*I heard of only one other prisoner doctor, also Polish, who was released from Auschwitz. One apparently had to identify oneself as an ethnic German to be eligible for release.

tors, and even more so that of the surgical victims, was overwhelming and decisive. The verdict was technically for Dering as plaintiff because of the inaccuracies in Uris's novel concerning the number of operations* and the use of anesthesia. But, in the British manner, the award was "one ha'penny"—a severe moral condemnation of Dering. Not long after the trial, he became ill and died.[7]

But, in terms of Dering's overall behavior in camp, Jacob R., as a Jewish prisoner doctor, made a simple, accurate observation: "Early in 1943, he was still very subservient. He was a servile *Häftling* ["prisoner"]. But . . . he changed: he became more of a comrade with the SS doctors."

Thus, Dering moved from terror to servility to identification with the Auschwitz environment and especially with medicalized power over life and death—a passage for the most part available only to non-Jews, especially so if they were strong anti-Semites, and still more so if ethnic Germans.

Physical Violence and "Evil for Evil's Sake": Zenon Zenkteller

Zenon Zenkteller was a Polish prisoner doctor who became notorious for physically abusing Jewish prisoner doctors working under him. The only one of this group legally prosecuted after the war, he was convicted and imprisoned.

Alexander O., a Jewish doctor who had to work under Dr. Zenkteller made clear that "there was never any colleagueship" and that "he was an enemy, a congenital enemy," and went on to say, with appropriately mordant humor:

> Some . . . like insects. I like cacti. . . . He [liked] to beat. . . . Dr. A. lived—I will use the German expression—*wie Gott in Frankreich* ["like God in France"], but he urinated every hour. We [a group of doctors made to do strenuous manual labor] were kneeling down or sitting down because we could no longer stand, famished and weak as we were. . . . He would go out and urinate on the wall of the block, usually on the left side. . . . He would urinate outside because, every time he would go out, we were busy working, seated or on our knees, and we would be kicked in the backside. Going and coming back from urinating, he would distribute his kicks. But those who were a bit out of his way did not get kicks because he did not go out of his way. He would only take two or three steps to kick. Otherwise, the others would only get such compliments as "Asshole!, Shitpig!" . . . I never saw Zenkteller go and urinate without kicking the backsides of those he could reach.

*The total of 17,000 used in the novel apparently stemmed from a prisoner doctor who had heard Dering boast of having performed that number of operations in Auschwitz, most of them not related to experimental sterilization. We may surmise, then, that the extremely incorrect number derived both from Dering's boast and from an Auschwitz environment so extreme that within it any number of harmful acts, murders, or criminal operations seemed plausible.

This Jewish doctor's judgment emerged clearly (Zenkteller "was the only [prisoner] doctor who would beat, insult without reason, . . . the only doctor who would eliminate, persecute, do evil for evil's sake"), and his rage was such that, encountering Dr. Zenkteller in a hospital soon after the liberation, O. seriously considered killing him ("I assure you it is the fear of being surprised and given away which kept me from strangling him").

Other prisoner doctors essentially agreed. They also understood Zenkteller to be psychologically disturbed: he was, as one prisoner doctor put it, "erratic" and "highly unstable," his beating of both colleagues and patients an aspect of his "episodes of violence." Part of that instability was the inevitable Auschwitz twist or contradiction—in his case, an occasional show of decency. When another prisoner doctor was critically ill with typhus, it was Dr. Zenkteller who first tried to place him on an "Aryan" block where he had a better chance to survive; though the attempt failed, the fact that he had been taken to the block rendered the ill doctor sufficiently "élite" that he was not sent to the gas chamber when a selection was made.

Fundamentally, however, as the other prisoner doctor went on to say, Zenkteller "was a faithful servant of the SS doctors." While Zenkteller himself "was powerful enough to decide on the life and death of any inmate, even the chief physicians among the inmates," in relation to the SS doctors "his submissiveness was one-hundred percent."

Zenkteller's story resembles, in many ways, the stories of Adam T. and Wladislaw Dering: the combination of Polish nationalism with anti-Semitism; early fear and near physical and mental breakdown in response to brutal treatment; adaptation by means of servile behavior to the Nazi hierarchy and murderous behavior toward prisoners; and then the development of a set of self-serving structural and psychological arrangements for perpetuating personal power and omnipotence. But Zenkteller differs from the other two collaborators in his extensive physical violence and generally sadistic behavior. I will argue later that such sadism is inseparable from a sense of omnipotence and has to do with overcoming one's own struggles with death and mutilation. But however we understand these psychological and social currents, we must recognize the extent to which the Auschwitz environment encouraged their coalescence into a self-process that rendered at least a few prisoner doctors activists in Nazi medicalized killing.

Jewish Medical Collaborator: Maximilian Samuel

The one Jewish doctor I know of who can be included here, Maximilian Samuel, had been a distinguished academic gynecologist in Cologne.[8] He had also been an ardent German nationalist, was awarded the Iron Cross for military service during the First World War, and was active in a movement against the French Occupation in Cologne. Probably for these reasons, he arrived in Auschwitz with instructions that he be afforded special consideration; and although then sixty-two years old, he was not selected for the gas chamber.

He first worked at Buna, where at least one prisoner doctor who became ill remembers him as rendering considerate medical help. But before long he was transferred to Block 10, where his gynecological experience was put to use as he became increasingly involved in the experiments on women conducted there. One of his major activities was the surgical removal of the cervix from a considerable number of women who were part of the "research project" conducted by Eduard Wirths on pre-cancerous growths (see pages 391–92). Some inmates claimed that he was a little more considerate than Nazi doctors who did the operation in that he removed less of the cervix, but most prisoner doctors were impressed by Samuel's extreme "diligence" in working closely with the Nazis. Furthermore, he denounced to Nazi doctors another prisoner physician who refused to continue to give anesthesia for his operations. There was also some evidence that Samuel made reports on inmates to the notorious Political Department.

Of the people I interviewed who knew Samuel, only one made a positive comment. A woman who had been subjected to sterilization procedures on Block 10 remembered him as having been "kind to us," as having spoken gently to the Jewish victims, and as having attempted to make whatever procedures he and others performed on them as painless as possible. But she may have *wished* to see a Jewish doctor in that favorable light. Certainly most former prisoners I spoke to, Jewish or otherwise, remembered Samuel as either arrogant or pathetic, or both.

They also recognized that he was a broken man. His wife had been killed upon their arrival in Auschwitz with their nineteen-year-old daughter. The daughter was selected for work, and there was a strong impression that Samuel's activities were part of his desperate efforts to save her life. He went so far as to write a letter from the camp to Himmler himself, pointing to his own First World War record and pleading that his daughter be spared. (The letter was left unsealed in the block office, where it was seen by another prisoner doctor.)

Then, in the middle of the experiments, Samuel was suddenly put to death. Speculations I heard from survivors about why he was killed varied greatly. Some stressed the extensive skin lesions or eczema he developed (which a few survivors attributed to his extreme tension and fear) as having rendered him too sick to be any longer useful, or caused his face to become "repulsive" to the SS. Other survivors spoke of his argumentativeness and conflicts with Clauberg; still others thought he had become superfluous with the arrival of a younger Jewish woman doctor, Wanda J., to take charge of Block 10. But most of all, inmates considered him to have seen and done so much as to have reached the dangerous status of "bearer of secrets." "He must have known too much or perhaps talked to somebody he should not have" is the way that one prisoner doctor put it.

With considerable personal pain, Hermann Langbein has described still another factor:

> One day the chief physician asked my opinion about Samuel. Even. earlier, Dr. Wirths had occasionally asked my opinion about functionaries in the infirmary, without ever giving a reason for his question. Afterward it always turned out that he had wanted to learn what I thought because he was considering the person concerned for a leading function. Since, from all I knew about Samuel, I had doubts about helping him acquire an influential post, I answered reservedly. Wirths replied that he too did not have the best opinion of Samuel, and [he] dictated something else. Soon afterward, Dr. Samuel was taken to Birkenau by the chief physician's sergeant, Friedrich Ontl. The office was ordered to prepare his death announcement.

Langbein claimed, "[On further reflection] I came to the conclusion that this was the only way I could react." He nonetheless continued to ask himself "whether I, too, bear unintended complicity in the death of this man."[9]

He went on to characterize Samuel as the kind of Auschwitz prisoner, found especially among the older ones, who "despite great intelligence and experience of life, despite knowledge of the Auschwitz extermination machinery, refused to accept reality and . . . nourished the insane hope of being able to create an exception for themselves."[10] The exception, as we know, had to do with the survival of his daughter. But also of great importance was Samuel's strong sense of himself as a German and, as such, a countryman of the Nazis and a colleague of SS doctors—an identity he could call forth in Auschwitz in order to try to save his daughter (who too was killed) and also himself.

If there is to be a last word about prisoner medical collaborators, it might best be Jan W.'s. This Polish doctor's cautious answer, when asked his opinion about the actions of Dering and Samuel, managed to convey some of the complexity of Auschwitz moral truths, along with his own considerable humanity:

> It is difficult to pass judgment on the behavior of inmates. It's difficult to accuse the Jews of the Sonderkommando of helping to kill their fellow Jews by pushing them into the gas chambers. It was done under pressure which deprived them of their will. But there were times when a man went over the border of what we could expect from him—did more than what was demanded or required—when he performed functions with sadistic satisfaction or even did certain things before he

received any orders and in that way anticipated the Nazis. These things we may consider as crimes. . . .

Perhaps the doctor's case is a little different because doctors are bound by their professional ethic, and physicians are people with higher education. But the cases of Dering and Samuel are different. . . . Dering obtained a certain position in the camp. . . . From Dering you could expect a certain ability to maneuver himself out of doing certain kinds of operations. . . . Samuel was a Jew, which meant a person 100-percent condemned to death in the camp. So he had the right to prolong his life—week by week, month by month.

Chapter 14

Killing with Syringes: Phenol Injections

> But then instead of doing it for medical purposes,
> it was for killing. . . . It was very much like a medical
> ceremony. . . . They were so careful to keep the full
> precision of a medical process—but with the aim of
> killing. That was what was so shocking.
>   —Auschwitz prisoner doctor

The most medical of all Auschwitz killing methods was the phenol injection, which was institutionalized during the relatively early phases of Auschwitz. A *patient* was brought to a *treatment room* and there administered a *drug* by a *physician* or (in most cases) his assistant, who wore a white coat and used a syringe and needle for the injection. In camp jargon, there were the active verb *spritzen* ("to inject, squirt, spray"), the passive verb *abgespritzt* ("to be injected off," or killed), and equivalent noun forms meaning "syringing" and "phenoling."[1]

Phenol injections were associated, in their early phase, with the direct medical killing of the "euthanasia" project. Thus Dr. Friedrich Entress, who organized the injections in Auschwitz, testified in 1947 that he had received what he called an "order on euthanasia" from Dr. Enno Lolling, chief of SS concentration-camp medicine, stating that "incurably mentally ill persons, incurable tuberculosis patients, and those permanently incapable of work" were to be killed. Later that order was expanded to include "sick prisoners whose recovery was not possible within four weeks." The order probably arrived in mid- or late 1941, when the Nazis were searching for efficient killing methods; in early 1942, at least two hundred prisoners with tuberculosis had been killed with phenol on Entress's orders.[2]*

---
*Entress remembered the first order as arriving in May 1942, but Langbein is convinced that he was in error concerning the date, since the phenol killings were under way in fall

That was approximately the time of the 14f13 extension of "euthanasia" into the camps, and phenol injections were a means of doing the killing "at home," at the same place where the selections were conducted, rather than sending victims to the killing centers established mostly for mental patients in Germany and Austria. As in the original "euthanasia" project, the killing of those who were seriously ill was extended to killing virtually anyone whose death was desired. In practice, "Aryan" prisoners usually received phenol injections only when severely debilitated (there were of course exceptions), while Jewish prisoners were vulnerable to them merely by being on the hospital block.

Phenol injections, then, anticipated the full development of the gas chambers and were used along with them where, because of relatively few people to be killed, gassing was considered uneconomical. For instance, two Dutch Jews who had been injected with blood taken from typhus patients, in experiments seeking to determine how long typhus patients were infectious, were killed by phenol injections.[3] And Dr. Wladyslaw Fejkiel described the "injecting off" of two young Gypsies as ordered by Mengele, possibly because they were twins whose post mortem was of interest to him.[4] But murder in Auschwitz was nothing if not flexible; and even when a small number of people was designated for phenol killing, "if by chance a transport was going to the gas chambers, then they went into the gas chambers."

Increasingly, from January 1943, children were killed by phenol injections. Early in that year, as many as 120 boys, ages thirteen to seventeen, from the Polish city of Zamosc—described as children whose parents had been killed—were murdered by phenol injection.* The children had made a powerful impression on prisoners, who gave them "the best they had," even somehow finding a ball for them to play with—until they were ordered to undress in the washroom, and cries of "Why are you killing me?" were heard, followed by "a muffled sound" of small bodies falling to the floor.[5]

Phenol injection also became standard procedure for secret political murders, whose victims included Auschwitz inmates as well as people brought from the outside to be killed in this way. As Dr. Jan W. put it, "The Political Department could issue orders for prisoners [in both of the preceding categories] to be executed on the hospital grounds, and the responsibility for carrying out the order rested with the SS physicians."

Medical killing by injection was by no means limited to Auschwitz—and, in one sense, went back to the injection of morphine and its deriva-

---

1941. Dr. Jan W. told me that "every day in 1942, twenty to thirty or more were killed this way." Most victims were Jews, but other prisoners were also murdered by phenol.

*There is some discrepancy about the number. In one source, Dr. Stanislaw Klodziński mentions two separate events—39 boys killed on 23 February and 80 on 1 March—which might account in part for varying numbers. Some could have been Jewish children who had been in hiding.

tives in the "euthanasia" of children and the later "wild euthanasia" of adults. Injections of phenol and other lethal substances were widespread in other camps. Early experimentation with phenol in Buchenwald was ordered by Mrugowsky, the overall Berlin chief of the SS Hygienic Institute, after it had been noted that tiny percentages of carbolic acid (phenol) preservative in serum was implicated in the accidental medical deaths of several German soldiers. Erwin Schuler (alias Ding), a camp doctor at Buchenwald who explained that "neither [he] nor Mrugowsky had ever seen a case of death by phenol," went ahead with the experiments considered "urgent for the fighting troops."[6] But in Buchenwald, too, phenol was mainly used to kill sick inmates, though it was also used for killing various kinds of political prisoner. Dr. Waldemar Hoven testified that on one occasion he was observed in the act by his colleague Schuler: "[He] said that I was not doing it correctly, [and] therefore . . . performed some of the injections himself."[7]* There would seem to be a certain psychological significance in the progression from claimed German military (life-death) requirements to mass murder of members of a "dangerous" group or "race."

Phenol and Jews as Spreaders of Epidemics

In Auschwitz, from about September 1941, phenol injections served mainly as the end point of selections. When patients became debilitated or a medical block was considered overcrowded, the SS doctor in charge "selected a row of prisoners who were immediately . . . killed by phenol injections." Those who had been on the medical block for relatively long periods were most vulnerable, as were tuberculosis patients (in accordance with the Lolling order). The euphemism of "euthanasia" or "mercy killing" combined with the principle of preventive medicine, and "Jews suspect of [spreading] epidemics" *(seuchenverdächtige Juden)* had to be, as Rudolf Höss said, destroyed. A prisoner doctor told how "Dr. Entress decided to fight the spotted fever [typhus] by means of phenol injections": an SS physician "decided whether the patient was to be admitted to the infirmary, given a phenol injection, or sent back to the camp."[8] Another prisoner doctor told how the camp doctor observed a group of emaciated prisoners and made a "lightning decision" by placing each patient's card in one of two piles.

*Hoven tried to imply that the only phenol killings he did were at the request of prisoners who asked him to help get rid of threatening inmates. There were such killings at Buchenwald, having to do with the struggles between political and criminal prisoners and various other factions. But Hoven and other SS doctors clearly did most of their direct medical killing (with phenol or sodium evipan) with sick inmates, including tuberculosis cases. Hoven himself was arrested by SS officers investigating corruption at Buchenwald—partly because he poisoned a material witness against the former camp commandant.

But rather than controlling epidemics, the widespread use of phenol injections had the opposite effect. Hermann Langbein, who worked as secretary to Wirths, told of informing the chief Auschwitz doctor that "most of those who come into the hospital are not healed but are injected [*gespritzt*]." Therefore, Langbein explained, "if one has a headache and fever [the early symptoms of typhus], he does everything not to have to go to the hospital. . . . That's how typhus stays in the camp." Langbein knew he would be listened to because he was aware of Wirths's determination to fight typhus epidemics, having been ordered to do so by Berlin. Langbein thought that Wirths seemed surprised and troubled by this information about phenol injections, and when Wirths sought an explanation from Entress, the responsible doctor, he was further deceived by the latter's claim that injections were being given only to incurable tuberculosis patients—a lie that Wirths was apparently willing to accept on the basis of the Berlin directive. Eventually Langbein was able to demonstrate the truth of the matter to Wirths; and as a result, Langbein suggested, the phenol injections decreased markedly and finally ceased altogether (see page 387).[9]

Other survivors have questioned during interviews how much influence these talks between Langbein and Wirths could have had. At the time (late 1942) Auschwitz's schedule of killing had been relaxed to keep a maximum number of prisoners working; and the increasing availability of the gas chambers and crematoria had largely supplanted phenol injections for mass killing.[10] While it is impossible to gauge the exact weight of these various factors, we can assume that Langbein did have a certain influence precisely because his message to Wirths (do something to stop mass phenol injections if you want to stop the typhus epidemics) coincided with Wirths's mission. (I shall have more to say about the chief doctor's healing-killing contradictions in chapter 18.)

The Injection Procedure

The choice of killing substance and the injection technique had a specific development in Auschwitz. There was considerable experimentation with other substances—benzine, gasoline, hydrogen peroxide, evipan, prussic acid (cyanide), and air—all injected into the vein. The prisoner pathologist, Dr. Miklos Nyiszli (see pages 350–51), thought he detected chloroform in his post-mortem examinations of four pairs of twins put to death by Mengele, and believed that it was injected into the heart.[11]

Initially, phenol was injected into a victim's vein, maximizing the medical aura of the entire procedure. A Polish non-Jewish prisoner doctor,

Marek P., vividly described how deadly injections were given in the same hospital room where he routinely assisted with surgical operations:

> This time there was a table prepared with syringes. The phenol was in a bottle. There was cotton—everything you needed for an injection. There was also alcohol, as with ordinary injections—and rubber tourniquets. There was just one table . . . and the right hand [of the victim] was put out on a kind of support table [to hold the arm steady], as with a regular intravenous injection, [and] the rubber tourniquet on the arm to apply the pressure to make the vein visible—all in the usual way. . . . Mengele [who performed this killing] then rubbed alcohol on the spot, just under the elbow, that he was using for the injection, and then injected the phenol. . . . He did it as though he were performing regular surgery.

Before long the technique was changed to injecting the phenol directly into the heart. Some witnesses thought that the change was made because the veins were sometimes hard to locate, but the real reason seems to have been the greater killing efficiency of a direct cardiac injection. Patients injected by vein might linger for minutes or even an hour or more. "It took them a long time to kill by intravenous injections, so they invented a faster method" was the way Dr. P. put it. (According to some testimony, many women prisoners continued to be injected by vein, after they were told that they were to receive "an inoculation.")

Then a place was decided upon: "Room 1," which became notorious; and later, as a Polish prisoner doctor told me, an innocuous-appearing room used as a laboratory by the Hygienic Institute ("It wasn't a special room [of] which the prisoners about to be injected needed to be suspicious").

The "concentrated aqueous solution of phenol" that was developed proved "inexpensive, easy to use, and absolutely effective when introduced into the heart ventricle," so that an injection of ten to fifteen milliliters into the heart caused death within fifteen seconds. The solution was put in a bottle resembling a thermos flask, and the person giving the injection poured it into a small bowl from which he filled the hypodermic. A large syringe and a long needle were employed, and the execution was performed by "driving the long needle into the fifth [rib] space."[12]

At the Frankfurt trial, Dr. Klodziński recalled the scene: "Sometimes it was still morning, sometimes noon, when those selected were taken to Block 20. Wearing a shirt, with a blanket and in wooden clogs, they were led into Block 20 through a side door. Those who could no longer walk were carried there on a stretcher. They were put in a corridor." Then the order to close the block was given (*Blocksperre*), and there was "dead silence" on the block: "All the patients on the block knew what was going on." Although Klodziński stated that "most of those selected themselves did not know what awaited them,"* many must have at least partly understood. The SDG then opened up Room 1:

> a room that was kept locked at other times and whose windows had been painted white. To the left of the door stood a small table; on it were a set of injection needles and syringes; next to these, a bottle with a yellowish-pink liquid—phenol. There were also two stools in the room, [and] on the wall [was] a hook on which hung a rubber apron.[14]

At that point two Jewish prisoner assistants brought a victim into the room (sometimes victims were brought in two at a time) and positioned him or her on a footstool, usually so that the right arm covered the victim's eyes and the left arm was raised sideways in a horizontal position. Sometimes one's right hand was at the back of one's neck, with the left behind the shoulder blade; and some victims were blindfolded with a towel. The idea was for the victim's chest to be thrust out so that the cardiac area was maximally accessible for the lethal injection, and for him or her to be unable to see what was happening. (There is also mention of a position in which the right arm was placed so that the hand was in one's mouth, not over one's eyes, so that one stifled one's own cries.) The person giving the injection—most often the SDG Josef Klehr—filled his syringe from the bottle and then thrust the needle directly into the heart of the seated prisoner and emptied the contents of the syringe.[15] Most prisoners fell dead almost immediately, but some lived for seconds or even minutes:

> The executioners used to boast about their records. "Three in a minute." . . . And they did not wait until the doomed person really died. During his agony he was taken from both sides under the armpits and thrown into a pile of corpses in another room opposite. And the next took his place on the stool.
>
> There was also substantial mechanization. . . . Approximately fifty people could be killed during one and a half to two hours. Thus, an average of two minutes and 22 seconds sufficed to murder one prisoner.

And finally, as Dr. Klodziński observed: "The corpses of those murdered with phenol shortly afterwards took on a pinkish livid color, small

---

*Because "phenol was . . . a secret of the camp hospital," and people risked their lives if they revealed it; because prisoner hospital workers realized that to tell the truth to the doomed people would cause them greater pain, and therefore tried to contribute to the illusion of "the injection as some normal administrative and medical procedure"; and because of the universal psychological need to refuse "to accept the idea that life is coming to an end." One could hold to that denial precisely because "everyone had for years [prior to Auschwitz] connected the idea of hospital, doctors, nurses, injections, medical treatment with the struggle for life—and not with murder."[13]

haemorrhages took place under the skin, the conjunctiva [exposed surface of eyeball] were bloodshot. Rigor mortis set in with a delay of several
hours."[16]

One of the Jewish assistants was a man named Jean Weiss, who described perhaps the most unbearable sequence I encountered:

> It happened on September 28, 1942. I don't know how many were
> lined up ahead of my father. The door opened and my father came in
> with a[nother] prisoner. Klehr talked to my father and told him: "You
> will get an anti-typhus injection." Then I cried and had to carry out my
> father myself. Klehr was in a hurry. He injected two prisoners at a time
> because he wanted to get back to his rabbits [which he raised as a
> hobby].

The next day, Klehr asked Weiss why he had cried, and Weiss told him.
Klehr said that, had he known who it was, "I would have let him live."
When a judge later asked Weiss why he had not told the SDG man at the
time, Weiss answered, "I was afraid that Klehr would make me sit down
next to [his father]"—and be killed along with him.[17]

Supplies of phenol were, like other medical drugs, kept in the Auschwitz pharmacy and were obtained as all medical supplies were obtained
—by means of requisitions to Berlin. According to a survivor who worked
in the pharmacy, the requisition would read *"Phenol pro injectione"* ("phenol for injection").

At first, relatively small quantities of phenol were ordered; but later,
between four and ten pounds (two to five kilos) per month. The chief
pharmacist, Dr. Viktor Capesius, explained to his underlings that the
phenol was to be used in eardrops in combination with glycerin, a legitimate medical preparation. As a judge in the Frankfurt Auschwitz trial
remarked, "With that quantity [of phenol] the ears of whole armies
could have been treated."[18] The medical pretense, if less than fully convincing, was nonetheless psychologically required, and was retained to
the end.

Phenol killing turned the hospital into a place for mass extermination.
Klodziński's estimate that twenty thousand people were killed in the
Auschwitz main camp (where most of the phenol killing took place) is
especially impressive in that these killings occurred during the twenty
months from August 1941 through April 1943—that is, over five hundred
days, since injections were usually not given on Sundays or holidays.
Killings averaged thirty to sixty a day, though on some days as many as
two hundred were done.

Doctors as Phenol Executioners

For a doctor, phenol injections were the most literal example of the entire healing-killing reversal. Although most of the injections were given by nonphysicians, SS doctors initiated them in Auschwitz, maintained responsibility for their administration, and sometimes continued to perform the injections themselves.

An early practitioner of phenol killing was Dr. Franz von Bodman, whom Langbein described as having shown considerable "initiative" in this form of murder. Although at Auschwitz only briefly, Bodman managed, as chief doctor *(Standortarzt)* during the summer of 1942, to inject many inmates by vein, resulting in slow and painful deaths. Once two girls who had been shot by SS men, one in the stomach and the other in the thigh, were brought to the medical block; Bodman prohibited anyone from treating the wounds and then personally injected both girls with phenol.[19] It is likely that this man's zeal in phenol killing was related both to especially strong Nazi involvement and to psychological inclinations toward omnipotence and sadism.

Josef Mengele injected phenol on several occasions—though not as regularly as Bodman—with his characteristic combination of detachment and flair (as I shall discuss on page 347). But the individual doctor most associated with phenol injections in Auschwitz was Friedrich Entress. Entress was a Polish ethnic German (from eastern territories lost to Poland after the First World War), who had been educated in German grammar and secondary schools and joined pro-German and pro-Nazi student groups at the university in Poznan. He entered the SS early and went quickly into the concentration-camp system immediately upon completing his medical training (indeed without having to write his dissertation), first at Gross-Rosen and then at Auschwitz, in December 1941, at the age of twenty-seven. Langbein, with considerable justification, characterized Entress as the "most notorious of all camp doctors."[20] In setting up the experiments with various substances that eventuated in phenol injections, into first the vein and then the heart, Entress was maximizing the murderous elements in the central directives he received. His interpretation of such directives generally followed that of the Political Department, and he was personally close to the extraordinarily brutal head of that department, Maximilian Grabner. Like Grabner, Entress was in conflict with Eduard Wirths, who arrived in Auschwitz in September 1942 and advocated a less draconian interpretation of these directives.

For instance, Wirths could accept the directive that tuberculosis patients had to undergo "special treatment" because they were a danger to others and could not be medically treated in Auschwitz, but wished to limit the policy to such patients, while Entress and Grabner "interpreted the order from Berlin as blanket permission to inject all *Muselmänner* and patients who were unlikely to return quickly to work." We recall Entress's attempt to deceive Wirths by claiming that the large number of patients he was having injected with phenol had all suffered from tuberculosis. Entress also conducted, on 29 August 1942, one of the biggest selections ever to take place on an Auschwitz medical block: he sent to the gas chambers not only patients ill with typhus but many who were convalescing, and also prisoner doctors and other medical personnel in no way ill.[21] Dr. Jan W. told me that "on that memorable day, Entress liquidated almost all of the patients of Block 20 because of typhus, as well as seriously ill patients from other blocks—with diarrhea, or who came from surgery or from the internal diseases block—as well as people who were convalescing. This was his . . . method for getting rid of typhus in the camp. . . . Entress did it all personally, with the help of SS orderlies."

Dr. W. estimated that Entress selected a total of one thousand to twelve hundred people that day, again with a sanction from Berlin interpreted in the most lethal way possible. One of those killed among the convalescing patients was Dr. Bujalski, former director of the Polish Ministry of Health. Dr. Bujalski had asked to remain on the medical block to work there and was said to have been told by Entress that he would be sent to a convalescent ward or sanatorium where he would receive a replacement for the stethoscope he realized he had left behind when entering the truck to take him to the gas chamber.[22] Entress was known not only to be especially "radical" in his selections behavior but also to be involved in experiments in which he infected prisoners with typhus in order to make medical observations on its communicability.[23]

He was ruthless in his pursuit of medical experience. He set up a tuberculosis ward for the purpose of learning the technique of pneumothorax therapy (the introduction of air into the pleural cavity in order to collapse a tubercular lung) under the tutelage of Wladyslaw Tondos, a Polish prisoner physician and lung specialist. Only after Entress had practiced that technique for some time did he order phenol injections for the entire ward. He also sought surgical experience under the guidance of Polish prisoner surgeons, causing harm and death to a number of patients. He particularly attached himself to Dr. Wladislaw Dering, an experienced surgeon and fellow Polish ethnic German, and "trained" with Dering during the latter's surgical removal of ovaries and testicles of Jewish prisoners as part of the sterilization and castration experiments (see pages 246–47).[24]

The phenol-injection project became a major outlet for Entress's medical "radicalism." For the most part, he supervised the project in a detached fashion. He did perform some early injections himself; but the general impression was that, in contrast to Bodman and at times Mengele, Entress preferred to turn over the direct killing function to others.

Polish prisoner doctors have provided a consistent picture of Entress (his tenure in Auschwitz [1941–43] was mostly during a period in which Jewish doctors were not yet permitted to work in the medical blocks). One Polish doctor spoke of him as "a very cold person, . . . without any expression. For instance, I never saw him laugh. . . . Actually for me he is one of the cruelest doctors I ever met in my entire life."

Dr. Tadeusz S. also stressed Entress's extreme coldness and distance ("He just didn't see me. I was like the air, not a person"), as well as the danger emanating from him ("I was extremely afraid of him").

Jan W. emphasized Entress's Nazi ideological intensity and his need to "shut himself off completely from his Polish influences"—the combination producing the "excess zeal" with which he treated prisoner doctors and other prisoners: "In camp he was eye to eye with former friends— Poles who were now prisoners. He would not help them or talk to them in Polish . . . and pretended that he did not know Polish. He was even aloof from former colleagues who graduated from the same university. He wanted to have his friends finished off as soon as possible."

Dr. W. thought that Entress had to "present this iron personality" in order to resist any suspicion of softness toward Poles, and that if he were to speak Polish "he might appear too friendly." This young Polish prisoner saw Entress as "completely true to his ideology," with an attitude toward Poles that "they either should be strong enough to work or if not should be liquidated instantly" and with "no psychological scruples."

To Dr. W., Entress was "an especially fanatical Nazi with the zealousness of the convert," a man who believed that Nazism "was the only path, and for that path it was necessary to sacrifice the lives of other people": "He treated Germans as *Übermenschen* ["supermen"]; Poles as *Untermenschen* ["subhumans"]; and Jews as not being humans at all."

Langbein suggested that Entress's "decidedly unathletic appearance, his sickly nature" might have contributed to his need to be " 'harder,' more cruel, than others." And Dr. W. believed that Entress's status as an ethnic German required him to "compensate for that deficiency by exaggerated, murderous zeal." Langbein and Dr. W. seemed to me to be psychologically accurate. For a man like Entress, the embrace of Germanism and Nazism can become so intense and so desperate as to be perceived as the only path to life itself—in his case to medical life as well. In addition, he had known no other assignment as a physician than the murderous one of concentration-camp doctor. He combined the absolute ideological passion of the healing-killing reversal with probably the most extreme numbing and doubling of any SS physician. He may well have consciously believed that his behavior in Auschwitz was the highest expression of the true Nazi physician. In 1946 Entress was tried and convicted by a United States court, and hanged.

The Doctors' Surrogates

The brutalized prisoners and the SS men who did most of the injecting tended to maintain the medical aura—in fact, to see themselves as doctors.

There was a hierarchy of phenol injectors, from a German political prisoner named Peter Welsch to four Polish prisoners to the leading SDG injector, Josef Klehr, and two others in his unit. Those in the sequence who injected most enthusiastically were likely to "play the doctor." A Polish prisoner orderly named Mieczyslaw Pańszczyk, for instance, who "bragged that he killed 12,000 people with his own hands," not only injected but "also liked to do smaller surgical operations although he had no medical training whatsoever. It didn't matter to him that he sometimes cut tendons and vessels when he cut open abcesses."[25]

Other prisoners, with good cause, considered such men to be psychopathic in their enjoyment of killing. They also, as a Polish prisoner doctor made clear, derived personal advantages from what they did: they had a "secure" job, did not have to work as hard as others, were given better food and generally preferential treatment. The injector "was under the protection of the Political Department, . . . the camp Gestapo," and "the other prisoners were afraid of this man."

Dr. W. told of one Polish injector who identified closely with Nazi anti-Semitism and "wanted the prisoners to be as frightened of him as of the SS people." One morning this man told Dr. W., "I had an interesting dream—a dream that after my death I would live in a special place where I would rule, where I would be sent thousands of people to kill personally with phenol injections. It was a wonderful dream." Jan W. commented that the dreamer thought it "a very positive dream—the murdering of people," and that the task "was not something imposed on him" but one "he chose for himself, and he enjoyed it." This dream epitomizes the ultimate Auschwitz vision: heavenly immortalization and absolute omnipotence via constant, institutionally arranged, medicalized (the dream mentioned only phenol injections) killing.

There were Polish prisoners who injected but had scruples: one man refused to kill a group of children and saved a number of sick people from injections before being enlisted to do them himself; and another man, despite injecting, continued to save the lives of people and also used his power as phenol executioner to do away with dangerous informers.[26]

Prisoner doctors besides Dering appear to have occasionally performed the injections. While German or Polish inmates were most likely to be called upon to perform phenol injections, Jewish prisoner doctors were asked to do them at times. One of Langbein's sources refers to a Dr. Landau, probably a Jew, who was said to have administered injections.[27] Further, a prisoner doctor injected mental patients with insulin,

(see pages 223–24)—a very different situation, but also a form of Auschwitz medical killing—and probably not unique. We recall as well Dr.
Michael Z.'s refusal to perform intracardiac injections by insisting upon
his technical inability, and Langbein cites a similar episode involving a Dr.
Mikluláš Korn who "had to fear the consequences of refusal much more
than any 'Aryan,' " but was not punished.[28] Dr. Jan W. also told of a
Polish doctor who was able to refuse and "got away with it."

At the time they were using prisoners for the task, the Nazis did not
seem to press those who were reluctant but preferred to seek out people
whose psychological and ideological inclinations made them willing or
even enthusiastic practitioners.

"Today I *Am the Camp Doctor"*: *Josef Klehr*

Sometime in 1942, phenol killing was essentially taken over by Josef
Klehr, who murdered as a delegate of Nazi doctors: "[Entress] left the
work to Klehr and then went away."[29] A semi-literate laborer and medical
orderly from Upper Silesia, he was intent upon killing *as a doctor*: "Klehr
put on his doctor's coat and told the girl: 'You have a heart condition.'
Then came the injection."[30] His nickname was "Professor," and his identification was not just with the doctor's role but with the latter's specific
Auschwitz killing role. Klehr conducted selections himself at times and
on Christmas Eve 1942, when told that the camp doctor could not appear,
replied immediately, "Today *I* am the camp doctor."[31]

Klehr took pride in his medical skills. He is said to have taken over the
phenol killings because one of the prisoners doing it had broken an
injection needle. He devised efficient ways of positioning prisoners for
injection into the heart, and was proud of his speed in killing people, two
or three in one minute. He even took up performing lumbar punctures,
or spinal taps—a demanding procedure, in which a long needle must be
injected between the vertebrae. He usually experimented on prisoners he
was to inject with phenol, and if they cried out (he took no measures
against pain), he "was reported to have hit these victims before their
death."[32]

Klehr was the ultimate caricature of the omnipotent Auschwitz doctor.
According to one account of a special execution of a Soviet political
"commissar," the victim, "covered with blood," was held down by four
prisoners while "Klehr . . . [stood] next to him in a white coat holding
a hypodermic, ready to kill." There are similar descriptions of Klehr
against a background of corpses turning to inject again, with his sleeves
rolled up and wearing either a white coat or "a pink rubber apron and
rubber gloves" and "holding a 20-cc hypodermic with a long needle" in
his hands.[33]

When there was no SS doctor present, Klehr would combine his image
of himself as doctor with that of oriental potentate:

To begin with, a prisoner immediately had to polish his motorcycle, on which he always came. Subsequently, he went directly into the doctor's room, had his boots taken off by a prisoner, and his feet washed. At the same time, another prisoner had to brush and polish his fingernails. He then sat in the middle of the room, smoked a pipe, had his feet in a tub, and sometimes had eight prisoners who were to read his every desire in his eyes, dance about him. He acted altogether like a Pasha. So, for instance, a prisoner tailor had to appear to take his measurements. He dictated some notes to another prisoner. Simultaneously, the Camp Senior of the Medical Block had to appear and give a report . . . on the events in the medical block. The prisoner pharmacist had to bring him medicines, which he [Klehr] took with him. . . . He did all this, however, only when the camp doctor was not present.[34]

As surprising as any other aspect of his behavior was a "medical" reversal he underwent upon being transferred, in the fall of 1944, to the outer camp Gleiwitz where he worked on a medical block and no longer did injections. A Czech inmate observed that "Klehr changed considerably. He was responsible for no more brutalities there and was generally decent." The same inmate overheard a conversation between Klehr and his wife, in which in response to her question about whether he was involved in any of the terrible things that went on in Auschwitz, he replied: "I am an SDG. I heal here and do not kill."[35] After his wife's visit, he was reported to have become even more insistent upon improving camp conditions for prisoners. This Czech inmate was also impressed with Klehr's wife and children (permitted to live nearby for a period of time) and seemed unable to understand how Klehr could have such a family.[36] He is believed to have killed by injection thousands of inmates.

Like the actual doctors, he was able to switch quite readily, at least for a time, from killer to healer, with the help of the influence of his family, especially his wife (who could visit more often in Gleiwitz). The deteriorating situation at the front might also have been responsible—that is, fear of facing enemy justice. But in his representation of himself at his trial, Klehr suggested the very opposite of repentance, and little of the healer seemed to be present in him in the courtroom. He was convicted at the Frankfurt Auschwitz trial and sentenced to life imprisonment and an additional fifteen years of hard labor.[37] (I shall discuss in chapter 20 this kind of contradictory behavior in connection with the Auschwitz self of the Nazi doctors.)

Klehr was estimated to have participated in the murder of between 10,000 and 30,000 persons (through selection or actual injections). Only 475 cases could be directly proven, plus complicity in about 2,000 more deaths. His sentence of 475 counts, for murders committed "on his own initiative (Eifer) with particular deceit (Heimtücke)," was the highest imposed at the Frankfurt Auschwitz trial. When the sentences were imposed, only Klehr immediately spoke up and said he would not accept the sentence; the other defendants were silent. In his closing statement, Klehr claimed to have had nothing to do with gassing or independent selections: "As a little man in Auschwitz," or "a soldier under orders," he "only carried out the orders of the doctors and only with deep inner reluctance."[38]

In sum, Klehr brought to Auschwitz enormous psychopathic potential, which the environment readily evoked (as it also did with some of the prisoners who regularly injected phenol). Every society has a pool of Klehrs to draw upon for its killing assignments, and the medicalized dimension gave particular form to his extreme combination of sense of omnipotence, paranoid sadism, and schizoid numbing. (As one prisoner put it, "[He] could kill a few hundred people the way a shoemaker rips a rotten sole off a shoe.") Klehr found a powerful *métier* in Auschwitz: while other SS men returning from leave would complain about having to come back to "this den of murderers [*Mörderhöhle*]," he seemed at home in the camp and his work in it.[39]

The Auschwitz Klehr was to a considerable degree a creature of the SS doctors, of Entress in particular: he was their psychological delegate who could perform the murderous acts they initiated. Because his hands were so dirty, the SS doctors could almost—but just almost—feel that theirs were clean.

"Decent" Killers

Two other SDG people, Herbert Scherpe and Emil Hantl, gave phenol injections but were seen by prisoners as very different from Klehr, as more or less "decent" killers. As one former prisoner nurse put it, they "behaved like saints compared with Klehr. They never beat anyone. . . . They acted politely. And most important of all, they said 'Good morning' when they came in, and 'Good-by' when they left. For us who had been so degraded, these were small tokens of humanity."[40]

It was these men who were assigned to the killing of the 120 Polish children from Zamosc between 23 February and 1 March. When the killing was completed, Hantl emerged "in a state of total collapse" and "completely went to pieces, cursed the war," and lost his SS demeanor. While prisoners were impressed with his breakdown, one commented that he had been "too cowardly to refuse to carry out the orders to kill."[41]

Scherpe reacted even sooner, emerging from the room in the middle of the killing muttering "I can't any more." The word in the camp was that he, too, had "broken down." He was observed, "pale and agitated," telling the chief doctor that he could not kill children, and was promptly transferred to an outer camp—and even promoted.[42]

Yet Scherpe and Hantl did a lot of killing: the court convicted Scherpe of complicity on at least 200 occasions of the killing of at least 900 people; and Hantl of complicity on at least 42 occasions in the killing of a total of at least 380 people. The court took account of their relative reluctance in the murders and of their friendliness toward prisoners and gave them startlingly light sentences: Scherpe, four and one-half years; and Hantl, three and one-half (served in full while he awaited trial), at hard labor.[43]

A show of revulsion, even among men who had done extensive killing, meant a lot in Auschwitz, as did the merest acknowledgment of the prisoners' humanity. But the real psychological point is that men much more ordinary than Klehr—men without his combination of omnipotence, sadism, and numbing—could be drawn into the phenol killings. Such men, to be sure, were more vulnerable to breakdown, especially when killing children (here resembling the *Einsatzgruppen* killers). The "decent" phenoler, because his killing was direct, had a more difficult time sustaining his work than did the "decent" Nazi doctor, whose responsibility was surely as great but who was able to place some distance between himself and the corpse. But the fact that there could be "decent" phenolers at all—that is, relatively ordinary, well-intentioned men who killed by injection—tells us much about the malignancy of the Auschwitz environment and the broad susceptibility of unremarkable men to becoming killers.

Chapter 15

The Experimental Impulse

I have no words. I thought we were human beings.
We were living creatures. How could they do things
like that?

—Auschwitz survivor

Nazi doctors are infamous for their cruel medical experiments. And no
wonder: those experiments killed and maimed; as tangible medical
crimes, they were given considerable prominence at the Nuremberg Medical Trial. Yet they were no more than a small part of the extensive and
systematic medicalized killing. And it is that aspect of the experiments—
their relation to the Nazi biomedical vision—that I shall mainly discuss.

Generally speaking, Nazi medical experiments fall into two categories:
those sponsored by the regime for a specific ideological and military
purpose, and those that were done *ad hoc* out of allegedly scientific
interest on the part of an SS doctor.

For example, extensive sterilization and castration experiments in
Auschwitz, conducted mainly by doctors Carl Clauberg and Horst Schumann, were encouraged officially as a direct expression of racial theory
and policy; the experiments with typhus contagion (injecting people with
blood from others with active typhus) and with the effectiveness of various preparations of sera (in treating experimentally induced cases of
typhus) were connected with military concerns about typhus epidemics
among German troops and civilian personnel in the East;* while the
study of pre-cancerous conditions of the cervix reflected a scientific interest of Dr. Eduard Wirths, the chief SS Auschwitz doctor, and his gynecologist brother Helmut. But the categories overlapped. (Mengele's research on twins, which we shall discuss in chapter 17, grew out of his
specific scientific interest but was also strongly affected by Nazi ideology.)
Here we shall focus on the extensive sterilization and castration experiments, in which Auschwitz more or less specialized, and which were a

*Typhus experiments were conducted only to a limited degree at Auschwitz, but on a
much wider scale at other camps.

direct extension of the biomedical vision, but also mention other forms of experimentation and scientific enterprise, including the establishment of a museum collection of Jewish skulls provided by Auschwitz.

Block 10

The center for these experimental projects was the notorious Block 10, a place that could be considered to be quintessential Auschwitz. Made up mostly of women prisoners, it was located in the men's camp, and the windows were kept closed and shuttered or boarded so that communication with the outside was totally cut off. One woman prisoner doctor who spent a year there described how, from the first night, she gained a lasting impression of having been transferred to a "horror place" that resembled both hell and a mental institution. And if one could peek out, one would witness executions, prisoners being shot to death in the courtyard of the infamous Block 11.

At the same time, inmates on the block were completely vulnerable to visits and surveillance of various kinds by SS doctors and, on occasion, by nonmedical officers: "A continuous coming and going of SS . . . [so that] we never felt safe." For any visit could mean new danger, and inmates therefore "awaited with impatience . . . the evening when we would be locked up as animals in a cage but . . . nonetheless felt freer."[1]

Another woman prisoner doctor, Adelaide Hautval, told of the five hundred women "guinea pigs," all Jewish, from various countries in Europe, who were usually selected directly from transports, according to the needs of the Nazi physician experimenters: "Some required married women, others young girls, a third a mixture of all the categories." Overall conditions were superior to those in the women's camp, because there the "guinea pigs . . . would have died before the results of the experiments could have been assessed." Inmates suffered from hunger, nonetheless, and from the constant uncertainty about "What will it be this time?" For they had absorbed the Auschwitz principle that *anything is permitted.* At the same time the women deeply feared a transfer to Birkenau, where they knew death was more likely, because in Block 10 there was at least a hope that "maybe they will still let us live after this," though few believed that possible.[2]

The block was divided into separate research areas: those of Professor Clauberg, Professor Schumann (both sterilizers), Dr. Wirths and his brother (who studied pre-cancerous growths of the cervix), and a special area for studies conducted by the Hygienic Institute.

Inevitably, there was a dimension of Auschwitz schizophrenia: in this case, the twenty-two prostitutes—mostly Germans, Poles, and Russians —the only non-Jewish residents of Block 10. On Himmler's orders, the SS opened bordellos at Auschwitz and other camps. Available to élite prisoners, mostly Germans, prostitutes were meant to be a work incentive and were also intended to help diminish widespread homosexuality among male prisoners (occasionally prostitutes were assigned to known homosexuals for that purpose, with predictable results).[3] The gynecologist Dr. Wanda J. told how prostitutes were instructed to visit her if they noticed any indication of venereal disease. Camp commanders frequently appeared on Block 10 to choose particular prostitutes for their subcamps. As Dr. J. put it in discussing the prostitutes, "that was a part of everything."

Extreme rumors spread through the camp about Block 10. Prisoners considered it a "sinister place" of mysterious evil. There were widespread rumors that Clauberg was conducting experiments in artificial insemination, and women were terrified of having "monsters" implanted in their wombs. Some survivors I spoke to believed that those experiments actually occurred. Another account had Clauberg speaking of his intentions to carry out artificial-insemination experiments in the future. There were also rumors of a "museum" on Block 10: "Skulls, body parts, even mummies"; and one survivor insisted, "A friend . . . saw . . . our *Gymnasium* [high school] teacher stuffed [mummified] on Block 10." Again, anything was possible, and whatever occurred there was likely to be a manifestation of the Nazi racial claim.

Sterilization by Injection: "The Professor"

Block 10 was often known as "Clauberg's block," because it was created for him and his experimental efforts to perfect a cheap and effective method of mass sterilization. He was Block 10's figure of greatest authority, "the main man for sterilization" as Dr. J. put it, and the one who "has the extras in equipment and space": in addition to the wards, an elaborate X-ray apparatus and four special experimental rooms, one of which served as a darkroom for developing X-ray films. As a civilian, Clauberg was an Auschwitz outsider who rented facilities, research subjects, and even prisoner doctors from the SS. He was a powerful outsider, holding a reserve SS rank of *Gruppenführer,* or lieutenant general. Höss and everyone else were aware that Himmler was interested in the work and had given the order that brought Clauberg to Auschwitz. He began his Auschwitz work in December 1942 in Birkenau; but after persuading the authorities that his important research required a special block, he transferred his experimental setting to Block 10 in Auschwitz in April 1943.

His method was to inject a caustic substance into the cervix in order to obstruct the fallopian tubes. He chose as experimental subjects married women between the ages of twenty and forty, preferably those who had borne children. And he first injected them with opaque liquid in order to determine by X ray that there was no prior blockage or impairment. He had experimented with different substances, but was very secretive about the exact nature of the one he used, probably intent upon protecting any

"medical discovery" from research competitors. Even the camp commandant, Rudolf Höss, who took a great interest in the work and witnessed
several injections, later wrote, "Clauberg informed me in detail on the
performance of the operation, but never revealed to me the exact chemical
composition of the substance he used." That substance is now believed to
have been Formalin, sometimes injected together with Novocain.[4]*

The injection was done in three stages over a few months, though some
women later described four or five injections. The goal of injecting the
caustic substance was to create adhesions in the fallopian tubes that
would cause them to be obstructed within a period of about six weeks,
as would be demonstrated by subsequent X rays. Clauberg had a prisoner
nurse, Sylvia Friedmann, observe the women after the injections for
symptoms of any kind.

Despite the terror induced in women victims, Marie L., a French prisoner physician, stressed that many so feared being sent back to Birkenau
(where one would be "awaiting death standing in frost, mud, and swamps
. . . without water or care") that they could view Block 10 as "a piece of
luck and the possibility of survival." Clauberg himself encouraged this
hope by his reassurances that he planned not to send them back to
Birkenau (meaning the gas chamber) but to take them to his private
research clinic at Königshütte, just a few kilometers from Auschwitz. That
could well have been true because Höss later reported that "after the
successful experiment, . . . Clauberg planned that everyone of the female
prisoners at the end of a year undergo sexual intercourse with a male
prisoner chosen especially for this purpose," in order to carry out a
practical test of Clauberg's sterilization method. This test, however, was
never performed "because of the course of the war."[5]

Clauberg eventually had as many as three hundred women under his
control on Block 10. The experiments were supposed to be highly secret,
and there was an attempt to isolate women who had been injected from
those who had not. Accounts differ about the fate of the women he
experimented upon. Those who refused to be experimented upon, or
who were considered for one reason or another unsuitable, were sent
back to Birkenau and usually gassed—as were those women who became
extremely debilitated. Most women experimented upon remained on
Block 10, though a considerable number developed fever and various
forms of peritoneal infection.

There was the constant fear of being killed because of knowing too
much. They also feared both sterilization and artificial insemination.
Clauberg is reported to have told prisoners he planned artificial-insemination experiments, and there is one report of his admitting to two
assistants that he had future plans for experiments in both natural and
artificial insemination.

*The formula was apparently developed by Clauberg and his assistant Dr. Johannes
Goebel, chief chemist with the Schering pharmaceutical firm.

Descriptions by women experimented upon begin to tell us in human terms what Clauberg was really up to. A Czech Jew named Margita Neumann told of being taken into a dark room with a large X-ray machine:

> Dr. Clauberg ordered me to lie down on the gynecological table and I was able to observe Sylvia Friedmann who was preparing an injection syringe with a long needle. Dr. Clauberg used this needle to give me an injection in my womb. I had the feeling that my stomach would burst with the pain. I began to scream so that I could be heard through the entire block. Dr. Clauberg told me roughly to stop screaming immediately, otherwise I'd be taken back at once to Birkenau concentration camp. . . . After this experiment I had inflammation of the ovaries.

She went on to describe how, whenever Clauberg appeared on the ward, women were "overcome with anxiety and terror," as "they considered what Dr. Clauberg was doing as the actions of a murderer."[6]

Survivors also mentioned his crude and cynical "jokes," as well as the resentments of him among other Nazi camp authorities who would like to have done away with Block 10, his protection of experimental subjects being seen by some as a way of maintaining his own enterprise.

Dr. L., who for a time took care of women in Block 10, observed Clauberg closely and described him as "short, bald, and unlikable." He was in fact about five feet tall, and several inmates referred to him as a kind of "caricature." In addition he had a history of violence: as a student, later toward his wife, and on still another occasion toward a mistress. As Marie L. said, in understatement, "I think that with him there was something quite unbalanced." Similarly, Dr. Tadeusz S. invoked Clauberg as evidence for his principle that "the greatest murderers were the greatest cowards," and described him as "fat and unpleasant looking, . . . a small, ugly, funny-looking, more or less deformed person. He wanted to imitate Prussian officers but he looked like a salesman in a general's hat. . . . He was absurd."

Yet Clauberg was also a professor and gynecological researcher and practitioner of considerable distinction. Long associated with the University of Kiel, his gynecological work there led to his *Habilitation* (qualification for lecturer-professorial status on the basis of advanced research and dissertation) in 1937 at the age of thirty-nine. The hormonal preparations Progynon and Proluton that he developed to treat infertility are still used today (in a letter written as early as June 1935, Clauberg discussed the former as useful for both maintaining and terminating pregnancy),[7] as is the "Clauberg test" for measuring the action of progesterone.

Clauberg's personal and ideological history, however, followed a familiar course. The oldest son of a rural craftsman who later established a weapons business, Clauberg was called to the military in 1916, saw action in France, and spent the last part of the war as a prisoner of the English. He joined the Nazi Party in 1933, became a committed Nazi who wore the Party's Golden Badge for meritorious service—while remaining personally and professionally highly ambitious—and reached his rank of reserve SS *Gruppenführer* (lieutenant general) in 1940.[8]

That same year a meeting with Himmler, arranged by a fellow SS officer, marked the beginning of a relationship based on a malignant blending of biomedical and political-racial ideologies—the initiative moving back and forth between the medical man and the SS leader, with the process culminating in "Clauberg's block" in Auschwitz. At this meeting Clauberg told Himmler of his intention to set up a research institute for reproductive biology, which would investigate both the causes and the treatment of infertility and the development of a nonsurgical means of sterilization. Himmler had first learned of Clauberg's work through the gynecologist's successful treatment of infertility in a high-ranking SS officer's wife. When Clauberg explained to the *Reichsführer* that such treatment required a preparation that could clear the fallopian tubes by softening any adhesions or substances blocking them, Himmler, whose real interest here was sterilization, was said to have suggested reversing that procedure by using agents that *produce* blocking. As a result of that conversation (whatever the sequence of who suggested what to whom), Clauberg redirected his research energies toward the explicit goal of finding an effective method of mass sterilization.

With financial support arranged by Himmler, Clauberg began animal experiments; found that a 5- to 10-percent solution of Formalin could produce the desired inflammation and blockage; sought out the highly viscous (resistant to flow) liquid that would, when containing Formalin, enable it to remain in the ovarian tubes after being introduced to the. uterus; and worked on X-ray tracing techniques for monitoring effects.[9]

A year later Himmler summoned Clauberg to confer and suggested that he conduct sterilization experiments at the Ravensbrück concentration camp. But with the help of Grawitz, the chief SS doctor now involved in the matter, Clauberg eventually convinced Himmler that Auschwitz would be more practical because of its proximity to Königshütte, where Clauberg already had his clinical facilities. On 30 May 1942, three days after their second meeting, Clauberg wrote a letter to Himmler remarkable in its expression of the German physician's *active*, indeed determined, effort to contribute to the deadly purposes of the Nazi biomedical vision.

Clauberg makes clever obeisance not only to Himmler's overall authority but to his "scientific" concerns, by stating that he (Clauberg) had been told that "the one person in Germany today who would be particularly interested in these matters and who would be able to help me would be you, most honorable *Reichsführer*." By mentioning proposed work on "positive population policy," Clauberg ingeniously alludes to the agricultural dimension so dear to Himmler ("The eventual or most probable importance of agriculture for the female capacity for propagation demands clarification") and then gets to the real point—the question of the "negative population policy," about which he makes the dramatic proposal that, having demonstrated the possibility of sterilization without operation on the basis of animal experiments, "now we must proceed to the first experiments on human beings." The letter goes on with this combination of flattery, slick scientific gloss, elaborate research projection (a laboratory for animal experiments, an experimental farm to investigate questions of "agriculture and fertility," etc.), and a pervasive medical focus ("The center from which all ideas start, all problems are raised . . . and finally turned over to practical use, is and remains the clinic") —all leading to the plan to "evaluate the method of sterilization without operation . . . on women unworthy of propagation and to use this method continually after it is finally proved efficient." He makes clear that Auschwitz is the ideal place for "the human material to be provided," and even proposes that it be named after Himmler as "Research Institute of the *Reichsführer* SS for Biological Propagation." The entire letter captures much of the ethos and corruption of the physician researcher within the Nazi biomedical vision.[10]

After a flurry of additional changes involving Himmler's adjutants and other SS doctors, and another visit with the *Reichsführer* himself, Clauberg's plan for Auschwitz work was approved in a letter in which Himmler (through his assistant, Rudolf Brandt) indicated that he would be "interested to learn . . . how long it would take to sterilize a thousand Jewesses," made some additional suggestions about method, and finally advocated as a test "a practical experiment [of] . . . locking up a Jewess and a Jew together for a certain period and then seeing what results are achieved."[11]

Himmler's enthusiasm for Clauberg's project had been independently nurtured by another physician correspondent, Dr. Adolf Pokorny, a Czech ethnic German who had retired with a high rank from a career in military medicine. In October 1941, Pokorny wrote a letter to Himmler that could also stand as a basic document in the ideological corruption of the healer. Pokorny's letter was written in response to the idea "that the enemy must not only be conquered but destroyed"; felt impelled to notify Himmler of recent work on "medicinal sterilization" in which the sap of a particular plant (containing *Caladium seguinum*) produced "permanent sterility" in both male and female animals; and advocated "immediate research on human beings (criminals!)" as well as extensive cultivation of the plant and absolute secrecy. Pokorny gloried in the vision of "a new powerful weapon at our disposal": "The thought alone that the 3 million Bolsheviks, at present German prisoners, could be sterilized so that they could be used as laborers but be prevented from reproduction, opens the most far-reaching perspectives.[12]*

---

*The letter earned Pokorny a place in the dock at Nuremberg. He defended himself by pleading that *Caladium seguinum* was so clearly unsuitable for human sterilization that he had written Himmler to divert him from considering more feasible methods. The court ruled that the letter, "monstrous and base as . . . [its] suggestions . . . are," did not justify a

The drug proved totally unfeasible for human sterilization, but Himmler made clear that he considered such experimental investigation of the greatest importance. He began to develop a file on what he called "sterilization by medicines," and a separate file on mass sterilization by X rays (which we will soon examine in connection with Schumann). Clauberg's project could thus be seen by Himmler as a newly scientific approach by a renowned professor to "sterilizations by medicines."

But despite the professor's high backing, the enthusiastic support and involvement of Höss, and the required sponsorship of Wirths, Clauberg had his difficulties at Auschwitz. He had considerable personal conflict with many of the other doctors there, and he experienced delays in acquiring the advanced radiological equipment he felt he needed. Most problematic of all, he was caught in his own contradictions concerning the efficacy of his sterilization method. He had always exaggerated that efficacy, both out of ambition and under pressure from Himmler to produce, and produce quickly, this revolutionary racial contribution to the Nazi project. On 7 June 1943, Clauberg wrote to Himmler attempting to justify his slow progress, referred to "temporary difficulties" including his long wait for an X-ray apparatus, and then engaged in some monumental double-talk: His method was "as good as perfected" (*so gut wie fertig ausgearbeitet*) but required a few "refinements" (*Verfeinerungen*), so that "even today it could be put to practical use . . . [for] regular eugenic sterilization"; indeed, he was now ready to reply to "the question which you, *Reichsführer,* asked me one year ago—namely, how much time would be required to sterilize one thousand women by this method?" There were still hedges ("If my researches continue to have the same results, . . . the moment is not far off when I can say") and finally the anticlimactic declaration (with his own quotations and italics): *"One* adequately trained physician in *one* adequately equipped place, with perhaps ten assistants (the number of assistants in conformity with the speed desired) will most likely be able to deal with several hundred, even if not 1000 per day."*[14]

The claim was still fuzzy, to say the least, and it turned out that "the main reason" for the letter was to request certain new arrangements (not clear from the letter but probably having to do with Clauberg's "sterilization race" with Schumann) and another X-ray apparatus he had located in Berlin but for which he needed Himmler's approval. The underlying significance of the letter is that combining Nazi political and biomedical ideologies, and living up to them medically, had contradictions and shortcomings—one might even say inevitable failures. These contradictions, together with Clauberg's general instability or "complexes," took their toll. Wirths, the chief doctor, was quoted to me as having said that Clauberg had "completely gone to the dogs" and had become a severe alcoholic and a "totally unscrupulous character." And Wirths's brother,

---

conviction, and concluded, "We find, therefore, that the defendent must be acquitted—not because of the defense tendered, but in spite of it."[13]

also a doctor, referred to Clauberg as "one of the worst characters I ever met."*

Clauberg's assistant in Auschwitz, Dr. Johannes Goebel, worked on producing the necessary caustic substance as well as improved X-ray tracing material and, although not a physician, was given the prerogative of performing many of the injections.[15] The number of women these two men are believed to have sterilized in this fashion has been estimated from seven hundred to "several thousand."[16] According to the nurse Sylvia Friedmann, when a woman died after injection Clauberg "showed absolutely no interest, no reaction, as though the matter didn't concern him at all." There were a number of such deaths.[17]

As Russian troops approached Königshütte, Clauberg fled to Ravensbrück and arranged for some of his research victims to be sent there as well; despite the extreme chaos, he continued with his sterilization experiments. But with the approach of the Allied armies three months later, he fled again, this time to Schleswig-Holstein, seeking to join the last group of loyal SS leaders surrounding Himmler, the only Auschwitz doctor to do so. But Himmler was captured and committed suicide; and Clauberg too was captured by the Russians on 8 June 1945. Imprisoned in the Soviet Union for three years before being tried, he was then convicted of war crimes and sentenced to twenty-five years' imprisonment. But following Stalin's death (in 1953), and various diplomatic agreements, Clauberg was repatriated with other Germans in October 1955. He was not only unrepentant but grandiose and bizarre: he listed on his professional card various Nazi medical organizations, including the "City of Mothers" he had run as part of his involvement in "positive eugenics," and advertised for a secretary under his own name. When interviewed by the press, he spoke proudly of his work at Königshütte and Auschwitz and claimed, "I was able to perfect an absolutely new method of sterilization . . . [which] would be of great use today in certain cases."[18]

After various pressures from survivor groups and others, Clauberg was arrested in November 1955; but for a considerable time, the German Chamber of Medicine, the official body of the profession, resisted action against him that would divest him of his title of doctor of medicine. A group of former prisoner physicians of Auschwitz issued an impressive declaration condemning Clauberg's actions there as being "in total disaccord with the sworn duty of every doctor," and bitterly decrying the fact that "such medical practitioners who . . . put themselves at the service of National-Socialism to destroy human lives . . . are today in a position to practice once more the profession which they have profaned in such a scandalous manner."[19] The German Chamber of Medicine finally did remove Clauberg's license. But when he died, suddenly and mysteriously, in his prison cell on 9 August 1957, the general belief was that he was

---

*He added, "It was said he [Clauberg] was a Jew himself [of course, he was not]: at any rate he looked like it. And [also] because he was extremely careful to obscure his traces."

in the process of naming names at the top of the Nazi medical hierarchy and that, consequently, medical colleagues helped bring about his death.[20]

It would be too easy to attribute Clauberg's criminal medical behavior to his physical appearance and resulting "complexes." While there is no doubt that he could be seen as a classical case of what Alfred Adler described as seeking extreme forms of compensatory behavior for deep-seated feelings of bodily inferiority,[21] I would also stress his intense relationship to Nazi ideology (stemming from a more or less typical historical experience beginning with the First World War) along with his extraordinary ambition within the Nazi system. A former student of his told how Clauberg, though "a frightfully ugly dwarf" and "full of complexes," nonetheless was friendly to students and took them on weekend trips, and added, "I liked him a lot then." Even with his psychological aberrations, that is, Clauberg might under a different regime have found a life pattern with a manageable mixture of accomplishment, arrogance, and corruption. Or, to put the matter another way, just as there are always Klehrs available for direct killing, so are there always Claubergs available for ideological and professional criminality and killing. Nazi institutions provided the ideal climates for nourishing Clauberg's compensatory grandiosity and psychopathic tendencies. Auschwitz drew also on his research talent, which was radically corrupted in the service of the "negative eugenics" of the biomedical vision.

X-Ray and Surgical Castration: Biomedical Patron and Political Doctor

Horst Schumann differed from Clauberg in being not a renowned specialist but a reliable "old Nazi doctor" (he joined the Nazi Party and the SA in 1930) who was available for ruthless medical enterprises. Schumann had been a leading figure in the "euthanasia" program as the director of the killing center at Grafeneck. When that center closed, he took over the one at Sonnenstein, subsequently became active in project 14f13 as a member of the medical commissions visiting the camps, and in that capacity had come to Auschwitz on 28 August 1941, and participated in the selection of 575 prisoners sent to the Sonnenstein killing center (see pages 142–43). His qualifications for Auschwitz X-ray castration were more political than medical.

In this case, Himmler played an even greater role in formulating the experiments, together with Viktor Brack, the Chancellery official active in both the "euthanasia" project and the establishment of the death camps. In early 1941, Himmler and Brack were already exchanging memos in which they shared a vision of "sterilization or castration . . . by means of X-rays" on a massive scale (see pages 274–76). Brack later claimed that the idea originated with Himmler for application to Jewish populations, especially in Poland, and also implicated Reinhard Heydrich, the most ruthless voice around Himmler, but at the same time admitted that Himmler's words "made a great impression on me." Brack in any case extended the shared fantasy to include assembly-line sterilization "quite imperceptibly" from behind a counter where the ignorant victim was required to fill in forms for about two or three minutes:

> The official sitting behind the counter could operate the installation in such a way as to turn a switch which would activate the two valves simultaneously (since the irradiation has to operate from both sides). With a two-valve installation about 150–200 persons could then be sterilized per day, and therefore, with twenty such installations as many as 3,000–4,000 persons per day. . . . As to the expenses for such a two-valve system, I can only give a rough estimate of approximately 20,000–30,000 RM (*Reichsmarks*).[22]

The idea was consistent with not only the larger Nazi biomedical vision but also the specific characteristics of Heinrich Himmler's thought. Himmler, Joachim Fest has accurately noted, wished to see himself as "not a murderer but a patron of science."[23] He was, moreover, a patron who took an active part in determining the concepts and methods of scientific enterprises under his auspices. In the Nazi movement, he was the pseudo-medical scientist par excellence, the personal and ideological epitome of the healing-killing reversal.* Trained initially in agriculture, he combined nature mysticism with a kind of biomechanics and fancied himself something of a medical visionary. He combined Rosenberg's racial vision with Walther Darré's agricultural mysticism: it is believed to have been Darré "who urged Himmler to transfer his attention from the breeding of herbs and the raising of chickens to human beings."[25]† And Himmler's wife Margarete, a nurse, is said to have interested him in "homeopathy, mesmerism, oat-straw baths, and herbalism." As Joachim Fest makes clear, Himmler's language was consistently biomedical: "There was talk of 'fields of racial experiment,' 'nordification,' 'aids to procreation,' 'the foundations of our blood,' 'fundamental biological laws,' 'the ruination of our blood,' 'breeding of a new human type,' or 'the botanical garden of Germanic blood'—truly the visions of a poultry farmer from Waltrudering!"[26]

*Himmler's vision had varying gradations of absurdity and pseudo science. For instance, he was an ardent believer (as were Hitler and Göring) in such expressions of mystical racism as the idea that the lost continent of Atlantis had been the original homeland of the Aryans, and that Aryans had not evolved from monkeys or apes like the rest of mankind but had descended to earth from the heavens where they had been preserved in ice from the beginning of time. Himmler, in fact, in 1937 established a meteorology division in the *Ahnenerbe* (see pages 284–87) to "prove" this "cosmic-ice" theory, though publicly the purpose of the new division was announced as developing new techniques for long-range weather prediction. Sympathetic to nature healing and an equally ardent critic of traditionalism and "Christian" prejudices of establishment doctors, he could view human experimentation in concentration camps as a form of liberation from these constraints in the name of bold scientific innovation.[24]

†Darré, the Reich farmers' leader and Reich food minister, was a "blood and soil" ideological theorist who glorified the German peasant as the driving force of history.

Underlings like Brack and physicians like Clauberg suggested projects they knew to be consistent with Himmler's ideas and policies. Brack's passion for sterilization and castration could also have been related to his own experience as a patient who had undergone X-ray treatment, and had consulted a medical authority about his fears that the treatment might have caused bodily harm, specifically to his genitals. Brack was also the son of a gynecologist, and a failed medical student with medical aspirations of his own. By June 1942, at the height of the German military penetration into Russia, Brack became more specific and programmatic. Referring to consultations with his superior and with the head of the area in Poland where the greatest number of Jews was concentrated, he spoke of the necessity of carrying through "the whole Jewish action [the Final Solution]" but estimated that two million to three million of the ten million Jews in Europe were fit enough to work and therefore should be "preserved" but at the same time "rendered incapable of propagating." Ordinary sterilization methods being used for hereditary diseases would take too much time and be too expensive, but "castration by X-ray . . . is not only relatively cheap, but can be performed on many thousands in the shortest time." He referred to "completed experiments"* and declared himself ready, even eager, to initiate such a project. But Himmler, ever the scientist, insisted that "sterilization by X-rays . . . [be] tried out at least once in one camp in a series of experiments."[28] Schumann was chosen for the task and, by late 1942, was at work on X-ray castration on Block 30 in Birkenau.

Schumann did not have Clauberg's extraordinary standing in Auschwitz, but his experiments were, if anything, even more sinister. Comparing the two, Dr. Tadeusz S. understood Schumann to have been "ordered by somebody to do . . . experiments . . . not original. Clauberg was the only one with his own ideas. . . . Schumann was inspired by . . . ideologists." Dr. Marie L. went further in declaring that Schumann's "manner of proceeding revealed a total absence of knowledge of gynecological anatomy."

Schumann's appearance was also the opposite of Clauberg's: tall, broad-shouldered, elegant in his *Luftwaffe* uniform, his face described by some as handsome and others as "brutish," and thought by Dr. L. to be "a representative of the new German racist ideal." Some inmates described him as "correct," but a prisoner secretary added that he was "cold" and "revealed no human feelings in regard to the prisoners."[29] Over all, these descriptions suggest a quiet, undistinguished version of Nazi-style hauteur, along with an attitude of detachment and absence of concern. His experimental policies were brutal and unrestrained. He

---

*In his Nuremberg defense, Brack claimed that, in referring to these nonexistent experiments, he had been manipulating Himmler by seeking to plant in his mind an alternative to the Final Solution as a way of stalling the whole process.[27] The evidence is that Brack was manipulating Himmler, but in order to press ahead at full speed with the castration-sterilization project. Such a kernel of truth could have enabled him to utter his false testimony with something approaching conviction.

worked on Block 30, in the women's hospital in Birkenau, in a large room containing two extensive X-ray apparatuses and a small booth for him, which had a window and was, of course, insulated with lead plates to protect him from radiation.

Experimental subjects—relatively healthy young men and women in their late teens or early twenties, who had been obtained by a previous day's order from the camps—were lined up in a waiting room and brought in one by one, often completely ignorant of what was to be done to them. Women were put between plates that pressed against abdomen and back; men placed penis and scrotum on a special plate. Schumann himself turned on the machines, which hummed loudly; and each "treatment" lasted "several minutes" according to Dr. Stanislaw Klodziński, "five to eight minutes" according to Dr. Alina Brewda, another prisoner physician. Many of the women emerged with what Marie L. called "substantial burns," which could become infected and take a long time to heal; and many quickly developed symptoms of peritonitis, including fever and severe pain and vomiting. Not long after the X rays, the women's ovaries were removed surgically, usually in two separate operations. This was the operation performed mainly by Dering (see pages 246–49), and the method often used—a horizontal incision above the pubic area as opposed to a median laparotomy (abdominal opening)—carried the greater danger of infection. The ovaries were sent to laboratories to determine whether the X rays were effective in destroying tissue.[30]

As Dr. L. wrote, "There were deaths, there were complications, there were aggravations of pulmonary tuberculosis, given the absence of preliminary examination. There were pleurisies, long endless suppurations." She observed also that the operations were performed "at a more and more accelerated pace," so that Dering could eventually perform ten within two hours.[31]

Dr. Wanda J. was ordered to comfort the young Greek women being operated upon ("Greek children, because they were between sixteen and eighteen, . . . [already] like skeletons") one after the other: the girls screaming and crying ("They called me Mother, [and] they thought I would save them but I couldn't") through the crude spinal tap and rough ten-minute surgery; the pathetic, childlike victim being carried out on a stretcher as the next one was brought in for the spinal tap. Dr. J. pointed out that Dering neglected to take the ordinarily obligatory step of applying a portion of the peritoneum (the membrane lining the abdominal cavity) as a flap to cover and protect the "stump" of the tube from which the ovary had been removed, and thereby contributed to later complications of bleeding and severe infection: "They were nine months in bed. I was doing the dressing all the time—and the smell, I can't tell you. They were in a big room—only . . . eight of them, because two died."

By then Schumann had lost interest in them (there was nothing more to find out concerning castration-sterilization), but Dr. J. had to go to considerable effort to keep them more or less hidden "because if Schumann knew that they [were] alive . . . [on] Block 10, he would kill them straightaway." They were known as "Schumann's girls."

The depth of these experimental victims' sense of violation and mutilation was evident during interviews I had with some of them thirty-five years later. A Greek-Jewish woman described her terror as she saw in a reflection "the blood pouring out as they opened my belly"; and then, after the two operations, "pus—like a pit from an infected wound, and a high temperature, . . . pneumonia. My body swelled up, and there were marks when I pressed my arm [edema]. They gave me medicine. I was paralyzed. . . . I couldn't move. My whole body was swollen up." In addition: "We knew we were like a tree without fruit. . . . The experiment was that they were destroying our organs. . . . We would cry together about this"; and, "They took us because they didn't have rabbits."

Schumann's experiments with men had a parallel course, as described by Dr. Michael Z. in a written report: First, the rumor that "Jews were being sterilized with X-rays" by "an air-force lieutenant-physician"; then a visit by Schumann to a male medical ward during which he ordered them to prepare for forty inmates on whom they were to keep records of medical observations; the arrival of the experimental victims with burn erythemas [red areas] around the scrotum ("From their description, we recognized the X-ray machine"); the victims' later accounts of their sperm being collected, their prostates brutally massaged with pieces of wood inserted into the rectum); their exposure to an operation removing one or two testicles, and in some cases a second operation removing the remaining testicle (conducted with "noticeable brutality" and limited anesthesia: patients' "screams were frightening to hear"); "disastrous" post-operative developments including hemorrhages, septicemia, absence of muscle tone from wounds, so that "many . . . would die rapidly, weakened morally and physically" and others would be sent to work "which would finish them." But "their deaths mattered little since these guinea pigs have already served the function expected of them."

Dr. Erich G. told of the psychological pain of experimental victims and of their questions to him ("Will I [be able to] be a father? Can I [have relations with] females?") but admitted that at the time that was not the greatest emotional stress ("To survive was more important than to be mutilated or even castrated"); and the fear was that experimental victims would be killed ("It was impossible to believe that they would allow people to live after the war to be a witness").

Schumann's callousness was reflected (as Dr. Tadeusz S. tells us) in the "little device" he constructed to insert into the rectum to stimulate the prostate and produce ejaculation, which was "painful and . . . humiliating so that the patients suffered a great deal." It also produced "terrible infections": "For Schumann it was nothing. . . . He was testing the results of his work."

One of the male victims told of the sequence from the X rays ("My genital organ, together with the scrotum, on a machine . . . the noise of a motor . . . from five to eight minutes," after which he "had a general ill feeling"); to the collection of sperm ("Dr. Dering came with a sort of club and put it into my rectum. . . . Some drops came out of my member"); to beginning arrangements for the operation ("I said, 'Why are you operating on me? I am . . . not sick.' [And Dering] answered, '. . . If I take not the testicle off you they will take it off me' "); to the painful spinal anesthetic and the operation itself ("After some minutes I saw Dr. Dering when he had my testicle in his hand and showed it to Dr. Schumann, who was present"). To another man asking the same question before the operation, Dering replied, "Stop barking like a dog. You will die anyway."[32]

Schumann's brutalization in Auschwitz is revealed by a lesser research project he conducted on a fungus condition of the face, a form of ringworm spread by large numbers of men being shaved with the same brush. Although experience had shown that the condition could be readily treated with various medicines, Schumann seized the occasion to try the efficacy of his X rays. These caused severe skin eruptions and infections, and in many victims impairment of salivary and tear-duct functions along with paralysis of face and eyes, which in turn caused a number of men to be sent to the gas.[33]

In addition to these Jewish victims, a group of young, healthy Polish men were subjected to the X-ray castration experiment. They were probably given an unusually high dosage because, as the former orderly in the ward reported, "Their genitals started slowly rotting away" and the men "often crawled on the floor in their pain." Ointments were tried, but the men did not improve; and after a long period of suffering, they were ordered by Thilo to the gas chamber.[34]

Dr. Klodziński writes of as many as 200 men being subjected to X-ray castration, and of about 180 of those to amputation of at least one testicle, 90 of these operations taking place on one day, 16 December 1942. While overall statistics are uncertain, the general estimate is that approximately 1,000 prisoners, male and female, underwent X-ray sterilization or castration, and about 200 of these were subjected to surgical removal of testicles or ovaries. Whatever statistics are available derive from the Auschwitz policy of keeping relatively accurate surgical records of these experiments.[35]*

Like Clauberg, Schumann continued his experiments in Ravensbrück, there victimizing thirteen-year-old Gypsy girls.

After the war he managed to live obscurely in Germany—although recognized at Nuremberg as a war criminal—until an application for a license for a hunting gun led to his being identified. He fled Germany

---

*At the Dering trial, the surgical register was summarized as follows: "There was a list of 130 numbered lines, each having a date between 5 March 1943 and 10 November 1943; an individual prisoner's number and name; and the nature of an operation in Latin, such as *castratio*, *sterilisatio*, *amputatio testis sin.* left, *amputatio testis dex.* right, *amputatio testis utriusque* bilateral, *ovariectomia sin.*, and *ovariectomia dex.* "[36]

precipitately, traveled extensively, and eventually settled in Khartoum in the Sudan as head of a hospital. There for about seven years he apparently became something of a Good Samaritan, working night and day treating Africans and conducting research into sleeping sickness; he described himself to a visiting journalist as having "found the serenity and the calm necessary for the moral balance of a human being."[37] But he was identified by an Auschwitz survivor on the basis of the photograph accompanying that article. He fled to Ghana, from where he was eventually handed over (in November 1966, after the death of Kwame Nkrumah who, as prime minister, had protected him for some time) to representatives of West Germany. By then, he had become weakened from chronic malaria and other illnesses. In custody for several years, he was convicted for his involvement in direct medical killing or "euthanasia"; but because of his heart condition and generally deteriorating health, he was released without having stood trial for his sterilization and castration experiments.[38] He died in Frankfurt in 1983.

There were some reports of his having shown regret and even contrition, and he was quoted as having admitted to his "euthanasia" activities at Grafeneck and his Auschwitz experiments and saying, "It was terrible what we did."[39] But at other moments, in the courtroom and elsewhere, he was much less than contrite, defending or denying his actions. It is doubtful that he ever morally confronted his own past actions, but it is possible that his work in Africa, though undertaken primarily to avoid justice, eventually served, in a partial psychological sense, as a form of penance.

Schumann has great importance for us because of what he did—intense involvement in both direct medical killing and unusually brutal Auschwitz experiments—and what he was—an ordinary, but highly Nazified man and doctor.

Anthropological Research: Specimens for a Museum

Block 10 played an important part in a form of "anthropological research" that was among the most grotesque expressions of the Nazi biomedical vision. Dr. Marie L. tells of its Auschwitz beginnings:

There appeared [on Block 10] a new protagonist of racial theories. He chose his material by having naked women of all ages file . . . in front of him: He wanted to do anthropological measurements. . . . He had measurements of all the parts of the body taken ad infinitum. . . . They were told that they had the extraordinary good fortune to be selected, that they would leave Auschwitz to go to an excellent camp, somewhere in Germany . . . [where] they would be very well treated, where they would be happy.

Dr. L. had seen enough of Auschwitz to suspect the terrible truth ("I told myself immediately, . . . 'They are going to a museum' "), though she and others refrained from saying so because they "lacked the courage," felt it would be more kind to remain silent, and could not in any case be certain of their suspicion.

These women were taken to the concentration camp at Natzweiler, near Strasbourg, which although not designated as an extermination camp, nonetheless possessed its own gas chamber with the usual false showerheads as well as one additional feature: a one-way mirror that allowed those on the outside of the gas chamber to observe those inside. This mirror had been installed because the gas chamber itself had been constructed as part of the necessary research equipment.

A prisoner doctor reported that the group of Auschwitz women (thirty-nine of them according to other records) were given a sham physical examination for reassurance, then gassed, and that the corpses were immediately transported to the anatomy pavilion of the Strasbourg University Hospital. A French inmate, who had to assist the project's director, SS Captain Dr. August Hirt, told how "preservation began immediately" with the arrival of bodies that were "still warm, the eyes . . . wide open and shining." There were two subsequent shipments of men, from each of whom the left testicle had been removed and sent to Hirt's anatomy lab.[40]

Hirt, a professor of anatomy, had under Himmler's instructions prepared the cyanide salts used to kill the Auschwitz prisoners in what was the inaugural use of the new gas chamber. He had originally advocated in a memo to Himmler the securing of skulls of captured "Jewish-Bolshevik commissars." The goal at that time was to "acquire tangible scientific research material" that would "represent . . . a repulsive but typical species of subhumanity." The memo recommended that "a junior physician attached to the *Wehrmacht*" first take photographs and perform various measurements and studies on subjects while still alive, make sure that the head is not damaged in the killing, and then take other specific measures for preserving the head and shipping it to the designated research institute where various studies could be performed on the skull and brain including those of "racial classification" and "pathological features of the skull formation." In locating two ultimate evils (Jewish and Bolshevik) in members of that group, and anticipating specific anatomical findings in their skulls or brains, the Nazis were acting upon the most extreme blend of racial-biomedical and political ideology.[41]

But there were apparently difficulties in rounding up "Jewish-Bolshevik commissars" and possibly in severing heads, so that it was decided to make use of full skeletons rather than merely skulls and to collect specimens in the place where any such task could be accomplished—namely, Auschwitz. It was said that 115 people were victimized in this way, all Jews (79 men, 30 women) with the exception of 2 Poles and 4 central Asians. The relatively high priority of the project is suggested by Eichmann's having been involved in its arrangements.[42]

The whole enterprise, bizarre even by Nazi standards, was sponsored by the *Ahnenerbe* ("ancestral heritage") office of the SS, which Himmler had created in 1939 to develop "historical" and "scientific" studies of the "Nordic Indo-Germanic race." *Ahnenerbe* brought mystical concepts to science ("the unity of soul and body, mind and blood") and combined the Gestapo mission of controlling Germany's intellectual life with Himmler's visionary ideas. It supported projects in archeology, German racial consciousness outside of Germany proper, and medical experiments in concentration camps. Under Himmler's orders, *Ahnenerbe* even came to sponsor a research program making use of Jewish mathematicians in concentration camps to work out theoretical problems of rocket production. Experiments in camps that it sponsored included Dr. Sigmund Rascher's notorious research in Dachau on the effects of high altitude, in which he wantonly killed experimental subjects; and the still more murderous work of Schuler in Buchenwald on typhus vaccines, in which six hundred people were killed.[43]

Hirt was said to have been brought into *Ahnenerbe* by a man who became his assistant in the Strasbourg project—Bruno Beger, an SS officer on Himmler's personal staff who had been sent to study anthropology in Berlin. Beger tended to embrace Himmler's wildest theories, and it was Beger who made the original arrangements in Auschwitz and perhaps wrote under Hirt's name the extraordinary memo I have just quoted.[44]

A former ardent Nazi, who remembered Hirt as a good friend and colleague during their days together as young instructors at a leading German medical center, described him as originally Swiss but a naturalized German, "a Nordic type with blue eyes and fair hair," an honorable and stable man even if at times "a bit impulsive," and an excellent anatomist with a promising academic career. A colleague of my own in the United States, however, who had studied under Hirt, remembered him as a very arrogant and threatening Nazi. In any case, there is no doubt about either Hirt's passionate Nazi involvement or the centrality of the Nazi biomedical vision in his participation in the "museum" project, even if Beger was its driving force. (Precisely that centrality was what Hirt's old friend wished to deny in his insistence that Hirt's entire behavior could be understood as an expression of the callousness of the anatomist.)

Toward the end of the war, there was apparently some confusion about whether and how much to continue with research procedures, and eventually the evidence was ordered to be destroyed. But that process could not be completed, and French forces liberating Strasbourg found in Hirt's dissection room "many wholly unprocessed corpses," many "partly-processed corpses," and a few that had been "defleshed . . . late in 1944," and their heads burned to avoid any possibility of identification—with "special care taken to remove the number tattooed on the left forearm." Hirt himself disappeared at that time and is now known to have killed himself shortly afterward.[45]

This museum project is remarkable for its merging of Himmler's racial vision with highly concrete, pseudo-scientific anthropological (Beger) and medical (Hirt) participation—all a logical outgrowth of the Nazi biological and political mentality.[46]

The Hygienic Institute: Sanctuary and Taint

What were perhaps the oddest and most benign of the experiments also took place on Block 10, in the section reserved for the work of the Hygienic Institute—and yet that institute hardly escaped Auschwitz evil.

Dr. Ernst B., whom I have frequently quoted concerning Auschwitz events and attitudes, confused prisoner doctors with his experiments relating dental infections to rheumatic and other bodily symptoms, and involving the injection of vaccines made from these infections in order to test a person's sensitivity. Dr. Michael Z. thought Dr. B. lacked focus ("[He] started a new project almost every day") and castigated him for having people's teeth pulled as experimental treatment. Another prisoner doctor similarly thought that Dr. B. was "amusing himself" with these experiments. But Dr. Wanda J., who could observe these experiments closely because of her position on Block 10, dismissed what Dr. B. was doing as inconsequential "stupidity." And referring to another aspect of his experiments, the rubbing of certain substances onto the skin, Dr. J. pointed out that it was easy to substitute plain water for the substance. More important, she went on to say, she was able to "choose girls" for these experiments instead of Clauberg's; to relieve their fear, she would rub the substance (usually just water) on herself "to show the girls that it's nothing."

Dr. B. made explicit his and his superior's intent, in creating the experiments, to rescue specific women (usually wives and relatives of male prisoners who worked in the Hygienic Institute) from Clauberg's unit, where they were likely to be harmed by experiments and then sent to the gas chamber. Block 10 was generally Clauberg's domain; and in order to be able to continue to occupy space there, the Hygienic Institute had to demonstrate to him that it was conducting "serious experiments." For that purpose Dr. B. arranged to produce by injection large inflammations in the upper thighs of these women; he did his best to explain to them that it was benign and necessary, but he was at the same time aware that "this created the impression in the general camp that I was involved in dangerous, life-threatening experiments." He confirmed that the experiments involved injection of vaccines made from tooth infections (of other people) in order to test for positive reactions; and when these were

found, to make dental X rays in the expectation of finding tooth infections. And he claimed that the women were later smuggled out of the
block by means of a system that included declaring them dead and bribing the "brothel *capo*" to let them make their exit with the group of
prostitutes who lived on Block 10 but left daily for work on other blocks.
When Dr. B. himself was on trial, women he had in this way experimented
upon testified to the life-saving nature of his actions, as did several prisoner doctors, male and female.

Yet Ernst B. was candid enough to describe, during our interview, the
multiplicity of elements that motivated him to do the experiments. There
was the satisfaction of getting individual people out of Clauberg's ward
and thereby "getting at Clauberg [whom he and his chief hated]." Also,
it meant helping "a relative of one of the inmates in my command with
whom I was good friends." In addition, he had heard that Clauberg's
experimental victims included "physicians and [other] highly qualified
women." It helped to discover that the brothel made "it not so . . .
difficult as we had thought to get them out."

But in addition to all that, Dr. B. had a motive similar to the motives
of many others doing experiments: "These experiments . . . interested
me." The opportunity to have available the necessary people for such
experiments "would have been most difficult . . . under any other circumstances." In other words, he too was drawn to the experimental opportunity Auschwitz provided—an admission confirmed by his having worked
with male research subjects, who were in no danger from Clauberg.

While we shall discuss Dr. B. at greater length in chapter 16, we can
say here that, for Nazi doctors in Auschwitz and other camps, the impulse
to experiment was powerful and many-sided; and so extensive was the
atmosphere of human experimentation that expressions of it, feigned or
partially feigned, could, at least on rare occasions, be used for the specific
purpose of saving lives.

Further Contradictions

The Hygienic Institute's small unit on Block 10 was a source of further
contradiction. It was generally thought of as a haven—no selections,
pleasant working conditions, and real medical duties having to do with
bacteriological and hematological problems. To some extent that unit
extended the generally benign atmosphere of the Hygienic Institute's
central Auschwitz location in Raisko, a town on the outskirts of Auschwitz. Thus Dr. Marie L. could commend the "very competent medical
staff, Jewish men and women work[ing] there" as "a great help to us
because they were "always ready to do secretly the analyses needed"—
by which she meant submitting reports, usually negative, that helped
patients. And considerable makework, very large numbers of blood and
urine analyses and fecal, saliva, and throat cultures, was carried on in the
Block 10 unit.

Yet there too harmful experiments were done. Bruno Weber, the chief of the Hygienic Institute,* determined blood groups on certain inmates and injected some with blood from different blood groups in order to study the degree of the resultant harmful agglutination of blood cells. More serious than these results were the consequences of collecting blood, whether for this or other experiments or for use in transfusions for German personnel. Not only was the blood at times collected from very weak inmates, but it was sometimes done cruelly or even murderously, by entering the carotid artery in a few prisoners and causing them to bleed to death. Dr. Michael Z. described one SS noncommissioned officer, "house painter by trade, [who would take] from each patient 700, 800 and up to 1,000 cc. of blood," and as a physician "doubted very seriously that any of these patients were able to withstand such bleedings."

Dr. B. explained, probably truthfully, that the intent was to take blood needed for producing the serum for the various blood groups; and while he seemed to defend his chief, he admitted that Weber told SS men to " 'go to the camp, fetch yourselves a few fat *capos,* and tap [*zapft*] them' " —with the result that the SS men did not limit themselves to well-nourished inmates but "tapped blood wherever they could get hold of it because it was much less work that way."

In addition, prisoner doctors soon discovered that the Hygienic Institute was using human, rather than animal, muscle for its culture media. Dr. Marie L. told how, hearing the sound of executions across the courtyard ("the muffled . . . shots we were all too familiar with"), she and others looked through the crevices of Block 10 windows and saw four women's bodies removed; then about a half-hour later, "the bodies came back to their place, but they were mutilated [and] . . . had cut [out of them] large areas deep into the flesh." Dr. L. could confirm what inmates working in a lab had already suspected after noticing "in the culture media pieces of meat with hairless skin." The simple conclusion: "Since the SS stole the meat used to produce the culture media, the chief SS physician of the Hygienic Institute found it very simple to replace it with human flesh." Dr. Michael Z. told how the same SS noncommissioned officer who brutally took large amounts of blood from inmates would accompany Dr. Weber to executions and "bring back trunkfuls of human flesh to prepare the culture media."

In Auschwitz, then, human flesh was more expendable than valuable animal meat; using it could seem an acceptable, even "sensible," expression of Auschwitz "medical science."

It turned out that Dr. Weber was involved in other fatal experiments, having to do with what Dr. B. described as "brainwashing with chemi-

*Langbein had the "impression that Weber was disgusted by the occurrences in Auschwitz, but nonetheless preferred stay in an extermination camp to service at the front. He constantly tried to emphasize the importance of his institute, for whose enlargement he invested all his energies."[47]

cals." He explained that the Gestapo was dissatisfied with its results in torturing people in the camp, mostly Poles, in order to extract confessions and information about comrades in the underground. "So the next question was, Why don't we do it like the Russians, who have been able to get confessions of guilt at their show trials?" Since it was thought that those confessions had been obtained by means of drugs, Weber was enlisted to investigate the matter; and he, according to Dr. B., "played along with them [the Gestapo]." Weber worked with Rohde and Capesius, the chief SS pharmacist, in trying out various barbiturates and morphine derivatives. On one occasion they were observed to feed a coffeelike substance to four prisoners, at least two of whom were known to have died that night, and the other two possibly later. Upon being notified of these deaths, Rohde is said to have commented that they had died a pleasant death—which, in that setting at that time, an ordinary SS doctor could well have said.[48]*

Dr. B's response to learning about his chief's experiments tells us much about the Auschwitz atmosphere. He said that his affection and respect for Weber changed "not at all" because, "within the context of Auschwitz,† what difference did two or three people make—people who were in the hands of the Gestapo and so already dead anyhow?" Dr. B. provided a "psychological explanation" for his chief's behavior: the latter's considerable ambition and high intelligence in a man seriously ill with kidney disease (from which he died soon after the war), which gave him the feeling "I must do everything now." Dr. B. added that Weber worked closely with Mrugowsky, the chief physician of the central Hygienic Institute of the Waffen SS in Berlin—an ideological and medical collaboration that may have been the more important influence. For Mrugowsky was a key figure in the planning and carrying out of destructive medical experiments in many concentration camps. The Nuremberg Tribunal found him guilty of planning fatal experiments with typhus vaccine in Buchenwald (carried out mostly by Schuler); of conducting fatal experiments with "poison bullets" in Sachsenhausen (together with Schuler and Dr. Albert Widmann, the SS chemist involved in T4 gassing); of assisting Gebhardt in fatal sulfanilimide experiments at Ravensbrück in which infections were artificially induced; and of planning and ordering of gas edema experiments, also fatal, in Buchenwald, including further experimentation with injected phenol. Mrugowsky undoubtedly coordinated many additional experiments as chief of all Hygienic Institutes. In that capacity, moreover, he was a central figure in the maintenance and distribution of Zyklon-B for use in Auschwitz and elsewhere.[49]

One of the more benign institutions in Auschwitz turns out to have

---

*Related experiments described at Nuremberg and elsewhere may have involved mescaline.

†Throughout our interviews, he repeatedly used this phrase—*unter dem Aspekt von Auschwitz*—to make similar points.

been a locus not only for the planning of murderous medical experiments but for the technology of mass murder in the death camps. And even in Auschwitz, that little Hygienic Institute laboratory on Block 10 was a frequent site for phenol killings (see chapter 14).

The Hygienic Institute on Block 10 is an especially concrete example of combined healing and killing. The same can be said of Wirths's relatively benign and yet dangerous experiments on Block 10, discussed in chapter 15. The unusually constructive arrangements among prisoner physicians and SS doctors saved many lives, even as the malignant central designs (of Himmler, Mrugowsky, and Grawitz) combined with Auschwitz medical authority (of Wirths and Weber) in lethal experimentation and in supporting the killing project.

Experimental Auschwitz

Auschwitz applied most of its energies to killing people, but its openness to virtually any form of human manipulation inevitably resulted in a wide variety of additional experiments. Eduard Wirths, as chief doctor, was the Auschwitz sponsor and facilitator of most of these experiments, particularly those in which there was interest from Berlin at a higher level.

An example here is the continuous experimental activity of SS Captain Dr. Helmuth Vetter, a key figure in pharmacological "trials" in Auschwitz and elsewhere. He was employed for many years with Bayer Group WII of the I.G. Farben Industry, Inc., Leverkusen, and, at Auschwitz, retained his connections. He ran medical trials for Bayer in Auschwitz and Mauthausen (and possibly in other camps) on several therapeutic agents, including sulfa medications and other preparations whose content is not exactly known.*

Vetter commuted between Auschwitz and Mauthausen in order to supervise the study of the effects of "ruthenol" and "3582" on many different serious medical conditions (typhus, typhoid, paratyphoid diseases, diarrhea, tuberculosis, erysipelas, and scarlet fever among others); but of the 150 to 250 patients he gave these medications to on the contagious disease ward in Auschwitz, about 50 were suffering from typhus. The impression of prisoner doctors was that these agents were of no therapeutic use, and some patients seemed to die quickly after receiving them. Vetter was reluctant to accept these negative findings, always insisting that better results had been obtained in other camps.[50]

Vetter drew other SS doctors into his research, including Eduard Wirths. The latter became not only what one observer called Vetter's

---

*Among these preparations were ones numbered 3582 (a nitroacridine preparation), V1012, and ruthenol (a combination of preparation 3582 and arsenic acid).

"official deputy" in Auschwitz but later actively pursued typhus trials himself, in which four Jewish inmates, artificially infected with typhus because there were no active cases available, were killed. These were apparently an extension of Vetter's work.

Vetter represents the Nazi research functionary, in whom ordinary medical vanities became lethal. He found in Auschwitz a testing area where he need not be restrained either by compunctions about harming —or killing—research subjects, or by rigorous judgments about therapeutic effects.

Fresh Samples and Numbed Detachment: Johann Kremer

The same was true of Dr. Johann Paul Kremer, who had intense career goals he attempted to achieve in Auschwitz. He was fifty-nine years old when he arrived there in August 1942, and thus belonged to an older generation than most camp doctors. Since 1935 an anatomy professor at the University of Münster, he was the only university professor to serve as an SS camp doctor.[51]

Kremer had a long-standing research interest in problems of starvation, which he pursued by seeking debilitated inmates selected for death, whom he later termed "the proper specimens." After he had a patient "placed on the dissection table," where he took a history focused on weight and weight loss, an SS orderly injected phenol into the person's heart: "I stood at a distance from the dissection table holding jars, ready for the segments [organs] cut out immediately after death . . . segments of the liver, spleen and pancreas."[52] On some occasions, Kremer arranged to examine these patients or have them photographed prior to their murder. We may say that he made maximally pragmatic use of the death factory for his own scientific aims. Dr. Jan W. told how, if Kremer spotted a prisoner whose cranial shape seemed unusual, or who interested him in any way, he would order that prisoner photographed and injected with phenol for his collection of "fresh corpse samples of liver and other organs," and concluded that "Kremer looked upon the prisoners as so many rabbits."

Dr. Kremer became notorious for a diary he kept (which was eventually discovered and published), with such sequences as:

> September 4, 1942 . . . present at a special action [selection] in the women's camp . . . The most horrible of horrors. . . .
> September 6 . . . Today, Sunday, an excellent dinner: tomato soup, half a chicken with potatoes and red cabbage (20 g. of fat), sweet pudding and magnificent vanilla ice cream. . . .
> October 10 . . . I took and preserved . . . material from quite fresh corpses, namely the liver, spleen, and pancreas. . . .
> October 11 . . . Today, Sunday, we got for dinner quite a big piece of roast hare with dumplings and red cabbage for 1.25 RM.[53]

Another theme in the diary is Kremer's sense of being victimized by the "medical establishment," which rejected his two pet scientific theories. One of those theories was constructed around his claim to have demonstrated the inheritance of traumatically acquired deformities, an idea at odds with all scientific evidence, then and now, and which especially violated the Nazi focus on pure heredity. He had in fact been reproached by the rector of his university for having published an article entitled "A Noteworthy Contribution to the Problem of Heredity in Traumatic Deformations." His second theory involved a claim that white blood cells and other phagocytes (cells that absorb and digest foreign bodies) are actually tissue cells (from other organs and areas of the body) that have undergone decay or "retrogression." Here he considered his Auschwitz research especially valuable because the "fresh samples" (taken just before death) he obtained there enabled him to study degenerative effects that could not be attributed to post-mortem changes.[54]

For while Kremer had been appointed titular professor, he had never been given an actual chair and brooded in his diary about "establishing a small laboratory of my own . . . once the war is over . . . [because] I have brought materials from Auschwitz which absolutely must be worked on." Auschwitz was to be the source of scientific breakthrough and revenge; and that anticipation, along with his general Nazification as well as his combination of overweening ambition and limited talent, contributed to his degree of numbed detachment, which was extraordinary even for Auschwitz doctors. Kremer was imprisoned for ten years in Poland, and again tried back home in Münster, where he was sentenced to another ten years, considered already served. He died in 1965.[55]

Male Experimental Block

A male experimental block was also created from part of Block 28, within the medical area of the main camp. Emil Kaschub, an advanced medical student, was also sponsored by Wirths, who brought him to the block and solicitously inquired about his research needs. Relatively healthy Jewish inmates were subjected to having toxic substances rubbed into their arms and legs, causing severely infected areas and extensive abcesses. The idea apparently was to gain information that would help one recognize attempts by German malingerers to produce such responses in order to avoid military service.[56] A prisoner who had worked as a nurse on this block identified some of the material used as "petroleum substances," which could be injected as well as rubbed into the skin, and gave rise to large inflammations and abscesses containing blackish liquid that "smelled of petroleum" and had to be drained.

The second series of experiments involved applications of lead acetate to various parts of the body, causing painful burns and various forms of discoloration. With both sets of experiments, specimens were sent to laboratories for study, and elaborate photographic work was done to create records of the conditions caused. The prisoner nurse discussed the large "black closet" used as part of the photographic equipment, within which experimental subjects had to remain still and upright for long periods, resulting in further suffering, moans of pain, and near collapse: "Often I had to carry inanimate beings to their beds."[57]

A third set of experiments required ingestion by mouth of a powder in order to study the symptoms of liver damage it caused: nausea, loss of appetite, jaundice, and discolored urine. This research was thought to follow upon Himmler's expressed interest in various forms of liver disease and jaundice because of problems they created for the German military.

This series of experiments on Block 28, then, reflects mainly official interest in conditions affecting the military but probably involved a certain individual "scientific curiosity" as well. Auschwitz provided a relatively technologized (in terms of the photography) research laboratory where a young neophyte physician was encouraged to serve the cause and make his medical name by means of experiments.

Finally, a series of surgical demonstrations were performed in various parts of the camp.

There was one report of the appearance, on Block 41 in Birkenau, of "three well-known German professors" to carry out vivisections in the form of exposing leg muscles followed by test application of various medications.[58] Another report involved medical students themselves performing experimental surgery on a female hospital block: the sudden appearance of "many young doctors in white coats (later identified as students) . . . [who] walked through the wards and looked us all over, who, through orders to the prisoner doctor, chose certain women, put anesthesia masks on them, and had them taken to an operating area, from which they returned hours later to wake up in their beds, each with wounds differing from the others." The women concluded that "each of the students performed an operation as an experiment in his specialty: throat, eyes, stomach, or gynecology," the last being the case of the woman who gave the testimony; and only much later did she discover that her uterus and ovaries had been removed.[59]*

We know of the SS doctors' tendency to gain surgical experience by attempting various operations, with or without the supervision of more experienced Jewish or Polish prisoner doctors, and often on prisoners who had no real medical need for surgery. The SS doctors systematically combined hospital files or identified at roll call prisoners with specific diseases or disease histories of a potential surgical nature—gallbladder, appendix, kidney stones, etc.—and had them report to the hospital. "If at a certain time a German doctor was studying gallbladder operations,

*Given the Auschwitz atmosphere, in which any kind of experiment was considered possible, descriptions such as these could include inaccuracies or distortions, but it is very likely that something close to what was described really occurred.

then prisoners suffering from this disease were placed on the operating table."[60]

Here again Auschwitz becomes a medical caricature: now of doctors hungry for surgical experience. In the absence of ethical restraint, one could arrange exactly the kind of surgical experience one sought, on exactly the appropriate kinds of "cases" at exactly the time one wanted. If one felt Hippocratic twinges of conscience, one could usually reassure oneself that, since all of these people were condemned to death in any case, one was not really harming them. Ethics aside, and apart from a few other inconveniences, it would have been hard to find so ideal a surgical laboratory.

Prisoner Doctors and Research

Inevitably, prisoner doctors were drawn into Auschwitz's experimental world. "I do not believe that there was one single SS doctor who did experiments without the help of prisoner doctors in some form or other, willingly or not" was the way that the French prisoner doctor Frédéric E. put it. Usually that involvement was no more than helping to treat victims "because they were sick after those experiments," but it could extend to performing the experiments or "research."

In the latter case, there were important distinctions to be made in the inmate professional's relationship to the work. For instance, Dr. Lottie M. referred to a Polish prisoner anthropologist, Teresa W., who took measurements for Mengele in his study of twins. Though Dr. M. and others thought highly of this woman, other inmates resented her because Mengele favored her (her own room, sufficient food, special treatment arrangements when she was ill) and also because "she did real work": that is, made accurate measurements in accordance with her own professional standards. In contrast, Dr. M. told of her own response to a request from Dr. König that she take blood from a particular patient every two hours over a twenty-four-hour period in order to follow the sedimentation rate. Because Dr. M. did not wish to be up every two hours during the night and was "not interested in his work," she simply drew the total amount of blood required, distributed it evenly into twelve containers, went to bed, and presented him with the containers the next day: "I didn't mind that this was not [authentic] and . . . just sabotage." That Teresa W. "did not have this attitude" suggests a morally problematic scientific integrity. An inmate was most likely to try to be accurate, as this Polish anthropologist did, when working regularly with an SS doctor (who might well be able to detect falsifications) in what seemed a relatively innocuous enterprise (and thereby inviting to one's own professional identity), such as W.'s measurements. At the same time, she claimed to know nothing about what was well known to many: namely, that Mengele would occasionally have one or both twins put to death so that he could obtain needed scientific information from post-mortem study (see also pages 349–54). Her later reluctance to testify against Mengele had to do not only with his having saved her life, which could be reason enough, but with her need for her own distancing and numbing in relationship to the "scientific" project she was part of.

Sometimes a prisoner doctor could cling to self-aggrandizing scientific accuracy at the possible expense of others' lives. For example, one Jewish professor insisted upon identifying as a special form of tuberculosis a syndrome of bone infection encountered in Auschwitz and (as Dr. Jacob R. described) tried to persuade everybody to agree with him, until colleagues pressed him not to because it was known that "at Auschwitz the diagnosis of tuberculosis was tantamount to death—at least for Jews."

More usual was the code among prisoner physicians that, even with straightforward clinical research—as in work done in the laboratories of the Hygienic Institute—one avoided reporting results that could harm inmates. Therefore, in the case of diphtheria, as Dr. Michael Z. tells us, a positive report would have meant selection for the gas chambers and therefore "signing their death warrant." He added, "How many tens of sputum specimens where Koch [tuberculosis] bacilli were swarming do we report as negative?" We may say that the true healing task of the prisoner doctor was to make use of his or her knowledge not only of medical science but of Auschwitz medicalized killing in making reports and diagnoses, whether accurate or falsified, that would best sustain the lives of prisoners.

The Noma Office: Berthold Epstein

That principle was very much at issue in one of the many examples of "research collaboration" between SS and prisoner doctors in Auschwitz.

One prisoner doctor described a sequence in which Mengele approached Professor Berthold Epstein, a distinguished prisoner pediatrician, proposing that, in return for "an extension of his life," he help prepare research that Mengele could publish under his own name. Epstein was granted a day to think the matter over. As an "old man" from an assimilated Czech-Jewish background in Prague who "had extravagant notions of honor," he was indignant that Mengele "wanted to rob him of his soul." But his colleagues quickly convinced him that "an attitude of this kind at a distance of three hundred meters from a crematorium was far from being realistic"; and that, "under the pretext of scientific research," prisoner doctors could do a great deal of good for other inmates and also enhance their own status.

Epstein then proposed research on the treatment of noma, a severe, spreading, ulcerative, gangrenous condition of the face and mouth, which is often fatal and was prevalent among Gypsy children and adolescents in the camp. Mengele agreed, and very quickly a "Noma office" *(Nomaab-teilung)* was established, where forty-five to seventy children were kept and given a special, nutritious diet, vitamins, and sulfa drugs, as requested by Professor Epstein and arranged by Mengele. The SS doctor also had the children photographed before, during, and after treatment and brought other SS doctors to the ward to observe the work. A considerable number of the children made good recoveries.[61] Whether or not every detail of this recollection is correct,* it shows that the SS doctor could, out of his own ambition, allow prisoner physicians to take research in a genuinely therapeutic direction (see also pages 360–61).

Ways of Resisting

I have discussed situations where prisoner doctors were pressured into participating in clearly harmful experiments that they could in no way view as legitimate research (chapter 12). Some, like Dr. Samuel and Dr. Dering, succumbed to those pressures; but other prisoner doctors resisted them, often indirectly and always cautiously.

Dr. Wanda J. called forth her status with Wirths, who respected and needed her on Block 10, in order to avoid involvement with Schumann and Clauberg. Concerning Schumann, she told me, "Not that I was a heroine [but] I wasn't his property"—which enabled her to make the false claim (which Schumann probably knew was false) that she was "not a surgeon." With Clauberg as well as Schumann, Dr. J. managed to limit her participation essentially to therapeutic help to victims. With Wirths she had to be more indirect and even vague, and when he suggested that she remove (as Samuel had done) the cervix of women thought to have pre-cancerous growths, she vacillated and stressed the fact that "first of all I organized the hospital" (see pages 237–38).

A French prisoner physician with strong Protestant religious convictions became known for her direct opposition to Nazi requests. Dr. Lottie M. remembered how Dr. Marie L. had shared the general view that none of them was likely to survive Auschwitz: "So the only thing . . . left to us is to behave for . . . the short time that remains to us as human beings." When pressed by Wirths to do culposcopic examinations of the cervix (to detect pre-cancerous changes), Dr. L. initially did so, but recognizing first that the examinations were entirely inaccurate, and second that the work had potentially harmful consequences (surgical removal of the cervix),

---

*Langbein corroborates the story, adding that the prize patient was a girl of about ten whose cheeks, through which her teeth had been visible, grew together with scar tissue. He also reported that before the noma was under control, Mengele had the heads of children who died of it severed and preserved in glass containers.[62]

she invoked a long-standing leg wound, which she said prevented her from participating in the research. But, not without fear, she was particularly afraid of making a quick second refusal, and so agreed to perform anesthesia for Dr. Samuel in an experimental operation (removal of an ovary) he did for Schumann. After that single experience, however, she refused to do any more of them.

When confronted by Wirths, Dr. L. and he had an exchange that has taken on legendary reverberations. She explained that such activities were "contrary to my conception as a doctor." He then asked, "'Can you not see that these people are different from you?' And I answered him that there were several other people different from me, starting with him!"

She also expressed resistance to Wirths's brother Helmut, who participated in his brother's research; and when Eduard Wirths subsequently asked her opinion about sterilization: "I answered that I was absolutely opposed, that it was a right we did not have to dispose in that way of people's lives and to sterilize them." She was transferred from Block 10 back to Birkenau without being otherwise punished, and was advised by knowledgeable inmates that, in her precarious situation, she should make herself more or less invisible. She also rebuffed two additional approaches: one from Dr. Samuel advising her to take part in experiments because "there are executions," to which she replied, "If I did them, I would commit suicide afterward." The second approach was from Mengele: "Of course I told him I did not want to do it"; afterward, "he told others that he could not ask me to do what I did not want to do."

Her resistance to experiments had been unusually firm; buttressed by her religious convictions, she was willing to die rather than violate her ethical code. While she undoubtedly had more leeway than a Jewish doctor in expressing these principles, her courage was no less impressive. An important element in the equation was the willingness of both Wirths and Mengele to give way rather than punish or kill her. SS doctors were committed from late 1942 to keeping prisoner doctors alive and functional; and in any case preferred to enlist for their dirty work those who were more malleable. Yet she too had to struggle with anxiety, and even she could not escape a brief involvement in experiments before succeeding in withdrawing from them completely.

Genuine Research

Prisoner physicians could themselves sometimes initiate genuine research, like the program in electroshock therapy developed by a Polish neurologist. Another prisoner physician who had been close to the situation, Frédéric E., told me that this man had been a renowned neurologist before the war, and that part of his motivation was the general knowledge that "German doctors liked to have extraordinary things happen in their camp that would give them considerable personal prestige," and were "very pleased when prisoner doctors would produce something scientifically interesting" which could then be published under their (the SS doctors') name. This was especially true of Hans Wilhelm König, who responded enthusiastically to the plan, arranging not only for male "schizoid" inmates to be brought to the hospital block for electroshock therapy but taking the unusual step of having female inmates brought there as well from Birkenau seven or eight kilometers away (see pages 227–28).

König, in fact, took a great interest in the work and regularly attended the shock therapy sessions. Dr. E., who attended some of them as well, felt that the process was genuinely therapeutic, and that it saved lives: "Those [inmates] with nervous disorders were never selected [for the gas chamber] by König because he was interested in the effect of the electrotherapy on them." Moreover, patients diagnosed as schizoid were placed "under the protection of Fischer and . . . König . . . [and] consequently . . . were treated . . . in a more favorable manner"—either permitted to remain in the hospital or, if sent back to the camp, not assigned to hard labor.

But no research or therapy escaped the Auschwitz taint. A prisoner who worked on a Birkenau hospital block later testified that "Dr. König did electroshock experiments on women," and added, "These women later talked about their treatment. I believe Dr. König carried out the electroshock experiments on sick women twice a week and that the women were later gassed."

In other words, the electroshock treatments could be seen as a prelude to the gas chamber, and on the basis of such testimony and other investigations the International Committee of the Red Cross in Geneva (in association with the International Tracing Service at Arolsen in West Germany) placed these "electroshock experiments" on the list of "pseudo-medical experiments" for which victims could be compensated.[63]

Frédéric E. was deeply troubled by this designation, which he considered to be a kind of mythology that developed because the "violent shock" involved caused "rumors that something terrible was happening." He initiated a correspondence with the International Red Cross authorities, insisting that the project had been genuinely therapeutic and asking that the designation "pseudo-medical experiments" be changed. The authorities wrote back that the electroshock had sometimes been given to people without mental illness and that it was "done in the utmost secrecy." Dr. E. ceased his protest only when told that the category "pseudo-medical experiment" meant that inmates could receive compensation as part of the indemnity to the Polish Government paid by the Federal Republic of Germany. Dr. E., in his last letter, made clear that he did not want to deny anyone such compensation, but nonetheless insisted that the designation was "an error" that should not be used in future publications. He was surely defending both his colleagues' integrity and his own. But the overall episode once more reveals the tendency for the Auschwitz environment to subsume virtually any medical effort to its relentless destructiveness.

Medical Witness

There is still another kind of research, much more rare, conducted solely by prisoners as a means of investigating what they were being subjected to—that is, as a form of medical witness. Frédéric E. and a distinguished prisoner colleague studied the blood of twenty-six other Auschwitz (Monowitz) inmates, falling into five groups ranging from new arrivals in relatively good condition to inmates in advanced states of emaciation and edema. These doctors eventually prepared a careful scientific report published in 1947, which Dr. E. told me with some pride was "the only published medical research done [by inmates] under the Germans."[64] He and his friend were interested in the deprivations of the diet and the physiological effects of these deprivations: "You see it was in 1944, and we could understand that Germany was going to lose the war, and we wanted to know what we were being fed." But in order to get König's approval, which they needed to do the research, they spoke of studying "inmates' weight loss from a medical point of view," rather than admit that they were evaluating the camp diet.

König probably let them go ahead because he envisioned the possibility of publishing the results "under his [own] name in the German medical literature": "It would have been perfectly possible for him to omit the fact that it had been done in Auschwitz. . . . There are always people who lose weight, who are in misery."

Just before evacuating Auschwitz, Dr. E. prepared two copies of a chart summarizing the results of the research, so that he and his collaborator could each carry one of them. His was lost through a search, but his collaborator managed to retain the other copy, and there was a discussion with a physician from the Hygienic Institute in Buchenwald of the possibility of resuming the work there. While that did not happen, the status achieved by E. simply through the discussions with the SS doctor was instrumental in preventing his being sent elsewhere and "may have saved my life."

In the paper itself, there are descriptions in dry medical language of "cachetics without edema," "moderate emaciation . . . with moderate edema," and "extensive edema [with] lowered plasma total proteins and albumin." But underneath those words is a passionate expression of the survivor mission of bearing witness and giving meaning to the Auschwitz experience by revealing some of its cruel medical dimensions. While even they might have had moments of self-questioning concerning whether they, too, were making other inmates into "guinea pigs" (all the more so since the work required the approval of an SS doctor), these prisoner doctors could undoubtedly see it primarily as contributing to the world's learning the truth of Auschwitz.

Removal of Limits

There is an additional Auschwitz research function: that of the camp as a constant source of victims for research done almost anywhere. Besides the Auschwitz prisoners taken to Strasbourg to be made part of Professor Hirt's skeleton collection, there are many other examples: eight prisoners from Auschwitz sent to Sachsenhausen for experiments with epidemic hepatitis, in which the possible death of the inmates was an accepted part of the arrangement; and the notorious sequence of twenty Jewish children, ages five to twelve, transferred from Auschwitz to Neuengamme in Hamburg, where they were subjected to injections of virulent tubercular serum and to other experiments, until they were removed from Neuengamme and secretly murdered just before the arrival of Allied troops.[65] Auschwitz was not just a medicalized death factory but a source of "raw materials" for everyone's deadly medical experiments.

Prisoner physicians could speak with bitter accuracy about the specific way in which their and other inmates' humanity was negated by Nazi experimenters. One observed that "man was the cheapest experimental animal. . . . Cheaper than a rat." Another declared that the experiments "had no scientific basis, and . . . that the main interest they had for those who performed them was to give Berlin, in their detailed reports, the illusion of important and continuous work, so that these brave 'researchers' might be kept far from the front in a position of sinecure."

We know that Nazi doctors partly justified the experiments by their sense that Jews were in any case doomed. While prisoner doctors made no such justification, their emotions were also affected by the Jewish death sentence. Dr. Jacob R. could remember a feeling that "the experiments were of considerably less import than the whole inferno I was viewing there."

The experiments represent, among other things, a removal of medical limits. Ordinary medical behavior is predicated upon maintaining life—and refraining from actual or potential killing or maiming one's patient in the name of enhancing the life of one's own group or people. Paradoxically, that medical vision of social cure contributed directly to using medicine to kill or injure. Hence the array of Auschwitz experiments, and others done elsewhere including artificially inflicted burns with phosphorous incendiary bombs; experiments on the effects of drinking sea water; experiments with various forms of poison, by ingestion as well as in bullets or arrows; widespread experiments on artificially induced typhus, as well as with epidemic hepatitis and with malaria; experiments in cold immersion ("in freezing water") to determine the body's reactions and susceptibilities; experiments with mustard gas in order to study the kinds of wounds it can cause; experiments on the regeneration of bone, muscle, nerve tissue, and on bone transplantation, involving removal of various bones, muscles, and nerves from healthy women. All of the experiments were related to the Nazi biomedical vision, whether they directly contributed to cultural genocide (as in the case of sterilization) or were the work of German physicians taking a leading role in biological and genetic purification.

In experiments in sterilization, of course, the ideological source and goals are clear. But all the other experiments as well reflect the Nazi image of "life unworthy of life," of creatures who, because less than human, can be studied, altered, manipulated, mutilated, or killed—in the service of the Nordic race, and ultimately of remaking humankind. One experiments without limit in order to "gather together the best blood" and "once more breed over the generations the pure type of Nordic German."[66] The task is never accomplished, so one must continue experimenting. All of Auschwitz becomes not only a vast experiment but an unending one.

Chapter 16

"A Human Being in an SS Uniform": Ernst B.

> His very first visit to the lab of Block 10 . . . was an
> extraordinary surprise for us. He came into the lab
> without force unlike the other SS, without a dog
> (Weber always came with a wolf dog), locked the
> doors behind him [so that his behavior could not be
> observed by other SS], said "Good day" and intro-
> duced himself, . . . offering his hand to my col-
> leagues and to me. . . . We were . . . long unused
> to anyone from among the camp authorities treat-
> ing us as people equal to himself.
> —Auschwitz survivor

I had heard and read a great deal about Ernst B. before meeting him, and
—amazingly for a Nazi doctor—all that I had heard was good. Former
prisoner doctors, in both their written and their oral accounts, constantly
described Dr. B. as having been a unique Nazi doctor in Auschwitz: a man
who treated inmates (especially prisoner doctors) as human beings and
who saved many of their lives; who had refused to do selections in Auschwitz; who had been so appreciated by prisoner doctors that, when tried
after the war, their testimony on his behalf brought about his acquittal;
who was "a human being in an SS uniform."

I did not have to track him down, as I had most other SS doctors, but
he was introduced to me by a German judge who had taken a deposition
from him in the Mengele extradition proceedings. Dr. B. had in fact
expressed enthusiasm about meeting me and discussing his experiences
with me in detail. I found him to be a neatly groomed man in his mid-
sixties, short and slight, pleasant in manner, generally likable. So pleasant
in fact that it made me a bit uneasy, and I reminded myself silently that,
whatever his virtues, he had been one of *them*: a Nazi doctor in Auschwitz.

Transition to Auschwitz

Ernst B. was a young general practitioner, just a few years out of medical school, when the war began in September 1939. By the following year, partly in response to the national patriotic enthusiasm surrounding early German victories, he began to develop an intense urge to enlist. As a young man, he felt, "I must take part," but had difficulty doing so because wartime medical planners in his region had declared him essential. Then, during a chance encounter on a city street, a friend from his medical school told him, "Heydrich [chief of the Reich Main Security Office] is a good friend of mine, and I'll arrange that for you." Dr. B. said that at the time he made no special distinction between the Waffen SS, in which the arrangement was to be made, and the army, except to consider the SS to be "like a good club." Months later the call came, and he was sent for a period of basic training followed by special officers' training. He tended to dismiss this sequence as essentially an orientation program for medical officers within the Waffen SS but acknowledged that there was some discussion of SS ideology and focus on the SS as an élite group.

Because of a background in bacteriology, he was assigned to one of the Hygienic Institutes, considered "a normal medical-military command within the Waffen SS." From there, after interviews in which his ideological views were explored, he was transferred to the special concentration-camp division of the Hygienic Institute. His impression was that those so chosen were considered "ideologically steadfast . . . [and] reliable." The high standing of his sponsor as a friend of Heydrich probably also played a part: when summoned to get his assignment from Professor Mrugowsky, the overall chief of all SS Hygienic Institutes, "I was a very small man but he received me as one of the inner circle . . . because of that [original] recommendation." Mrugowsky paid him the high honor of assigning him to Auschwitz, telling him almost jauntily, "There you will find a good friend."

Though Ernst B. had heard of Dachau "and maybe one or two camps in northern Germany," he claimed to know "nothing about Auschwitz. . . . and nothing about the extermination of Jews" at that time. Certainly he was completely unprepared for what he encountered upon arriving in Auschwitz in mid-1943, his relative innocence attested to by the fact that he had with him his wife (who had joined him at a duty assignment not too far away just before his transfer). When driven through the camp in an open vehicle, they were shocked by what they saw: "Starving people working, . . . a great number of them, . . . everywhere guards. . . . Far off in the distance, a large fence. . . . It was very bad."

They were taken to the office of Bruno Weber, the "good friend" Mrugowsky had promised him, a man Dr. B. had liked and respected as his superior at the first Hygienic Institute to which he had been assigned. After he and his wife had both expressed their horror at what they had seen (his wife said specifically, "This is not for us!"), Weber took him aside, told him to send his wife home, and asked him how he could make such a disastrous blunder in bringing her there.

Alone with Weber, Dr. B. continued to express his desire to leave, but, in his confusion, felt "fortunate to have Weber [there] as my friend." Weber urged him to stay and serve there as ordered and stressed that his leaving would cause embarrassing "complications" for their common SS sponsor as well as uncertainty concerning B.'s own future.

Weber then laid out to B. "almost with irony" the central Auschwitz truth, invoking the official term the "Final Solution of the Jewish question": "He [Weber] said, 'If you want to see how it works, go look out of the window. You will see . . . two large smokestacks. . . . The normal kind of production of this machine . . . is a thousand men in twenty-four hours.' "

Weber then added what Dr. B. called "the most important thing to me" —an explanation of how the autonomy of the Hygienic Institute from the camp and its medical hierarchy would enable them to keep their own hands clean and "stay out of this whole business." Weber added that they were responsible only to their Berlin chief, Mrugowsky, who encouraged the Auschwitz unit to employ capable prisoner physicians in its laboratories to produce work that could be published under his name. That arrangement contributed to the group's advantageous situation, as did its important role in combating the danger of typhus epidemics. Weber added that if B. stayed ("If you and I can stick together"), the institute's position would become even stronger. B. was immediately convinced and made no effort to leave.

In moving from "hearing . . . the [Auschwitz] story and seeing the smoke on the one hand and being directly confronted with the actual machinery on the other," he had two enlightening lessons. The first began with a sudden visual impression he had during his first days at the camp, an image he is still not quite sure how to evaluate. He observed a miserable-looking group of prisoners from the "outside *Kommandos*" (*Aussenkommandos*) marching back from their work, bunched together six abreast, in humiliating rapid cadence, all of them emaciated and dressed in the same Auschwitz clothes: "Then all of a sudden I . . . thought—I don't know whether it was true or whether I imagined it—I still don't know. . . . I thought I saw a schoolmate of mine. . . . Immediately after . . . I talked to Weber and said, 'I'm sure that was Simon Cohen.' "

A Jewish classmate from a well-to-do family, Simon Cohen had been a good friend during the early 1930s, when anti-Semitism was already widespread in Germany. The two boys were drawn to one another partly by their common lack of interest in schoolwork and would take long vacation trips together on their bicycles. Upon returning from a year abroad in 1933, Ernst B. found that the Jewish boy "wasn't there any more." He had sometimes wondered what had happened to his friend.

When questioned, Weber told him that there were large numbers of

Cohens, that in any case prisoners were registered not by name but only by number, and that there was simply no possibility of finding the man. When B. persisted, he encountered an evasiveness that seemed Kafka-esque and sinister: the SS man responsible for the building Dr. B. had seen the group of prisoners enter passed the question "Do we have a Simon Cohen?" to the *capo*, who in turn spoke to another prisoner, who more or less did the same, until the query was itself bureaucratically dissolved.

Dr. B. began to realize that everyone considered his question strange, highly inappropriate, and possibly dangerous; prisoners feared that an SS officer seeking out one of their number "couldn't mean anything good for that person." But for a few days he was obsessed with finding Cohen and "making some human contact." He did not succeed but in the course of his quest did make such contact with a different Jew. A former prisoner physician, Michael Z., who had worked in the Hygienic Institute, told me how taken aback he was when Ernst B. burst into the laboratory "look[-ing] for a Jewish friend. He asked me, speaking quite loud . . . : 'Do you know Cohen?' I told him, '[Please] be quiet, you do not have the right to speak like that.' " Dr. Z. explained why he felt it necessary to protect Dr. B. by quieting him down and, by implication, to protect himself as well. He told B. that "tens, thousands of Jews . . . come through," that "many of them were named Cohen," and that it would be impossible to find any such person. But at the same time Z. was deeply moved by SS doctor's quest: "I understood that he was indeed a man who had a different kind of mind, . . . that he was capable of human feelings. . . . Yes, it did impress me . . . because it was unheard of to see an SS pronounce the name of a Jewish friend."

The incident made Dr. B. realize that in Auschwitz "it was a completely different existence" and that he had to "comprehend the whole mentality of the place." Immediately after the unsuccessful search, he began to have recurrent dreams about Simon Cohen—at first frequent, then less so during his stay in Auschwitz, and still occurring occasionally up to the time of our interviews:

> He was always a very attractive young man. And now [in the dream] he had really deteriorated. . . . And he looked at me with a reproachful, beseeching expression [*vorwürfsvollen, bittenden Blick*] . . . sort of [say-ing], "It can't be possible that you stand there and I am . . . [like this] . . ." or more like a disappointed expression: "How can you belong to those people? That can't be you [*Wie kannst du zu denen gehören? Du bist doch der garnicht*]."

Dr. B. went on to tell me, "The older I get, the less I think it was really Simon Cohen and the more I believe it to have been a mirage, . . . an invention . . . of the imagination." He even wondered whether he "only dreamed it"—though we know from what the prisoner doctor recalled that the impression was strong enough for B. to embark upon a real search. We can say that the illusion (as it probably was) and the dream were insistent assertions of Ernst B.'s humanity, and of his discomfort and guilt at being part of the Auschwitz machinery. In their questioning of his personal camp reality ("It can't be possible that you stand here. . . . How can you belong to those people? That can't be you"), they expressed his resistance to succumbing, or at least to succumbing completely, to the very "Auschwitz mentality" he was in the process of discovering. At the same time, they charted his transition from ordinary man to Auschwitz doctor.

His second lesson was the direct confrontation with the way in which SS doctors functioned, or what he called the Auschwitz "system of treatment":

> The SS doctors . . . supervised the work of the prisoner doctors, . . . mainly . . . seeing that the work was done economically. In other words, the person . . . who cannot be expected to work any longer will be selected for the crematorium. It was a terrible shock to me to see this procedure. . . . Each day, whenever one went through the camp, one saw . . . groups that had been sorted out [selected] . . . [and] were waiting for the truck to depart [for the crematorium].

Dr. B. made clear to me that these two sets of images (of a victimized Simon Cohen swallowed up by the death factory and of groups of inmates who had been selected by his own colleagues and subjected to the same fate) were part of a profound psychological shift. The nature of that shift, of the Auschwitz transition period, was reflected in his analogy of the slaughterhouse (in which one first experiences horror but after a time adapts sufficiently to enjoy one's steaks [page 197]). For him as for others, heavy drinking was a central element in the process of numbing and usually took place at the Officers' Club, to which Weber regularly accompanied him, introducing him to other officers "and above all the . . . doctors with whom [he] had to work." Under alcohol, Dr. B. could express doubts about Auschwitz to which his drinking partners responded with statements of nonresponsibility and resignation (see page 196). The doubts themselves, as he explained further, were "romantically [melodramatically] overplayed" *(mit Romantik überspielt)*—fantasies of escape rather than serious moral questioning. When drinking heavily, for instance, "I could think of nothing other than, 'How did I come to be here? . . . How can I . . . go to Switzerland with my wife and four children?'" Then "one drank even more" toward a state beyond any thought: "And the next day one was very sober and had a painful headache and kind of realized that what one had thought about the previous night was in a practical sense impossible."

His transition was aided by his strong desire to cease being an "outsider" and to become, as soon as possible, an Auschwitz "insider"—a goal to be achieved by "harmonizing" with fellow SS officers and men as well as with significant inmates. While Ernst B. found most other SS doctors disappointing as people (much less than the élite, in terms of intellect and family background, he had expected), two of them took on special meaning for him: Weber, in ways already mentioned; and Josef Mengele, whose name Dr. B. brought up spontaneously as "the most decent colleague [anständigste Kollege] that I met [there]," a relationship we will return to. In addition, B. was impressed by a nonmedical SS officer, who ran Auschwitz agricultural operations in a way that B. thought was fair and saved lives, providing him with a model of how one could work in Auschwitz constructively and "differently" from most others.*

To become an "insider" among prisoner physicians, he made systematic efforts "to make contacts, to meet people, and to overcome the barrier" between them and himself. His method, as recorded in the epigraph to this chapter, was in the Auschwitz context nothing short of sensational.

Within a few weeks, he felt he had gained the confidence of this prisoner group, felt accepted by SS colleagues, and found himself becoming reasonably comfortable in the camp in general. But that comfort was shattered after about six months by a request from Wirths that B. begin to perform selections. Wirths could not order him to do so ("I was not his subordinate") but, as chief doctor, could and did apply considerable pressure on him to comply. This was the summer of 1944, when enormous numbers of Hungarian Jews were arriving, making it virtually impossible for the relatively small number of camp doctors to handle all of the selections. B. had the impression that the camp commandant suggested that some of the selections function be taken over by his own nonmedical officers but that Wirths insisted the process remain medical and turned to the Hygienic Institute, ordinarily outside of his jurisdiction, as the only source of additional available doctors. Wirths was successful in persuading Weber to select. But B., when repeatedly approached by Wirths, gave a series of reasons for refusing: that he had too much work, found it incompatible with his assignment, and simply could not—was unable psychologically to—do it. He illustrated the last reason by telling Wirths, "I . . . observed it [selections] and . . . could stand it for only half an hour [and then] had to vomit" —to which Wirths replied, "That will pass. It happens to everyone. . . . Don't make such a fuss about it."

When the pressure mounted to the point where Dr. B. felt he might not be able to maintain his resistance, he abruptly boarded the night express to Berlin to seek out Mrugowsky, and told him he was simply unable to

---

*SS Lieutenant Colonel Dr. Joachim Caesar had a degree as an agronomist. According to Dr. B., Caesar had been close to Himmler, but as the result of a disagreement over SS methods had been sent to Auschwitz as "ironic punishment." Nonetheless he was put in charge of all agricultural operations at Auschwitz, which, as Langbein says, was a position of great importance to Himmler.[1]

do selections. B. remembered Mrugowsky answering, "I myself could not do it either. I also have children." Then the chief of the Hygienic Institutes, also indignant that "his" doctor had been pressured by Wirths, picked up the phone and made the calls necessary to reassert his authority in protecting B. from selections: "In a few minutes it was all done." B. insisted that Mrugowsky's actions were more than mere assertion of authority, "I must say, it was also humane [*menschlich*]"; and his further comment that this was "the same man who was later hanged as a war criminal" suggested either contradictions in Mrugowsky's behavior or possibly B.'s sense that the Nuremberg verdict had been unfair.

While Dr. B. was never again asked to do selections, the episode had certain uncomfortable ramifications for him. As a compromise, Mrugowsky provided a young doctor named Delmotte, whose Auschwitz assignment specified that only one half of his time would be at the Hygienic Institute and the other half as a camp doctor—which meant he was to do the selections instead of Ernst B. An ardent member of the SS in his mid-twenties and from a family with high Nazi connections, Delmotte had just emerged from one of the first classes of a special SS cadet training course made available for doctors; he had wished to be sent to the front but agreed to Auschwitz because of having been promised that he could write his doctoral dissertation there.

At the first selection he was taken to, Delmotte became nauseated and returned to his room quite drunk; what was unusual, however, was that he did not leave his room the next morning. Dr. B. heard that Weber, upon visiting Delmotte, found him "catatonic . . . completely blocked"; Weber thought at first that the young doctor had been stricken with a severe illness but concluded that he had simply had too much to drink. When he finally emerged in an agitated state, he was heard to say that he "didn't want to be in a slaughterhouse" and preferred to go to the front, and that "as a doctor his task was to help people and not to kill them." It was an argument, Dr. B. said, that "we never used" in Auschwitz: "It would have been totally pointless." Indeed, no other Auschwitz doctor I came upon in the research expressed that truth so clearly and repeatedly. B. thought that Delmotte spoke in that way only because of "his ingenuousness, his youthful inexperience, his total ignorance of the work in this respect." B. also stressed that Delmotte approached the medical profession "with high ideals and great enthusiasm," that he had "grown up in an SS cadet camp" and was "determined not to betray his SS ideals," and that he had declared (though this only when drunk) that he would never have joined the SS if he had "known that there was such a thing as Auschwitz." At the heart of Delmotte's resistance to selections, in other words, was his SS idealism.*

*Langbein confirms B.'s version of these events, reporting that it was the morning following the outburst that he realized that alcohol had not played the primary role. He also observed that Delmotte's appeal to his superior had been "diplomatically very awkward—he told us that later—in that he had officially refused and said he requested either to be sent to the Front or he himself should be gassed. But he could not do it [select]."

Upon learning that he had been brought in to replace Ernst B. who had refused to do selections, Delmotte angrily confronted him, more or less suggesting he had been hypocritical ("On what grounds do you do [what you are doing]?"), and insisted, "If you are not going to select, then I am not going to select either." B. "didn't feel good about the whole situation": "Of course I didn't tell him about my visit to Mrugowsky." In speaking of Delmotte's subsequent resentful withdrawal from both B. and Weber for not supporting him, B. admitted that there could have been ways to do so: "I have to say this to my shame."

In taking his case to the new commandant, Arthur Liebehenschel (Höss's temporary successor),* Delmotte encountered a "therapeutic" attitude ("I can certainly understand this. One must first get used to a new environment"), according to what Dr. B. was told about the conversation. Indeed, Liebehenschel—with the probable collaboration of Wirths, with whom he was on good terms, and the cooperation of Weber—arranged for a "therapeutic program" that had three specific components.

First, Delmotte was assigned to Mengele's mentorship. Mengele, speaking from a similar commitment to SS loyalty and ideology, could convey the message that even if one thinks that extermination of the Jewish people is wrong, or is being done in the wrong way (Delmotte, according to Dr. B., believed that "Jewish influence" had to be combated but disapproved of the Auschwitz method), "as an SS man [one was] bound to participate." Mengele could also claim that, since prisoners became sick and died terrible deaths, it was "more humane to select them." And he could ultimately fall back on the combined patriotic, nationalistic, racial, and biomedical argument that, during this wartime emergency, one should do nothing to interfere with the great goal being sought: "the triumph of the Germanic race." Mengele, that is, could appeal to the same SS idealism that had originally contributed to Delmotte's refusal, and, within two weeks, had him selecting.

Second, Weber, as a "good psychologist," made highly unusual arrangements for Delmotte's wife to live with him in Auschwitz. She was, according to Dr. B., extraordinary in both her beauty and her amorality ("no heart, no soul, no nothing"), her only discernible interest in Auschwitz being two enormous Great Danes she kept at the Hygienic Institute and constantly fondled. The strong implication was that Delmotte's regular sexual access to her made him, as B. put it, more "quiet."

---

*Höss was replaced in November 1943, following the arrest of the Auschwitz political leader Maximilian Grabner. Grabner was implicated through an SS anticorruption investigation, originally aimed at profiteering, although it also charged him with murders beyond those authorized, notably of Polish prisoners. Grabner's exit was supported by Dr. Wirths, with whom he had had confrontations over killings. Although implicated in Grabner's misdeeds, Höss was, in fact, promoted into the central concentration-camp administration. According to Langbein, the change was made because the outside world had learned too much of what was happening at Auschwitz; the change was, then, apparently cosmetic, although Liebehenschel did carry out some reforms in the direction of fewer arbitrary procedures and less harsh punishments. Of course the main business of Auschwitz continued as before.[2]

The third element was the making available to Delmotte as intellectual mentor (for the research and writing involved in his dissertation) a distinguished older Jewish prisoner physician, a professor and widely acclaimed scientist who, according to Dr. B., became a "father figure" to Delmotte. The two men became extremely close, and it was B.'s claim that the professor even advised Delmotte to go ahead with selections because "he would be severely punished if he refused." B. had the impression that the professor "contributed the most toward helping Delmotte out of his [difficulties]—let's say, to motivate him." Because of his own psychological needs, B. may well have exaggerated the professor's role in regard to the selections question—I would give greater emphasis to Mengele's influence and to that of the overall Auschwitz environment—but I have seen letters from the professor confirming his closeness to Delmotte.

Delmotte selected without further incident until selections were discontinued in Auschwitz in the fall of 1944. After the evacuation of Auschwitz, Ernst B. met him briefly in Dachau—after which Dr. B. "never saw him again." Delmotte tried to flee to his home area but was soon caught; when taken into custody (or about to be) by American troops, he shot himself.

Dr. B. thought that Delmotte had killed himself because of having violated his own medical principles in performing selections, and because he could, in any case, expect the death penalty from the Americans and wanted to spare himself and his family the pain and humiliation of conviction and execution. But what had actually gone on in Delmotte's mind continued to trouble B., remaining "a key problem" that he felt a need to "trace further." He did make some inquiries but did not succeed in learning any more. He added, with a quality of feeling unusual for him: "I had . . . hoped that I could be of some assistance to him, because I have a bad conscience toward him. . . . He had to do the job which I had succeeded in getting out of. . . . Maybe I could have been more honest with him, but it was very difficult in that situation."

Background

Who was this unusual Auschwitz doctor? A not very unusual man, an exploration of his past suggests, but one with certain preoccupations and abilities that contributed to his Auschwitz behavior.

Ernst B. came from an upper-middle-class professional family, his father a university professor distinguished in his scientific field, a man with whom he "had no personal contact, no personal relationship." B. nonetheless "respected him very much" because of the intensity of his commitment and his combination of personal integrity and tolerance for his children's idiosyncrasies. B.'s mother "was the opposite"—affectionate and close to him, and insistent on her beliefs and on the virtues of her own family traditions, which were strongly nationalistic, with two of its members being distinguished physicians.

His early memories include images of merging with the rural landscape, extreme isolation from other human beings, and fear close to
terror of wild beasts, fed in part by jungle tales his parents told him. He
associated the fear and isolation with the First World War—both with the
increasingly difficult living conditions caused by the war, and then with
the sense of humiliation experienced by his family in an area occupied by
the French following the German surrender (at which time he was a small
boy).

But one particular war-related event took the shape of an ultimate
family tragedy: the death of his uncle, who had been critically wounded
while serving as a military physician. The uncle was described as possessing qualities that lent readily to legend: a "completely model doctor" who
was also gifted in the arts, "a man who died in his late twenties but had
already produced a standard medical work still highly regarded."

A central theme of Ernst B.'s early life, carried through into adolescence and adulthood, was his struggle to make what he constantly referred to as "contact" *(Kontakt)* with other people. He felt difficulty in
doing so with other children, including his younger sister and brother.
He sought it in vague religious stirrings having to do with what he called
"religious communication," as exemplified in his experience by Christmas feelings and sermons of "harmony and peace" and a subsequent
belief that one should belong to some religion—feelings that went beyond his father's post-Protestant atheism and his mother's concession to
the need for some religion while being antagonistic to both Catholics and
Protestants. He had a similar attraction as a schoolboy to the utopian
thought of Thomas More and even to the communist ideas of the 1920s:
for a short time "the basic connection was made for me between early
Christianity and communism."

As he entered adolescence, however, he was influenced by his mother's
fiercely nationalistic opposition to such ideas, and by her allegiance to
anti-revolutionary groups on the right that stressed "national and military activity" and were "very, very emotionally German." Her group, the
Jungdeutscher Orden (Young Germans' Order), drew upon the earlier romantic back-to-nature youth movement or *Wandervogel* (literally, "bird of
passage"), in which his mother had been strongly involved. He went to
political gatherings with her, where he did not especially enjoy the marching, "but the drinking afterward was very good."

Drinking, in fact, had become important to Ernst B. from about the age
of fifteen—in his view, "very early in comparison to others" though "not
really very unusual." He drank "to have contact" with his peers at a time
when life seemed to be a series of defeats. At school he was "a very bad
. . . very lazy pupil." At home he was removed emotionally from his father
—and his mother "sort of overdid it in the other direction"—while feeling himself inadequate in relation to the "very high standard" of culture,
especially music, in his home. "So all I could do was drink with . . . young
people." Of this period in his life, he said, "I had problems in general

in making contact with people," and "unless I had a few glasses of wine I was not able to establish contact with that person." Also, his rejection by his first love made him feel "like shit!"

He was to have one additional defeat before his life could be turned around. The young Ernst, who had an interest in art and painting, thought he "could become something," rather than the nothing he felt himself to be, by studying art abroad. He did that for one year; and although he made a certain progress in his work, he felt isolated, had great difficulty with the foreign language, and began to drink heavily, again in search of contact with others. "It was simply a completely primitive difficulty in [making] contact" was the way he put it.

Upon returning home, he was ready to make a new commitment: "I saw very clearly . . . that I had to become a doctor." Indeed his parents, on the basis of family tradition, especially as represented by the physician uncle killed in the First World War, "had this idea from the time I was a baby." His father now approached him Socratically and asked whether he thought he could become "one of the top ten painters" in Germany (as would be necessary if he were to support himself). It was to Ernst B. "an illumination" (*eine Erleuchtung*), and "everything became clear." Feeling angry at himself for not having thought of it that way, he plunged back into his academic work, passed his *Abitur* (crucial qualifying examination for admission to a university), and gave up painting for studies leading to medicine.

Kept on a small allowance by his father ("He was afraid that I might start drinking again") and needing money, Ernst B. learned about a job hosting foreign students and that applicants would be tested for their knowledge of such cultural areas as theater and opera. Knowing nothing about the latter, he hit upon the "trick" of going to the library and reading carefully through all newspaper reviews of recent performances of all the major operas, so that when examined he could say, "Yes, but the performance in Hamburg fell through completely because the conception of the producer was such and such"—and thereby appeared to possess complete mastery of a field about which he knew very little. The nature of the job helped solve his long-standing problem: the (mostly) "American students were only interested in making contact during the beer drinking," which then became his "responsibility as well." He did well in his studies, and his life came into balance: upon returning home, "I could tell my father I don't need the allowance any more and . . . could show him a good examination [result]." More than that, the experience provided him with a rush of "self-confidence in my life" and the feeling that "I am very fit for [able to manage in] life [*ganz lebenstüchtig*]."

He continued to demonstrate that adaptability by joining the Nazi student organization during the early days of the regime (when only about 20 percent of students belonged to it) as he realized that he had to do so if he was to hold on to the job. He felt it necessary to conceal that membership from his mother, an ardent anti-Nazi. Indeed, at the beginning his family viewed the Nazis as more or less disreputable, the worst element of the society. But by the mid-1930s, the "spectacular" economic successes of the regime began to change that impression, along with the emerging "enthusiasm of . . . young people." His father moved grudgingly toward approval of Hitler in a tortuous, not uncharacteristically German, manner, asking, "How is it possible that such a primitive man can reach such an influential position?" and concluding, "It can only be that he isn't so primitive but just pretends to be." Ernst B. himself reacted with parallel convolution: always antagonistic and yet respectful toward the Prussian military culture, he was struck by the fact that "the conservative, Prussian military men, especially the young ones, started to become very National-Socialistic," which led him to think that "there must be more to it [National Socialism] . . . something more there."

But he was to develop a much stronger bond with the Nazis in a way that was both serendipitous and calculated. When completing his medical studies in the middle and late 1930s, he gained the impression that one had to take part in an officially sponsored organization. Wishing to avoid the paramilitary ones, he joined a student "scientific society." He was immediately drawn into a competition the group sponsored for finding an indigenous German product (rather than having to bring one in from the outside) that could be used for a culture medium in bacteriological work. Partly perhaps on the basis of his knowledge of nature, B. "got a good idea," located the indigenous product, and suddenly found himself in the extraordinary situation of "a student having a laboratory, two assistants, and a prize." He was now "a scientist who received strong praise from the Party," a man with a "good start" who had "the good fortune to get political support even though my topic . . . was not political." Now he was in the position of "not just receiving commands" but of taking leadership in advising scientific teams on what could be grown in certain Bavarian forests, and what must be cut down in order to make room for such growth. He received an additional prize in a more public ceremony, which caused him only one problem: his wife-to-be thought him a "top Nazi" and avoided him for some time. He completed his medical studies with a flourish, proud of the fact that his thesis on his discovery of the local culture medium was a "fine thing . . . about twenty lines, I think, no more."

This special *Erlebnis,* or "experience" (his term for the entire sequence), undoubtedly influenced his decision to join the Party at the time: "Not only because in a practical sense I had to [for getting an assistantship at a clinic] but with a positive feeling . . . [and with] no obligation, no force." He did, in fact, obtain a coveted assistantship and a good hospital connection at his university while retaining his position in the bacteriological department and even, in 1939, being awarded a two-year scholarship for study abroad—thwarted only by the outbreak of the war.

He began to observe less positive features of the regime during two years of subsequent medical work: important medical positions came to be "occupied by political people," and even his father's professional eminence did not protect him from close scrutiny by Nazi-appointed assistants on the lookout for potential political deviance.

Dr. B. did not consider himself a Nazi ideologue but, like many Germans of the time, held "a positive attitude toward [the Nazis'] economic successes and toward the possibility of reform [of society]." What made him uneasy was the idea of people looking on him as someone who has been able to get ahead because he "has [politically] cooperated," and he was especially intent upon convincing his mother and his future wife that such was not the case. When the war broke out, that conflict contributed to a sense of shame—sometimes aggravated by casual remarks people made—that a healthy young man like himself was not "among the soldiers" fighting for his country.

Helping Prisoner Doctors

Once over his selections crisis, Dr. B. had no major difficulties in Auschwitz. He consolidated a remarkable set of relationships with prisoner doctors, about a hundred of whom were assigned to the Hygienic Institute. While their situation was relatively benign for Auschwitz even prior to his arrival, he went further than anyone else in concern for their well-being. When they were sick he made provisions for their medications and general care and visited them himself. He helped them send messages to, and arrange visits with, wives and friends in other parts of the camp. He contributed to their survival by keeping them closely informed about various Auschwitz currents and plans. And he directly saved lives in additional ways: by protecting prisoner doctors from selections, by finding them and rescuing them from the gas chamber when they had been selected, and by the benign experiments discussed in chapter 15.

Prisoner doctors came to view him as a very special figure—"perhaps the only one," according to Dr. Erich G., "mentally . . . consciously opposed to [Auschwitz and the Nazis], . . . the only one who really behaved [in a] friendly [way] to doctors." Another prisoner doctor thought Dr. B. "oddly out of place in the SS," was moved by both his concern when he was severely ill, and B.'s later insistence that he not go back to work too soon but "just lie outside in the sun and rest." While a third doctor considered Dr. B. "an educated research worker," a fourth thought him "a very kind man" but not especially bright: "We decided that . . . he was stupid . . . because he was so nice with us."

That decency had a powerful impact on inmates ("Anyone who has never experienced the camp cannot know how much real value such things have for morale"), according to one doctor. And seeing Ernst B. as a man out of place in Auschwitz and the SS in general, they searched for explanations of his being part of both. While they were reasonably accurate in seeing him as "ordered there" (to Auschwitz) by the SS (as

Dr. Tadeusz S. stated), the doctor just quoted went further and said, "He himself . . . often repeated [the point that he] had not enrolled voluntarily in the SS, but only under coercion, which in 1944 was possible." And a third doctor said similarly, "He told me he was not considered kosher by the SS [because his wife was related to a German officer who defected to an Allied nation] so that is why they put him in this position in the Hygienic Institute . . . where they could keep close watch on him." I suspect that these falsehoods (he was, in fact, eager to join up and acknowledged volunteering for the Waffen SS) resulted mainly from his need to achieve maximum acceptance by the prisoner physicians. Possibly also they exaggerated and distorted it out of a need to believe that this SS doctor, who treated them humanely, was not a genuine SS officer— not really "one of *them.*"

Ernst B. tended to romanticize his integration with the inmates: "After half a year [in Auschwitz], I discussed all personal . . . [and] all possible questions openly with the prisoners. [There was] no difference in my social contact with them from with other personnel"—in terms that suggest how far that integration actually did proceed.

He could then attribute what he called a "perverse reaction," in deciding not to take advantage of an opportunity to be transferred from Auschwitz, to his having become "integrated into the whole thing." Prisoner doctors to whom he talked about the opportunity of course urged him to stay, and he was referring to his relationship with them within the overall Auschwitz situation when he added that "the situation was so extraordinary that you . . . could not get out."

He remembered asking himself, "Is it right to stay, or would it be better to leave?," and deciding that he should stay: "Here I had impact [*Resonanz*]* and I felt I could accomplish something positive [in comparison with other possible assignments]. . . . At least I could do something humane here." He enumerated other ways in which he could contribute to the lives of prisoners: by turning over to them meat given him for testing and telling SS officials that large "samples" were required; and helping in a project to distill spoiled marmalade to produce orange brandy, which could be, in turn, exchanged with SS men for meat from the slaughterhouse and bakery products, all for inmates. Over time he realized that these maneuverings were safe "because every person there was also corrupt."

Dr. B. had another dream that expressed his conflicts and the depth of his integration with prisoners—a dream so dangerous that he can remember having had it only after leaving Auschwitz, though I gained the impression that fragments of it may have occurred there as well. The dream involved a young Jewish woman laboratory assistant in the Hygienic Institute who had a talent for making drawings from photographs of the

_____

*The choice of this word—literally, "resonance"—suggests the idea of human interaction rather than mere influence.

families of the SS officers and men; she had been placed there by a noncommissioned officer who made a little business from her drawings. Having had her make a drawing from a picture of his wife and children, B. was fascinated by this very "primitive" young person who was able to alter her drawings from crude ones for crude SS men to "marvelous" and "tasteful" renditions for more cultivated SS officers like himself. She was from the nearby Beskid Mountains, and on one occasion when B. spoke of driving into them she warned him not to because "there are too many partisans there."

> I dreamed that I fled with her into the Beskids to the partisans. . . . I'm sure that there was nothing . . . in any way erotic. . . . There are various versions. . . . [Mostly] we are in a primitive Beskid house, and then the partisans arrive, and we go with them [join them], and so on. . . . There are no further details that I can remember.

He thought the dream might be related to his seeing the drawing again upon returning to Germany (he had apparently sent it from Auschwitz to his wife), a drawing he both treasured (keeping it sometimes in his office and sometimes in their bedroom) and was made anxious by (taking it down because "I had too many bad dreams"). The eroticized tie with this young female prisoner in connection with fleeing to join the Nazis' enemies suggests an ultimate integration and an image, however fearful, of transcending and erasing the Auschwitz taint.

Former inmates tended to exaggerate and simplify Ernst B.'s conflicts, as did one doctor who stated that Dr. B. "confessed that . . . he was drinking more and more in order to react less to what was happening around him." He was asked whether he believed Hitler would win the war, and is said to have answered, "If justice exists on earth, then Hitler should lose the war, but is there really justice on earth?"—the kind of enigmatic answer that prisoner doctors could experience as very heartening.

Only one prisoner doctor noted "emotional problems" in Dr. B., observing that he would at times become tearful and had a variety of psychosomatic ailments and "the pattern of a heavy drinker." While confirming that B. was decent to individual Jews, this doctor said that he was "hostile to the [Jewish] population"—the only inmate to make this claim about B.

But Dr. B.'s conflicts in no way interfered with his fundamental adaptation to the place. As he said to me, "I must—this now really sounds—one cannot understand it if I say . . . I didn't really mind being there." For his need for contact was satisfied there. He was "really touched" by the fact that "as soon as one had a little contact with an inmate, . . . the most important thing then was—almost more important than eating— . . . that [he] could talk to someone about [his] family." He even claimed that *because* he was an "outsider" they could talk more readily to him about their families than they could to their fellow prisoners—again a dubious claim but one that says something about the terrain Dr. B. inhabited in Auschwitz. And he had proof of that shared terrain in warm letters from inmates received after the war.

One reason he could adapt so well was that his assignment there kept him separate from the killing process, which is partly why he could say that "we are pulling the wrong string" in talking so much about the killing: more "in the foreground for . . . doctors is the problem of starvation." But even that could be overcome "if one had . . . or at least believed . . . one had a task to fulfill and friends for whom . . . one could do something . . . good."

He did describe moments when misery, which usually "one would overlook a lot," would be suddenly revealed by "a certain, special glance" of a prisoner that would break through one's "protective cover" (*Schirm*; literally "umbrella"), and one would feel "the experience of misery or despair in such a situation." He added that, just as small details move one in connection with beauty, so do "small idylls" of a negative kind, and then "one has to become very active" to overcome the feeling.

Yet his Auschwitz dream recurred: "To me . . . the most dreadful thing during the whole time . . . was again and again the look of this very good friend," of Simon Cohen who "probably . . . was a hallucination." That periodic self-accusation was absorbed by, and perhaps served a function in, his relatively comfortable overall adaptation. What he derived in particular from his relation to prisoner doctors was suggested in a phrase in a handwritten letter he sent to me, the only one in English, concerning his relationship with the older prisoner professor who had served as mentor to Delmotte: "I adored [the professor] as a father and I believe he also accepted me as a son." Allowing for Dr. B.'s possible exaggeration, we are nonetheless struck by these two young SS doctors looking to a Jewish prisoner professor as a father figure and possibly experiencing a measure of sibling rivalry in the process. That the feeling was reciprocal was confirmed by warm letters from former prisoner doctors, including those from the professor himself. After reading one of them to me, Dr. B. began to muse about "the duty to stay in Auschwitz" and his capacity "to feel quite comfortable there." He spoke of having in the camp an active sense of the "special calling in me to be a physician." This statement represents his own relationship to the Auschwitz schizophrenic situation; it could have been made by no other Nazi doctor.

Dr. B.'s Family: "I Never Told Her the Full Truth"

Ernst B.'s relationship with his wife and young children was crucial to his Auschwitz life, but indirectly and from a distance. One of his first

Auschwitz reactions was "I had done something wrong, especially in relation to my wife." He was referring to the fact that his insistence upon joining the military, which she had opposed, had taken him to Auschwitz, even though "I really hadn't wanted what I had ended up doing." After their bizarre arrival there together, "it took half a year before I met with [her] again"—because of duty requirements and, one suspects, a certain ambivalence about seeing her. About Auschwitz activities, he told her, "I have nothing to do with the whole business—I am only in this institute." And in fact, "I never told her the full truth." As he began to see her more frequently—he and Weber arranged for him to spend a week at home every two or three months—he "had a good feeling and a bad feeling." He wanted to see his wife and children ("I was of course very happy to be there") but was aware of a feeling of guilt ("I . . . hoped to make things good again"). He felt the need to keep his wife and Auschwitz separate.

He described extreme "inner resistance" to the thought of her visiting him there ("I never would have considered the idea"). During those first days when they were there together, she asked questions about the camp and was given some of the usual fictions (in such a large place it was inevitable that many people died, so that a crematorium was needed, and the smoke was due to the fact that it was not working properly); and although over time she inevitably learned much of the truth, he did not wish to expose her to "a closer look at things." Upon returning from each visit, he was also troubled by the "contrast" Auschwitz presented to the peaceful family scene, creating in him strong feelings of "how lucky one could be not to be stationed there."*

In 1944, one of their children died a crib death at the age of eight months. Dr. B. described his wife's reaction as one of "great shock," but his own as less intense because he had seen little of the infant, and since "the future did not look very bright . . . dying as a baby might not be so tragic." But he added that it also could be a "reasonable indication of what was to come"—possibly an indirect way of expressing the sense that they were being punished, perhaps by God, for Auschwitz.

Dr. B. associated thoughts of his wife and children with his inclinations to help inmates, but he attributed those inclinations even more to his "bond" *(Verbindung)* with his parents, especially his father. He spoke of the latter's "life of integrity" and "refus[al] to make any concessions" of a kind that would have improved his financial situation. And then Dr. B. expressed an additional thought: "If they both [his father and mother] were to find out that I had come to do these criminal acts [*zu kriminellen*

---

*One prisoner doctor remembered what he thought to be a visit of Ernst B.'s wife: "She was an attractive young woman who greeted us when passing with 'Good day' [*Guten Tag* —an extremely polite greeting in Auschwitz] but otherwise avoided areas where we were." Either he was referring to B.'s initial arrival or she actually made a visit that B. did not remember or care to discuss. In any case, this prisoner doctor thought that B. was sufficiently buoyed by seeing his wife that he began painting soon afterward.

Handlungen] in this manner, it would have been almost unbearable for them." He was being a bit ambiguous about whether he actually saw himself as having performed "criminal acts" or as merely being exposed to them or to the potential for performing them. But it is of some significance that it was in relation to a parent-centered conscience that he came closest to associating his own behavior with the idea of criminality.

SS Colleagues

A remarkable aspect of Dr. B.'s adaptation was that his closeness to prisoner doctors did not seem to interfere with his integration with SS colleagues. He tended to defend their behavior and to minimize differences between them and himself, despite glaring evidence to the contrary.

A case in point was his attitude toward his chief, Bruno Weber. Most inmates feared Weber, who seemed to them unfeeling, a stickler for regulations, and dangerous. But Dr. B. claimed that Weber had a very "bad press" with inmates because "he appeared to be cold . . . and a . . . good SS physician" but, "in fact, in a practical way he helped more inmates than I did . . . because of his higher position." The kernel of truth in B.'s claim is that the beneficent atmosphere of the Hygienic Institute would have been impossible without a certain amount of "closet decency" from Weber. But B. needed to go further, to see differences between himself and Weber as no more than differences in "bedside manner" (see page 195). He explained that Weber "played this role . . . of the stern SS physician" because he was "fearful" of being caught violating SS rules—and that, because of his "ambition . . . to make a career in the SS." Whenever I would point out criminal actions of these other SS doctors—for instance, Weber's participation in selections and in lethal human experiments—B. would neither deny nor condemn that behavior but simply attribute it to the "Auschwitz atmosphere" or "Auschwitz mentality." I believe he was trying to tell me that he was no different from them; that he too was part of that "Auschwitz atmosphere" and "Auschwitz mentality"; that he lived and worked as part of their community and in considerable measure thought like them. His exaggerated claim to sameness was undoubtedly a measure of his integration into *that* group as well.

During the interview in which he told me about SS doctors' contribution to technical problems in burning bodies, I asked him whether he himself would have considered helping with that kind of task and his answer was clearly affirmative: if a "hygienic catastrophe" could have been avoided, he would have certainly "as a matter of course contributed [his] knowledge as with any other problem": "I also was . . . for me it was also everyday living, you see." He was saying to me again and again: I, too, was one of them.

Friendship with Mengele

How much he was one of them is revealed in his relationship to Mengele, which leads us to the heart of Ernst B.'s own moral and psychological ambiguity. During our first interview, while discussing the intensity of his involvement in Auschwitz to the point of his not acting on an opportunity to leave, he spontaneously said to me, "I had very good contact with Mengele. Have you ever heard the name Mengele?" And that was when he declared, "I really must say that he was the most decent colleague I met there." During our five interviews together, over a two-year period, Dr. B. retreated not an inch from that startling judgment. He always warmed to the subject, intent on correcting what he took to be widespread misunderstandings about the man and what he represented in Auschwitz. It was wrong to talk about Mengele as the "typical SS doctor," B. insisted; rather, Mengele was "the exception," separate from the older group long associated with the camps, independent in attitude, and "on principle opposed to the system of the concentration camps." B. pictured Mengele, Weber, and himself as having much in common: Weber critical of the extermination of the Jews; Mengele equally critical of the extermination of the Polish intelligentsia; and B. becoming aware that Mengele's "general evaluation of the camp was quite similar to [B.'s own]."

Dr. B. and Mengele had much else in common—as doctors in their early thirties with a similar upper-middle-class family background, and as Bavarians with traditional antipathy to Prussians. More than that, Dr. B. remembered Mengele as "helpful," "a really fine comrade" *(sehr kameradschaftlicher*; literally, "very comradely"), and admirable in his open expression of "outspoken antipathies and sympathies [for people]."

When I brought up the question of Mengele's human experiments, B. sprang to the defense of his friend: human experiments were "a relatively minor matter" in Auschwitz; children (who made up most of the twins Mengele studied) had little chance to survive in Auschwitz, but Mengele made certain they were well fed and taken care of; Mengele sought a better diet for patients on medical blocks and fought the corruption that siphoned off their food; wild rumors and fantasies developed about Mengele because he worked in a special room that others were forbidden to enter. And when I asked B. whether he would change his views if I presented him with extensive evidence of Mengele's practice of occasionally sending one or both twins to the gas chamber, B. answered unhesitatingly in the negative "because under the conditions of Auschwitz one must always say that Mengele's experiments were not forms of cruelty." In defense of Mengele, he repeatedly invoked the "conditions of Auschwitz" or the "Auschwitz atmosphere." That is, since one had the opportunity to perform "kinds of experiments that could not be made in a normal world," Mengele "did just the type of scientific research that was possible under the specific conditions of the camp." Moreover, Mengele "assured" his friend that he "*most* [B.'s emphasis] carefully prevented them

[the children] from finding out about their future fate of being gassed."
But the larger point was always that, as long as a man acted in accordance
with the morass of Auschwitz, we cannot judge him negatively now:

> One must be aware that in the Auschwitz milieu, where thousands
> were being killed continuously, such a thing [Mengele's killing a few
> twins] was nothing at all extraordinary. Absolutely nothing that might
> be particularly noticed or come especially to his or anyone else's mind.
> . . . But as an outsider one cannot understand this.

Further, Dr. B. rejected evidence of Mengele's cruelty: "I can't believe
that. . . . It would be contrary to the . . . personal impression that I have
of him through my close intimate association with him [and] through
doing work with him alone in . . . genuine professional contact." In slight
qualification, B. admitted that he could not observe Mengele in all situations, so that concerning "how he behaved in his own camp and . . .
concerning the selections . . . I can say nothing." But B.'s general message
was: What I saw was commendable and collegial. What I did not see I
cannot comment on. If people say he did bad things, they are exaggerat-
ing or fantasizing and I cannot believe them. Mengele was merely acting
consistently with Auschwitz principles, whatever he did. And, no one who
has not himself experienced Auschwitz can understand or judge these
things.

In his overall attempt to restore Mengele's "good name," Dr. B.'s
organizing principle was integrity. Mengele behaved according to his
convictions. Mengele also did valuable scientific work. Perhaps there was
a certain loss of humanity (Dr. B. admitted under my prodding), but "if
somebody is as convinced as he was that the Jews had to be exterminated
. . . then one can imagine how this restraint [associated with ordinary
humanity] does not exist"—and "always, again, has to be seen under
Auschwitz conditions."

Mengele was no hypocrite, that is, and showed initiative and a sense
of responsibility in several ways. As an example, Dr. B. told how Mengele
"was the only one among the SS doctors who concerned himself with the
practical [aspects] . . . of gassing"; the "overburdened" facilities and
"technical . . . mistakes" made the whole process "even more inhuman,"
so that "as perverse as it may sound, he took the trouble to look into these
matters . . . for humanitarian reasons."

Contrasting Mengele's constructive energies with the usual Auschwitz
attitude of "that's not my business," Dr. B. on several occasions told how,
at the time of the evacuation of Auschwitz toward the end of the war,
when everyone was preoccupied with personal problems, only Mengele
had the presence of mind and sense of responsibility to organize the
dynamiting of the gas chambers. The task was really "under the jurisdiction of the commandant, not the SS doctor," but the commandant
"would have been willing to leave the whole stinking mess [*Sauerei*, slang

often used in the camp] standing." Each time Dr. B. spoke of it, he praised the act, though he gave it different meanings: an expression of Mengele's "disapproval of the entire annihilation structure as a disgrace to SS principles and to his own religious beliefs"; to conceal the "filth" from the occupiers as an expression of his "belief in the German race"; and because he "didn't want to leave anything behind that would make the SS look bad."

In our last interview, Dr. B. spoke again with intensity about the "utter chaos" at the time, with everybody fleeing and "Mengele . . . the only one who noticed [the SS command] left the crematoria standing," and returned with a few underlings "to blast them as thoroughly as possible."

If Mengele followed a pattern (which I could demonstrate to B.) of alternating between civility and cruelty to prisoners or of relegating a healthy twin to the gas chamber for experimental purposes, then "for *him* [Mengele] there was no discrepancy." Here B. invoked Rudolf Höss, "who . . . made Auschwitz what it was" but, at the same time, "was in his private life a person of absolute integrity." (For a discussion of the principle involved and of distortions in B.'s example, see page 201.) B.'s point seems to be that a genuine believer in the Nazi project could engage in cruelty and murder with "absolute integrity."

To Dr. B., Mengele was a free spirit of "optimistic character," who acted on his own beliefs even when contrary to official Auschwitz policy. As an example, B. spoke of Mengele's strong stand against the annihilation of the Gypsy camp. Set up as a family camp, the Gypsy unit rapidly deteriorated and became extraordinarily filthy and unhygienic even for Auschwitz, a place of starving babies, children, and adults. B. insisted that there were "sufficient rations . . . delivered to the camp for all of them to survive," but that certain adult Gypsies of high standing kept most of the food, thus denying it to all others, including hungry children. The Auschwitz leaders, "shocked" by the situation, came to the conclusion that it was virtually impossible to change it and that the only solution was to "gas the entire camp." According to B., Mengele strongly opposed that decision, made several trips to Berlin to try to get it reversed, and went so far as to declare to other Auschwitz authorities that annihilating the Gypsy camp would be "a crime."

Ernst B. himself told of becoming deeply interested in the Gypsy situation, and was appalled by what he described as scenes of fathers and mothers eating while permitting their own children to starve: conditions "were atrocious, . . . worse than in all other camps," and constituted "a very great problem." He added, "Since I survived [*überlebt*] that Gypsy camp, I have developed the worst possible opinion of Gypsies. And when I see a Gypsy I make sure to get away quickly. . . . I can't stand to hear Gypsy music."

The phenomenon of blaming the victim is at the center of Dr. B.'s perception of the event. The intensity of his involvement and of his aversion to Gypsies, suggests that he struggles with guilt feelings nonetheless—as also perhaps does his arrogating for himself the term "survivor." He expressed considerable sympathy for the camp officials faced with the intractable problem of the Gypsy camp, even as he both admired Mengele for "boldly" opposing its annihilation and thought it natural for him to join actively in that annihilation once the decision was made. Mengele remained for Dr. B. a profound source of connection to the Auschwitz atmosphere.

Dr. B. gave an elaborate description of Mengele's "early SS ideology": the main currents of European culture taking shape from such "Germanic" groups as the ancient Greeks as well as the Normans and Vikings; that emerging culture undermined by Christian morality of Jewish origin, culminating in a vast historic threat posed by Jewish influence to the Germanic race; the need to revert to ancient German myth in creating a contemporary SS Order at the heart of the Nazi movement, a major goal of which was the elimination of Jewish influence. In Dr. B.'s recitation of all this, there was an intensity, perhaps even enthusiasm, suggesting that it invoked the presence of his friend and that something in him [B.] was drawn to the message. Indeed B. claimed that Mengele "didn't preach," and that all these matters were discussed between the two men "very objectively." B. had a way of domesticating Mengele's wildly visionary ideas, both because they were not entirely alien to himself and because he could invoke Mengele the scientist and "researcher on racial matters."

Dr. B.'s psychic struggles with what Mengele represented were reflected in his contradictory descriptions of Mengele's views on exterminating the Jews. He sometimes spoke as though Mengele strongly opposed the Auschwitz killing project, and quoted him as terming it a form of "absolute idiocy" and "stupidity," and even declared that "Mengele would never have joined the SS if Hitler had announced in advance that we shall let the Jews go through the smokestacks as soon as we have triumphed." Yet later Dr. B. stressed that Mengele "was fully convinced that the annihilation of the Jews [was] a provision for the recovery of the world, and Germany," the only open question being the method to be used. The latter view is undoubtedly closer to the truth. But my point here is that Mengele became something of a mouthpiece for Dr. B.'s own inner contradictions about the "Jewish problem": at times B. could refer to the overall issue of annihilating the Jews as though it were a serious question for men of good will to contemplate, disagree upon to some extent, but approach with an open mind and with "rational discussion." And when he summed up the traits of character he so admired in Mengele ("a good soldier, . . . no phony ambitions within the SS," and "did not hesitate to oppose . . . openly [whatever] . . . he felt was wrong"), these were the qualities that B. had been brought up to admire and found in his father, and that, ironically, he believed gave him the strength to behave decently in Auschwitz.

In that vein he attributed something more to Mengele—a genuine leadership principle. In contrast to Höss, whom Dr. B. saw as "a perfect soldier" because he carried out orders to the letter, Mengele was a "leader of men." For B., he was a man in the heroic mold. He was intellectually ahead of his time, getting at the "biological basis" for political behavior and leadership in ways that scholars are now beginning to address. And he had an "absolutely firm 'life principle' [*Lebensprinzip*] for which he stood up more than anyone else I knew [and] took risks to an incredible degree in order to carry forth his convictions." B. added "Very few have done that. Mengele was one of them."

Dr. B.'s testimony in the extradition case against Mengele is consistent in many ways with the patterns I have discussed. He described Mengele as having been convinced that the Jews had to be exterminated; that selections in Auschwitz were imperative and even "humanitarian"; and that Auschwitz was "only a . . . partial anticipatory final solution" in terms of what was to come. Although he portrayed Mengele as a man of conviction and said he knew of no fatalities in Mengele's research with twins, Dr. B.'s detailed testimony on Mengele's relationship to selections could have been legally damning to his former friend. Now B.'s "harmonizing" was with the German court.

At one point, I asked Dr. B. how he would feel, considering the different paths taken by himself and Mengele, if they had a chance to meet in the future. His reply, while cautious, made clear that he would be glad to see his old friend and to resume their relationship on an even more "rational" basis than before: "And there would result—as I know him—completely emotionless talk. Talk without emotions. Emotions, they remained at Auschwitz. For all of us."

Evacuation of Auschwitz and Dr. B.'s Trial

In preparing for the evacuation of Auschwitz in January 1945, Ernst B. tried to arrange for "his" doctors to survive, whether they were among those making the forced march or those who would stay. A doctor who had been among prisoners able to march out in the regular evacuation noted, "When we passed the laboratory the SS staff was waving us good-bye and wishing us good luck. They seemed to give us a strange sense of 'We are in this together.' "

It was decided that the Hygienic Institute should reassemble itself at Dachau; and while "everybody tried to save his skin," Dr. B. did his best to help organize that laboratory. Though there was talk of preparing for a German "counteroffensive," it is likely that this focus on rebuilding the Hygienic Institute was in the service of demonstrating to the Occupation the benign nature of Nazi medical activities in the camps, as well as maintaining the medical "as if" situation to the end. In the midst of very bad conditions at Dachau, prisoner physicians there who had formerly worked in the Hygienic Institute were enormously relieved to see Ernst B. and Weber and to hear from them: "We want you to work with us again." While at this time most SS doctors anticipated the forthcoming power reversal and became newly considerate toward inmates, Dr. B. went considerably further. With Allied armies approaching, he discussed with prisoner doctors possible arrangements for their escape from Nazi control, including the idea of providing them with SS uniforms. He then shook hands with them and "said goodbye in a very friendly way," and as a last act took a pistol out of his drawer and gave it to one of them for their protection. While he admitted to an element of a self-serving motivation, he also later explained, "There existed the . . . likelihood that another massacre . . . could happen. . . . I had a few pistols—why should they lie around?"

During the last days of Dachau, Dr. B. was advised by prisoner friends to go into hiding for a short period because the atmosphere immediately after the Nazi defeat would be such that "anyone in an SS uniform [would] be beaten to death"; afterward he could emerge and clear himself with the inmates' help. He did that briefly, was taken into custody under a false name by the Americans at Dachau, and for a time protected by former inmates who, when brought in to identify SS personnel, intentionally "didn't see me."

After about a year in custody his identity was discovered, and he was put on trial. He told me that, at that time, "I personally did not feel guilty." B. spoke of his sense of "togetherness" toward SS officers in prison with him; and of his "macabre" feeling when some were given the death penalty. He began to be worried when it became clear that the Russians were in charge and might want to create a show trial.

Former prisoner doctors rallied behind Dr. B. with impressive testimony on his behalf. Women doctors from Block 10 notably validated his claim that the experiments he did there harmed no one and saved many lives. The professor who had been so close to him and Delmotte organized testimony from many who had worked in the Hygienic Institute, and testified himself that Dr. B. "stood up for the rights of all prisoners . . . with admirable bravery . . . [and] with truly cordial helpfulness . . . far beyond the usual laws of humanity." The professor told how B. had saved his life after a severe stomach hemorrhage, and how "among the inmates of the Hygienic Institute a veritable 'Dr. B. cult' came into existence, which accorded him not only reverence and respect but also sincere gratitude and love."

This professor expressed similar sentiments in a personal letter to Dr. B., which included a warm and detailed account of the former's experiences during the two years since the end of the war, and stated, "You know very well what I owe to you. I am convinced that without you I would not have stayed alive." In addition, he wrote of his chagrin at finding the Hygienic Institute destroyed when he went back with an investigative commission to inspect the area, along with his pleasure at discovering that scientific records were still intact. In a later letter he asked Dr. B. about additional scientific data from the Hygienic Institute and suggested their publishing a joint article with the possible institutional attribution "From the Hygienic Institute of the Concentration Camp Auschwitz." Years later, after the professor had died, I was able to talk to his daughter, who knew a great deal about her father's relationship to Ernst B., especially how he had saved her father's life on three separate occasions. Dr. B. had taken on, as a result, an almost mythical quality in her mind: she thought of him not as an SS doctor but "as my father's savior," imagined meeting him sometime in Germany, and went so far as to say that when her father died Dr. B. seemed in certain ways to replace him in her feelings.

She was puzzled, however, by one aspect of the relationship. She had seen the warm correspondence between the two men, including Dr. B.'s grateful letter following his acquittal. After that, her father wrote back saying in effect (in her words), "You saved my life—I saved your life— now we are even." She noted that the two men then stopped corresponding; and when she asked her father why he did not write the German doctor again, he told her, "Well, we saved each other's life. That's all. What more could we talk about?"

I suspect that her father did experience the matter as a true exchange. First, he had mobilized full energy and influence on behalf of acquittal and liberty for a man who had previously been within the category (but not the mentality) of the professor's own concentration-camp jailor. Then he must have needed to step back from the Auschwitz-derived dependency on and gratitude toward Dr. B., as well as from his own Auschwitz involvements and compromises, in order to assert finally an unbridgeable area in the separate terrains of prisoner physician and SS doctor in Auschwitz.

Dr. B.'s "Auschwitz Confession"

Ernst B.'s most powerful prison experience had to do with "a roomful of files" from the Hygienic Institute, which the examining judge, by now favorably disposed toward him, asked him to examine. B. plunged into a study of such questions as how long an ill prisoner and prisoners in general could survive in Auschwitz on the diet provided them. He went about the task energetically and methodically, studying nutritional components of diets for various kinds of prisoner, including those suffering from different diseases, and concluding that seriously ill inmates had a life expectancy of no more than fourteen days and the general life expectancy of an ordinary prisoner was no more than three months. His findings, which were used by the court and by other researchers, were published. He stressed to me that, beyond these statistics, "What is important is that for months I was alone in a room [cell] with these files and nothing else," and that "through dealing with these papers I established a special contact with Auschwitz." Before that, in a group cell, "one used every opportunity to suppress these memories," but in that room, "confronting the problem . . . in a different way, . . . one could deal with those thoughts without the need to push them back." He then compared his situation to that of Rudolf Höss, with whom he had briefly shared a cell and talked just days before Höss was hanged. He found that, after Höss "had written his confession [*Bekenntnisse,* which could also mean 'confessional memoirs'], he felt "relieved . . . of a great burden." Dr. B. felt himself comparably relieved: in effect, his scientific study of life-death factors was his "Auschwitz confession."

The intensity of that experience was reflected in dreams that began at that time and have since continued: "Whenever I have a dream related somehow to Auschwitz, those papers will appear too." The psychological work of that study of Auschwitz files took him as close as he ever came to a conscious sense of guilt concerning his relation to Auschwitz:* "I continuously occupied myself, . . . subconsciously and in my dreams, with finding out how one could make things edible, usable for human beings. . . . In my dreams the hunger [of inmates] kept me much . . . occupied, [because] we ourselves lived very well and the others, the prisoners, were starving."

After being acquitted, a former prisoner now in a high position offered to arrange for Dr. B. to re-enter academic medicine and university life. But he preferred to return to the area where he had practiced in the past, because "this human oasis meant more." In general, "I did not want to make any kind of experiment . . . [but] wanted to use the safest method," and "told myself that only human values in themselves matter."

He wanted to avoid "experiments" either in medicine or in life. Like many former Nazi doctors, his impulse was to retreat from situations of intensity and cultural disability and to find a safe and reliable path—in his case to spend much of the rest of his life both absorbing, and moving away from, the Auschwitz experience. People in his area accepted him, apparently knowing something of his background and looking upon him as someone who had served with the Nazis but had been cleared of accusations of criminal behavior.

The Course of the Interviews

Certain patterns developed in Dr. B.'s attitudes and relationship to me over the course of our five virtually day-long interviews, totaling about thirty hours. During our first interview he was, compared with other former Nazi doctors I met, extraordinarily enthusiastic and ingratiating. He seemed to pour out all he could about almost anything I asked him, and volunteered a great deal on his own. He did, like others, seem most comfortable as a fellow observer of his own earlier experiences; and he sought to construct a narrative of his life that minimized his encounters

---

*As opposed to his guilt toward Delmotte, which had to do with personal decisions and personal consequences rather than with being part of Auschwitz evil; or even to B.'s particular guilt toward Simon Cohen, which he experienced periodically.

with such troubling matters as Jewish persecutions, his early SS training, and some of the more sordid details of the Auschwitz transition period. Nonetheless, his rendition of Auschwitz in that first interview was remarkable in detail, candor, and psychological atmosphere. Though I was not without a certain restraint, the tone of the interview was friendly. Later my assistant who did the interpreting expressed his amazement at how two people like Ernst B. and myself, whose lives had been so antithetical to one another, could communicate so well at a first meeting.

Because of Dr. B.'s continuing enthusiasm I was able to schedule a second day-long interview later the same week. He then made clear his wife's reservations about our meetings, having to do with her association of Auschwitz with his subsequent imprisonment and her sense that the interviews could cause him subsequent harm. She in fact made two appearances during the interview, in which she expressed these feelings and more. During one she said haltingly in English, "I am not against you— just against Auschwitz." And a short time later, with B. absent, having been called away briefly to see a patient, she again came in, lit the Advent candles on the Christmas tree (it was the third Sunday of Advent), and more or less lingered in the room without saying anything. My assistant and I had the impression that she wished to draw us into a modest religious ritual, a kind of spiritual communion; but although there was beauty in the scene, framed as it was by a wooded landscape at dusk in the distance, I was aware of my own sense of not being at all ready for an experience of communion with her at that moment.

That second interview was the longest and most detailed of the five. Notable was Dr. B.'s willingness to expose increasingly his vulnerability and conflict: in connection with the Delmotte episode and his "bad conscience" toward the other SS doctor, and his Auschwitz dreams with their element of self-condemnation.

The third interview was an important turning point. He began by complimenting me on the clarity of case studies in a book I sent him in response to his request to see earlier work of mine. But he then emphasized how people were likely to reconstruct past events in a way that was favorable to them. He made clear he was referring to himself, and was telling me, in effect, that I should not accept what he told me about his Auschwitz experiences as the full or only truth. He was struggling for candor and perhaps at the same time expressing a new version of one of his consistent themes: that Auschwitz was so complex and paradoxical that it was not really graspable or recoverable to memory.

But now his insistent return to Mengele's virtues began to reveal the extent of his own Nazi involvement. His stress on the "rationality" of his and Mengele's discussions of the far reaches of SS ideology was part of a new emphasis on the extent to which he, Ernst B., really belonged to that group of SS doctors. I could sense he was penetrating further into the Auschwitz atmosphere as he coolly delineated ways in which SS doctors would help with "technical problems." As he stressed the Auschwitz principle of everyone's having "dirt on his walking stick," he moved closer not only to the heart of Auschwitz but also to his own connection with the camp and its functions. In other words, by probing more deeply and becoming increasingly candid, he was forced to reveal aspects of his involvement that would no longer fit into the comfortably controlled narrative a part of himself wished to construct. That is why he seemed more tense during this interview than in others; and at the end he tried to retreat from his own impasse by focusing on the issue of Auschwitz overcrowding: on how there were as many as 140,000 prisoners in the camp at times, and how scientific experiments with mice in crowded cages revealed extreme behavior, including cannibalism.

The fourth interview took place nine months after the third, the delay caused by a number of factors, but mainly by reluctance on his part, apparently due to his wife's continuing objections. As a compromise we met in a small university office I had access to in Munich, requiring that he drive several hours to meet me. Although still affable, his tone was significantly different. He told me that his attitude about Auschwitz and related issues had "hardened." He now insisted upon recognizing what was good about the Nazis as well as what was bad, and upon looking at other forms of cruel behavior in history and thereby seeing the Nazis as by no means unique.

He had in fact hardened toward me and the interview situation as well, becoming increasingly assertive in expressing the Nazi point of view at the time in ways that left doubt about how removed he was from that point of view, then and even now. There was an element of contempt in his dismissal of any possible comparison between violent contemporary cults (in particular the one led by Jim Jones, which culminated in the mass suicide-murder of more than nine hundred of its followers in 1978) and the Nazi Auschwitz structure. And there was a tone of defiance in his stress on the "logic" of the Nazi killing in Auschwitz for those doctors who believed in the vision of National Socialism as a "world blessing" (Weltbeglückung) and Jews as the "fundamental evil" (Grundübel). His language became more crude—for instance, in his use of the term "home-baked problems" (hausbackene Problemen) to describe routine problems. He seemed assertively unapologetic, at times almost enthusiastic, as he took me on a journey through the foulest Auschwitz realms. And in stressing that Nazi doctors saw such tasks as offering advice on the burning of bodies as "not an ethical problem at all—just technical," he seemed to be rejecting any moral perspective on Auschwitz. At the end of the interview, when comparing Nazi times with the present, he said that, despite the "full liberation" today, there is an absence of "ideals for youth," a "lack of commitment," which leads to "chaotic conditions" and the absence of "a coherent community." The Nazis "overdid it" in the opposite direction, he acknowledged, but in Hitler's admittedly "primitive methods" there was "something right," something that "was good with the Nazis."

Now it was I who became tense, as I found myself appalled by what I was hearing and aware of my declining sympathy for this man, who had been a hero to people in Auschwitz who most needed him. But toward the end of the interview, he spoke positively about our whole sequence of meetings, because "through specific questions one is forced to fully think something out" and "in speaking about it, it becomes clear." I came to believe that he had experienced a certain relief at making a stronger representation of his earlier Auschwitz self, perhaps better able to do so because he was outside of his house and on more or less neutral ground. Probably a more important factor was the expectation that this would be our last interview. Earlier he had gone quite far toward collaborating with me as a critic of Auschwitz and the Nazis, and thereby expressing his postwar German (non-Nazi) self. But that became increasingly difficult for him to do as he dug more deeply into the Auschwitz experience with a continuing candor that he himself required for his own psychological struggles. In that sense his own conflicts might have been as important as his wife's objections in bringing about his increasing resistance to the meetings. But he had at the same time become involved with them and me, and his candor in conveying his resurrected Auschwitz self was something of a last gift in the form of potential insight.

He also offered to respond to written questions I could send him by mail. But when I did, he failed to carry out his promise, eventually writing to explain that not only was he distracted by other things but that the simplest question, to be answered truthfully, required an elaborate delineation of the Auschwitz schizophrenic situation. Moreover, he found that impossible to do when "not . . . in personal contact during [that] conversation"—that is, when not in a face-to-face interview situation. Still clearly involved in the exchange, he agreed to see me one more time during my next visit to Germany.

We talked in a hotel room, and the impersonality and unconnectedness of such rooms could have been a factor in the freedom and intensity of his responses. He went still further in pressing the "logic" of the mass killing, though he remained evasive in answering the question whether most Nazi doctors really favored Auschwitz mass murder. Nor was it fully clear where *he* stood on the issue: he had frequently declared himself against that policy, but now an element of himself seemed able at least to go along with it. In general he seemed to speak still more from within the ideology of the time, reasserting his relationship then to the internal SS Auschwitz structure. Yet he was also more active than ever in associations and a continuous rush of information and insight. That was his final "last gift."

Now that we were really parting, he had more aggressively asserted his claim to be his own man, no longer bound by what he took to be requirements of our interviews or of my approval. I too was more aggressive in vigorously probing many issues initiated earlier, no longer concerned about the danger of losing him for future interviews. We had both made an effort to find sufficient common ground to enter into something on the order of humane dialogue. We had each made compromises, and the process was valuable for us both, but we could only sustain it temporarily. In parting, each of us felt a certain relief in returning to what he really was and is. Which is not to say that Dr. B. returned to being a Nazi, but rather that he overtly reclaimed Nazi-related elements still important to his sense of self.

Consistent to the end, he made no moral statements. He did make clear that, despite the late hour, he would drive the several hours back to his home so that he could enjoy the winter sunshine and skiing the next day. He had valued our interviews. But now he was eager to leave the hotel room, to leave Auschwitz and the conflicts that had been engendered by our dialogues.

Dr. B. and the Jews

Ernst B.'s achievements and ambiguities are reflected in his attitude toward Jews. The basic consideration here is his remarkable record in Auschwitz of treating them as human beings in need. His Simon Cohen dreams, moreover, suggest sufficient openness to a Jewish friend to internalize him as a kind of conscience, and also an expression of humanity in German-Jewish relations. But when I asked whether he had previously been concerned about his friend's fate, he answered vaguely, "Perhaps [on a] subconscious [level] [*Vielleicht unterbewusst*]," upon becoming aware of the "Jewish emigration," and added that he and his friends had the impression that Jews were emigrating under "relatively good conditions because they were unwanted, because they had no opportunities to remain here longer." He could place the Cohen family in that category because it was well-to-do and influential, but the image is essentially a Nazi one and covers over early victimization of Jews.

Then, reaching for candor, he added that his friendship with Simon Cohen "was not especially intense," and that in his mainstream group of German friendships, "we didn't have any Jews." He added also, "I am convinced that I, like many others, suppressed that . . . [in a] conscious [way]." That theme of having repressed or suppressed what was happening to the Jews recurred throughout our talks. As he said, "That was at a time when general prosperity was developing for most people, and of course it was much easier simply to suppress unpleasant things." But we may also assume a certain degree of awareness, and acceptance, of that victimization.

The subject came up in a direct way during our second interview. At the time his wife made her statement about not being against me, only against Auschwitz, she also asked me, "Why don't you help the Jews?" adding (in relation to Israel and a Middle East impasse then occurring) that "they are still the most hated people in the world" and that they needed to be helped in some way so that they would not be in a situation where they were so hated. Dr. B. commented that the Germans and the Jews were now the two most hated peoples in the world. While none of this was overtly anti-Jewish, it was consistent with the earlier German attitude of viewing the Jews as "the problem." What both of them said was also probably related to their impression that I was Jewish. If so, her meaning was probably something like: "Why don't you help your fellow Jews—who are still the most hated of peoples and therefore need the help —and leave my husband alone?" While we cannot identify Dr. B.'s views precisely with those of his wife—she had always been more anti-Nazi than he—his words at the time suggested agreement and were also consistent with tendencies we have observed in him of blaming the victim. The suspicion that I was a Jew could also have contributed both to his intensity in seeking an accommodation with me during the interviews and to his reactive ambivalence once he had done so. And it could have contributed as well to his wife's worries.

Dr. B.'s attitudes toward Jews included espousal of "understanding," if not sympathy, for advocacy of the Final Solution, as well as for the Nazi polarity of National-Socialist "world blessing" and Jewish "ultimate evil." Those draconian attitudes were intrinsic to the Nazi context he shared, but were much less operative in him than was his capacity to respond humanely to individual Jews. Whatever these conflicts and contradictions, this capacity, when expressed in an institution whose purpose was the annihilation of Jews, was exemplary and, for many, life-sustaining.

Dr. B.'s Postwar Self

An important part of B.'s post-Auschwitz self and worldview is his unfinished business with Auschwitz. His conflicting needs are both to continue to explore his Auschwitz experience and to avoid coming to grips with its moral significance. His insistence that Auschwitz was not understandable serves the psychological function of rejecting *any* coherent explanation or narrative for the events in which he was involved. He thus remains stuck in an odd post-traumatic pattern: unable either to absorb (by finding narrative and meaning) or to free himself from Auschwitz images.

Yet he does require psychological maneuvers to fend off the extremity of Auschwitz evil. One of these is equating Auschwitz with other collective examples of hypocrisy and failed ideals, such as the schizophrenic situation of the Christian church in doing "things that had nothing to do with 'love thy neighbor.' " Auschwitz is thereby reduced to something historically ordinary, and he is enabled to acknowledge a little more of his Auschwitz self.

His language and style of discussion during the interviews was consistent with that kind of maneuver, especially in its exclusion of the moral domain. While intelligent and articulate, he avoided almost completely expressions of feeling, would laugh or giggle uneasily when dreadful issues were raised, and (as German assistants noted) would leave out verbs and even adverbs in avoiding specific statements—that is, avoiding responsibility for his words, often resorting to clumsy forms of speech.

Over the course of the interviews I had the sense he had taken on the postwar self of a pleasant, conservative-democratic German of advancing years, while inwardly retaining a strong sense of his personal history as part of the Nazi generation. A connecting link between these two views of himself were the writings of certain contemporary biologists. He often had books by Desmond Morris and Konrad Lorenz on his desk and would sometimes initiate a discussion with me about the biological sources of aggression and imperialism. In that way he could be both a contemporary man and retain a biological worldview that had for him a degree of continuity with the Nazi period. Lorenz, prominent both as a Nazi and as a postwar German-Austrian biological scientist, could particularly serve as that kind of link. Ironically, Dr. B. seemed to require some affirmation of his Nazi-related self (after all, that was *he* as a young man) for him to muster the strength and candor to probe it and Auschwitz as intensively as he has.

Overall Life Patterns

Finally, Ernst B.'s overall life patterns may help us to understand his special combination of Nazi affiliation and life-saving decency, and particularly his avoidance of selections—even though, in the collective historical structure I am discussing, themes from an early life can do no more than reveal certain individual tendencies within that structure.

The most persistent theme in Dr. B.'s life, beginning in earliest childhood, has been his quest for human connection, for contact. I suspect that the German family structure does much to create that hunger, and that it was expressed and fed in the Nazis' extraordinary focus on unity, on collective merging (the slogan: "One people, one party, one leader!"). But for Dr. B. it has meant a highly personal search for acceptance, recognition, belongingness, and intimacy—requiring some or all of these in order to feel alive. Inseparable from that quest has been an ideal associated with his father (or his admired uncle) which he called "integrity" and had to do with holding on to one's life project, to one's sense of self, whatever the pressure to yield or dissemble. Much of his life has been a struggle to balance these two fundamental, and at times seemingly incompatible, aspirations.

Dr. B.'s family shared much of the German nation's experience of the First World War in terms of abject humiliation, isolation, and—above all —loss. The national regenerative impulse was reflected in his being assigned a "survivor mission" of carrying on the unfinished work of the gifted uncle killed in the war. In his swing from rebellious artist to compliant physician, Dr. B. acted out a host of frequently encountered German polarities having to do with defiance and submission, romanticism and science, distant vision and pragmatic task. Whatever B.'s (and his countrymen's) journeys through Christianity, traditional utopian thought, and nationalistic movements, it was finally the Nazis who provided the path to revitalization along with a way of balancing, or at least absorbing, those polarities. He developed an impressive talent for maneuver on behalf of group acceptance and standing, but the hunger for connection could overwhelm him, as in his insistence upon sharing the transcendent national experience of war and victory.

Once in Auschwitz, his powerful need for group affiliation could hold him there, and he characteristically sought reliable connection with inmates no less than colleagues. But when asked to do selections, he could resist the kind of doubling that would have been necessary for that task. While we cannot be certain how, psychologically, he was able to do that, he probably called forth elements of the affiliative as well as the integrative inclinations within his self-process. The first, the group need, could well have helped him in a paradoxical fashion: more fluid than fixed in his style of connection, he was probably less bound than others to the kind of absolute loyalty and obedience that would have carried him over the threshold of doubling into the selections. At the same time an aspect of integrity (modeled on his father originally perhaps, but now his own), having to do not only with nondissembling but also with decency, help, and healing, had become part of his self-process. His Auschwitz dreams reflected that humane dimension and kept him aware of it in opposition to the ethos of the camp.

To be sure, he called upon the hierarchical support of his institute, and stressed, as one had to, his personal inability to meet the requirements without contesting "the objective validity of ideological orders and the call of loyalty to obey them."[3]* In that act he called forth both his talent for group maneuver and his ideal of integrity of the self.

Avoiding selections this way did not mean giving up Nazi affiliations, as we know; but it did mean that his doubling in Auschwitz need not be as great as that of other doctors: his Auschwitz self, however, allowed him to adapt to shared SS requirements in that murderous environment; while his prior, more humane self, reinforced by frequent contact with his wife and children, remained reasonably intact. Unlike most other Nazi doctors, he could remain essentially a physician-healer and, in that sense, may have been partly correct in saying that his medical calling contributed to his decency toward prisoners.

That achievement was admirable, even extraordinary. Yet Auschwitz has continued to confuse him over the years, and we now have a better idea why. By not doing selections, he separated himself from the camp

*One could also effectively agree with an order but raise appropriate practical objections, or just say nothing and evade the order.

and its functions; but as a Nazi affiliate and a man hungry for group acceptance, that old Nazi bond is still necessary to him. Similarly, his sense of integrity requires that he both stand critically apart from Auschwitz mass murder and at the same time affirm the truth of his involvement with his Auschwitz colleagues and with overall Nazi camp life. Simon Cohen and Josef Mengele reverberate within him as alternative modes of moral being—just as they did in Auschwitz.

Chapter 17

Dr. Auschwitz:
Josef Mengele

The SS man from *Mein Kampf*—very righteous and puritanical.

—Auschwitz prisoner doctor

He was capable of being so kind to the children, to have them become fond of him, to bring them sugar, to think of small details in their daily lives, and to do things we would genuinely admire. . . . And then, next to that, . . . the crematoria smoke, and these children, tomorrow or in a half-hour, he is going to send them there. Well, that is where the anomaly lay.

—Auschwitz prisoner doctor

My work on the Nazi doctors began and ended with Josef Mengele. It was initiated by legal documents on him and was completed in the summer of 1985, just at the time a team of scientists declared bones discovered in a Brazilian grave to be his.

Although I had originally considered focusing my study on Mengele, I soon realized that such a focus could further the cult of demonic personality already surrounding him and thereby neglect the more general Nazi phenomenon of medicalized killing. Not that I aim to debunk this exemplar of Nazi evil: while he is obscured by his demonic mythology, he has in many ways earned it. Rather, my task is to try to understand how his individual psychological traits fed, and fed upon, the Nazi biomedical vision, and to learn what he has to tell us about medicalized killing and corrupted medical science. For the fact that Mengele seemed to thrive in Auschwitz says much not only about the man, but even more about the psychology of the institution.

Mengele did not become an infamous public figure immediately after the war. He was of course known to Auschwitz survivors, was the object of testimony given in 1945, and was mentioned occasionally during the Nuremberg investigations, but he was not among the accused either there or in subsequent medical trials during the 1940s. It was only in 1958 that he began to reach a status of public infamy, partly through the efforts of the German writer Ernst Schnabel, who learned about Mengele's Auschwitz activities in the course of research for a book on Anne Frank.[1] Survivors from all over the world began to speak out and provide testimony for developing German legal inquiries. And as Mengele moved through various parts of South America to prevent capture or extradition, these testimonies of survivors continued unabated, along with more dubious reports and claims emanating from those less qualified to speak. While he is known to have spent considerable time in Argentina and Paraguay, his long stay in Brazil has been less recognized: his legend has been extended by reports of encounters in those places, including even a false claim of someone's having killed him.

Surely no Nazi war criminal has evoked so much fantasy and fiction. In a 1976 novel, made into a widely distributed film, *The Boys from Brazil*, Mengele is portrayed as a brilliant, fiendish scientist engaged in the cloning of Adolf Hitler. A little over a decade earlier, in a more serious dramatic exploration of Nazi genocide, the play *The Deputy*, Rolf Hochhuth created a Mengele-like character known only as "the doctor" who "has the stature of Absolute Evil, far more unequivocally so than Hitler." In a play that generally renders a character sensitively in terms of moral and psychological conflicts, Hochhuth goes on to claim that this Mengele figure so contrasts with "anything that has been learned about human beings" as to resemble an "uncanny visitant from another world," so that there is no point to exploring his "human features."[2] Thus, inadvertently, Hochhuth too has contributed to the cult of demonic personality. And on a leading American television news program, Isser Harrel, who headed the Israeli Secret Police at the time of the Eichmann capture, told an interviewer that "the moment the name of Mengele was mentioned, Eichmann went into a panic"; on that same program, Mengele's power was reflected in the statement of a man who claimed to see him regularly in Paraguay and lauded his Auschwitz effort "to rid ourselves of society's cripples,"[3] but in a way that "didn't do anything more than scratch the surface." We need to take a step back from the legend and look at the man, at what he did in Auschwitz.

Background

What we know about the thirty-two-year-old man who arrived in Auschwitz on 30 May 1943 is not especially remarkable. He was the second son of a well-to-do Bavarian industrialist—not from an "old" German family but from one that could be considered *nouveau riche*. The family is described as "strict Catholic," and Mengele identified himself as a Catholic on all his official forms, rather than using the more favored Nazi category of "believer in God." He is remembered from his youth as a serious student, a popular and enthusiastic friend in whom one could recognize "a very distinct ambitiousness," a young person with intelligence but more or less ordinary.[4]

His early right-wing nationalism was reflected by his joining the *Stahl-helm* (Steel Helmet, a nationalistic war veteran's organization) in 1931, at the age of twenty. He subsequently became enthusiastic about the Nazi movement, joining the SA in 1934, and applying for Party membership in 1937 and for SS membership upon being admitted to the Party the following year. There are rumors that, while studying in Munich, he met such high-ranking Nazis as Alfred Rosenberg and even Hitler himself— rumors that, in the absence of evidence, fit well with his mythology.

What does seem clear, and what Ernst B. emphasized to me concerning his friend, is that these Nazi leanings had considerable influence on his intellectual choices. Matriculating at the universities not only of Munich but also of Bonn, Vienna, and Frankfurt, Mengele came to concentrate on the physical anthropology and genetics of his time, eventually working under Otmar von Verschuer at the Frankfurt University Institute of Hereditary Biology and Racial Hygiene: the model institute mentioned earlier in connection with the quest for a "biologized" society by means of a national system of files on individual genetic characteristics. Verschuer's son much later remembered Mengele as "a friendly man," so kind that women at the institute referred to him as "Father Mengele"— a nickname that could of course have other connotations.[5]

Mengele produced three publications prior to his Auschwitz arrival. The first, completed in 1935 but appearing in 1937, was his dissertation in the Anthropological Institute (in the department of philosophy) at the University of Munich, and was entitled "Racial-Morphological Examination of the Anterior Portion of the Lower Jaw in Four Racial Groups." In this study he was intent upon demonstrating structural differences in a portion of the lower jaw in old Egyptians, Melanesians, short-skulled Europeans (mostly Eastern and Dinaric [Adriatic coast of Yugoslavia]), and long-skulled Europeans, primarily Nordic. He insisted that a previous investigator's failure to determine differences was due to deficiencies in method; and that "wherever a distinction is possible, it must be made." In following the practice of his time and place, he depended upon extensive measurements precisely rendered. He concluded, not surprisingly, that these anterior segments of the lower jaw "show clear differences well suited for racial distinctions." But his division of the two European racial groups is both cavalier and vague, especially in his undefended assumption that the long-skulled European material "represents primarily the Nordic element."[6]

His medical dissertation, published in 1938 and entitled "Genealogical Studies in the Cases of Cleft Lip-Jaw-Palate," prefigured his Auschwitz work on genetic abnormalities and indirectly on twins (he did not use twin studies but referred to their importance). He was sufficiently deferential to his teachers to confirm prior work by Lenz and Verschuer on the existence in this area of an "irregularly dominant hereditary process," and associated the deformity studied with a wide variety of additional deformities and anomalies in the same families. His method was essentially genealogical.[7]

His third publication was entitled "Hereditary Transmission of Fistulae Auris" (an abnormal opening in the cartilage of the ear), identified as a publication from the Frankfurt Institute for Hereditary Biology and Racial Hygiene directed by Verschuer, and published in a journal *Der Erbarzt* ["The Genetic Physician"] edited by him. This is a brief case report on hereditary transmission of this kind of fistula, again by means of the Lenz-Verschuer principle of "irregular, dominant hereditary process." Mengele also makes a point of the simultaneous occurrence of these fistulae with dimples of the chin (he himself was said to have had such a dimple).[8]

All three studies are consistent with hereditary emphases supported by the Nazis but by no means intellectually initiated by them. The studies are full of charts, diagrams, and photographs that claim more than they prove, but could probably nonetheless be considered relatively respectable scientific works of that time even outside of Nazi Germany. What they all suggest is Mengele's commitment to bringing science into the service of the Nazi vision.

Mengele was apparently headed for an academic career, and was looked upon favorably by Verschuer, who in a letter of recommendation praised his reliability, combined background in anthropology and medicine, and capacity for clear verbal presentation of difficult intellectual problems.[9] Mengele's choice of a professor's daughter as wife was also in keeping with his academic aspirations.

His military experience loomed large in his life: six months in 1938–39 with a specially trained mountain light-infantry regiment in the Tyrol, then considered a rather elegant form of service, including skiing and mountain climbing; and from 1940, service in the reserve medical corps, and then three years with a Waffen SS unit, mostly in the East including action in Russia with the Viking division; a wound that led to his being declared medically unfit for combat, and four decorations, including the Iron Cross First Class and Second Class. He was said to have "acquitted himself brilliantly in the face of the enemy during the Eastern Campaign," and was promoted to the rank of captain *(Hauptsturmführer)*. The only doctor in Auschwitz to possess that array of medals, he was enormously proud of them and known to refer frequently to his combat experience as a source of authority on various matters. In a semi-comical incident, one of the Iron Crosses fell from his uniform while he was riding through the camp on his bicycle, and was recovered only after a frantic search by a group of prisoners.

In talking about his friend, Dr. B. made clear that Mengele came to Auschwitz with a special aura because he arrived more or less directly from the front ("because he was wounded") and because he apparently chose Auschwitz: asked to be sent there because of the opportunities it could provide for his research. We now know that, upon Mengele's being sent to Auschwitz, Verschuer applied for and received from the German Research Society *(Deutsche Forschungsgemeinschaft)* financial support for his student's work there.*

What did Mengele actually do in Auschwitz? Some prisoners thought him unimportant there and have wondered at his later notoriety. A former SS man, for instance, who spent more than four years with the Political Department testified that among the SS doctors he knew he had never encountered Mengele and in fact had "never heard [his] name . . . during the whole time I was in Auschwitz."[11] And Dr. Jacob R. told me, as did a few other prisoner doctors, that Mengele did not seem exceptional: "At the time I just saw him as one of the many SS doctors." But more frequent was the opposite impression, expressed by Dr. Henri Q., that Mengele was a key Auschwitz participant "whose role was very important, more than that of the others"—and who was seemingly ubiquitous: "He had a reputation, it was a name that was heard the most. He was everywhere. He was seen the most often—the others were less prominent—which means he was the most active among them." That quality of being "everywhere," and everywhere active, was at the heart of Mengele's impact in Auschwitz and of his mode of being in the camp.

He also committed real crimes, murderous crimes, direct murder. The Frankfurt Court, in indicting him for extradition, spoke of "hideous crimes" committed alone or with others "willfully and with bloodlust." These crimes included selections, lethal injections, shootings, beatings, and other forms of deliberate killing. And this list was distilled conservatively from the testimony of hundreds of survivors. But by the SS's standards at Auschwitz, Mengele was an admirable, indeed outstanding, medical officer. In recommending him for promotion in August 1944, Eduard Wirths spoke of his "open, honest, firm . . . [and] absolutely dependable" character and "magnificent" intellectual and physical talents; of the "discretion, perseverance, and energy with which he has fulfilled every task . . . and . . . shown himself equal to every situation"; of his "valuable contribution to anthropological science by making use of the scientific materials available to him"; of his "absolute ideological firmness" and "faultless conduct [as] an SS officer"; and of such personal qualities as "free, unrestrained, persuasive, and lively" discourse that rendered him "especially dear to his comrades."[12] Allowing for excesses in any

*Mengele arrived in Auschwitz on 30 May 1943, and the grants were approved on 18 August 1943. The confirmation described the work for one grant obscurely as concerning "specific albuminous matter" *(spezifische Eiweisskörper);* the other was to study "eye color." Verschuer later wrote that the work had "the authorization of the *Reichsführer* SS (Himmler) and consisted of "anthropological examinations"; further, "blood tests are sent to my laboratory."[10]

recommendation for promotion, this remains, to say the least, a rousing endorsement. It could even be seen as a contribution to the Mengele legend from the side of the SS.

We can look more closely at Mengele's Auschwitz existence by examining his involvement in selections, in "scientific research,"* and in his varied relationships (with his SS colleagues and with prisoner doctors), and also his overall psychological characteristics and continuing significance for others.

Mengele on the Ramp

For many inmates, Mengele embodied the selections process. As one prisoner doctor put it, "I . . . think that Mengele developed an *idée fixe*: selections, selections, and more selections." He tended to be identified as (in Dr. Peter D.'s words) "the chief of those who did the selections." Or as another prisoner doctor said, "Everything in Auschwitz was under . . . Mengele. . . . Mengele was the one who was present at all the transports. Usually he alone, himself, stood on the ramp and he made the selections. When he couldn't do it, he sent another clever . . . SS doctor [to do it]."

The strength of that impression is conveyed by a witness in the Frankfurt Auschwitz Trial who had worked in the "Canada Kommando" unloading prisoner transports, and who remembered only the name of Mengele. When the judge commented, "Mengele cannot have been there all the time," the witness answered, "In my opinion, always. Night and day."[13] Dr. Olga Lengyel, speaking less specifically, caught the overall feeling of inmates in her description of Mengele as "far and away the chief provider for the gas chamber and the crematory ovens."[14]

Actually, the evidence we have is that Mengele took his duty turn on the ramp like everyone else. But the impression that he did all, or almost all, selections was fed by at least two factors: he frequently went to the ramp when not selecting in order to see that twins were being collected and saved for him; and he brought such verve and energy to the selections task that his image became most associated with it.

Former inmates described him as an elegant figure on the ramp—handsome, well groomed, extremely upright in posture. They sometimes misperceived him as "very Aryan-looking" or "tall and blond," when he was actually of medium height and had dark hair and complexion. His attractiveness hid Auschwitz truths: he "conveyed the impression of a gentle and cultured man who had nothing whatever to do with selections, phenol and Cyclon B."[15] A survivor described him to me as "the false front for the crematorium."

He had an easy rhythm in his conduct of large-scale selections: "a

---

*In subsequent discussions, I refrain from using quotation marks with "research," but it should be understood that I view Mengele's work as always lacking full scientific responsibility (see especially pages 365–69).

nice-looking man with a stick [riding crop] in his hand . . . [who] looked at the bodies and the faces [for] just a couple of seconds [and said], . . . *'Links* ["left"], . . . *Rechts* ["right"], *Links, Rechts.'* " And another observant inmate contrasted Dr. Franz Lucas's deliberate manner on the ramp with Mengele's "graceful and quick movement" (see pages 194–95).

Some described a quality of playfulness in his detachment, his "walking back and forth . . . [with a] cheerful expression on his face, . . . almost like he had fun, . . . routine fun. . . . He was very playful." But observant survivors could see that he was playing a role; noted the prominence with which he displayed at least one Iron Cross, and the intensity with which he seemed to wish to contrast his own elegance with the prisoners' barely human state; and spoke of him as "like a Hollywood actor," "like Clark Gable," or "a Rudolph Valentino type."

At the same time, prisoners were struck by the contrast between what he looked like and what he was. One survivor, describing him as "good-looking, . . . very cultivated," declared that "he really didn't look like a murderer," but immediately added, "He hit my father with his stick on his neck and sent him in a certain direction [to the gas chambers]." Or, "He was brutal but in a gentlemanly, depraved way." For Mengele's studied detachment could be interrupted by outbreaks of rage and violence, especially when encountering resistance to his sense of the Auschwitz rules. For instance, an arriving teenager, directed by Mengele to the right while her mother and younger sisters were sent to the left, "begged and wept" because she did not want to be separated from them: "[Mengele then] grabbed me by the hair, dragged me on the ground, and beat me. When my mother also tried to beg him, he beat her with his cane [riding crop]."

In another, similar case in which a mother did not want to be separated from her thirteen- or fourteen-year-old daughter, and bit and scratched the face of the SS man who tried to force her to her assigned line, Mengele drew his gun and shot both the woman and the child. As a blanket punishment, he then sent to the gas all people from that transport who had previously been selected for work, with the comment: "Away with this shit!"[16]

He could also express cruelty and violence in response to signs of orthodox Judaism. A woman described how he ridiculed her mother's wig (the *Scheitel* worn by orthodox Jews) and "picked it [off her head] with his stick." And there were endless stories of his smooth deceptions: a promise to a woman, who asked to do her father's work for him, that "father would be very well and the air would make him healthy": "In that same night my parents were gassed." And deadly sarcasm to a man asking for "light work": Mengele answered, "You'll get light work," and sent him to the gas chamber.[17]

He could occasionally break his own rules, on what appeared to be a whim: saving, for instance, a mother and eleven-year-old daughter because he was struck by their beauty, and reportedly commenting, "That certainly is a painting."[18] Allowing for retrospective exaggeration and fantasy, there is the reliable consistent impression of a man on the ramp at home with his task, with both fierce adherence to the rules and almost casual solipsism.

On the Hospital Block

On the hospital blocks he could also be flamboyantly casual and comfortable in his selections activity. Dr. Lengyel called him a selections "specialist" who "could show up suddenly at any hour, day or night, . . . when we least expected him."[19] According to one prisoner doctor, "he had no problems—not with his conscience, not with anybody, not with anything." For, as Dr. Magda V. said, "he was absolutely convinced he was doing the right thing." Prisoners would "march before him with their arms in the air," Dr. Lengyel tells us, "while he continued to whistle his Wagner"—or it might be Verdi or Johann Strauss. It was a mannered detachment: "like an automaton, a gentleman carrying out indifferent functions,"[20] and (according to Dr. Marie L.) "very cold . . . in German, *sachlich* [meaning 'businesslike, matter-of-fact']."

According to Dr. L., he would change signals (thumb up instead of thumb down) to indicate those being sent to the gas chamber. And he always bordered on sadism: "He had a special kind of smile, . . . even joking, that bastard!" More overtly, there are many stories of his striking people with his long riding crop, in one case running it over tattoos on the bosoms of Russian women, as a Polish woman survivor described, "then striking them there," while "not at all excited but . . . casual, . . . just playing around a little as though it were a little funny."

Most of all, his ward selections were done with relentless conscientiousness and "responsibility." It mattered to Mengele that, among people he thought should be selected, every last one be tracked down—"like a bloodhound" was the way another survivor put it.

One might expect that someone so intent upon absolute personal control would disdain the involvement of prisoner doctors in selections, but that was not the case. Mengele encouraged or demanded their participation, and by so encompassing them broadened rather than diminished his own control. Dr. Marek P. stated that "Mengele would not listen to the Polish doctors at all"; and Dr. Magda V., who became skilled at handling SS doctors, said of Mengele, "I don't think that for a moment I could manipulate him, ever, ever."

Among inmates on the medical blocks, Mengele inspired both intense up-close observations and the most elaborate fantasy, or combinations of both. People focused on his eyes: he was "a very bad person, . . . and you saw it . . . in his eyes, . . . brown and bloodshot," according to one survivor; or he violated the principle a woman survivor described having learned from her mother, that "whoever has nice eyes has a nice soul";

or his eyes had a "cruel expression" or were "the eyes of a fish," or "dead eyes," "wild eyes," or eyes that never looked at one's own.

Some survivors spoke of his odor. One described him as "young, . . . elegant, . . . smart, . . . smelling of eau de cologne," and as "very sensitive about bad smells": "Before his arrival the doors and windows had to be opened." And more generally, Marianne F., who worked on the medical block, spoke of his "white coat over his uniform—shining new white" and characterized him as "Clean, clean, clean!"

Mengele's passion for cleanliness and perfection carried over into a selections aesthetic: he would send people with skin blemishes to the gas chamber or those with small abcesses or even old appendectomy scars. "My two cousins were sent in front of my eyes by Mengele to their deaths because they had small wounds on their bodies," was the way one survivor put it. Limited evidence of scabies, or rashes or scars from scarlet fever, or even rubella (German measles) on the skin of children could have the same effect.

Specific prisoner responses to Mengele's selections were dominated by a special quality of fear and helplessness. Dr. Gisella Perl wrote, "We feared these visits more than anything else, because . . . we never knew whether we would be permitted to continue to live. . . . He was free to do whatever he pleased with us."[21] It was significant that many survivors who had witnessed the annihilation of the Gypsy camp considered that decision to have been Mengele's—an understandable assumption, both because the policy seemed consistent with the man and because Mengele was relentless in tracking down Gypsies, especially children, who tried to escape their fate. Though the assumption was factually wrong, its psychic truth lay in Mengele's inexorable commitment to the Nazi principle of murder-selection.

Dr. Lengyel speaks of prisoners' rage: "How we hated this charlatan! . . . How we despised his detached, haughty air, his continual whistling, his absurd orders, his frigid cruelty!" She described the temptation on one occasion, when seeing lying on a table his briefcase whose contours clearly revealed the revolver inside, to "seize the gun and slaughter the assassin."[22] While full awareness of that rage might not come for many inmates until their liberation from Auschwitz, it was certainly building while they were there.

Mengele could also be perceived, almost in the manner of Hochhuth's portrayal of him, as a nonhuman evil force. Dr. Wanda J., in commenting that she never spoke to him because he never addressed her or her colleagues, added, "The devil should speak to him." And another prisoner doctor spoke of Mengele as "the lord of life and death." Such figures of speech meant more in Auschwitz than in other places. The perceived ratio of Mengele's beauty and evil could become a mystical indicator. Marianne F., observing Mengele on the medical block, describes how she "played this little game": "If the sun rises red you'll live this day, because it's beautiful and you detach the image of [Mengele] from what you knew he was." Mengele's beauty, she was saying, and her capacity to detach that beauty from his actions, provided magic sustenance.

Mengele fed his legend by dramatizing murderous policies, such as his drawing a line on the wall of the children's block between 150 and 156 centimeters (about 5 feet or 5 feet 2 inches) from the floor, and sending those whose heads could not reach the line to the gas chamber. One survivor theorized that this preoccupation with height had to do with Mengele's own relatively short stature.

One prisoner doctor thought him "deranged" after having witnessed Mengele's rage upon hearing that an arriving group consisted of *psychiatric* patients and nurses. Rage at Jews' surviving the Nazi "euthanasia" policy of killing mental patients could have been enough to explain this action, but one suspects a more general attitude toward all things psychiatric.

Inmates who were not subject to his deadly whims could gain perspective on the man. One prisoner doctor said that Mengele "existed in a paradise of illusions"; and another prisoner, observing Mengele in the SS doctors' general office where "I didn't have to be afraid of him," went on to say, "I didn't notice any special elegance in him."

But noting his energy and vitality, inmates saw him as a man who thrived in Auschwitz. One wrote that "Dr. Mengele had the air of a man who took great satisfaction in his work and was pleased with his calling."[23] This observation is consistent with that of Ernst B., the SS doctor, who said that he never talked with his friend about inner conflicts because "Mengele had no problems."

We can put the matter another way and say that Mengele's harmony with Auschwitz rendered him unique unto himself, *sui generis,* as a former prisoner tells us: "You see a handsome, tall man coming. Do you know if he is a doctor or not a doctor? You know it is Mengele, nothing else."

A man who assumed Mengele's level of omnipotence was inevitably seen at times as a savior. Contributing to this image were his whimsical decisions to let people live, as well as his insistence that those judged young and strong enough to work stay in the correct line even when they resisted doing so. A typical account was that of a woman of twenty-five who was directed to the right but, when Mengele turned away, "got back to my mother's side" (on the left), was observed by Mengele and sent to her original line, only to once more "run to my mother's side," and once more be sent back by Mengele. Only he, and not the person in question, could decide upon death; and to be granted life in the face of one's own insistence (however inadvertent) upon remaining with the doomed could be perceived as a godlike form of rescue.

Or on a medical block, precisely because Mengele was so cold and unyielding, the few occasions when he responded to a plea were rendered almost mythic. One survivor, for instance, believed that in the case of people who were "young and beautiful, maybe a spark . . . *of* human being was evoked in him," and told of two girls for whom she successfully intervened with him. Mengele undoubtedly derived psychological satisfaction from such incidents—all the more because he did not necessarily have to alter his basic policies: the two girls in question were sent to the gas chamber a short time later.

Another woman, in her teens when she arrived, told of a sequence of one of Mengele's acts of rescue: her responding to her mother's plea to join her in the line of the living; becoming sick on the hospital block, where "Dr. Mengele visited me daily" and "gave the order to treat me well"; and finding out additionally from the prisoner doctor that "Dr. Mengele was very interested in me and I should definitely return to my block the next day [and that] there he wouldn't look for me [for selection]."[24] Undoubtedly with the help of distortions and imagined attitudes, this woman saw Mengele as a combination of omnipotent rescuer and concerned physician. (On occasion he even examined and treated prisoner patients, rare for SS doctors.)

Or one could be rescued by the God figure's own cough: a woman remembered that Mengele's slight cough had come just at the moment he was to evaluate her, permitting her to move quickly ahead to what she had perceived to be the line of the living.[25]

Direct Killing

Mengele could also kill directly. He was observed to perform phenol injections, always with a correct medical demeanor. He seemed to Dr. Marek P. to be always intent upon improving the killing system and upset at others' inefficiency: "He was infuriated by seeing the whole long line of people waiting [and] would take the syringe and show them [SDG personnel or prisoners performing the phenol injections] how to do it faster." Mengele himself administered the injections "without speaking," and "as though he were performing regular surgery . . . without showing any emotion at all."

Mengele also shot a number of prisoners and was reported to have killed at least one by pressing his foot on a woman's body. And there were additional reports of his having thrown newborn babies directly into the crematoria or open fires.[26]

In selecting for death or in killing people himself, the essence of Mengele was flamboyant detachment—one might say disinterestedness—and efficiency.

Research on Twins

Though usually cool and detached in his killing, Mengele was passionate in conducting his research, particularly his study of twins.

Indeed, he probably came to Auschwitz for that purpose. He had apparently worked with twins under Verschuer at the University of Frankfurt a few years earlier: Mengele's teacher was the man who in late 1935 had insisted, "What is absolutely needed is research on series of families and twins selected at random . . . with and . . . without hereditary defects." One could then achieve "complete and reliable determination of heredity in man" and "the extent of the damage caused by adverse hereditary influences," as well as "relations between disease, racial types, and miscegenation."[27] No wonder that Verschuer supported Mengele's research so enthusiastically, or that Mengele regularly sent specimens to his teacher and visited, while stationed at Auschwitz, the latter's research institute in Berlin.

In Auschwitz, Mengele found a way to live out this intellectual dream derived from his mentor. While he could not always have the family data going back over several generations that Verschuer wished for, he could arrange to his heart's content what his teacher called "a fixed minimum of examinations . . . in all cases."[28] Indeed, Mengele could exploit the unique opportunity Auschwitz provided for quick and absolute availability of large numbers of these precious research subjects, especially identical twins.

Mengele did not merely issue orders that twins be rounded up: he was a central, even fanatical, figure in the rounding-up process. Teresa W., who was sometimes in a position to observe ramp selections from close up, told how Mengele, looking "strange," would plunge into the "river" of arriving Hungarian Jews, "going quickly, . . . the same speed [as] the crowd and [shouting] only, *'Zwillinge heraus!'* . . . with such a face that I would think he's mad."

Once he had selected the twins, Mengele made them part of an elaborate research structure, Auschwitz style. Besides the general SS doctors' unit (used by all SS doctors), he had three additional offices, mainly for his work with twins: one in the men's camp, one in the women's camp, and one in the Gypsy camp. In all these places, twins had special status. They were given a special number sequence, and in many cases "ZW" (for *Zwillinge,* or "twins") was made part of the tattooed number. They were frequently permitted to keep their own clothing and sometimes their hair. Twins, mostly children, had special blocks, usually within medical units and often together with other research subjects of Mengele, such as dwarfs or inmates with other abnormalities. An older child or an adult from among the twins, generally known as the *Zwillingsvater* (literally, "twins' father") would be put in charge and would become, in effect, the block chief. In each area, then, there took shape an extraordinary twin-dominated world of Mengele's "odd" research subjects.

As one of them, Simon J., describes:

> We were very close. . . . There was a little fellow, . . . two-and-a-half, . . . the darling of the . . . block. . . . We had all sizes and shapes . . . a pair of eighteen-year-old strapping, magnificent boys from Hungary, excellent football-soccer players, . . . completely identical. We

had a pair of seventy-year-old Austrian gentlemen. . . . And then there were the dwarfs. . . . A very macabre sort of ship of fools.

The prisoner anthropologist, Teresa W., who did measurements on the twins, estimated that the influx of Hungarian Jews during the spring and summer of 1944 led to the accumulation of about 250 individual twins in Birkenau, mostly children but some adolescents. As she pointed out, "It is very difficult [under ordinary conditions] to find twins in such a number." And in the men's camp, Simon J. described "a collection of about one hundred of us . . . from the ages of three to . . . seventy . . . singles and doubles, males only." Mengele's main inner sanctum, where he kept his records, was in Birkenau, where he was chief doctor. Ernst B.'s observation about the mystery surrounding this room was confirmed by several survivors. One, for instance, told me that prisoners knew of it, but "had no approach to this room," and that he kept his research records there: "How or in what manner we don't know, because we never could come near this room of his."

Because they helped in mailing arrangements, prisoners confirmed that Mengele regularly sent reports and specimens to Verschuer's Berlin-Dahlem Institute of Racial Biology. (On pages 357–60 I discuss Mengele's method and his scientific aspirations.)

He permitted mothers of young female twins to stay on their block with them, apparently out of his concern that the children remain in good physical and mental condition. But as another twin went on to say, "there always came a day when the mothers would be sent back to the regular camp," which usually meant their deaths. While fathers of twins were studied much less frequently, there was at least one notable exception: a physician who himself became both a research subject (undergoing the usual tests and measurements) and an assistant to Mengele (preparing reports on geographical distribution of Hungarian twins).[29]

Identical twins, Mengele's most treasured research objects, were often examined together, and comparatively, as two of them* described:

> It was like a laboratory. First they weighed us, then they measured and compared. . . . There isn't a piece of body that wasn't measured and compared. . . . We were always sitting together—always nude. . . . We would sit for hours together, and they would measure her, and then measure me, and then again measure me and measure her. . . . You know, the width of, say, our ears or nose or mouth or . . . the structure of our bones. . . . Everything in detail, they wanted to know.

These twins insisted that Mengele did virtually everything himself. Since they were in Birkenau, where his anthropological assistant was

---

*These two women, still profoundly identified with one another at the age of fifty-one, insisted upon being interviewed together, and their voices on the tape are not distinguishable from one another.

known to do her measurements, it is possible that they may be expressing some confusion between his *control* of the situation (which was virtually absolute) and what he actually did. But Mengele undoubtedly performed some examinations, perhaps especially with identical twins. They described him as very methodical: "He concentrated on one part of the body at one time. . . . Like [one day] he measured our eyes for about two hours." They stressed that, although they were always examined nude, Mengele was proper and "never rude," approaching them detachedly and more or less professionally. They spoke of being examined as frequently as twice a week for a period of five months in late 1944 and also remembered vividly a special visit to the Auschwitz main camp to be photographed. (Mengele seems to have varied the frequency according to the interest particular twins held for him, again undoubtedly giving much more attention to identical twins.) During these examinations a certain amount of family history was taken, involving sicknesses of all kinds; but "mostly he wanted to know if there were more sets of twins . . . in the family." And, like other twins I spoke to, these two were impressed by the amount of blood taken from them—an estimated ten cubic centimeters at every session. Given the inadequate Auschwitz diet (though theirs was better than ordinary prisoners), "We were wondering where [the blood] came from"; and toward the end they remembered it as being difficult to draw: "It wasn't coming any more . . . from our arms."

The more sinister side of Mengele's twin research emerged in his elaborate arrangements for pathological examination of corpses. For Dr. Miklos Nyiszli, his main prisoner pathologist, Mengele prepared a special dissection room, including a "dissecting table of polished marble," a basin with "nickel taps" and "three porcelain sinks," and windows "with green metal screens to keep out flies and mosquitoes." The adjoining working room had a large table, "comfortable arm chairs," three microscopes and "a well-stocked library, which contained the most recent editions." The overall arrangement, as Nyiszli later wrote, was "the exact replica of any large city's institute of pathology."[30]
Nyiszli's earlier deposition (made in July 1945) reveals Mengele to be a direct murderer of his twins:

> In the work room next to the dissecting room, fourteen Gypsy twins were waiting [about midnight one night], guarded by SS men, and crying bitterly. Dr. Mengele didn't say a single word to us, and prepared a 10 cc. and 5 cc. syringe. From a box he took evipan, and from another box he took chloroform, which was in 20 cubic-centimeter glass containers, and put these on the operating table. After that, the first twin was brought in, . . . a fourteen-year-old girl. Dr. Mengele ordered me to undress the girl and put her on the dissecting table. Then he injected the evipan into her right arm intravenously. After the child had fallen asleep, he felt for the left ventricle of the heart and

injected 10 cc. of chloroform. After one little twitch the child was dead, whereupon Dr. Mengele had it taken into the morgue. In this manner, all fourteen twins were killed during the night.[31]

The dissection of corpses, then, could be the final step in Mengele's twin research. While this was by no means the fate of all twins (most had a much better chance to live *because* they were twins), it nonetheless epitomizes Mengele's combination of relatively ordinary scientific procedure with literally murderous scientific fanaticism.

But Auschwitz was unique not only in the numbers of twins it could provide, but in what it enabled one to do with the twins: each one of a pair of twins could be observed under the same diet and living conditions and could be made to "die together . . . and in good health"—ideal for post-mortem comparisons.[32]

Sometimes Mengele killed twins simply to resolve a dispute over diagnosis. Dr. Abraham C., a radiologist who did work for Mengele, described to me one such situation: a pair of Gypsy twins, "two splendid boys of seven or eight, whom we were studying from all aspects—from the sixteen or eighteen different specialties we represented." The boys had certain joint symptoms which, according to a belief at that time, could be linked to tuberculosis. Mengele was convinced that the boys were tubercular, but the various prisoner doctors, after careful clinical study, found no trace of that disease. Still unconvinced, Mengele shouted at the prisoner doctors, especially at Dr. C., telling him, "All the others could make a mistake, not the radiologist. . . . It must be there." Mengele then left, ordering C. to remain there, and returned about an hour later, now speaking calmly: "You are right. There was nothing." After some silence, Mengele added, "Yes, I dissected them." Later C. heard from Nyiszli that Mengele had shot the two boys in the neck and that "while they were still warm, began to examine them: lungs first, and then each organ . . . [doing] some of the work himself." The two boys had been favorites with all the doctors, including Mengele: "[They] were treated very well, spoiled in all respects. . . . These two especially, . . . they fascinated him considerably."

Other research was done on twins, some of it difficult to evaluate from their reports. For instance, a survivor twin told me how shocked he and others were to discover a fully equipped laboratory right next to their block, as well as "dark rooms . . . [with] all kinds of lights, . . . different lights . . . [which] literally blinded us." He spoke of Mengele's supervising "a lot of research with chemicals," sometimes applied to the skin to see what color or reaction they would cause. He stated that Mengele's assistants "started with . . . the cervical area, then drew blood from behind the ear," and of how they "might stick a needle" in various places from behind, including the performing of spinal taps—all this done to young children and sometimes resulting in deafness, collapse, and, among the smaller ones, death. He and his twin sister, twelve years old, would be placed together, separated by a burlap sheet, and both then subjected to these various examinations and tests, including injection of material into the spine and the clamping of some part of the body "to see how long you could stand the pressure."

This particular description could well include procedures one was subjected to, those thought to have been applied to other prisoners, and those unclearly seen or feared. Given the nature of the Auschwitz environment, however, virtually any detail described could have considerable truth; and even those less than fully accurately rendered, considerable psychic truth.*

Within the Auschwitz twins' subculture, there was an odd atmosphere that combined sanctuary with terror. As Simon J. put it, twins got the message "If we do what is wanted from us, . . . we would come to no harm, because we are the subject of an investigation headed by Dr. Mengele." That is, "We were not allowed to be beaten" because the word was out "not to ruin us physically." J. could even say that twins felt themselves "completely elevated, segregated from the hurlyburly of the camp." Even a twin who was caught in such an ordinarily "ultimate sin" as stealing food would, instead of being severely beaten or sent to the gas chambers, be merely rebuked or punished mildly. The twins became aware that, unlike most other prisoners, their lives had existential value: "A single thing kept us [alive]: . . . his experiments," is the way Tomas A. put it. Their existential value was immediately apparent in the matter of hair: they could retain theirs for the research reason that hair characteristics, including color, had to be recorded.

Hence they were given desirable jobs that did not expose them to the most severe kinds of physical abuse; children among them could serve as a "runner" (Laufer) or messenger, or sometimes simply as a helper. Many were permitted to move relatively freely about the camp, and therefore had valuable opportunities for "organizing" (buying and selling, mostly food), to be privy to useful information, and to create what one of them called a "thriving economy" on the twin block.

They were rewarded for their cooperation, as A. tells us: "[After being] measured and measured, . . . we had white bread and . . . milk with Lukchen [a macaroni-like mixture, considered a great delicacy in the camp]," for the ostensible purpose of compensating for the blood that had to be taken from them. In the Auschwitz context, that was "marvelous," and was combined with other advantages: "the best clothes . . . through Mengele"; and as a survivor twin explained, "We had our hair . . . [so] they [other prisoners] said, 'At least, you look . . . human.' "

It was equally clear, however, that this sanctuary was more than a matter of Mengele's whim: "We should count [ourselves] as very lucky

*But most descriptions by survivors could be in general terms confirmed, and unless otherwise indicated, I consider them to be essentially accurate.

that he's interested in us [as Simon J. put it]. Mengele is God—we found it out very fast."

Both protector and potential destroyer, he had "terrifying power around him [as] the person who, with his left eyelash, could rub us all out," in J.'s words. As he went on to explain: "He [Mengele] always carried around him an aura of . . . some terrifying threat, which is, I suspect, unexplainable to . . . normal . . . human beings who didn't see this. I [have] found . . . [it] literally impossible to transmit the edge of this terror."

Mostly Mengele kept twins alive for his research. Teresa W. claimed never to have been aware of his killing any of those she had measured; and while she might have resisted learning the full truth, it would have been "impossible [for her] not to know." Similarly, the "twins' father" (or prisoner leader) of the male group also stated, "As far as I know, none of the twins was gassed or burned." He pointed out that, in January 1945, the older male twins were evacuated but the smaller children stayed with him and were with him when the Russians entered the camp.[33] But another inmate, who assisted Teresa W. in her anthropological measurements and made wider observations, claimed that "about 15 percent" of the twins were killed, some as a consequence of experiments performed on them, including surgical operations.

Generally speaking, then, Mengele kept intact his two main "data bases" in Auschwitz and Birkenau; killed individual twins (especially when the other had died) or pairs of twins living outside of the twins' blocks (notably Gypsy twins at the time of annihilation of that camp) for post-mortem examinations;* and subjected twins on the children's block and elsewhere to fatal operations.

The irony remains that, among children, one almost had to be a twin to stay alive. As a survivor stated, "Virtually no one from my school survived, and no one from there of my age except another twin." The proof of that survival could be seen in the documentary Russian film made at the time of the liberation of Auschwitz.[34] In a moving scene, a hundred or more children emerge from inside the camp, most of them twins, including some older ones who had originally been ordered to evacuate but, in the confusion, had been able to hide themselves safely. Simon J. told me proudly, "I'm in that group—I remember that very well."

Mengele's relationship to his main professional assistant tells us much about his sense of the project. When Teresa W. was severely ill with typhus, she told Mengele about her anthropological background and

---

*Certain twins, not on any of the regular twins' blocks, were subjected to extensive examinations by Mengele's team of prisoner doctors. One prisoner doctor, in discussing Mengele's killing of an individual twin for the purpose of the post-mortem findings, told me that he and his prisoner colleagues "knew all these cases because they passed through our hands." They would receive the post-mortem report—"enormously detailed—all of the organs described in all particulars"; and "every twin in this group had his own file, and the post-mortem examination was the twin's last document in the file." The twin had to be killed, at least in certain cases, in order to complete his or her research file.

mentioned having been the assistant of a world-famous Polish anthropologist. Mengele arranged for her to have the best treatment available, and with her beginning recovery sent for her even though she was
"so weak that [she could] not really walk," because he was "in such a
hurry" to put her to work for him.

As did the twins, W. felt that the work offered her a sanctuary from
more dangerous alternatives, and that in Auschwitz "Mengele was a
god." She said that Mengele never had a "private conversation" with her
or even talked about her professor, was polite but distant, and would only
discuss the work. He would sometimes gently question her descriptions
of bodily characteristics, all the while taking pains to provide her with the
most comfortable arrangements available to prisoners. An attractive
young woman with an elegant cultural background, she inspired rumors
in Auschwitz that she and Mengele were having an affair. They almost
certainly were not, but the rumors were probably fed by Mengele's pattern of both appreciation and generous reward of those who could contribute to his passionate involvement in twin research.

Partly because of her overestimation of the quality and legitimacy of
the research, Teresa W. made a jarring discovery one day in Auschwitz.
Asked by Mengele to carry a box to another part of the camp, she felt an
impulse to open it and see what was inside, only to discover "that it
contained glass jars, in which were human eyes." She was "deeply
shaken": "At that moment I realized that Mengele was obviously able to
kill people, in order to obtain some sort of research results."

Yet so much did she believe in the research that she made copies of all
the forms she filled out in order to preserve her own record of the work;
she buried these forms in jars under the block "until such a moment
[when] I can dig them up"—but she never recovered them. She contrasted what Mengele would do with the material with the more objective,
statistical approach of her professor. Mengele, she thought, would have
kept alive his "stud" (groups of twins and their offsprings) in order to
study the inheritance of a variety of characteristics from intelligence to
capacity for certain kinds of knowledge to susceptibility to illnesses—all
of which she thought could give Mengele "a quite interesting result."

During her talks with me (spread out over a couple of years) she
became more critical of Mengele as "fanatical" and "murderous," but
remained confused by him partly because of her continuing respect for
the work. She was one of the few prisoners I know of who remained loath
to make definitive judgments about him and was reluctant to testify about
him in legal proceedings. Her attitude was surely influenced by his having
saved her life but also by his professional approach to her and his having
convinced her of the validity of the work with twins.

Mengele's own attitude toward the twins research was fiercely enthusiastic. Dr. Lottie M. stressed how passionately involved Mengele was with
"his genetic idea," and a Polish woman survivor told how he "rushed

through [his duties on the medical block] in order to have more time for his twins." That passion made him "totally blind to" the general misery of the camp. When he found identical twins in any transport, this woman went on to say, "Mengele beamed—he was happy, . . . in a kind of a trance." When deprived of possible twins—as on one occasion when he was not notified about the arrival of a transport—he was observed to become enraged and threatening.

As he also did when children, out of fear or fatigue, interrupted the examinations, or, as another survivor put it, "if something didn't go right in experiments" or even if a temperature reading was not recorded on a twin's chart. Once when a child screamed that he felt like passing out, Mengele "became enraged . . . [and] knocked the whole table down." His attitude, according to this observer, seemed to be that if he could not complete the work immediately, he "might not be able to achieve it." He also became "furious," according to another survivor when a girl twin died at the wrong time—as in the case of one who succumbed to diphtheria while he was following her syphilis. He was attentive to and provided special care and medications for the surviving twin, who also developed diphtheria and whom he was said to like very much—until she recovered, at which time he had her killed so that her syphilis could be confirmed at post-mortem examination.

This duality—a confusing combination of affection and violence—was constantly described to me. The Polish woman survivor, for instance, described him as "impulsive . . . [with] a choleric temper," but "in his attitude to children [twins] . . . as gentle as a father . . . [who] talked to them . . . [and] patted them on the head in a loving way." He could be playful with them as well and "jumped around" to please them. Twin children frequently called him "Uncle Pepi"; and other twins told how Mengele would bring them sweets and invite them for a ride in his car, which turned out to be "a little drive with Uncle Pepi, to the gas chamber." Simon J. put it most succinctly: "He could be friendly but kill." And two other twins described him as "like a dual personality, like Dr. Jekyll and Mr. Hyde, I think."

Twins felt Mengele's appeal. One believed that Mengele liked him: "[He] immediately referred to me as his friend" and said that he was "very fascinated with something in the Jew" and was generally pleasant and "very human." This man believed that Mengele protected the twins from Heinz Thilo, an SS doctor who wanted them killed, so that the latter was the "devil of death" (an evil murderer) while Mengele was the "angel of death" (who still had a little bit of feeling). But this survivor admitted that Mengele, in the laboratory, "became a different person entirely, . . . a fanatic, . . . [and] if he didn't see blood on his white uniform, he wasn't content." Tomas A. remained still more troublingly bound to Mengele: "For twins Mengele was everything, . . . just marvelous, . . . a good doctor, . . . our backing [support]. If [it hadn't been for] him, we wouldn't be alive." For a long time after liberation, A. found it impossible to believe the evil things he heard about Mengele, and he still struggles with the contradiction. He can now sum up the situation: "For us, for the twins, [he was] like a papa, like a mama. For us. On the other hand, he was a murderer."

While several of the twins came to the conclusion that Mengele had been nice to them only to maximize their participation in his research, others had difficulty ridding themselves of the sense that his affection for them had been genuine.

Apart from his research, the relationship Mengele sought with the twins, and with all of the environment, was one of *absolute control.* That form of omnipotent quest again combined Auschwitz realities with Mengele's individual-psychological inclinations. Simon J. captured the tendency when he said that "Mengele was judgment day," and had the further association of an image of an inmate, among a group walking slowing toward the crematorium, shouting out a verse chanted on Kol Nidre night (the beginning of Yom Kippur, the Day of Atonement). Mengele sought control not only over life and death but over all behavior and all criteria of value, scientific and moral.

Hence J. could add, "As far as we knew, there was Mengele—then one half a light-year, . . . and then the rest of them [other doctors and SS officers and personnel]." That same aura of omnipotence led to impressions on the part of various twins that Mengele was "the main show," an "on-the-floor presence," and "always in charge."

Unlike others in Auschwitz, Mengele continued his research with twins until the very end. A few months before his hurried departure, he insisted upon inviting Dr. Lottie M. into his inner sanctum to look at "the results of [his] anthropology research work." She could make little of them from superficial glances at charts and statistics, but remembered him saying with some feeling, "Isn't it a pity that . . . this falls into the hands of the Bolsheviks. Isn't it a pity?" While he apparently took most of the records with him, Dr. M.'s impression was that he recognized the imminence of the German defeat and was mainly preoccupied with what would happen to that material.*

One survivor contended that Mengele had to "get a lot done quickly" because of his conflict with Thilo and others who wanted the project shut down. A survivor, who claimed to have intelligence connections and special knowledge, went further in describing Mengele's research as having been in bad repute with Nazi officials, so that his entire Auschwitz standing was in jeopardy "if he did not submit results." While those claims find little support elsewhere, Mengele's "race against time" could have been generated from within himself as part of a need to see himself —and be recognized—as a great biological and racial scientist. Certainly his research with twins was central to that aspiration.

---

*It is possible that a significant amount of this material did fall into Soviet hands, as they are believed to retain—or at least to have retained originally—large numbers of Auschwitz documents that they have not made available to others or even publicly acknowledged.

Method and Goals: "There Would Never Be Another Chance Like It"

Mengele's method was a product of his scientific training and earlier experience, his Nazi ideology, and the peculiarities of the Auschwitz setting.

His anthropological prisoner assistant, Teresa W., considered Mengele's method more or less standard for the time, the norm for anthropological work. She recognized it as the same approach she had been trained in at her Polish university under a distinguished anthropologist with German pre-Nazi academic connections. That professor stressed "the biological foundation of [the] social environment" and the delineation of "racial types" (although her professor strongly rejected Nazi theories of racial superiority), making use of statistical methods he had introduced.

Mengele's approach differed only in being "terribly detailed," more so than she thought necessary. It included measurements of skull and body, and various characteristics of nose, lips, ears, hair, and eyes. His anthropological assistant was given quality Swiss instruments, a white coat "like the physicians," a secretary to write down observations, and a prisoner anthropology student to help her. Teresa W. told me that Mengele never discussed his research aims with her, but she considered the work scientifically legitimate and had testified earlier that "in the area of recognized anthropology, [work with twins] constitutes a very important part of research, in which especially the aspect of heredity plays a great role." And as W. said to me, "If he would like to have a false statement, than [why] all this trouble to do such . . . detailed research?" She did, however, recognize that Mengele might "twist [his findings] a little bit to his aims" if it would demonstrate German racial superiority; and also that "maybe if something was not . . . according to . . . Nazi wishes, . . . he [might] not publicize it." She was also aware of what she owed to the research: "In a way, his anthropology really saved my life in Auschwitz."*

The relative number of identical twins (those developed from a single ovum) as opposed to non-identical twins (from different ova) among Mengele's research subjects is unclear. Also unclear is the extent to which he maintained this crucial distinction, since non-identical twins are genetically similar only to the extent that ordinary siblings are. The fact that a few ordinary siblings are known to have successfully masqueraded as twins gives us reason to doubt the reliability of Mengele's research findings.

Mengele remained in close contact with Professor Verschuer throughout his stay in Auschwitz and regularly sent him research results and specimens at the Kaiser Wilhelm Institute of Anthropology and Human Heredity and Eugenics in Berlin-Dahlem that Verschuer then headed.

---

*Mengele also used twins as subjects for more general anthropological interests. In the Gypsy camp, according to Dr. Alexander O., Mengele "kept . . . samples of hair [and] eyes [from twins], equipment to take fingerprints, handprints, and footprints," and "compared the various Gypsy ethnic groups."

There is also recent evidence that, during his Auschwitz time, Mengele periodically visited his professor and was received by the latter's family. Verschuer destroyed all of their correspondence shortly after the war and, despite this incriminating act, claimed ignorance about Auschwitz and about any potentially criminal ways in which Mengele might have gathered the material.[35]*

Dr. Lottie M. could thus say of his interest in twins: "That was his question . . . genetics . . . genetics and environment. I think he did as he could have if he worked as assistant of Professor Verschuer." And Teresa W. also emphasized his opportunity to study hereditary principles which, whatever her and others' criticism of the work, rendered it "undoubtedly of the highest value for anthropology."

Ernst B., his Auschwitz friend, described the work as "pure scientific research," making use of twins to study questions of identical inherited dispositions (selbe Erbanlagen) Mengele had begun to investigate under his professor at the university. The research could take advantage of "the extreme conditions of the camp": one could, for instance, give protein to one twin to observe its effect in preventing disease in comparison to the other twin to whom it was not given; and one could pursue investigations with a "potentially fatal outcome." Dr. B. knew that Mengele was "in constant touch with his old institute," but thought he told people there little about Auschwitz conditions because "he was ashamed to talk about this with his former colleagues." Mengele nonetheless expressed to Ernst B. pride in his colleagues' encouragement and "used that as justification" for pursuing scientific work.

Dr. B. said something else of great importance, not generally appreciated: Mengele had begun work on his Habilitation, the academic presentation necessary for a formal appointment as university lecturer and ultimately professor; and the clear implication was that his Auschwitz research with twins was to constitute a major portion of that "Habilitation work." Mengele's academic ambition, that is, was bound up with his passion for Auschwitz research—as was his feeling, again quoted by Dr. B., that "it would be a sin, a crime, . . . irresponsible [toward science], not to utilize the possibilities that Auschwitz had for twin research. There would never be another chance like it."

All that seems clear enough, but the prevailing opinion in Auschwitz about Mengele's research was quite different. Most inmates believed, as Dr. Abraham C. put it, that Mengele "wanted to find the cause of multiple pregnancies in order to be able to repopulate Germany, which had been subjected to considerable losses." Dr. C. even claimed that Mengele "spoke of it very freely." And as "Mengele's radiologist" (C.'s own term), he was in a position to observe and hear a great deal. Dr. Miklos Nyiszli,

*Dr. Helmut Verschuer, the professor's son, also remembered his mother's reporting that she once asked Mengele whether what he had to do was demanding; he answered, "It is horrible, I can't talk about it."[36] That memory is difficult to evaluate and should not in my view be taken as clear evidence of Mengele's having been uncomfortable in Auschwitz.

who worked still more closely with Mengele, said similarly, "To advance one step in the search to unlock the secret of multiplying the race of superior beings destined to rule was [for Mengele] a 'noble goal.' "[37]

Teresa W. was aware of that view, and expressed skepticism about it because she "did not hear anything from Mengele" that suggested this goal. But I had the impression that she was no longer quite certain about Mengele's goals. There was still another rumor, that Mengele "wanted to pair up female twins with male twins, and . . . they should have sexual relations . . . to see if twins would be born of twins." A related rumor was that twins' sperm would be used to impregnate "German ladies," so that they could have twins in turn; or that twins' blood would be injected into the veins of German women, ostensibly for the same purpose.

Over all, most prisoner doctors were more skeptical than Teresa W. about the quality of Mengele's work with twins. Dr. Jan W. thought him very "superficial" as a researcher and, after looking at fragments of notes from the research kept in the Auschwitz Museum, said that "no scientist would take [them] seriously." (The notes consist only of a few columns of figures, and it would be difficult to draw from them conclusions of any kind.) One prisoner doctor put the matter simply and absolutely: "He wanted to be God—to create a new race."

In evaluating these various views, there is no doubt about the truth of the first position: namely, that Mengele was continuing work with twins initiated by others and possibly himself in the Frankfurt and Berlin institutes, stressing genetic determinism. Earlier in my work I thought that this perspective, along with Mengele's scientific and academic ambition, accounted for his twin research, and that the vision of learning the secret of multiple births was the fantasy of others. Now I am not so sure. The evidence seems to me consistent with at least the possibility that Mengele had the ambition of extending his genetic determinism toward some form of racial application: the use of knowledge of genetic factors that influence the formation of twins to stimulate that formation in particular situations.

He also might have wished to use what he learned from twins for the genetic cultivation of superior individuals, not necessarily twins themselves. While these purposes fall far short of the grand vision of "repopulating Germany," they would be consistent with German national goals at the time and certainly with Nazi ideology. They would also be consistent with something else his friend Dr. B. told me: that Mengele's work had bearing on selecting national leaders "not [on a] political basis but [on a] biological basis." In other words, Mengele might have wished to use genetic insights derived from twin research both for "breeding" desirable leaders (Teresa W. saw him as "like a stud owner") and for selecting them from among existing contenders.

But we cannot be certain about Mengele's precise motivations. W., who worked so closely with him, said to me at one point: "To hear his confession—his answers to different questions people might put to him—would be interesting." It would have, indeed, though even he might not have been entirely clear about his exact motivations. But I believe they would include his characteristic combination of exaggerated scientific claim and related ideological fantasy.

Dwarfs, Noma, Eye Color, and Other Areas of Research

Though nothing compared with his interest in twins, Mengele could also be passionate about his work with dwarfs, and was once described as "beside himself with joy" upon discovering an entire family of five dwarfs. Such a family of course was a panacea for his genetic focus, while at the same time satisfying his interest in the abnormal: his wish, as his anthropological assistant put it, "to have as much a characteristic [of abnormality] as you can give him."

Nyiszli told of doing his first post-mortem examinations on people selected from transports because of some abnormal physical development. He and others took measurements of them; then an SS noncommissioned officer shot them; afterward, Nyiszli did the dissections, prepared a protocol, and then treated the corpses with calcium chloride and "put the clean bones together in packages, which were then sent to the . . . institute in Berlin-Dahlem."[38] Also, Dr. Lottie M. told of a sequence of Mengele's enthusiasm at receiving a family of dwarfs, his extremely intense study and seemingly generous treatment of them, and then their disappearance: "A fortnight and . . . the study is finished, . . . so [to] the gas." (As in the case of twins, a number of dwarfs did survive, including two described by Tomas A. as talented musicians who lived among his group of twins and frequently played for the SS.)

But inmates understood the dwarfs to reflect Mengele's obsession with *Jewish* abnormality. As Dr. Magda V. put it, "I think Jews must have been freaks to him—like the dwarfs." And a friend of Teresa W. saw him as "fascinated by all sorts of freaks of nature, . . . dwarfs, hunchbacks, imbeciles of all nations, . . . hermaphrodites"—all of them Jews. Another prisoner doctor noted his interest in giants as well and, more generally, in "growth disturbances" and "growth indicators" in children and young adults. Dr. Erich G. mentioned Mengele's "preconception" and even "religious feeling" that among Jews there is a greater "heredity of bad qualities" than among other races. In that way, Mengele's interest in dwarfs connected with his general attitude toward Jews: it is not surprising that ordinary inmates feared his freak hunting. As another survivor tells us, "I was a little afraid of him. Everyone was afraid. Maybe he will ask you, 'Come here,' and he will find something on you interesting."

Mengele's third interest was noma, an area of research that he may have more actively chosen than was suggested by the prisoner doctor's description of his approach to Professor Epstein (see pages 296–97). In any case, we can be reasonably sure that Mengele was seeking to further his own scientific name, and that he would have published results under that name alone.

This gangrenous condition of the face and mouth is known to result from extreme debilitation, and prisoner doctors had no doubt that such debilitation or cachexia (a general wasting of the body) from Auschwitz diet and general conditions was the fundamental cause of the frequent occurrence in Gypsy children of this ordinarily rare disease. Mengele did not entirely dispute this assumption, as he permitted Professor Epstein to give at least one lecture on noma in which the importance of cachexia was stressed. But Mengele was clearly more interested in a genetic or racial source, so that a prisoner doctor who was given the task of bacteriological work on the condition, could ask, "But why did the German physicians not think, . . . as we thought ourselves, that this noma epidemic was to be attributed to the misery, lack of hygiene and nutrition, to which these children were submitted, rather than to another cause?"

Eva C., the artist who worked with Mengele, recalls an incident in which he took her to an extremely debilitated Gypsy boy moribund from advanced noma—"a little bundle of bones"—and asked her, "Would you believe that this kid is ten years old?" C.'s sense was that Mengele was not so much commenting on how much younger the boy appeared as implying that "this is that kind of race, . . . like he didn't realize that he did it to that kid." This pattern of blaming the victim was especially blatant in Mengele's noma work.

Mengele again killed for science. One prisoner doctor told me how Mengele one day brought in "two heads . . . wrapped in newspaper . . . children's heads . . . smelling of phenol." It was clear that Mengele had had the children killed in order to make possible their post-mortem study, and he was bringing the heads to this doctor for bacteriological examination.

Mengele's work on eye color was a particularly strange and revealing episode in his Auschwitz research career. Characteristically, it began with a scientific basis. He regularly sent eyes of Gypsies back to the Berlin Institute, where a study was being conducted of hereditary factors in eye color, with special focus on a condition known as heterochromia of the iris, in which the two eyes of a person are of different colors. A woman physician named Magnussen who worked at the institute was in charge of the eye project. Dr. Nyiszli reports the occurrence of heterochromia, with one blue and one brown eye, in six of eight Gypsy twins he was ordered on one occasion to dissect. His dissection showed that these twins had been killed by phenol injection, though he also found evidence in all of hereditary syphilis and in some of tuberculosis. Mengele said that, because of the syphilis and tuberculosis, they "would not have lived in any case"—a comment Nyiszli took as a signal to write in these diseases as the cause of death. He preserved the eyes of the six heterochromic twins and prepared them for shipment to Berlin.[39]

A bizarre story told to me by Dr. Alexander O. made clear that aspects of the project could be less than scientific. After Mengele had demonstrated heterochromia in a few members of a Gypsy family, he instructed Dr. O. that, "when things have taken their course," he was to extract the eyes and put them in containers with preservative to be sent to Berlin— Mengele adding ominously, "*All* of them, do you understand?" Dr. O. understood perfectly; and as one by one the family members died of their extreme debilitation (Mengele apparently did not think phenol injections were required), he would be notified and would excise the eyes from the corpse, prepare them for shipment, and hand them over to the block scribe. One day the scribe called him angrily and said that Mengele had a record of eight family members and, "You've given me only seven pairs of eyes. We are missing two eyes!" When Dr. O. began to protest that he had been notified only about the seven, the scribe said that the eyes of the last family member "have to be sent today! You know what that means—they have to go today!" O. understood that as a signal to plunder substitute eyes from random Gypsy corpses, and after stumbling about among a group of them, did succeed in finding the correct colors, a blue eye from one corpse and a black eye from another; he then excised and packed them in the usual manner.

Mengele had an added project: that of actually changing eye color in an Aryan direction. Dr. Abraham C. wondered why Mengele was devoting so much attention to a few seven-year-old boys who seemed unremarkable, and then realized that "those children had one odd characteristic: they were blond and had brown eyes, so Mengele was trying to find a way to color their eyes blue." Mengele actually injected methylene blue into their eyes, causing severe pain and inflammation, but "their eyes of course did not change." Dr. C. had the impression these children were gassed, but he may have been wrong: a former block elder told of thirty-six such children who apparently survived. There is a record, however, of a little girl named Dagmar, born in Auschwitz in 1944, who died after Mengele's eye injections.[40] Of the children subjected to the eye-color experiment, at least one child became almost blind; the eyes of most of the others, after considerable pain and infection, gradually returned to normal.

Concerning the study of heterochromia, Hermann Langbein reported having an opportunity after the war to meet with Professor Verschuer, who told him about the "enormously interesting specimens" of different-colored eyes Mengele had sent him, and seemed "surprised and upset" when Langbein told him they had come from Gypsies Mengele had ordered killed because of this abnormality. In Verschuer's attitude we encounter a hypocritical academic accessory to Mengele's characteristic pattern of killing for science.

But the methylene blue injections are of a different order, not in their cruelty (which was usual) but in their extraordinary scientific naïveté—or, one might more accurately say, their scientific corruption.

Mengele was thought to have done further research in a variety of areas, but unclear accounts make it difficult in some cases to distinguish what actually took place from distortions or even fantasy. Yet, in each case, he *could* have been somehow involved.

Eva C., for instance, on the whole an accurate and earthy observer, told me with uncharacteristic hesitancy and confusion of a vast research unit she was taken to, a special block in the Auschwitz main camp where people were being experimented upon, some of them wearing a diver's suit and lying in water with ice in it. Mengele walked about quickly and somewhat agitatedly, giving orders in a way that showed that "he was very definitely *the* top dog in there, too." Other inmates were convinced that Mengele performed sterilization experiments; and although he was clearly not a major Auschwitz experimenter in this area, there were enough reports to suggest he might have had some peripheral relationship to it. One survivor told me that Mengele "cut off the balls" of a very young twin, and that he (this witness), in fact, saw the testicles "lying on our table." A Greek survivor, one of whose testicles had been removed, appeared in court against Schumann but held Mengele equally responsible and told of the latter's supervising the crude method of collecting sperm from males involved in sterilization experiments. Other survivors told of injections Mengele gave or ordered given in the abdomen that left one sterile.[41] One woman told of an injurious substance being injected into her back by an assistant of Mengele, resulting in loss of her menstrual periods and inability to conceive. A survivor, whose fiancé worked on Block 10, spoke of "medical research and experiments by the notorious doctors Mengele and Clauberg" on that block."[42] Another survivor told of bone-marrow experiments, involving several operations on her thigh, with removal of material for bone-marrow transplants. An international commission confirmed that this woman had been subjected to medical experiments, and she was able to locate another survivor victimized by the same kind of procedure.

My belief is that each of these reports stems from some form of actual abuse, usually experimental, even if there was some confusion in details, including the question of which Nazi doctor was involved. Mengele's unbridled research interests, special Auschwitz energies, and extraordinary absence of moral restraint made him a candidate for real acts that sound fantastic no less than for unbridled fantasy.

Mengele set up an Auschwitz caricature of an academic research institute. Doctors, mostly Jewish, with varied clinical and laboratory backgrounds, were called upon to contribute to his work by diagnosing and sometimes treating (when consistent with Mengele's interest) his research subjects. Key figures in confirming diagnoses were Dr. Abraham

C., the radiologist, and Dr. Miklos Nyiszli, the pathologist. Nyiszli in particular attained enormous prestige in the camp and could move about as he wished by invoking Mengele's name. Before being taken on, he was given an "examination" by Mengele on his knowledge of pathology and forensic issues. The extent of his work with Mengele made him a controversial figure in the eyes of some other prisoner doctors. But the point here is the fact that the most important man on Mengele's team was the dissector of corpses.

Mengele even organized a series of colloquia, usually involving about fifteen doctors working with him and ten or fifteen brought in from other camps. Mengele would select the topic and run the meeting, while prisoner doctors would be asked to discuss particular cases from the standpoint of their specialties. Their discussion was tempered by their awareness, as one put it, that "any of us could be sent off [killed] at the slightest sign of displeasure on Mengele's part." While reluctant to disagree with Mengele, they also had to consider the danger of being associated with a false diagnosis (even if Mengele favored it) that could be confirmed as false by post-mortem examination.

Mengele was a *collector.* In accumulating dwarfs, as Dr. Lengyel put it, Mengele had "the mania of a collector, not of a savant."[43] Other prisoner doctors similarly saw him as an endless collector who served as an instrument of his professor without possessing any special qualities of his own as a scientist. (He was said to have collected doctors as well. One prisoner doctor told a story of a large group of Hungarian doctors [thought to be about 380] that Mengele gathered in late 1944; most of them were sent to a harsh working camp in Germany, where the great majority became severely ill and debilitated, and many died.)

Mengele's impulse to collect could be directed at any kind of specimen —fetuses, as we know, and "very beautiful gallstones," as Dr. Nyiszli tells us. Encountering the gallstones while dissecting a corpse, Nyiszli immediately thought of Mengele as "an ardent collector of such items": whether or not he had presented Mengele with such a gift before, he knew it would be appreciated. He carefully washed and prepared them, and Mengele's response was not only pleasure but the recitation of lines from a comic ballad of the warrior Wallenstein:

> In the Wallenstein family
> there are more gallstones than precious stones.
> [*Im Besitze der Familie Wallenstein*
> *Ist mehr Gallenstein, wie Edelstein.*]

The gallstones put Mengele in such a good mood that Nyiszli could successfully request permission to go about the camp to look for his wife and teenage daughter.[44]

Mengele as Scientist

In exploring with me Mengele's attitude toward his research and toward science in general, Teresa W. said: "In his scientific research he was honest . . . and fanatic. He was a strange man." The word "honest" expressed her sense of the legitimacy of his method and of his having been a man with a genuine "scientific background" who was "absolutely capable of doing serious and appropriate scientific work." His fanaticism was evident to her in his behavior not only at the ramp but when attempting to preserve his "research findings" at the time the camp was about to be liberated. He became "completely mad-looking," went desperately to his equipment and papers, and "put everything—instruments, all [there] was, in this trunk . . . paper, stationery, everything—pack, pack, terrific speed, not a word spoken to us—nothing, no expression, . . . just shuffling everything." His assistant remembered him looking "like the man who is flying under fear of something happening," his face distorted and seeming to have changed color, so that it was now "a very dark color, like brown."

As she probed the matter she became increasingly aware of his potential for research distortion, and we have noted her sense that he might "twist [results] a little bit to his aims." Although she insisted upon distinguishing him from a completely antiscientific racist like Hans F.K. Günther—because Mengele "wanted to be . . . [and] *was*" a scientist who "loved" scientific work—she realized that he was "a little bit . . . limited" by his fanaticism. That "little bit" turned out to be a great deal:

> If you think that [the] German race, or any race, is absolutely superior, and that means it has the right to destroy a weaker race, that is already a limitation. . . . He [did]n't like to think [about or] . . . go deeply in[to a] problem [that] contradicts his own. [He was like] a religious man . . . absolutely so committed that he will only consider the people going to church as the right people—or [those who] have the same face as he has.

Struggling with the idea of such scientific distortion in an intelligent anthropologist and "educated man," Teresa W. could only attribute it to Mengele's conviction "that Hitler [was] doing something absolutely incredibly good."

Mengele saw himself as a scientific investigator at large, ever on the alert for "interesting" or "important" medical or anthropological material. Gisella Perl tells of his strong interest in obtaining dead fetuses for study. On one occasion, when she and a few friends were surprised by him while eating illegally obtained food, she handled what she knew to be a situation of grave danger by immediately calling his attention to an unusually intact preserved fetus: *"Herr Hauptsturmführer* may be interested in this specimen." Mengele's rage diminished, and he said, "Good! . . . Beautiful!" and spoke of sending it to Berlin.[45]

Similarly, when he learned that one identical twin had an undescended testicle, he not only studied the other twin from the standpoint of evaluating possible genetic factors, but also sought to learn all he could about the phenomenon of the undescended testicle. And he pursued a hypothesis concerning the low hairline of Gypsies as an identifying characteristic to the point of insisting, against all evidence, that a group of French nomads were of Gypsy origin. Dr. Alexander O., in relating this story, commented, "Such a learned stupidity, so ingenious," and thought this "level of sophistication in stupidity" to be characteristically German.

Mengele, according to Marek P., would follow his "usual hospital routine" in the morning, checking on the medical blocks, participating frequently in various aspects of the killing, and later going to his pathological laboratory in Birkenau in order to obtain the results of post-mortem examinations. In this way, Dr. P. concluded, "he combined his interest in killing procedures with his research interests."

And he behaved in specific ways like a research scientist. Prisoner doctors observed his intensity, ambition, and apparent seriousness of purpose, his being a "work addict" as opposed to the relative laziness of other SS doctors. We know their impression of his being "all over the camp," and Nyiszli refers to his energy in rushing back and forth between the ramp, where he selected, to the pathology unit, where he spent "long hours" and would insist on having Nyiszli show him various tissues under the microscope.[46] Dr. Abraham C., Mengele's radiologist, thought that his greatest pleasure was to "spend hours and hours in Nyiszli's autopsy room" because he "seemed to have a genuine passion for medical questions, which, of course, could be best resolved in the autopsy room." Prisoner doctors observed how Mengele would rush from the medical wards to his beloved research areas, would come early in the morning to the Gypsy block to study noma cases, despite his great fatigue from having slept little because of having been most of the night directing people "toward the gas chamber." And he was indeed unusual in coming in on Sundays to make measurements and work on his records.

Mengele's constant collecting was equated by Teresa W. with the anthropology of that time, but researchers have always questioned any scientific policy of endless accumulation and measuring. A young German scientist wrote in 1935: "It is not useful to take as many measurements as possible; one must restrict oneself to the most significant ones." The young scientist was Josef Mengele; and in the same doctoral dissertation he spoke critically of a previous researcher who had "lost himself in details."[47] In Auschwitz that critic seems to have done the same, but, given his equation of Auschwitz with opportunity, he considered all details there to be "significant ones."

Everyone was aware of the extent of Mengele's scientific ambition, but W. went further in her impression that what he was doing was part of a larger plan in which "one day he will have a big research station . . . [probably there at Auschwitz], and he will have human material [there] . . . prepared, measured . . . ready [for] further investigation."

Toward his research subjects, Mengele's detachment could border on the schizoid. Dr. Lottie M. described him as "the coldest cynic I have ever seen," and his attitude toward inmates as "the same as [toward] mice and rabbits." Similarly, Nyiszli told how, after one of the crematoria had been blown up in the rebellion of the *Sonderkommando,* and he suggested a possible transfer of the dissecting room because "this environment is highly unsuitable for scientific research," Mengele answered coldly, "What's wrong? Getting sentimental?"[48]

In addition to Mengele's frequently mentioned "German mentality," Eva C., the artist who worked with him, saw him as an imperialistic researcher concerned not about people but about their disease: among the Gypsies, "he was like a white doctor in a jungle situation with natives, unconcerned about the individual but concerned about eradicating tropical disease, . . . where natives mean nothing because . . . a lion [will] eat . . . them anyway." In addition, he seemed to her "not aware of worldly things" and "very strange, . . . a stranger to the world." The same schizoid quality may have been responsible for a prisoner doctor's observation that "he was a very difficult man to trace . . . [and] would disappear and reappear, . . . would be gone and reappear again." There was the suggestion that much of his activity could have been false motion, partly in the service of creating his aura of omnipotence—the man who could appear from nowhere, be in control of everything.

Mengele did experience awe, perhaps even something like love, for "science," but his way of being a scientist was to seek absolute control over his research environment. As with those whose "dedication" was so obsessive, small interferences could unnerve him—as in the case of his outburst toward Nyiszli for getting some grease on records of his dissection: "How can you be so careless with these files, which I have compiled with so much love!"[49] Here we recall Dr. B.'s recollection of Mengele saying that not to utilize the possibilities Auschwitz offered would be "a sin, a crime" and "totally irresponsible" toward science. Dr. Marek P. could say to me, with some sadness, "He seemed to combine so much caring with so much killing."

We know of the variation in evaluations of Mengele as scientist. For Ernst B., Mengele was a gifted, even prophetic scientist, to be commended for his ability to adapt *as a scientist* to the special conditions of Auschwitz. Among inmates, that judgment was essentially reversed. Even Teresa W., who alone spoke of authentic scientific work with twins, had her qualifications about Mengele's interpretation of it. Most inmates went further: Dr. Jan W. thought Mengele only "pretended to be a scientist," flamboyantly collecting and labeling materials while lacking the intellectual coherence to do anything more with them. Similarly, Dr. Abraham C. thought Mengele had some ability but that what he did was "not real science" because he held certain ideas that he "considered absolute" and then "he . . . would simply look for proofs to support them."

That attitude was reflected in Mengele's colloquia, which "came out of the questions he asked, the instructions he gave, and the whole body of research he had us do." After prisoner doctors answered Mengele's questions, "he would comment, criticize, but not discuss [them] with us." Dr. C. had the impression that Nyiszli and Professor Epstein were exceptional in that Mengele would occasionally discuss ideas with them, and that Epstein was the only one "who dared contradict him and discuss with [Mengele . . . various] ideas." But Epstein, too, avoided going beyond a certain point. Mengele's essential pattern was to create intellectual interest and a demand for scientific opinion while remaining impermeable to that opinion if it contradicted his views (sometimes he would be quiet in order to wait for the X rays and post-mortem—and if proven wrong, he would be quieter still), all the while maintaining total control over the lives and deaths of prisoner scientific participants. Eva C., the artist, told how Mengele would strain to find "proof" of his views. In his search for Aryan versus non-Aryan qualities, he would attempt to observe whether Gypsies "had a darker area around the waist" (although "a two-piece bathing suit could get the same result") and, with some agitation, would insist upon demonstrating that blue eyes found in Gypsies "had little brown freckles . . . so . . . they are not pure Aryan blue eyes." Yet she thought him "earnest and sincere in going about these pursuits."

Dr. Frédéric E. was more blunt. Referring to an experiment in which Mengele tried to determine whether one twin was more susceptible to poison than another, this doctor called it "a crazy idea of a man who understood nothing about real scientific problems but . . . had the possibility . . . to experiment . . . without any control or restrictions." Another prisoner doctor called Mengele "a megalomaniac who wanted to become a great scientist and to reach this aim it was best to experiment with human beings." And still another thought Mengele's scientific work to be "garbage," and Mengele a man who "never applied judgment." Dr. Alexander O. characterized Mengele as "a fanatic . . . possessed by his pseudoscience." "Possessed" is an apt term here, suggesting Mengele's combination of fierce energy along with his mystification in what he did.

There might well have been a third component to that "possession" —the specter of inner doubt. Mengele required of himself the belief that what he did in Auschwitz was warranted by its claim to science. Among the more knowledgeable and intellectually superior prisoner doctors he surrounded himself with, we may suspect that he experienced some inner question about those scientific claims. Part of his desperate motion in Auschwitz might well have come from a struggle to cover over those doubts, to hide them from others capable of making scientific judgments, and above all from himself. Mengele's combination of science and pseudo science, of omnipotence and doubt, were probably shared widely among Nazified German scientists, and his serving as a personal connection between the *anus mundi* of Auschwitz and the German medical-academic establishment would seem to have been completely appropriate. In leaving the camp at the end, Mengele fled to the Berlin-Dahlem Institute to which he had sent his specimens. It is unclear whether he left new material there (destroyed later by Verschuer) or took from it old material he had earlier sent. In any case he was said to have gone there to make his report on his work.[50]

Mengele and His Fellow Nazi Doctors

Mengele's relationships with SS medical colleagues also show contradictions as well as discernible patterns. We know of Dr. B.'s lauding him as "the most decent colleague I met there." Ernst B.'s description of Mengele's close professional and personal relationship with Weber suggests the existence of a "medical-intellectual élite" at Auschwitz.

A survivor, who had had opportunities to observe SS doctors together, thought Mengele somewhat removed and "quite arrogant" toward other SS doctors, but also said he had "a strong personality and could influence people." We have heard of some of that persuasiveness in Mengele's manipulation of Lolling for the sake of maintaining support for his research and apparently countering Wirths's opposition to some of it, perhaps that portion of the work that required having children in the camp.

Considering these tendencies, as well as Dr. B.'s recollection of the impressive "rationality" with which Mengele could spin out his wildly Nazified racial-historical concepts, Mengele's position with other SS doctors in Auschwitz may well have depended upon his talent for *rationalizing the murderously absurd.* He could be persuasive because, perhaps more than any other SS doctor, he could make "good sense" of Auschwitz.

Deadly Colleagueship: Mengele and Prisoner Doctors

Much confusion about Mengele stemmed from his solicitude toward prisoner doctors which, while not without contradictions, could be impressive and life saving. More than merely needing them for his research purposes, Mengele placed doctors in a special category: as Dr. Lottie M. put it, ordinary prisoners (Jews especially) "were the rabbits and mice," while the doctors were "the human beings," so that even Jewish doctors could become his "colleagues." She told the story of how, when the Czech camp was annihilated, Mengele made up a very small list of those who were to be spared, which included his twins, his artist Eva C., and several Jewish doctors. When one of the doctors said to him that he would not go with Mengele unless his wife and daughter were spared as well, Mengele permitted both of them to survive. Despite his coldness, Dr. Lottie M. considered him more intelligent than the others, and more direct and pragmatic. So much so that he could chide her for having attempted to help Jews ("How could you hope to have been successful?") when she told him why she had been arrested and even to tell her that she must have been "a little schizoid" for having made these attempts.

Dr. Magda V. also said that "you could talk to him" and "give a more or less intelligent answer" when a medical issue arose: "We had a working relationship up to a point." That relationship involved a certain degree of mutuality: on the one hand, "He knew I would not do anything not one hundred percent correct," and she could count on his protection. Dr. V. was convinced that, during the last days of Auschwitz, only Mengele's protection prevented her from being shot for knowing so much about the camp's inner workings; yet also that "if he [had been given] the order to shoot me, I think he would have done it without thinking." Even the control he exerted over her was within a context of relative friendliness ("The joker knew me better than I knew myself"), and she remained grateful to him for having treated her with a measure of respect and for having kept her alive.

Women prisoner doctors seemed to have observed Mengele more closely and perhaps understood him better than did their male counterparts, but two men had what were probably the most excruciating relationships with him. One was Dr. Nyiszli, the pathologist, who described such moments of closeness as: "A long afternoon in deep discussion with Dr. Mengele, trying to clear up a certain number of doubtful points [during which] I was no longer a humble . . . prisoner, and I . . . defended and explained my point of view as though this were a medical conference of which I were a full-fledged member." Friendly gestures from Mengele came to mean a great deal to Nyiszli, as they seemed to transport the two men out of the master-slave relationship into one of colleagues: "I know men, and it seemed to me that my firm attitude, my measured sentences, and even my silences were qualities by which I had succeeded in making Dr. Mengele, before whom the SS themselves trembled, offer me a cigarette in the course of a particularly animated discussion, proving he forgot for a moment the circumstances of our relationship."[51] Also, one survivor observed Nyiszli and Mengele to have been "very close to each other" and "very comfortable together."

But Nyiszli was anything but comfortable in describing that relationship, along with some of Mengele's crimes, in his deposition of 28 January 1945 and his later book (published in 1960). That discomfort probably contributed to certain discrepancies between the two documents. But Nyiszli's most powerful suggestion of the ambiguity of his function as Mengele's pathologist was his later declaration that "I would begin practicing, yes, . . . but I swore that as long as I lived I would never lift a scalpel again."[52] In other words, while Mengele had been good to him in Auschwitz, Nyiszli felt that the price of that friendliness had been his own medical integrity.

Dr. Alexander O. spoke animatedly of his first encounters with Mengele ("One could not have a better impression") who showed himself to be cultivated, pleasant, and knowledgeable in discussions not only on medical subjects but about literary questions, even Flaubert. "He forgot who I was," so that when the two men were together, "it was just one doctor confiding in another." Dr. O. thought he had made a friend, but "then he disappointed me." When Mengele questioned him about his family, Dr. O. said that his wife had come to Auschwitz with him (which Mengele undoubtedly understood to mean that she had been killed) but that his small children were still in France. Mengele then sprang to his feet and asked, "Why [did] they not come here as well?" O. looked at me gravely and added, "Do you know what that means? . . . That means, why did they not come here to be gassed?" Mengele expressed even greater anger on learning that the children had been hidden by French priests, and at that point, as O. said, "he disappointed me forever."

Eva C., the artist, characterized her relationship to Mengele by saying, "I was a pet!"—by which she meant someone useful to him and also pleasant (as a charming, intelligent young woman) to have around. Mengele was also to discover that his "pet" had her own pet, a puppy given her by an influential male prisoner. Upon discovering the creature, Mengele first expressed anger: "What is the meaning of this!" But when told it was hers, he softened and said that it resembled a shepherd, "like a puppy from Germany"; he even petted it, and left without saying anything more. Mengele also made pets of two babies born in Auschwitz, and his appearing every morning to play with them was "a highlight" of his day—though everyone knew the babies would have to be killed. C. carried the metaphor further, likening the situation to an inspector (Mengele) visiting a city dog pound to check up on the keepers (prisoner professionals) and the other prisoners (the dogs):

> And he [the inspector] would point out maybe a pile of dirt or something in the cages . . . and admonished the keeper [to] wash up that excrement there, . . . to keep it clean, to keep the dogs healthy, to keep them well fed. Look, this one doesn't have water, you'd better give them some food. . . . And he inspects . . . these chambers where they [the dogs] are killed, you know, and sees that they are working well, and says, "How many are you? Well, it's too crowded. You better put in two more [chambers] today."

Eva C. went on to explain that most people consider that "what is going on in the city pound is sane and normal and can't be done in any other way," which is the way that the SS, and especially Mengele, felt about Auschwitz. For Mengele, above all, "everything has to be controlled . . . to the point of killing," and "everythings that's out of control is wrong." She was saying that Mengele was not only the "medical keeper" in Auschwitz but the keeper of the Auschwitz norm. He liked to be amused by pleasant and useful "pets," but they and everything else had to be under absolute control. She did not think Mengele extraordinary but "just a very charismatic man"—with the implication that only in Auschwitz could he develop that charisma and become "Mengele." For C. thought he had "star quality": "Marilyn Monroe flashed through my mind," here referring to his fetish about appearance and his eroticizing the contrast between his own physical perfection and the impaired state of inmates. She did not speak bitterly of him—he had on the whole been pleasant to her and had enabled her to thrive by Auschwitz standards—but at the end she said something characteristic in regard to Mengele and his control: "I was going to ask you not to reveal my whereabouts because I know he's still alive, and he might not be very happy knowing that I was."

There was much sexual speculation about Mengele among the inmates. There were many stories of women prisoners finding him extremely attractive, but Eva C. told me that "he had no sense for women." Although he did sometimes manifest prurient interest in sexual details when questioning pregnant women (according to Dr. Lengyel, he "never missed the chance to ask the women indiscreet and improper questions"),[53] he seemed to others distant and puritanical. C. told of an incident when, seeing a hefty prisoner from the rear stripped to the waist in front of a block, Mengele called angrily, "What is that man doing there?" Then the prisoner, turning around, revealed herself to be a woman (she was a German lesbian). Despite the fact that she spoke arrogantly to him, Mengele "just got terribly, terribly red, . . . blushed, and said, 'Oh, carry on,' and turned away and marched out of there." Dr. Lottie M. similarly recalled Mengele being much more concerned than the other SS doctors about lesbianism in the women's camp as well as about homosexuality in the men's camp.

Prisoners varied in their impression of whether Mengele could be influenced and whether he was corruptible. A group of them officially congratulated him upon learning that his wife had given birth to a son, but neither becoming a father nor the congratulations seemed to change Mengele's attitudes. It was widely believed that, like most SS personnel, he had enriched himself in Auschwitz (contrary to Ernst B.'s emphasis on his complete integrity) but that (as one survivor put it), while most of the SS doctors would "both take and give," Mengele would "only take." His attitudes often confused prisoners because, as Dr. Marie L. observed, "Nobody understood what he wanted."

Despite Mengele's apparent overtures of colleagueship, most prisoner doctors maintained no illusions of equality. The relationship was exemplified by an incident in which he carefully examined the wounded buttocks of a Polish prisoner physician and prescribed medication for washing and treating the area—after he himself had ordered that the man be given twenty-five lashes for an alleged infraction, and then observed the punishment.

Though generally thought of as being in control of others and himself,

Mengele could also explode with condemnation and rage. His form of blaming the victim was usually a matter of blaming the inmate "colleague." In his agitation about the annihilation of the Gypsy camp, Mengele called together a group of prisoner doctors and berated them for wrong diagnoses, threatening, "You'll pay for it!" should autopsies reveal further mistakes. As one prisoner doctor commented, "That is when he ceased to be a colleague, since he called us dogs and pigs." At that time Dr. Marek P. remembered Mengele saying specifically that "it was our fault" that he had to liquidate the Gypsies. P. believed that Mengele was upset because he had taken such pains with work on Gypsy twins and "suddenly it was all liquidated," creating a need in him to "find a group on whom he could release [project] his feelings of being responsible for it."

Similarly, Dr. Lengyel told how, just before the camp's liberation, Mengele came to the women's medical block and "declared that because of our negligence, the typhus epidemic had reached such proportions that the entire region of Auschwitz was menaced." In the subsequent rush to prepare serum and vaccinations, Mengele "accused us of sabotaging the vaccinations," and "in fact discontinued them." He would sometimes accuse prisoner doctors of "not seeing enough patients" and at other times of "giving the sick too much care and wasting scarce medicines."[54] While the pattern of blaming the victim was present in many SS doctors, with Mengele both the accusation and the anger were especially required for his way of interpreting and experiencing.

Thus, Dr. Gerda N. told how Mengele, in a sudden rage, "nearly wanted to choke this lady doctor—actually put his fingers around her neck, accusing her of treating patients poorly and shouting: 'They will die. Then we Germans will be responsible!' " Dr. N. added, "He wanted to give us a show . . . [so] that we should believe that the Germans are really caring . . . for the people here"—and also, I would add, so that his imagery of Nazi virtue could be sustained.

Dr. N. also spoke of Mengele's brandishing a pistol as he entered a room to talk to the chief prisoner physician of a women's medical block, demanding that she select a large number of typhus patients for the gas chamber. She added that, even without a drawn gun, whenever Mengele went into her room with a prisoner doctor, he was metaphorically holding a gun to that person's head. He could make his threats, direct or indirect, while mostly maintaining the illusion of colleagueship by behaving considerately toward prisoner doctors.

Another prisoner doctor expressed the anguish of being manipulated by Mengele in a series of cruel deceptions. He asked her to make a list of pregnant women so that he could "feed them milk" and get them to a better camp so they could have "healthy babies"; after she had acceded to the request despite a certain skepticism, they were transferred to the "H-block," or "Heaven block" *(Himmelblock)*, from which they inevitably went either to the crematorium or to a research block. An example of what she called Mengele's "diabolic" attitude was his appearing on a Jewish holiday and announcing, "This is *Tishahb'av* [the commemoration of the destruction of the First and Second Temples]," and "We will have a concert." There was a concert, then a roll call, and then an enormous selection, causing her to ask bitterly, "Why should we listen to music while we are being cremated?"

She stressed that Mengele's behavior was carefully planned: "He must have written it down: music; sit down; *Zählappell* [roll call]; crematorium." All this was part of his "sadistic play," she believed, because "every step Mengele [took] was a psychological basis for torture." And compared with other SS doctors, Mengele was "more sadistic, . . . more *raffiniert* ['sophisticated, tricky, sly']. He [was] more elaborated . . . because he must know psychology."

Sometimes the psychological sadism could be naked, as when he spoke to a Jewish woman doctor pleading unsuccessfully for the life of her elderly father, also a doctor: "Your father is seventy years old. Don't you think he has lived long enough?" Or, to a sick woman: "Have you ever been on the 'other side'? What is it like over there? . . . You will know very soon!"[55]

Mengele maintained these forms of deadly "colleagueship" until the very end. A prisoner doctor describes encountering him in the infirmary of a camp in Czechoslovakia after Auschwitz had been evacuated. Mengele referred to a patient who was mentally deficient, and said, "If you were intelligent . . . she could have fever, she could need medication," meaning that "he wanted to find . . . a reason to get rid of her [or a means of doing so] because she was an idiot, . . . and [implied] we were so stupid we did not understand." She added, in amazement, "Just think . . . he was already at the time a cornered beast, and that did not mean anything. He still had to find a way to kill someone."

The "Double Man"

Prisoner doctors found themselves struggling with Mengele's extraordinarily deep-seated contradictions—with his overt doubling. Dr. Abraham C. felt compelled to raise "the big question which we ask ourselves: Was he a kind man, good with children, good in general, who was only driven to do the things he did by his passion for research? Or was he a monster who only plays a role with the children to hide his game better, to get his ends more easily?" While very few prisoners would adhere to the first characterization, the second does not satisfy either. Dr. C. himself seemed to reject both, as he went on to articulate the principle of unfathomability I quoted at the beginning of this book (page 13). Mengele was for Dr. C. the source and epitome of this principle of unfathomability, though he meant it to apply to much that happened in Auschwitz.

Dr. Magda V. similarly spoke of Mengele as "a split personality." She was aware of others' reports of his brutality and had "no doubt" about his capacity for it, but added, "never in my presence." When she went on to wonder whether she might not have had a "humanizing effect" on Mengele and other SS doctors because "I treated everyone [inmates and SS doctors] like a human being," she was expressing another principle of doubling: the importance for each self of being confirmed by others. The word "double" (or its French equivalent) was actually used by Dr. Alexander O. in his excruciating struggles to come to terms with Mengele:

> The double man [*l'homme double*]. The double [*le double*], that is to say he had all the sentimental motions, all the human feelings, pity, and so on. But there was in his psyche a hermetically closed cell [*une cellule hermétiquement fermée*], impenetrable, indestructible cell, which is obedience to the received order. He can throw himself in the water to go and save a Gypsy, try to give him medication, . . . and then as soon as they are out of the water, . . . tell him to get in the truck and quickly off to the gas chamber.

Dr. O. identified not only the doubling itself but the central role of Mengele's ideology (though only hinted at) in the process. As O. went on to explain, "Mengele liked the Gypsies a lot. He loved the Gypsy children, who called him 'Uncle Mengele.' " But he knew that the *Reichsführer* SS [Himmler] had ordered a slow death of the Gypsies, and Mengele was "the kind of man . . . to believe that orders had to be executed." Without such a concept, one who, like Teresa W., was exposed to Mengele's decency but at the same time accepted the truth of reports about his experiments and cruel behavior, has to end up declaring painfully, "I can't understand him!" Or prisoners might develop their own racial theory to explain his contradictions: for instance, the rumor that he was kinder to Gypsies than to others because "he himself was of Gypsy origin"—a rumor that was consistent with his dark non-Aryan appearance.

Eva C. told, with considerable sensitivity, how her own psychological experience as an inmate helped her understand Mengele. She pointed out that prisoners also began "to behave like that . . . with a shell around us," and how she herself watching grotesquely weak women on the sick block stretching their arms out and pleading, "Help me! Help me!" made her "somewhat embarrassed" because of her feeling "We're here to die. What do you mean, 'Help me'?" Then she could add, "The fact that these people actually had retained their sanity [in asking for help] and I was nuts . . . never entered my mind. You know, I was already touched with [affected by] that whole [Auschwitz] mentality." C. explained further that both the SS doctors and the prisoners "were being processed—so I could understand Mengele." Auschwitz was "a different planet" whose rules totally reversed those of ordinary society: according to those rules, "we were there to die and not to live." And "to be able to accept being where we were, we had to switch . . . to a different kind of mentality, to a different kind of attitude." SS doctors had to make a similar switch, in their case much helped by prior immersion in Nazi ideology: "They were well prepared." She was able to grasp something of the murderous doubling in Nazi doctors by recognizing more limited and benign forms of a related process in herself and other prisoners.

While all Nazi doctors underwent doubling in Auschwitz, Mengele was special in the seemingly extreme incompatibility of the two components of his double self, along with the extraordinary energy he could mobilize within that adaptation. His doubling was enhanced by certain psychological traits. I have in mind three dominant features of his self-process: his schizoid tendencies, his extraordinary capacity for numbing, and his impulse toward sadism and omnipotence (which turn out to be closely related). Eva C. puts us in touch with those traits by means of an artist's description of the man, one that turns the tables on Mengele and makes him an anthropological subject:

> He looked like Peter Sellers, but better. . . . His head was like a cat's head. It was wide at the temples. He had a widow's peak, dark brown hair, brown eyes. His eyebrows made a kind of accent circumflex, like a cat. Using Mengele's own terminology, I would say he had an M-shaped mouth; a straight, short regular-medium nose; a wide, broad head; a mark on his left ear—a flat round disk on his ear cartilage. . . . His eyes were like Peter Sellers's eyes—as though only half of the iris would show. They were dead eyes.

The "dead eyes" were part of his schizoid pattern, as was perhaps behavior associated with the rumors that he had been "shell-shocked" or that his war injury was a concussion; and also consistent with C.'s observation that "he seemed to be from a different planet and had just come down in a space ship."

Mengele's withdrawn state is also reflected in Dr. Marek P.'s description of him as a man who "never looked into your eyes . . . [or] show[ed] any signs of enjoyment . . . [but] seemed always . . . [to have] something else on his mind other than what he was doing, even when he was speaking to you." A related trait was one prisoner doctor's observation of his "lightning-fast change from being, on the one side, attentive and jovial . . . and then, within a fraction of a second, cynical and brutal."

One expects considerable psychic numbing in a schizoid person, but with Mengele the numbing was extreme. As Dr. Lottie M. put it, "The main thing about him was that he totally lacked sentiment, lacked feeling" concerning the horrors of Auschwitz in which he was participating. As she further explained, "It's that he didn't ever see a *person* . . . [in] his contempt for everybody—except the doctors." And so he seemed to have "no personal ties." Dr. Alexander O. said he had "indifferent eyes . . . indifference to pain." Teresa W. said he was "without emotion on his face." And the rumors of his impotence, the impression that he had "no sense for women"—whether or not true, these reflected the prisoners' strong impression of his general lack of human feeling.

Sadism suggests pleasure in causing pain, and we have seen many different expressions of that tendency in Mengele. Even his style of dress and display could be understood as something close to sadism in that environment. It is also what is frequently called "narcissism"—in popular usage, extreme self-absorption, as opposed to the psychoanalytic technical meaning of sexual energy (or "libido") directed at one's own body or person. Of Mengele one has the impression that both his "narcissism" and sadism were bound up with his profound impulse toward omnipotence, toward *total* control of his environment, and specifically the kind of life-death control available to an SS doctor in Auschwitz.

Indeed, the importance of the Auschwitz environment in activating all of these traits—schizoid tendencies, numbing, and the sadism-omnipotence combination—cannot be overemphasized. Several prisoner professionals emphasized that, were it not for Auschwitz, Mengele could undoubtedly have followed a successful academic career. As Dr. Magda V. put it, "In ordinary times he could have been a slightly sadistic German professor."

None of Mengele's behavior—least of all his capacity to inflict pain and feel nothing for victims—can be understood separately from his involvement in ideology. Unlike most SS doctors, Mengele was a true ideologue: a man who understood his life to be in the service of a larger vision. He undoubtedly viewed himself as a Nazi revolutionary, a man committed to the bold task of remaking his people and ultimately the people of the world. He and those like him differed from previous revolutionaries in their invocation of biology: *Mengele exemplified the Nazi biological revolutionary.* He was part of a vanguard that saw its mission as noble and viewed courage and cruelty (or "hardness," as the Nazis were fond of saying) toward enemies or impediments of any kind as personal virtues. For a man like Mengele, the ideological mission justified everything.

That is why Dr. V. could call him "the most absolutely convinced Nazi among them"; Dr. Lottie M. could speak of him as an "intellectual true believer," capable of complaining about stupidity of individual SS personnel "and yet believe in absurd . . . [racial] theories"; Eva C. could say that "next to Hitler he was the most convinced"; and Dr. O. could call him "Hitler's robot."

As his friend Dr. B. constantly stressed, Mengele was an extreme anti-Semite. He viewed the Jews as a highly gifted people who were locked in a life-and-death struggle with Aryan Germans. His anti-Semitism was part of the broad ideological sweep of racial theory: Dr. B. put it clearly when he said that "Mengele was fully convinced that the annihilation of the Jews is a provision for the recovery (or cure) of the world, and Germany." And Dr. Jacob R. understood Mengele as an SS mystic who believed that "if all the Jews were annihilated, victory would come [of] itself."

Mengele's anti-Semitism was both sweeping and immediate. Among SS doctors, according to Dr. B., Mengele would speak derisively of catering too much to Jewish inmates and of Auschwitz becoming a "Jewish sanitorium." Dr. Magda V. said, "I think really he hated us" and "treated Jews like laboratory animals—not quite human" because "we were really biologically inferior in his eyes."

Ideologues like Mengele can appear to be "cold cynics" in that they need not feel others' pain if it is in the service of a "higher purpose." They can also have pockets of pragmatism for the same reason—certainly the case with Mengele. Nor is ideological fanaticism incompatible with personal ambition. While Mengele might have been a "good soldier" for the SS (as Dr. B. put it), one who lacked "fake SS ambitions," we know him to have had very real ambitions that had to do with his ideology and with his overweening desire to become recognized as a great scientist.

Few would question Dr. Nyiszli's observation concerning "so much cynicism" and "so much evil" in Mengele, or his verdict on him as "a criminal doctor."[56] But that cynicism and criminality, the numbing and the omnipotence—all these were bound up with what all too many people in Germany and elsewhere at the time experienced as a compelling, even ennobling vision of the future.

The Ultimate Auschwitz Self: Physician-Killer-Researcher

More than any other SS doctor, Mengele realized himself in Auschwitz. There he came into his own—found expression for his talents, so that what had been potential became actual. Intelligent but hardly an intellectual giant, Mengele found expression and recognition in Auschwitz *beyond his talent.* The all-important Auschwitz dimension was added to his prior psychological traits and ideological convictions to create a uniquely intense version of the Auschwitz self as physician-killer-researcher.

Mengele took hold of and maximized the omnipotent authority held by any SS doctor in Auschwitz. He could give a forceful and flowing performance in displaying that omnipotence because it blended so readily with the traits and ideology he brought to the camp. In Auschwitz, Mengele was the "right man in the right place at the right time." His energies no less than his ambition were galvanized by this Auschwitz synchronization of all his faculties. Hence the comment by a prisoner (quoted earlier) that "he always had the air of . . . [a] man . . . doing his job and doing it well and [who] hasn't got the slightest doubt about the job." Or as Dr. Jan W. put it: "This was his big thing there, his Auschwitz, and he enjoyed doing it."

However atypical for an SS camp doctor, Mengele became the spirit of Auschwitz, the one most in tune with the place, an example for others. That is why he was chosen by Wirths and Weber (despite his conflicts with the former) to be Delmotte's mentor, the person who could convince this reluctant doctor of the virtue and necessity of doing selections. And that is why he could help Dr. B. adapt to Auschwitz and be an "inspiration" to him despite their ideological and characterological differences.

Above all, Mengele could combine his ideology and medical energies to impose a logic on the entire Auschwitz killing process. Observing his "fit" with the place and the energies it released in him, other SS doctors, and to an extent inmates as well, could not help but feel that Auschwitz "logic." Mengele himself of course experienced that logic even when he objected to specific policies (the destruction of the Polish intelligentsia and the annihilation of the Gypsy camp). For these objections were based on an *ideal* Nazi vision, which he wanted Auschwitz to live up to (and he apparently considered these two groups to be essentially "Aryan"). His ideological dedication and discipline were such that his objection to aspects of the larger Nazi-Auschwitz vision never diminished—might even have intensified—his allegiance to the whole of it. In brutally tracking down for the crematorium the same Gypsy children on whom he had lavished so much affection, he was demonstrating not merely his obedience to orders but his loyalty to a higher truth whatever the lesser errors within it. The Auschwitz logic he disseminated had to do with the *conviction* of his performance there, and it was "medical" logic.

The conviction in turn was a manifestation of his talent for doubling, having greatly to do with his schizoid tendencies and inclinations toward numbed detachment—a talent that Auschwitz as an institution strongly nurtured. There was, then, a mutually reinforcing process—a vicious circle—in his proclivity for doubling, the Auschwitz demand for it, and his energetic expression of it there. Dr. Tadeusz S.'s characterization of him as "the perfect SS man" might well be changed to "the perfect Auschwitz SS advocate and physician-mentor." Mengele could become the quintessential Auschwitz pedant because his actions so well articulated the camp's essence.

It was precisely this special vitality achieved in Auschwitz that Dr. B. referred to as Mengele's "strong life principle"—a life principle that included omnipotent-sadistic impulses of rare intensity to which he could all too easily give vent in Auschwitz. Whatever the self-absorption and brooding in his "dead eyes," Mengele was probably the most alive Nazi doctor in Auschwitz. In speaking of him as a doctor "playing God" and then reversing that image to "God playing doctor," one prisoner doctor touched upon Mengele's sense of being the embodiment of a larger spiritual principle, the incarnation of a sacred Nazi deity—whether that deity was itself an ideological vision of the future or the Führer himself.

Evil Deity or Evil Human Being?

This demonization process, initiated in Mengele's mode of functioning in Auschwitz, helps us to understand his aura and his significance for Auschwitz inmates as well as for ourselves today. Here we return to the Mengele legend: the image of Mengele as an evil deity.

When Hochhuth wrote of his Mengele figure as "only playing the part of a human being," he was trying to simplify Nazism by constructing a figure of such pure evil as to no longer belong to the category of human being. Such an exemplar distills and clarifies evil, and we know enough about Mengele to affirm his qualifications for the category. But even Mengele has shown too many familiar facets of human behavior for one to leave him in that legendary role and, with Hochhuth, "[refrain] from any further effort to plumb [his] human features."[57] I have made clear my rejection of the legend of pure ahuman evil, clarifying as it may be, in favor of a commitment to probing motivations and behavior. I return to the legend now only to explore more about Mengele's function as the ideal candidate for this cult of demonic personality.

At moments in Auschwitz, prisoner doctors felt it necessary to divest Mengele of his physician's status: "He was a monster, period, no more doctor than anything else," was the way Dr. Abraham C. put it, "a monster and . . . only evil or calamities could come from him."

A woman survivor conveyed some of Mengele's aura when she said, "He represents what this [Auschwitz] represents to us": that is, Mengele is Auschwitz. Another spoke of him as "so terrifying" that he was "more like an abstraction." To convey Mengele's meaning for her, she read to me a short story she had written, based on a childhood memory, and involving her unsuccessful attempt, as a little girl, to placate and please the male bully who had been terrorizing her and other Jewish children. Afterward she concluded, "Mengele was feared, . . . was admired. We tried to please him, . . . almost like seducing [someone]." Mengele's style of omnipotence, then, produced both terror and a measure of admiration, a combination that serves a legend well, but from which individuals have great difficulty extricating themselves.

Adding to Mengele's aura was the mythology of his escape. There was the false rumor that he "had caught typhus when the camp was liberated.": "While he was convalescing, he escaped."[58] Actually he left before the liberation, but the mythology continues in relation to the places where he is thought to have been seen after leaving Auschwitz—Ravensbrück, Dachau, a small camp in Czechoslovakia—whatever the accuracy of any of these identifications. The escape legend is extended by his apparent contempt for postwar authority—and for justice, in living for years in his home in the vicinity of Günzberg where he was protected by local officials and family influence; by his subsequent exploits in South America, including practicing medicine under various names in different places, disappearing just in time to prevent extradition from Argentina to West Germany, advising dictators (such as General Alfredo Stroessner of Paraguay, who is of German descent) on such matters as annihilating their local Indian populations; by his outsmarting a youthful female Israeli spy who attempted to seduce him in order to lure him into death or capture, and was herself found murdered; by rumors of his involvement in an extensive drug trade run by Nazis throughout South America; and by various reports of people meeting and talking with him in Paraguay, reports that suggest he still had influence in a German, if not Nazi, community there, and also that he was preparing his own memoirs defending his actions over the course of his life. Whatever the mixture of truth, exaggeration, and falsehood, the legend grew.

For many survivors, Mengele had so come to represent Auschwitz evil that meaning in their lives could be restored only by his capture and trial. "I would like to live and see this trial and then I could die," is the way one prisoner doctor put it. In adding that "a human being should know, . . . should be told that his deeds are evil [because], after all, there is not only heavenly, but also earthly justice," he was struggling to move beyond the legend to the man. The twin Simon J. made the point more directly: "I would wish to have a good front-row seat and listen to the proceedings [because] I fear him totally. . . . To me he is the key to my sense of fear from everything that is German." And then the crux of the matter: "I would be very interested to hear the details and to see him pass [through] this metamorphosis of turning back into a person instead of God Almighty." Another survivor expressed a similar need for Mengele to come to understand that "this is what happened," and then added, "After that I hope I can make peace with myself."

Mengele's imagined trial, then, involved both the legend and the man: justice for Mengele came to represent a restoration of a just cosmos—a means of overcoming a vast "wound in the order of being," in Martin Buber's phrase, that Auschwitz has represented. It also came to signify the desacralization of a terrible deity: the god must be rendered not only human but vulnerable to truth and retribution. Only then, for many survivors who were rendered helpless to the point of feeling their humanity virtually annihilated—only then could they regain freedom from his control, experience a sense of vitality, feel alive. A few of those survivors, while exploring Mengele's meaning for themselves, insisted on thinking beyond him. Dr. Henri Q., while well aware of Mengele as "a terrible man" and "the name one heard most" in Auschwitz, nonetheless warned me against concentrating too much upon him because Auschwitz had to be understood as "a collective enterprise." Another prisoner doctor had the same message: "There's not only one Mengele. They are all part of Mengele—all the doctors." She was saying that what was so glaring in Mengele, morally and psychologically, was present, perhaps more muted, in all of the SS Auschwitz doctors. We can say, then, that, while Mengele qualifies as the exemplar for "medical Auschwitz," we should use him to help us unlock, and not ignore, the broader evil of Auschwitz truths.

Other survivors invoked the character of Dorf (in the 1978 television film *Holocaust*[59]), an intelligent careerist who rises in the SS hierarchy until he becomes a key figure in the planning of the annihilation of Jews. Dr. Lottie M. said that Mengele, like Dorf, was "very cool," "clean-cut," a "pretty boy"; and that, although Mengele was more ideological, she could well imagine him doing what Dorf did in the film, providing the euphemism *Endlösung,* or Final Solution, for mass murder. Dr. Magda V. was struck by Dorf's similarity to Nazi doctors: "He wasn't a monster— . . . none of them [the Nazi doctors] were, you know"—but merely a fallible and corruptible human being. Mengele was closest, but, she concluded, "I think they [Nazi doctors] were all Dorfs."

Recognizing Mengele and other Nazi doctors in this believable fictional character also helped the metamorphosis from deity to human; Mengele could have been seen as a man with talent for maneuver whose ambition had been fiercely aroused, and who sanitized the killing project he so effectively served.

The revelations that emerged in 1985, at the time of the discovery of his corpse, concerning Mengele's postwar life in Europe and especially South America change little in this evaluation.[60] From the son who was born when Mengele worked in Auschwitz, and a few people who lent him support or shelter, we gain a sense of a man increasingly on the run: at first, effectively manipulative and successful in avoiding pursuit but, over the years, more and more alone, despairing, frightened, fearful of being hunted by "the Jews," at times even suicidal. He no longer had his Auschwitz stage. Rather than absolute control over others, he had virtually no control over his own destiny. Not surprisingly, he remained a fanatical ideologue; but as his diaries lapsed into rantings about science and religion, he became increasingly an ideological caricature of a caricature. Yet he had been capable of affection: toward his son, who at the age of twelve encountered him briefly as the "nicest of uncles"; toward his brother's widow, who became Mengele's second wife in what his son described as a "love marriage"; much later toward a housekeeper whom he asked to live with him but who refused because he would not marry her; and finally toward a pack of mongrel dogs he enjoyed spending time with and providing with medical and surgical treatment.

He was reported to have died in 1979 as a result of a heart attack while swimming and to have been buried under the name of another man in Brazil. The identification was made from a study of his remains, especially bones and teeth; now it was his corpse that was being dissected, rather than the corpses of his Auschwitz victims.

Yet that resolution was psychologically unsatisfactory, especially for Auschwitz survivors. The need was to capture him and put him on trial, to hear his confession, to put *him* at *their* mercy. Failing that, many survivors refused to believe that the remains in the Brazilian grave were Mengele's. Soon after that identification, a twin whom Mengele had studied told me that she simply did not believe that the arrogant, overbearing figure she had known in Auschwitz could have undergone a "change in personality" and become the frightened hermit in Brazil. She was saying, in effect, that she and others had not been provided with a psychological experience of that "metamorphosis" from evil deity to evil human being. But we do have a story of metamorphosis after all—that of a man divested of his power for evil, gradually disintegrating in life, mentally and physically, and then rapidly and visibly as a corpse. That metamorphosis will inevitably over time take hold in the minds of survivors and others.

Mengele's many-sidedness in Auschwitz was both part of his legend and a source of his desacralization. In the camp he could be a visionary ideologue, an efficiently murderous functionary, a "scientist" and even a "professor," an innovator in several areas, a diligent careerist (like Dorf), and, above all, a physician who became a murderer. He reveals himself as a man and not a demon, a man whose multifaceted harmony with Auschwitz can give us insight into—and make us pause before—the human capacity to convert healing into killing.

Chapter 18

Healing-Killing Conflict: Eduard Wirths

> I can say that I have always done my duty and have
> never done anything contrary to what was expected
> of me.
>
> —EDUARD WIRTHS

Eduard Wirths lived out most directly, and most extremely, the Auschwitz healing-killing conflict and paradox. A man with a strong reputation as a dedicated physician, and described by inmates who could observe him closely as "kind," "conscientious," "decent," "polite," and "honest," he was the same man who established the camp's system of selections and medicalized killing and supervised the overall process during the two years in which most of the mass murder was accomplished. Because of that dichotomy, he was one of the few Auschwitz doctors frequently spoken of as not only criminal but "a tragic figure." Hermann Langbein, the political prisoner who served as his secretary in both Dachau and Auschwitz, believed him to be the only Nazi doctor in Auschwitz who refused to succumb to its ubiquitous corruption and in no way enriched himself there. From the time of his first encounter with Wirths in Dachau, Langbein was struck by his medical conscientiousness and considered him "completely different from other SS doctors."[1]

He differed also in the story of his death—not in the way that he died (a considerable number of Nazi doctors committed suicide) but in what transpired just before his death. It is claimed (probably accurately) that a British intelligence officer, a member of the group to whom Wirths surrendered himself, greeted him and then said, "Now I've shaken hands with a man who . . . bears responsibility for the death of four million human beings." That night Wirths hanged himself; although cut down, he died two or three days later, in September 1945.[2]

I was able to learn a great deal about Dr. Wirths from a wide variety of sources: from interviews with two close family members, with other SS doctors who knew him in Auschwitz, and with prisoner doctors and other inmates who had contact with him there; from his own writings, mostly in the form of revealing letters he wrote to his wife and other family members from Auschwitz, and a desperate autobiographical apologia he prepared just before being taken into custody; and from various other SS records and trial materials. Finally, Langbein—in his writings and our talks together—has been an important source of knowledge about Wirths.

Recently a Dutch documentary film has explored the chief doctor's life and Auschwitz activities on the assumption that he is a key figure for our understanding of Auschwitz and of Nazi functioning in general.[3] Wirths provides the specter of a "good man" becoming a leading figure in a project of unprecedented evil.

Background

Eduard Wirths was born in 1909 in a village near Würzburg in southern Germany, the oldest of three boys. His father, a stonecutter from a craftsman tradition, had developed a successful stoneworks and become a notable figure in the area. Wirths senior had served as a medical corpsman in the First World War, from which he emerged in a depressed state with pacifist leanings, which were undoubtedly expressed in his (as one son put it) "making doctors of us all." (Another son also became a doctor, and the third probably would have had he not died of cancer as a child.) This strict and revered father had liberal views, which contributed to a family atmosphere of humanism and democratic socialism.

Among the boys it was Eduard who came most under the father's influence in becoming meticulous, obedient, and unusually conscientious and reliable—traits that continued into his adult life. He never smoked or drank and was described as compassionate and "soft" in his responses to others.

Eduard was always a good student and apparently became a very good doctor. He did special work in gynecology under a well-known professor, Hans Hinselmann. Although he had shown talent as a surgeon, he settled into a general practice in a rural area near his birthplace partly out of the need to support a family, having married the first and only woman with whom he was ever involved.

Drawn to nationalistic and *völkisch* ideas during his student days, he joined the Nazi Party and the SA in 1933 and applied for admission into the SS the following year. An ardent and idealistic National Socialist,* he volunteered to serve in the Thuringian State Office for Racial Matters

---

*Langbein points out that Wirths had some initial difficulty with the Nazis because of earlier Social Democratic sympathies. But there is no doubt about Wirths's subsequent Nazi enthusiasm.

(*Thüringisches Landesamt für Rassenwesen*) in Weimar because, as he wrote on an SS form in 1936, "I was particularly interested in human genetics and racial hygiene." He wrote also of his "love for the biological tasks set by the SS." Although brought up as a Catholic and initially identifying himself as such on official forms, he later reverted to the Nazi-preferred category of "believer in God."[4]

From the late 1930s, he divided his time between his country practice (in which he was said to be so conscientious that he sterilized his own instruments), state medical positions (where one was close to the regime), medical work with ethnic Germans being "resettled" in Germany from Eastern areas, and military service for which he volunteered. He entered the Waffen SS in 1939. He served in Norway and saw combat on the Russian front until, in April 1942, he was declared medically unfit for combat duty because of a cardiac condition and possible additional ailments.

Wirths's early attitude toward Jews was contradictory. His family was not anti-Semitic, and he not only had Jewish patients but continued to treat them even after it became illegal for Aryan doctors to do so. With no Jewish doctors in the area, Jews would sneak into his consulting room at night, sometimes for injuries sustained in Nazi persecutions. At the same time, Wirths clearly embraced some of the broader Nazi anti-Semitic worldview, came to believe that "the Jews were a danger to Germany," and apparently retained this *ideological* anti-Jewishness until his death.[5]

Chief Auschwitz Doctor

Wirths spent short periods of time at Dachau and Neuengamme, two concentration camps within Germany, before being sent to Auschwitz in September 1942. He was probably sent there as chief doctor because of his medical reputation, as others before him in that position had failed to stop persistent typhus epidemics that increasingly affected SS personnel. Langbein later described Wirths as "a competent physician with a strongly developed sense of duty and extremely conscientious and careful"; and even Lolling, his antagonistic and incompetent superior, described him as "the best physician in all the concentration camps," to which Commandant Höss added: "During my 10 years of service in concentration-camp affairs, I have never encountered a better one."[6] While Wirths's medical humanity—concern about and friendliness toward prisoner patients—was certainly *not* a reason for his appointment to a high post in Auschwitz, it did, according to Langbein, come to mean a great deal to many inmates there.

Wirths lived up to expectations in stopping the typhus epidemics by means of widespread disinfection procedures and enlisting the cooperation of prisoner physicians in identifying, isolating, and treating typhus patients. He also improved conditions on the medical blocks, extended the work of Polish prisoner physicians who had been in Auschwitz for some time, and began to permit the large numbers of arriving Jewish physicians to do medical work as well. All this was consistent with overall SS policies of maintaining a work force in Auschwitz; and Langbein found it possible to appeal to Wirths on policies that could save lives by presenting a case "from a purely medical point of view."[7]

For instance, he persuaded Wirths to take steps to end the fatal phenol injections by pointing out that they made it impossible to maintain antityphus medical measures because prisoners, becoming fearful of the sick block, avoided it even when afflicted and thereby infected others (see page 257). Once convinced, Wirths had the two people most responsible for the injections transferred from the medical block: Entress, the SS physician who ordered most of them; and Klehr, the noncommissioned officer who performed more of the injections than anyone else.[8]

Wirths was also protective of prisoner doctors and other prisoners doing medical work. On one occasion he was heard to castigate Irma Grese, the notorious woman SS officer, with the words "Do not beat my people!" when he found her whipping a prisoner who worked on the medical block. And when a prisoner chief of Block 10 insisted upon beating other prisoners, Wirths not only removed her but gave unprecedented authority to the Jewish prisoner doctor he had appointed to run the medical block.[9]

Wirths exercised his medical autonomy in a confrontation with the Auschwitz Gestapo head, Maximilian Grabner. Grabner's Political Department maintained a prison in the basement of Block 11, periodically had inmates shot at the "Black Wall" in the courtyard between blocks 11 and 10, and would then officially report those victims as having died of some illness in the infirmary. Upon learning of this system (with Langbein's help), which considerably elevated the recorded death rate in the medical blocks, Wirths got angry and declared, "The Political Department has to take responsibility for its own dead." Since it turned out that Entress and Klehr had again been part of the arrangement, especially through Entress's close connection with the Gestapo, their transfer helped solve this problem as well. The matter emerged during Konrad Morgen's celebrated SS investigation of Auschwitz corruption (see pages 138–39): the judge backed Wirths since killings at the Black Wall, unlike those in the gas chamber, were not considered legal. Morgen also supported Wirths in opposing Grabner's urging that pregnant Polish women be killed. In these struggles against Grabner and other Auschwitz enemies, Wirths anchored himself in medical propriety but at the same time scrupulously adhered to rules and regulations.[10]

Wirths used his medical authority in other ways to save lives. At Gestapo trials held in Auschwitz, he frequently testified to the medical capacity of an accused, usually a Polish civilian, to perform useful work, thereby arguing for the prisoner to be allowed to enter the camp as an ordinary inmate rather than be shot at the Black Wall. He also gave psychiatric testimony that similarly served the accused.

Wirths clearly felt most comfortable when dealing with actual medical matters, and Höss testified to his "constant struggle with the Construction Department because he always urged improvements and new construction in the medical facilities." Wirths in fact devoted much of his time during 1944 to the planning and construction of a new SS military hospital. In September of that year, with the war completely lost and the Soviet armies not far away, there was a ceremony marking the opening of the hospital and Wirths was promoted to *Sturmbannführer,* or major—the whole scene epitomizing the fantasy element in this claim to healing. But as Langbein observed, "It was a purely medical task and he was glad to do it."[11]

Wirths conveyed an aura of moral scrupulousness: for instance, he alone among Auschwitz doctors kept to wartime food rations. He consistently took stands against brutality and random abuse of prisoners, was generally antagonistic to the ordinary criminals who took part in that abuse, and was much more sympathetic to Communist political prisoners such as Langbein, in whom he could sense the kind of integrity he respected.

The two men developed the kind of tie that Langbein spoke of as "deepen[ing] into a human relationship."[12] Indeed, a chief camp doctor or an otherwise prominent SS doctor was likely to develop a close relationship with a prisoner secretary, as in parallel situations in Buchenwald and Mauthausen. The necessary elements seemed to include an SS doctor who retained a kernel of medical humanity; official SS encouragement of a certain amount of medical help to prisoners to maintain a work force; a prisoner secretary who was intelligent, reliable, and in his own life morally or ideologically committed (often a Communist political prisoner); and German cultural ties between the two men. Bonds between chief doctors and prisoner secretaries could also be reinforced by their common capacity to adapt to bureaucracy.

Wirths's conflicts and character traits made him vulnerable to influence from "a powerful personality" (in Dr. Tadeusz S.'s words) such as Langbein, and the latter consistently utilized the relationship to better the situation of inmates in general and of the Communist prisoner underground in particular. The relationship enabled Wirths to retain a humane sense of himself. Langbein and a few other inmates (including Karl Lill, who remembered the incident after the war) apparently had a sufficiently warm relationship with Wirths and his wife to come into their home in Auschwitz during the time the family was living there, and play "horsies" [*Reitpferdchen*] with two of their small children. Despite their very different situations, both Wirths and Langbein probably experienced a sense of shared struggle within a death-saturated environment.[13]

The emotional conflicts in Wirths we shall shortly discuss were clear to prisoners around him, as was his strong desire at times to leave the place. Langbein and others tried to dissuade him from doing so on several occasions, and pointed always to the good he had done for prisoners as contrasted with the fearful uncertainty of a potential replacement. These efforts culminated in a Christmas card Langbein arranged to have hand-lettered for Wirths and delivered by a camp messenger. The card included two lines from Franz Grillparzer, the Viennese nineteenth-century dramatist, which read:

> One human life, alas, is so little,
> One human fate, however, is so much!

There followed: "In the past year you have saved here the lives of 93,000 people. We do not have the right to tell you our wishes. But we wish for ourselves that you stay here in the coming year." The card was signed: "One speaking for the prisoners of Auschwitz." Knowing that Wirths "was not able to escape the influence of the murderous atmosphere at Auschwitz," Langbein feared "that he [Wirths] might get discouraged," and wrote the card in order to encourage him to stay and continue measures on behalf of inmates. The figure of 93,000 was drawn from the difference in mortality rate among prisoners in 1943 as compared with that during the summer of 1942.[14]

The relationship between Wirths and Langbein could not escape the Auschwitz paradox operating in all such relatively humane relationships between prisoners (including prisoner doctors) and the SS: while contributing to the saving of many lives, it helped the SS doctor adapt to his central function within the death factory.

Prisoner Doctors' Recollections

Most prisoner doctors and other inmates who had contact with Wirths remembered him favorably, and he had directly saved the lives of several. Dr. Tadeusz S., for instance, admitted that his views were colored by "personal feelings" because Wirths saved him on two occasions, once from the punishment bunker which usually meant death. He characterized Wirths accurately as "very intellectual . . . and broadly cultivated, unlike the other SS people who were primitive, but . . . a Nazi ideologist . . . who did not like the methods of the gas chamber, . . . [who] wanted the Nazis to win but not in this way. . . . Surely a Nazi in spirit but not a cruel one."

Dr. Wanda J., installed by Wirths as head of Block 10, was grateful both for his sponsorship and protection and because "everything I asked Wirths to do he agreed." That patronage had saved her from the bunker as well and had helped her to save a number of young women by keeping them on her block as "maids." Her ultimate judgment of him had to be ambivalent: "He was a Nazi . . . from head to toe [as well as] a criminal . . . because he was choosing women . . . and men for the gas." Yet he had saved her life: "I must say that toward me he behaved like a gentleman."

Another prisoner doctor was aware of Wirths as a man "from a decent family, who had some moral fiber," and described his having been given the nickname of "Dr. Unblutig" (Dr. Unbloody), after the trademark of a corn-plaster product showing an old white-haired doctor urging that corn plaster be used in place of surgery. The nickname could imply killing without bloodying one's own hands, but this prisoner doctor felt that it had more to do with Wirths's personal mildness and constructive efforts in a "bloody" environment.

Wirths cultivated friendly relationships with certain inmates. Dr. Tadeusz S. told of appearing at Wirths's office to bring some reports and of Wirths continuing to dictate letters to family members in which he expressed sympathy toward prisoners and unhappiness about the war: "He wanted me to listen to those letters." Dr. S. believed that, in addition to "wanting to be liked," Wirths was thinking ahead about what his personal situation would be after Germany's defeat.

Langbein described a power reversal in these relationships during the last year of the war. In mid-1944, a BBC broadcast, making use of information provided by the Auschwitz underground, included Wirths's name on a list of Nazi officers involved in the murder apparatus and passed a death sentence on them. Aware from documents that it was the time of his wife's birthday, Langbein, after discussing the matter with underground colleagues, arranged for flowers (acquired by inmates who did gardening) as well as a painting of her and the children (done by a prisoner artist from a photograph) to be delivered to the chief doctor. The next day, Langbein explained to Wirths that the gift, and especially the family picture, "is to show that the death sentence has been revoked," and added, "I'm not saying this on my own." It was the underground's way of declaring its presence to him at an appropriate time. Langbein later recalled that he had written, "Now you are our tool, Chief physician!" But beyond their wish to increase their final influence over him, Langbein and his friends also wished to establish a process that could lead to actually saving the lives of Wirths and his family.[15]

In late 1944 or early 1945, Karl Lill—a Czech Communist who, with Langbein, served as Wirths's prisoner secretary—sent a note to Wirths (which Lill later described in a letter to Wirths's father) asking the chief doctor to prevent a Nazi plan (that Lill and others had heard of and that actually did exist), originating in the Political Department, to kill all prisoners. Again with a combination of threat and compassion, Lill declared that, if Wirths were to stay and help, it could then be concluded that "in this unprecedented morass one man, a German officer of the Waffen SS, acted like a human being until the end"; he urged Wirths not to waiver: "For your and your family's and a far mightier One's [meaning God's] sake." In another letter Lill told how, at their last meeting, Wirths urged him "with tearful eyes" to join the prisoners' evacuation because he was convinced that should Lill remain in Auschwitz the Russians would kill him.[16] At that point Wirths's emotions were undoubtedly affected by his own confusion, guilt, and anxiety about the future.

Experimental Research

But prisoners' views of Wirths depended upon their individual vantage points, and some were extremely critical of him, especially of his experimental research.

Wirths's main research concerned pre-cancerous growths of the cervix (the outer portion of the uterus). It involved, first, use of a then-new instrument, the colposcope, which was inserted through the vagina, so that the cervix could be viewed first in its natural state, and then after the application of certain substances (acetic acid and an iodized compound). When certain changes were observed (questionable cases were to be considered positive), the cervix was surgically removed and sent to his brother's laboratory in Hamburg-Altona (under the supervision of Hinselmann, Wirths's old professor and one of the first doctors to use the colposcope) where the tissue was studied for pre-cancerous growths. Wirths's brother, an already noted gynecologist, was involved in the work, and since he did the surgery and held demonstrations for others, was considered by some inmates to be its initiator.[17]

While, as Dr. Marie L. explained, "at first sight this experiment appear[ed] relatively harmless," that turned out to be far from the case: the colposcopic examination was unreliable; moreover, it was unnecessary to remove the entire cervix (a biopsy could have been done); and the poor condition of Auschwitz inmates made for many complications, including infections and hemorrhages, some of which either caused deaths or else left patients sufficiently debilitated to be selected for the gas chamber. This prisoner doctor was later to declare that Wirths's project "equals the other experiments in its arbitrary nature and utter contempt . . . [and] originate[s] . . . from Nazi minds without scruples."

Several survivor physicians condemned Wirths to me for the killing of Dr. Samuel, the Jewish surgeon who combined pathos and arrogance in his close collaboration with Wirths and other SS doctors under the illusion that it would enable him and his daughter to survive (see pages 250–53). Both were killed, and Samuel's death in particular has been looked upon as a betrayal on the part of Wirths in either giving the order or acceding to it. Thus Dr. Jan W. insisted, "The liquidation of Dr. Samuel said something about his [Wirths's] character because Samuel collaborated with him for quite a long time, and he made use of Samuel's knowledge."

Langbein condemned Wirths's typhus experiments, which resulted in two fatalities; and it was, in fact, the chief doctor's secretary who made this surreptitious episode more widely known (see pages 291–92).[18]

As physician survivors evaluated the larger Auschwitz experience, their view of Wirths tended to become more critical. Dr. Wanda J., despite being protected by him, spoke of him as having been "more clever" than the other SS doctors in that "he never did [anything] with his [own] hands, but always ordered somebody to do [things] for him. He never operated himself, . . . never did . . . anything . . . not injections, nothing." When Dr. J. concluded, "I have to say to you that he was probably as bad as the other ones," it was with a touch of reluctance. Dr. Jan W. was less reluctant to declare, "From the formal point of view, Wirths was responsible for everything that happened in [the medical sections of] the camp from September 1942 until the end of the camp's existence, so he must have accepted, ideologically, everything that went on in the camp. . . . Millions were destroyed."

A "Correct" Bureaucrat

Wirths combined bureaucratic skill with a quality of "correctness" (a concept of proper, controlled, relatively impersonal behavior that infuses German culture and character) and reliability in ways that enabled him to help inmates while succeeding within the SS. His organizational loyalty was always clear to other SS observers. Ernst B. looked upon him as little more than a representative of Nazi authority, a man one would do well to stay away from because of his demanding "spirit of the bureaucrat." Rudolf Höss, observing Wirths more closely, spoke of him as a man with "a strong feeling of duty," who was "extremely conscientious and . . . obeyed all orders and directives with painstaking care." Also "correct" with inmates, the commandant went on, Wirths's only fault was frequently to be "very soft and good natured" with them and to treat prisoner physicians "as colleagues." But he was "a good comrade . . . very popular"; he "helped everyone who came to him," and "everybody trusted him."[19]

For "everybody" to trust Wirths required that he largely accept the Auschwitz situation—as Höss implied in commenting that Wirths never objected to the use of an ambulance marked with a red cross to transport those selected for death to the gas chamber, despite the fact that he "was usually very sensitive about such matters." Indeed Wirths himself drove about in a car flying "a white pennant with a red cross."[20]

There is a similar implication in a comment made by Helmut Wirths, concerning a horrible scene of extremely emaciated corpses he and his brother had viewed outside of a medical block: "What really bothered me was his [Eduard's] telling me that these were the dead from natural causes." Wirths meant of course that they were not victims of the gas chamber or any other means of direct killing—but in calling *any* deaths in Auschwitz "natural," he was going quite far in his identification with the institution.

Wirths's ideological anti-Semitism contributed to his bureaucratic adaptation to Auschwitz. He could permit Jewish prisoner doctors to do more medical work, but said it would be "impossible" for them to treat any Aryans and insisted that the medical blocks be set up to prevent that from happening. His concept of the "correct" was probably involved here no less than his ideological anti-Semitism.

His bureaucratic integration also undoubtedly contributed to his typhus experiments. Langbein told me that he estimated Wirths's thought processes to be as follows: Typhus was still a problem for SS personnel; a new medication or serum had to be tested; and since there were no typhus cases at that time in Auschwitz: "These are anyhow only Jews, they would die in any case, but now I can try out a drug [on them] which could be important for many [German] people."[21]

Perhaps Wirths's organizational loyalty was most revealed when he invited Langbein to win his freedom by joining the SS. Wirths had been excited to learn that this policy, occasionally applied to Aryan prisoners, could be implemented with Langbein in a way that would permit him to continue the work he was doing in the camp, but from within the SS. Wirths was upset when Langbein gently refused ("His face los[t] its friendliness"); but upon hearing Langbein's explanation that since the inmates were his comrades, he would not be able to do the things SS men in Auschwitz were commanded to do, Wirths commented, "Your view does you honor," though sounding "a bit disappointed."[22]*

Selections

Selections were the crux of the matter—for Auschwitz as an institution, for its chief doctor, and for understanding Wirths's inner contradictions. Significantly, he was, at least initially, strongly opposed to selections in general and to doctors performing them. Höss noted this opposition to the mass killing of Jews, and Langbein referred to another SS officer who remembered Wirths telling him that the task of physicians was to treat patients and that selections were not a proper activity for them.[23]

But rather quickly Wirths found himself fighting hard to bring selections under the control of physicians, which meant under his control. A close friend and SS physician colleague later testified that, before the spring of 1943, selections were conducted by the camp commander and his subordinates; and that Wirths was convinced that they sent many people fit for work to the gas chambers and was at about that time able to arrange for physicians to take over (see also chapter 8).† The official

---

*What Wirths did not know was that the man he was recruiting for the SS was half-Jewish, a secret that Langbein (as he later explained) guarded carefully in the camp, since its becoming known could have greatly endangered him.

†This sequence resembles that of a physician I interviewed: a distinguished academic specialist who had displayed some courage in speaking out against experiments on human beings at a meeting of military physicians, only to take part (though in a somewhat indirect way) in such experiments later on. He had been politely summoned by Conti, with whom he had a "fair discussion," during which his superior apparently convinced him of the importance of the experiments for saving the lives of German soldiers. He too had the need to remain loyal to the tasks put forward by the Nazi project, while clinging to the belief he could improve upon what was being done by participating in it.

policy (set by Berlin) of doctors performing selections had been, as in the case of many such policies, largely ignored in Auschwitz. Wirths could demonstrate his bureaucratic correctness in insisting that Auschwitz adhere to established policy. Moreover, as Dr. B emphasized, control over selections was an important source of power in the camp, and Wirths consolidated his own power by having physicians conduct them. In accepting both motivations, one must also say that Wirths's advocacy was *a way of insisting that killing be medicalized.* This advocacy parallels the slogan mentioned in connection with direct medical killing, or "euthanasia": "Let the syringe remain in the hand of the physician."

Wirths also insisted upon taking his own personal turn in doing selections, rather than merely delegating them to physician subordinates. The attitude was one Langbein "respected to a certain degree," in that Wirths refused to shirk what was generally considered an onerous task.[24] Here Wirths's attitude, as the "humane doctor" combating primitives, was in effect: "Let the syringe be in *my* hand. If anyone kills, let it be me as well." Once more conscience gave way to conscientiousness, and saving lives became associated with killing.

More than just asserting medical control of selections, Wirths became their organizing authority, their "responsible person." It was he who discussed with SS leaders whether camp needs dictated higher or lower percentages of transports selected for the gas chamber; or whether more people should be selected for death from within the camp in order to diminish overcrowding and the danger of epidemics. And it was he who was responsible for policies during selections (again probably on the basis of discussions with camp leaders as well as with other doctors), such as whether or at what point mothers and children should be separated from one another, etc.

Thus, when large numbers of Hungarian Jews began arriving in Auschwitz, it was Wirths who exerted pressures on the SS doctors from the Hygienic Institute to select, even though that was not part of their camp assignment. He also (with Mengele) pressured a reluctant Franz Lucas (see pages 194–95) to select and brought him to the ramp so that he could participate in his first large selection, which Wirths himself conducted. Not only did he angrily rebuke Lucas for subsequent efforts at avoidance, but he threatened the dentist Dr. Willi Frank, who also showed some recalcitrance, with the principles of "Führer order," of equivalence to front-line duty, and of refusal as desertion. And on another occasion, Wirths berated a subordinate for reluctance to remove fillings from corpses "during the fifth year of war!"[25]*

While lacking Mengele's flair and posturing, Wirths was himself a commanding figure at selections. Tall and "Aryan-looking," he was described

*Even Wirths's once taking the reverse attitude and saying—of a noncommissioned officer who objected to participating in selections—"At last a person with character!" is another example of his extraordinary capacity to manage inner contradiction in Auschwitz.

by one survivor as "the most handsome of all in his uniform." Wirths too had a sense of his SS bearing, so that, the same survivor tells us, he always "exaggerated his own perfection [in contrast to] the riffraff down there."[26] In other words, Wirths's dignified, authoritative demeanor gave a certain legitimacy, even "grandeur" to the selections.

Wirths's control of selections ultimately controlled him. Dr. Tadeusz S. told me of a revealing incident in which he and Langbein intervened with Wirths after Entress had selected two thousand Jewish patients for the gas chambers. They argued that the patients were healthy and could do good work for Germany. "Wirths was close to crying," and helped Dr. S. to arrange for first eighteen hundred, and finally even the last two hundred, to remain alive. But a few days later, Wirths selected two thousand other people in a different subcamp. Dr. S. concluded: "That was his way of legitimating his work for his bosses, but not in front of Langbein and myself, which was very characteristic . . . for his behavior." Wirths strongly resisted seeing himself (and having others see him) as one who participated in killing. But in fact he did participate in killing, while diligently overseeing the entire killing structure.

What selections epitomized—Wirths's participation and entrapment in the healing-killing paradox—applied to his entire Auschwitz experience.

Personal Experience: Love Letters, Family, and Home

In addition to others' observations on Wirths's behavior, important evidence about what he was *experiencing* at the time, psychologically and morally, is provided both by documents—his own letters to his wife and his father, and his apologia at the end—and by family members who observed him closely.

Like most Nazi doctors, Wirths underwent conflict in Auschwitz but adapted sufficiently to do his work there. A tortured man who efficiently ran the Auschwitz system of medicalized killing, he was remarkable for both the intensity of his conflict and the murderous significance of his work. His doubling, while certainly extreme, was also significantly different from that of other SS doctors, in that there coexisted within him not so much an Auschwitz self and a prior self as two contending Auschwitz selves. On the one hand, he was a loyal and dedicated Nazi with a profound commitment to Nazi versions of the German state and the Germanic race; on the other, a staunch advocate of medical humanity and improved conditions for prisoners. His Nazi-Germanic self committed him to loyal participation in the Auschwitz project; his physician-humanitarian self rendered him a prisoners' advocate. He had to keep the two selves separate from one another, even as he tried desperately to unite them. The wonder—and the general misfortune—is not that his internal structure eventually broke down but rather that it held together for so long.

To an extraordinary extent, Wirths's capacity for any psychological
equilibrium depended upon his ties to close family members, especially
to his wife. She and their first three children, then very young, were with
him in Auschwitz for some months, perhaps almost a year, in late 1943
through September 1944. Before and after that time, over the remainder
of his two-and-a-half years in Auschwitz, he wrote frequent long letters
to her, letters that were passionate, imploring, and often desperate. He
invested his wife and children—and that part of himself bound to them
—with a quality of absolute purity and goodness. And he clung to that
purity and goodness with the special intensity of a man being consumed
by evil.

In his first letter, written on 7 September 1942, just a day after his
arrival in Auschwitz, he immediately connects his love and duty toward
wife and family with his work in Auschwitz. Referring to the "superhuman" task he must accomplish there, he says that all he does is "for you,
my life, my heart, for you and the children"; and that "nothing is impossible as long as I have you, my beloved." Indeed, he renders his Auschwitz
task an immortalizing project: dealing with a "wild country that requires
much work to be done, much German spirit, energy, and German work."
It will be the work "of pioneers, not easy, but it must be done for our
children, my angel, for our children."[27]

He struggles to suppress initial shock and horror and quickly invokes
destiny and duty. He associates her "immensely great love" with the
"protective inoculations" he requires for the assignment.[28] That is, their
love is to inoculate him against what he sees and does at Auschwitz.

And once the ordeal is over, "then we will be allowed to be true only
to ourselves, my love, and this will be worth the trouble."[29] At that time,
he will have earned the full joy of their love by completing this Auschwitz
responsibility. *Auschwitz becomes associated with an ennobling sense of German
mission on behalf of the absolute purity of his wife and children, an immortal mission
on behalf of the future.*

In subsequent letters, he pours out an endless series of endearments,
including every kind of diminutive of her name: "most beloved wife,"
"dear soul," "you my whole heart," "beloved little treasure," "little
birdy," "little Father Christmas," and "Almighty One." His intensity is
accompanied by a certain formality of structure (confirmed by German
readers): his endearments are absolute, but his style and phrasing are far
from uninhibited. The endearments are accompanied by, and in fact
greatly contribute to, his struggle for control.

During the last half of 1943, a major theme in his letters is his joyful
anticipation of his family's joining him in Auschwitz. Emanating from the
death camp is an almost coy tone of preparation as he describes the
removal of piles of débris and the ruins of an old cellar, and tells his wife
that "for the last two days a large *Kommando* has been working in our
garden," and that he has found an architect "who makes very nice draw-

ings [and] good suggestions."[30] In later letters he looks forward to the roof being put on, the floor being laid, the windows installed, a special plan for the garden; and still later, with the tone of a thoughtful bourgeois husband, he mentions his purchase of "2 whiskbrooms, 1 meat-pounder, 1 children's table, 4 matching chairs, a little footstool, a hobbyhorse." He speaks of feeling "embarrassed" by all the preparations necessary for the house—in regard not to Auschwitz victims but to other SS doctors because three of them have to team up in a single house.[31]

When he writes of his "request to erect the fence soon because of the children,"[32] one wonders how high the fence was to be: only high enough to keep the children in, or much higher so that little or nothing could be seen of the Auschwitz world outside?

He refers delicately to his sexual longing and aims his one expression of violence at anyone who would take house, happiness, and beloved from him ("I would bash in his skull"). It is striking how far he has removed their relationship from his Auschwitz world as he inquires tenderly about her condition, urges her to do the prescribed exercises, and expresses concern about what was apparently a postpartum depression (after the birth of their fourth child) in which she spoke of dying.[33]

Ever the family man, there is exuberant mention of pictures of the children, of the appearance of the first tooth in one of them, and of prayerful concern about his mother-in-law's health. As if to preserve and contrast that family purity, he speaks of "a disgusting fellow" who has impregnated a woman and refuses to marry her.[34]

A touch of tension emerges as Wirths's wife seems to resist moving to Auschwitz; and apparently referring to her requirements, he explains that it would be impossible to remove the "dirt and disorder" even after the house has been finished. He then quotes a slightly bitter little joke: a comment by his friend Horst Fischer that the house would be ready "probably only when the war is over,"[35] a joke that turned out to have its own prophetic truth. Their daughter later suggested that, in spite of these urgings, "he did not want her [his wife] to be dragged into this." The Auschwitz side of their relationship was problematic to both, and Wirths's wife later claimed that, when there witnessing her husband's pain at performing selections, she wished to leave but did not because of being told by a confidant that her presence was crucial "if you want to save your husband."[36] Each was ambivalent about being there, and about the other's being there. But he stayed, and she came.

After she has finally left, there is patter about family events and rituals and much about the vicissitudes of his dogs: Basco who "escapes" through a passage created by a bomb crater under a fence; then a second dog "I just had to acquire"; and still a third. And when the two new acquisitions become ill, "my little room at home is . . . a sick ward." In late November 1944, in the midst of German military disaster, he refers to the goose he has been raising to send to her for Christmas as "fat and big."[37] His tone moves back and forth between that of a rural landowner and a boy away from home rhapsodizing about the delicious cake sent to him.

Finally, in December 1944 and January 1945, his gifts to her become more practical: a "dynamo flashlight," which he tells her how to use, along with other emergency equipment; but also a bottle of champagne as well as hard-to-get food and oil. He asks her to send him his ski boots (for skiing—or for fleeing the advancing Allied armies?).[38]

Now fearful about the future, he nonetheless speaks of the "good pineapple punch" at his quiet New Year's Eve dinner at the home of Richard Baer (Liebehenschel's replacement as commandant), pours out his love with added intensity, along with mounting anxiety ("I can only sincerely implore the Almighty to let me keep our happiness . . . to preserve us for us!"). And with the Russians approaching, his main concern is that he is unable to get through to her by telephone. Now there are suggestions of death imagery from both sides as he implores (probably in response to her depressed thoughts): "Really, you must not leave me, my all," and adds, "I . . . almost have to die with love and pain of longing."[39] With everything collapsing, he clings to a still more totalized love and family immersion to buttress his threatened existence.

In a mid-January letter he drifts into a fantasy of future arrangements for their rural German home: a consulting room separate from living quarters "so that you are less bothered," the telephone placed in the hall with an extension line under the bedroom door. While he seems to be wishing away his plight, he is sufficiently focused on it to go into hiding. On 24 May, after the surrender, he begins to express "my greatest guilt" —not to Auschwitz victims but to his wife and children for having led them "into misery and situations of want." Auschwitz is there but fended off in a claim of moral ignorance: "What is it that I have perpetrated? I do not know." And in early July, from Hamburg, a similar theme, but now restated to suggest he is being persecuted because of the very strength of his love: "Is it a sin that I love you so much . . . ? Has it been hubris that I long for you, my all, my life, and that I bound your fate to mine at any price?" In all this—at least in what he writes to her—Auschwitz is either ignored or at most is no more than an unfortunate source of their pain. In his last letter to her, written on 15 July 1945, he reasserts their love as conquering the death he now anticipates even as that love displaces conscience: "The essence of our life . . . a love that glorifies, understands, knows and overcomes everything."[40]

In Auschwitz too his family had shielded him from everything else. He had written in December 1944 that "when you and the little ones were with me in Au[schwitz], one could feel nothing of the war!"[41] We can be certain that "war" included Auschwitz itself. When enmeshed in family love, that is, Wirths needed feel nothing of killing.

His daughter, whose earliest memories are of Auschwitz, recalled his playing warmly with the children and being "always terribly kind to us."

Reflecting back on the situation as an adult, she spoke of "these two worlds, his family and this . . . job of his." She felt that his family "was the only thing that kept him going," and that "he desperately needed his family there to keep his sanity." There were certainly problems for Wirths and his wife when she was there: according to Kremer, a confidant of Wirths viewed him as a man who "had all sorts of trouble with his wife and children."[42] There was always a conflict between his "having his job there and his family who weren't supposed to notice anything." Of course, with his family present, he was able to notice less of Auschwitz. While it is also probably true that there were moments when their presence intensified his awareness of his killing function, even then he could, as we have seen, deflect the target of his potential guilt onto his family, especially to his wife for exposing her to such a place.

Over time, Auschwitz became a kind of home for Wirths, even a sanctuary. Only at Auschwitz could he live with his wife and children, at least for a time; only there could they have a "family home." Commenting on his "sniffling and coughing" in the cold of the camp in late November, he once wrote: "In summer one ought to live in Auschwitz, but in autumn and winter one ought to be at home." In the same letter, he expressed sadness that "a piece of wild romantic life" near Auschwitz would be lost because of the reconstruction of a riverbed.[43]

He maintained his own domesticity in Auschwitz and wrote sadly to his wife of the death of their dog Basco, who "suffered a lot so I gave him Mo [morphine]," adding, "It is good that he died; he was in the end blind in both eyes."[44] If one asks how it was possible for Wirths to describe that incident without in any way associating it with Auschwitz selections, the answer is that the psychological function of his "euthanasia" of the dog provided an alternative source of moral concern and thereby increased his numbing toward selections.

And about two weeks before the appearance of Soviet troops, he invoked Auschwitz's advantages as a way of sympathizing with his wife's sense of isolation: "You are right, my love, that here one is in the midst of life, and that you at home . . . can gather no experiences." He then urged her to "come again to me in Auschwitz when the Soviet offensive has ended."[45] He had also written to his brother Helmut to come to Auschwitz "because it would be more [safe] than in Hamburg." While there was geographical and military truth to that claim (Hamburg was largely destroyed by Allied bombing, and Auschwitz hardly touched), the psychological theme is that of the perpetrators' sense of sanctuary in the place where they have been wielding absolute power over life and death.

Father and Younger Brother

Other family members, especially his father and his younger brother, were also of great importance to Wirths in connection with Auschwitz. The latter, encountering Wirths in Berlin soon after the latter had arrived in Auschwitz, remembered him saying that he had "seen such terrible things, things that were unimaginable, [that he could] never go home again and look into the eyes of [his] children." Eduard told his brother of dreadful scenes of thousands of dead bodies lying in shallow ditches, but said nothing at the time about selections.

We know that Helmut Wirths later went to Auschwitz to collaborate with his brother on cancer experiments. But although Eduard did want help with the cancer studies, Helmut later stressed (possibly partly for reasons of self-exculpation) that he went less for that reason than to offer him personal support: "I knew of his immense misery": "My personal view is that my brother didn't want . . . me there for those materials [the research] . . . [but] only needed . . . a human being to speak with." Helmut said "[At least at first] I admired him [because] I would not have been able to do it [stay at Auschwitz and perform selections]. . . . I would have run amok."

There was a painful interplay in Auschwitz between the two brothers concerning selections. Eduard asked Helmut to accompany him to selections, for the ostensible purpose of seeing the full horror of the place. Helmut, who by this time had learned what they were, said he just could not do that. Since, when Eduard had talked about leaving Auschwitz, Helmut and their father had urged him to remain and do whatever good there he could, he now replied angrily, "You tell me I have to stay here [and be here] every day, and you will not [come even] one time to see [a selection]." Later Eduard (according to Helmut) said that he did not really want to take him there but just wished to see if he would agree to go with him. That kind of confused exchange could well have occurred, though many other things were undoubtedly said. One suspects not that Eduard was determined to leave, but rather that he stressed to his brother and father, almost petulantly, the negative side of his ambivalence about staying, and in so doing could also deflect the Auschwitz problem and place it on family psychological terrain.

Helmut, who had planned to stay about two weeks, said that he left after only a few days because he was so revolted by the place. He described getting into difficulty with an SS officer when the latter, at the casino the first night, asked him how he liked their *Sommerfrische* (vacation; literally, "summer air"), and he angrily answered, "Shame on you to say such a thing in this place!" According to Helmut, Eduard had to calm the situation, and shortly after advised his brother to leave.

Helmut has confirmed that he and his father did urge Eduard to remain there, and claimed that they thought that he could help people by doing so—"but it was theoretical," Helmut added regretfully, meaning that the advice did not take into account the concrete horrors of Auschwitz.

Their father's advice to Eduard to remain undoubtedly had great weight. We know the father to have been a demanding but respected patriarchal figure, and Eduard to have been the older son who almost always obeyed and followed the straight and narrow path. The father, who had visited Eduard first in Dachau and then in Auschwitz, later described the latter visit in uneasy, defensive terms. He remembered seeing prisoners who seemed to be "semi-free," and two young Jewish women working in his son's office who were "basically cheerful," and noted of inmates that "in the morning they went out singing and came back at night singing"; he claimed to have learned only later on that "they *had* to sing!" Even after coming to understand much of the truth of Auschwitz, including "how the people died there of . . . sicknesses and . . . were exterminated," he declared to his son, "There is no place in the whole world where you can do as much good as in Auschwitz. Endure."[46]

Whatever good they hoped Eduard could achieve in Auschwitz and whatever their own relationship to Nazi ideology, his brother and father were caught up in the same German commitments to duty and obedience that affected Eduard himself. Their advice gave his Auschwitz stay a family sanction, and at the same time furthered the kind of moral displacement we have been discussing: the issue became more a struggle with family values and family obedience and less with Auschwitz mass murder.

Moral Crusade: Rectitude and Compromise

Important to Wirths's adjustment in Auschwitz was his sense of being on a continuing moral crusade. The purpose of the crusade could be amorphous—the transformation of the primitive Auschwitz environment with "German work"—but was always in the context of war and survival ("Yes there is war, and it is a hard, the hardest, time"). His crusade could become more concrete, and more inwardly credible, when it focused on a version of "medical humanity." In his apologia, he speaks of "my difficult struggle," which was against disease and especially typhus epidemics, and on behalf of better medical care for prisoners, including accurate medical reports depicting true conditions at Auschwitz, expanded facilities and improved equipment and supplies, utilization of a division of Jewish prisoner doctors, replacing brutal ordinary criminals with more decent political prisoners, eliminating fatal phenol injections on the medical blocks and cutting down on selections there, and bringing about a significant decline in the death rate among those living in the camp. The Auschwitz command's frequent opposition to him gave this crusade further meaning for him, as did the slogan "Manpower" [*Arbeitskräfte*] he claimed to have stressed. In his apologia, he went so far as to claim that he was doing God's work (he had "a sign from above [that] I should and must fight on") in preserving Jews, and that "it probably can be credited to me that Jews are alive in Europe at all today."[47]

One reason Wirths could almost believe this was that *in his feelings* he did oppose—as was known to Höss and others—the very mass killing of Jews he supervised. On 29 November 1944, Wirths wrote to his wife: "Can you imagine, my dear, how wonderful it is that I am no longer

forced to do this terrible work, yes, that it no longer exists."* In correspondence with his parents, he corrects the elder Wirths's mistaken impression that he, Eduard, had been actually responsible for the changes,
but does relate his personal crusade to their achievement ("I pointed out
at every opportunity that offered itself to me . . . the inhumanity, impossibility and genuine indignity of the whole procedure"). His way of doing
so was to stress how "they [those advocating the killing] have burdened
. . . our entire people, . . . particularly at the time of such a terrible war"[48]
—an approach that met with acceptable Nazi standards of opposition as
well as his own loyalties. He could still, however, understand his crusade
to be on behalf of family and future—that is, on behalf of his "decent
self."

His crusade, then, was on behalf of maintaining acceptable standards
within the Nazi movement. It could extend to such petty matters as telling
a man on the medical staff under his command (as Wirths describes in
a letter to his wife), that if he does well in a course he was leaving to take,
he would get fourteen days of special leave, while adding that along his
travels this man would purchase some wool, a valuable wartime commod-
ity, and bring it to her[49] (hardly a notable vice by Auschwitz standards,
but suggesting that Wirths was not above bending his rectitude slightly
in order to please her).

His sense of moral crusade was significantly maintained in the struggle
against Grabner and the Auschwitz Gestapo. Here he could denounce
their corruption and "illegalities" in murdering and foisting their murders on his unit. Within the Auschwitz structure, his crusade against
Grabner might well have demanded a certain real courage, but it also had
the enormous psychological value to Wirths as a crusade against evil as
symbolized by Grabner.

Wirths's combination of rectitude and compromise enabled him to feel
relatively comfortable in Auschwitz. From the beginning, he pitted "only
one thing, the straight path," against the ultimate corruptions of Auschwitz. In terms of personal arrangements, he could say, "I asked for nothing," and reveled in his friend Horst Fischer's reassurance that he deserved the house being built for him and everything else: "If I hadn't
created [what I have] here, Auschwitz would not be . . . what it is now."[50]

Yet it is Wirths who complained of Fischer's rectitude, seeing him as
"always straightforward and honest, thus making some things difficult
for himself and me"—rather than doing things "diplomatically," which
meant making compromises even as one "keep[s] to one's straight path."
Wirths's development of his Auschwitz self enabled him to adjust to the
camp, to (in Helmut's words) "g[e]t used to it." (Wirths could still claim
rectitude for his Auschwitz self by taking such stands as objecting—in
early January 1945, with the Russian armies close—to nurses living in the

*This was the time when, with Russian troops approaching and most available Jews
already killed, a decision was made to stop large selections in anticipation of closing the
camp.

officers' club after having been bombed out of their own quarters: "The proximity of the men there is no good at all.")[51]

When in hiding after the war's end, Wirths's crusade took the form of mobilizing relatives and friends to look out for his family. And as he began to sense that his existence as a fugitive was his family's greatest burden (his only future being trial, conviction, and death), his suicide can be viewed as the final act in his crusade.

A Loyal Nazi

Whatever his conflicts connected with that crusade, Wirths never ceased to be a leading figure and a respected physician within the Auschwitz SS subculture.

In a letter to his wife of 27 November 1944, he gushes his pleasure ("Isn't this a fine thing. I want to kiss you, my love with my deeply felt love.") at 599 men being decorated with the Iron Cross because of their "bravery"[52]—referring, it turns out, to the revolt of the *Sonderkommando*, during which one crematorium was set on fire and a hand grenade was thrown into an SS group; the revolt was quickly put down by SS troops whose bravery consisted of slaughtering everyone remotely suspected of having participated in it.* His letters are full of newsy references to gala social occasions: a special dinner in the *Führerhaus* for department heads, with half a wild duck for each; a hunt in early January 1945, where he shot six hares and was permitted to keep one ("You, my all, get that one tomorrow"); a Christmas party in 1944 at which a talented SS sergeant sang "As a Small Boy at the Mother's Breast" (*Als Knäblein klein an der Mutter Brust*) and included a comic sequence of Santa Claus bestowing on Wirths "[not] a medal but a liverwurst" (suggesting that the good physician was a sufficiently important member of the group to be made an object of affectionate fun); and lunches and dinners at the home of Baer, the commandant with whom he was friendly—to the point of becoming the mediator in the Baers' extreme marital discord.[54]

He in fact remained a committed Nazi throughout—one who, as Helmut Wirths pointed out, really believed that "the Jews were a danger to Germany"; who supported Hitler's 1939 warning that if the Jews began a war they, not Germany, would be destroyed; and who could say of the arriving Hungarian Jews during the summer of 1944, "They are the worst of them." Helmut went on to explain that [Eduard] believed in National Socialism . . . [but] never believed that Hitler himself could know [about the killing of the Jews]"—and that Eduard would tell Helmut, "I must try to go to Hitler [and tell him about this]. He *can't* know . . . [about these]

---

*Filip Müller, a prisoner eyewitness, described how "about 450 of our comrades . . . had fought bravely and died honorably, refusing to resign themselves meekly to their fate. . . . A few SS men had died, a few more had been wounded. . . . It became known later that when awarding the Iron Cross to several SS men the *Lagercommandant* had mentioned that this was the first time concentration camp guards had prevented a mass break-out, a feat of bravery for which their *Führer* had decorated them."[53]

cruelties." Helmut said that until the end his brother "believed [in] Hitler as a good man" and "couldn't believe that they [the Nazis] wouldn't win."

Earlier, Wirths had shown Langbein a plan for extensive expansion of Auschwitz "after the victory." Langbein commented that Wirths "feared a defeat of National Socialism even though he had become familiar with its true face at Auschwitz more clearly than anybody else"; Wirths held to the Führer's ignorance about the extermination camps because "he probably needed this [thought] construction in order to justify for himself his membership in the National Socialist movement." When Langbein, in their last conversation toward the end, stated that the war had been completely lost, Wirths said, "That's horrible," and when Langbein said, "That's good, doctor," Wirths responded, "How can you say that? You're a German too."[55]

In his apologia, Wirths exaggerated his alienation from others in the Auschwitz hierarchy and the degree to which he took "refuge in . . . illness." His heart and kidney problems did undoubtedly intensify under the stress of his conflicts, and we know that actual antagonisms with other SS officers led him to suggest to Höss that he wished to be transferred,[56] though he apparently never made anything on the order of an all-out effort to leave. His later claim that he "worked for the Polish Resistance . . . movement" is a falsehood built upon the tiniest kernel of truth (his having worked supportively with Poles and others whom he suspected or knew were part of the Resistance); and his probably accurate claim that toward the end he was accused by the Gestapo of "demoralization of the people," when he made a statement that the German armies could no longer resist, was the kind of experience Karl Brandt also had (see footnote on page 115) and one typical for a "decent Nazi" at the end.[57]

And though he went into hiding after the surrender, he held to his duty virtually to the end, long after others (like Mengele) had fled. He could thus write to his wife on 13 January 1945, with considerable truth (defending himself against negative allegations made by Grabner): "I can say that I have always done my duty and have never done anything contrary to what was expected of me."[58]

Wirths's Medical Self

Beyond his crusade from within and his Nazi loyalties, Wirths adapted to Auschwitz by clinging to the sense of himself as a physician. The healing image of the physician helped him deny his and other Auschwitz physicians' actual killing. He could attribute that killing to "the camp authorities" who, he wrote in his apologia, would appear secretly "without notifying the physician or at times when one knew the physician was absent, or at night" and then have "the sick and weak removed from camp in order to kill them with poison gas." In defending that falsehood, Wirths articulated the healing-killing paradox with exquisite accuracy: "It was insane that people whom one has saved through the efforts and art of the physicians [though he did not here credit prisoner physicians], who because of treatment, improvement in diet, personal hygiene, etc. were now forcibly killed."[59] Because a part of him, as a physician, opposed the process, he could see himself as one combating the killing, even while actually orchestrating it.*

He could thus later claim that he had acted in accordance with his "Christian and medical conscience" and that "my work as a physician was purely that of offering care": "I took the point of view that I was employed in Auschwitz only as a physician and could not act contrary to my conscience."[60] While the absurdity of these claims are partly a function of his immediate postwar desperation, they also reflect an actual self-image of a man who understood himself to have struggled to maintain his medical conscience.

No wonder he conveyed such excitement in announcing to his wife (on 23 July 1943), "Just think, I have come up with an entirely new delousing preparation, already tried it out on 500 people, and with excellent and above all 100% success"; he added, "I hope to have a degree of success in this respect such as the world has never seen before [so that] in one fell swoop I could do away with all of the typhus and above all, my little one, nobody has helped me with it . . . on the contrary." Now he is a lonely medical spirit who can point to a real epidemiological achievement, even if because "it is done with a strong poison it is naturally not without danger."[61] The delousing preparation was cyanide gas, or Zyklon-B.

We can understand why he found it important to hold an "office hour" for SS families, and to serve as marriage counselor and personal advisor to them. He was a healer among them, even if (as he later claimed with some truth) they looked upon him suspiciously as an unreliable intellectual and part of the "academic international"; he and they had a functional stance toward one another. Also understandable is the intensity of his involvement in work on a new military hospital, so that his greatest sadness in acknowledging to Langbein at the end that Germany had lost the war was that "the work on the [new SS] infirmary will have been totally in vain."[62]

By claiming for himself this stance as healer, Wirths could place his Block 10 experiments in the dignified and technical medical category of "colposcopic mass examinations of the uterus for early detection of cancer with the active support of Professor Dr. Hinselmann." He could even put a medical face on selections by claiming that he "demanded of the camp authorities that physicians would have to be consulted for a decision regarding the ability [of inmates] to work"—though adding (and thereby half acknowledging the killing element), "I had to burden the physicians subordinated to me with this terrible fact." His apologia also contains a visionary plan for "a large field hospital for sick prisoners with a capacity for 30,000–40,000 sick people" which would service other

---

*Wirths's apologia had the purpose of exculpation—he was trying to save his own life —and he was willing to bend the truth considerably to that purpose.

concentration camps as well and "eliminate the influence of the camp authorities." He did not say, of course, that those expanded medical facilities were part of the general Nazi vision of a vast expansion "after the victory" of Auschwitz killing and slave labor.[63]

There is a final key to the adaptive value of Wirths's medical self in his brother's characterization of him as "a good doctor" who "tried to do what he could do" on the assumption that "if anybody must be killed, . . . a doctor has to be a witness, . . . guilty or not." In the middle of death, even death he is bringing about, a healer has the noble function of bearing witness—because he is a healer.

Adapting to Evil

Wirths's pattern illuminates the crucial distinction between conflicts and actions: in the absence of a basic decision to change one's actions (cease doing selections, leave, etc.), the tendency is to absorb conflicts and mold them to one's adaptation. Wirths's depression and even his change in demeanor (according to his wife, from an outgoing, happy man to a deeply troubled and reclusive one) were a way of maintaining his adaptation—as, of course, was his opposite tendency, remembered by his daughter in Auschwitz, toward tenderness and gaiety with the children.

Reportedly somewhat depressed while in Dachau, then more so in Auschwitz, Wirths exclaimed to his brother Helmut, "How can I go on living?" After the war Wirths wrote of having been "so emotionally burdened that I saw suicide as the only way out of these grave conflicts of conscience [Gewissenskonflikten],"[64] but he implied that his psychic state was improved by being able to travel to Berlin and obtain permission for medically constructive steps in Auschwitz.

Wirths clearly experienced guilt feelings, a sense of self-condemnation, but his brother Helmut made it clear that those feelings of "not being able to live in peace with his conscience" were greatest "[at the] beginning and in the end"—as were all of his conflicts. During most of the time between, Wirths could see Auschwitz, as Helmut put it, as "a task" (the "crusade" for improvement I have spoken of). The messages of gratitude he received from prisoners also helped allay guilt; and even when he "fell into despair," as his brother put it, because he realized that Auschwitz evils were not diminishing but "became more and more," the despair was partial and by no means incapacitating.

His expressions of guilt toward the end were still ambiguous. In a letter to his parents, but particularly his father, of 13 December 1944, he declared, "The guilt cannot be denied" (including his own, we must assume), "but surely our people has atoned for much by its heroic conduct, by its immense sacrifices, particularly among women and children" (an expression of mitigation but also of retained loyalty not only to the German people but, we suspect, to their cause) "which in my opinion could have been avoided if one had stayed away from such things from the beginning"[65] (partial criticism of Nazi policy, especially perhaps of mass murder). And also affecting that kind of statement was his sense of other possible readers: prisoners to whom he wanted to convey opposition to Nazi excess, and Nazi authorities before whom he did not want to appear disloyal or treasonous. The letter too was a means of adaptation.

The letters to his wife at the end became more desperate because the adaptation could no longer be maintained: approaching Soviet and American troops were associated not only with danger to his life but with a kind of judgment day. He began to invoke God (his brother said that "he became a religious man in Auschwitz") and also wishful pictures of a quiet, harmonious family and medical future. Threatened with losing everything, his need to merge with his wife intensified ("I *only* live in you"). And, after leaving Auschwitz, his affirmation of his "good conscience before God and before man"[66] seems wish rather than conviction. He was then, in his brother's words, "completely broken, a man without hope," not only because Auschwitz had been his downfall but because he had lost the entire structure, including Auschwitz and the Nazi movement, to which he had been adapting. Only guilt toward his family was manageable, which is why he called it his "greatest guilt."[67]

During those last days, he questioned the behavior of his superiors in not having "the necessary courage" that might have enabled them to ease his situation. He was still a man with a crusade, now more tortured, this time to save his own life and his family's future (getting "the other side" to "understand . . . [the] strong constraints on me and all the things that . . . tormented my brain and still torment it"). He was also saying goodbye when he referred to himself as "your Eduard [who] wishes to live and fight only for you and the children and he will be here and with you, with God and you."[68]

In contemplating death, he came a little closer to exploring his Auschwitz behavior. He spoke of the suffering of their people "which had to come after all these years of evil." About himself he was more convoluted, acknowledging profound error and perhaps guilt but still justifying his behavior and invoking a guilt-denying form of religious resignation.[69]

Although his brother Helmut and others had offered to hide him longer, Wirths was apparently ready to go into British captivity in the hope, as he wrote, that "the way I have now begun is righteous in the eyes of God and of my conscience."[70] The apologia he composed at the time for presentation to Allied authorities was, as we have seen, a mixture of truth, half-truth, distortion, and falsehood, presenting the picture of a man unwillingly called into the SS concentration-camp system where he fought the good fight but was always himself being victimized and "robbed of the fruits of my work." But the claim was in direct conflict with the high evaluations he had always received from his superiors: the Auschwitz commandant's office had praised him for his "soldierly tenacity"; and Lolling, for filling his position "to the most complete satisfaction of his superiors." On the basis of such recommendations, Wirths had been promoted in September 1944.[71]

Now he ruminated on passages from Nietzsche, such as "Oh, demolishing is easy, but building!"—and on how "finally painful experiences, sad events, lead our heart back to the faith of our childhood."[72] But he was essentially without hope, spoke frequently to his brother of suicide, and during a last smuggled visit with family members, his brother and wife found him manifestly suicidal. At this point he was in what would clinically be called an agitated depression, accompanied by extreme despair, in which the necessary components for suicide were present: the sense of entrapment and futurelessness, the existence of a prior image of suicide as a possible option in one's life, and the desire to convey an enduring principle best expressed by killing oneself (in his case affirmation of love for his wife and family together with a solution to the tormenting question of guilt).

The British officer's statement that he was shaking hands with a man responsible for the death of four million people activated all three of those components of suicide. Wirths had reason to feel hopeless about any future and to call forth existing suicidal imagery to perform a final act that would spare his family the pain and disgrace of a trial while neither acknowledging nor denying the dimensions of his guilt.

Perhaps the main point to be made about Wirths's suicide was that he committed it *after* all that he had done in Auschwitz. While there, despair was part of his adaptation, part of what has been called a "life of suicide" —a life in which the possibility of killing oneself enables one to avoid genuine confrontation with questions of meaning.[73] While Auschwitz lasted, nothing in his conflicts prevented him from carrying out his functions in that death camp. In this way his story represents, however exaggeratedly, the overall experience of Nazi doctors in Auschwitz.

Evaluations

We get a deeper sense of Wirths's moral and psychological contradictions—and of their larger significance—by noting the difficulties others had in evaluating both the man and his suicide.

Hermann Langbein, the prisoner closest to him, was said (in a 1946 letter of Lill's about Wirths to Wirths's father) to have "loved him very much and called him his 'fairytale prince' whom, after the war and in a different uniform, he wanted to see again—as a friend."[74] But Langbein also came to juxtapose Wirths's extremely valuable help to prisoners with the fact that "for two years he had a decisive SS function in the extermination apparatus." Langbein criticized Wirths less for his role in selections, which he considered imposed upon the chief doctor, than for his last-hour, fatal typhus experiments, which Wirths chose to do himself.[75] In discussing these with me, Langbein spoke of Wirths's actions as reflecting "the total demoralization of all people who worked in Auschwitz in an SS uniform"; and in summing up what Wirths did in Auschwitz, Langbein declared, "All I can say is that for us it was good, for him it was probably bad." He told me that he believed Wirths killed himself "because he had a conscience." In public commentaries, Langbein stopped short of definitive moral evaluation, saying on one occasion, "Who wants to be the judge? Who wants to condemn? Not me." Unlike Langbein, Lill was unqualified in his favorable judgment of Wirths, sought to locate him in 1945 in order to help him, and wrote to his wife the following year praising Wirths's "courage and great astuteness" in helping prisoners. Lill called Wirths "our best ally" and declared, "Your husband fought the good battle and he was alone."[76]* That would have been Wirths's own idealized version of his personal crusade.

Other prisoners were considerably less complimentary. Dr. Tadeusz S. told me that "Langbein said he would defend Wirths, and I like Langbein but I said I would testify against Wirths." Dr. Marie L. spoke of Wirths with something approaching disdain. Dr. Jan W., who appreciated Wirths's help but insisted he be included among "the mass murderers," said that Wirths killed himself not as an act of conscience but "because he couldn't face the responsibility [of what he had done]." And Dr. Wanda J., grateful for his help but judging him "a criminal," summed up her view by saying, "Anyhow, he did the decent thing. He killed himself."

Two SS doctors I spoke to considered him an SS bureaucrat. One described him as "correct" and "under the control of the camp commandant." The other considered him a man without much imagination, "rather sterile . . . [and] factual."

And an additional judgment was expressed during a television documentary, by a childhood friend of Wirths trained in law and theology, who was a bitter anti-Nazi. He spoke warmly of Wirths as "among us the most good-natured, softhearted, most capable of pity," but had broken early with him because of their radically different response to the Nazis. In judging father and son, the old friend, who had left the law for theology under National Socialism, put the matter sadly but clearly: "To defend his father I would be the right lawyer. To defend Eduard I would have inhibitions."[78]

Wirths's family members have had to make the most troubled evaluations of all.

His widow tried to cling to a sense of his virtue, avoided any discussions about Auschwitz with the children, and told them "only about personal things." As it became necessary to speak about the subject, she emphasized that Wirths "could do a lot of good, and that they would not have

---

*In the same correspondence with the family, Lill spoke of Wirths as a man of "rare nobility"; and in one extraordinary letter to Wirths's wife in 1976, Lill, as a dedicated Communist, imagined ideal "human beings of the future" as possessing "the courage, the astuteness, and the self-control" of Wirths, whom Lill "half-jocular[ly]" characterized as "an 'educated Marxist' . . . a *comrade* Albert Schweitzer."[77]

to be ashamed of him." Later in the documentary, she came to the idea that "if you were among them . . . that is the guilt." And she told Langbein that her husband's suicide "was probably for the best"—a statement that might have referred to her husband's despair, the hopelessness of his legal case, and the pain a trial would have caused everyone, or was perhaps an acknowledgment that, despite her commitment to his goodness, he had to be judged guilty.

His two sons struggled more directly with the issue but no less ambivalently. The older son, who had warm childhood memories of playing with his father, said, "I do not know whether it is right to defend him," and ended, "I wish to leave the question open." The younger son, with no such childhood memories, seemed to come closer to a judgment in his sense that his father's suicide meant that "he must have felt guilty," and that "I don't know why he didn't refuse right at the beginning because he knew what happened there." But then he denied that his father had commited crimes, and said, "I don't know."

Wirths's elderly father struggled with his own role in having advised the son to stay at Auschwitz, and, in a long and carefully worded letter to the Frankfurt Court, told of having "entreated [his son] . . . to save lives where he could" but that "he should not execute inhuman orders"—an admonition that sounds dubious at all levels for everyone. The father listed in detail ways in which his son did save lives, and characterized his activities in Auschwitz as "sacrificial." Yet in the very last words of the documentary, he held his own original advice up to question: "But he had to become guilty there, did he not? I ask you only: was that [my advice] right?"[79]

Wirths's daughter, a married woman in her early forties, recalled being told by her mother virtually nothing about her father except that "he was dead from the war"; and also that "he was a good man and a really good father," which was consistent with a few loving memories she had of him. With the family decision to cooperate with a Dutch film maker on a documentary about Wirths, her mother began to tell her more, including details of selections, while emphasizing Wirths's despair, wish to leave, and decision to stay "in order to prevent an even worse situation." In books the daughter was now reading, "all of a sudden there is a totally different picture [of him], a totally different [person]." She found this "very hard" and "difficult to believe," "wanted to apologize for him . . . to understand him . . . to find justification." She tried to see him as "a soldier in war who shoot[s] people [as] his work," and as having stayed in order to "save his family" (that is, to prevent repercussions). Struggling to get inside of her father's pain, she believed that only his family ties prevented him from killing himself earlier; she considered him at the end "a broken man" who, "knowing that he had killed people, . . . could not live with this."

She said that, after repeated discussions with her younger brother, "in the final analysis neither of us condemns him. . . . We cannot condemn him, *him* himself." But her ultimate question about her father reflected both her profound doubts and her difficulty comprehending how far his ideology had taken him. That question was: "Can a good man do bad things?"

Eduard's brother Helmut, the family member most consistently involved in the issue, was apparently motivated by two powerful incentives: to convey his brother's struggle and in some measure to clear his name; and to illuminate more generally this episode of Nazi mass murder as a way of bearing his own constructive witness. His "mission" was complicated by his own involvement in some of those events. He was in frequent touch with Hermann Langbein, read extensively about Auschwitz, and attended the Auschwitz trial in Frankfurt, bringing with him at times his son, a younger colleague, and the childhood friend of Wirths mentioned earlier. Helmut and his son were in pained dialogue: "There was a time when he [the son] doubted that anybody at all during that time [the Nazi era] remained correct [*noch korrekt geblieben;* by implication, did not become guilty]—including me."

Helmut strove for a broadly humanitarian perspective, declaring that he "could understand" and had no animosity toward the British officer whose statement about shaking hands with a man responsible for the death of four million Jews preceded Wirths's suicide; and claimed to have told his brother before leaving Auschwitz, "If I were a Jew, I would, after the war, hang every German man, child . . . old men, everybody." But his simultaneous need to defend his brother led to a stress on the latter's good deeds to the point of erroneous idealization, as in his claim that Wirths persuaded Höss to permit children to remain with their parents at selections and thereby survive.

Helmut tried to regard his brother as "an extraordinarily misused [*missbrauchten*] person," as "a very good human being . . . the best father, a good doctor . . . [who had the] terrible fortune [misfortune, fate] to [be brought into] this situation." And, "if you [got into] this machinery of murder, you are forced to become guilty." But he went further in admitting, "Sometimes it is hard for me to believe all those things about my brother—how he would do those things, . . . selecting children for the gas chamber." He was also extremely troubled about Langbein's account of his brother's participation in typhus experiments, wondered whether Langbein could be mistaken, and added, "I struggle against [believing] it." He seemed to view the incident as a more direct Hippocratic question than any other, and admitted that, if the description were true, he would have to "feel differently" about his brother because such experiments "would almost certainly mean death for a human being." He also admitted he had no reason to doubt Langbein's account.

In discussing his brother's record, Helmut raised the central question of the healing-killing paradox: "Can you murder in order to save another?" And later: "Whichever way you turn . . . you must become guilty." At some level he was probably including himself in that judgment as he was by no means without conflict over having advised his brother to stay and having himself actively participated (however he minimized that participation) in his brother's cancer research.

He had come to considerable truth about Auschwitz, which he could state with something approaching eloquence, as in the epigraph to chapter 7. His eventual judgment of his brother was repeatedly that of "tragic guilt . . . inescapable guilt," as described in classical Greek drama. He meant that circumstances create a destiny that leads inexorably to guilty actions—but he too understated his brother's *active* Nazi commitment. Helmut stressed his brother's youth and inexperience at the time, along with his own, and wished that he himself could have been at the time "a mature man . . . able to judge [things] better." Then he would have been able to take "an unconditional stance against these events," for he had come to the conviction that "the only thing to do in a situation like that is to say, 'No, I won't do it.' "

What can be finally said, then, about the psychological fit between this "good, conscientious doctor" and the Auschwitz killing project?

The beginning key is Wirths's unique combination of passionate Nazi ideology with impressive medical talent—a combination that could propel one quickly into a position of medical leadership, or leadership in medicalized killing. He was significantly immersed in Nazi ideology in three crucial spheres: the claim of revitalizing the German race and *Volk;* the biomedical path to that revitalization via purification of genes and race; and the focus on the Jews as a threat to this renewal, to the immediate and long-term "health" of the Germanic race. While Wirths did not absolutize these convictions in the manner of a Mengele—they were in him combined with a strong current of medical humanism—his commitment to the Nazi cause was probably no less strong.

Wirths had another trait insufficiently noted by commentators: a combination of moralism and obsessiveness that under ordinary conditions contributes much to making one a "reliable professional," and in Auschwitz contributed to the efficiency with which Wirths set up and maintained the entire structure of medicalized killing. It enabled him to be always both "correct" and meticulous about rules and regulations, whether in trying to limit Auschwitz evil or (more importantly, as it turned out) in serving it.

In Auschwitz, Wirths was thrust into the ultimate *atrocity-producing situation.* He encountered a set of conditions so structured organizationally and psychologically that virtually everyone entering into the situation committed atrocities. In that sense there is some truth in Helmut's claim that, once sent there, his brother *had* to become guilty—but only if one remained there. And powerful psychological forces bound Wirths to Auschwitz and overcame his ambivalent desire to leave.

"Enduring" in Auschwitz—staying there, whatever the duress—was a moral position not only endorsed by his family and by his own feelings of duty but by his deepest sense of self and world. Into that principle of "staying the course" went a young lifetime of filial, national, and ideological piety: strong immediate inclinations to obedience as well as a transcendent commitment to what he perceived as his immortalizing racial, national, and cultural substance. That immortalizing pull could prevail over whatever horror the humanist in him experienced, and contribute greatly toward his remaining the physician-manager of the very atrocity-producing situation so much of him abhorred.

However unusual Wirths was, he was at the same time all too representative of the physician's corruption in Nazi Germany. He was a partially willing implementer of the most visionary of all Nazi projects of healing the Aryan race by killing those seen as threatening it. He was what his father called a "sacrifice" only in the sense that, in embodying the most extreme reversal of healing and killing, he took on a large measure of the taint and guilt of his profession if not of his generation.

He was both a self-motivated implementer of his fate and a man acted upon by forces greater than himself. That is, he first seized upon the medical role of cultivator of the genes offered by the Nazis; was then propelled into a sequence of unsavory environments culminating in Auschwitz, environments that offended him but called forth his loyalties; and ended by providing skilled and reliable professional service to the killing project he had morally come to oppose. He was both brutally "misused" (in his brother's word) by a murderous regime and his own architect of that very misuse.

Whatever Wirths's pain and ambivalence, his form of doubling was in many ways ideal for the overall Auschwitz function. His Nazi-Auschwitz self, with its attachment to racial purification and national revitalization, could serve the killing project with extraordinary efficiency; his humane medical self, so strongly supported by loving family relationships, helped maintain his general function and contributed to his "decency" in his own eyes as well as those of other prisoners and many SS colleagues and fellow officers as well. Wirths was very much what William James called a "divided self," but the division was functional for Auschwitz. His was the doubling characteristic of the general phenomenon of the "decent Nazi"; and true to that phenomenon, Wirths got the job done.

Wirths was extreme in his involvement in both the healing and the killing functions. In that way his doubling resembled that of Kurt Gerstein, the SS officer who, in strange and as yet insufficiently understood ways, behaved as an ardent SS activist; who took over much technical responsibility for Zyklon-B gas and its delivery to Auschwitz; but who also had an impressive record as an anti-Nazi, claimed to have infiltrated the SS in order to understand its killing operations, and tried desperately toward the end to inform the world of Nazi mass murder. Unlike Gerstein, however, Wirths never stepped out of his Nazi role to denounce to others the evil project he himself was part of. Both Gerstein and Wirths demonstrate that doubling can enable a man to be a passionate advocate of both killing and healing (see footnote on pages 161–62).

Wirths's suicide did not result from a breakdown in the doubling itself, or from resistance to the killing project. Rather it was a *consequence* of both the doubling and the project. Dr. Jan W.'s claim that Wirths killed himself because he "couldn't face the responsibility" for what he had done was therefore true. Suddenly stripped of his official-medical place in the immortalizing Nazi project, Wirths was vulnerable to the inevitably harsh consequences (trial, condemnation, death) of his actions.

Yet Langbein may also be correct in saying that Wirths killed himself because he "had a conscience." He had more of a conscience than most Nazi doctors and possibly most human beings. But that conscience had been harnessed to the Nazi movement itself, to which he gave devoted service; it could not be dislodged from that movement even in Auschwitz, and even though a portion of that conscience was applied to saving the lives of prisoners.

His message to the future via his suicide also contains an expression of conscience: the principle that he who becomes involved in mass killing must himself pay with his life; and the accompanying principle, more dubious in our eyes but strongly felt, of maintaining the "purity" of the future of one's family by destroying its tainted component—oneself. Yet there may have been still a third principle, related to the other two: the reassertion of the healing ethos by destroying the physician (himself) who had become tainted with killing.

PART III

THE PSYCHOLOGY
OF GENOCIDE

Introduction to Part III

The behavior of Nazi doctors suggests the beginnings of a psychology of genocide. To clarify the principles involved, I will first focus systematically on the psychological pattern of doubling, which was the doctors' overall mechanism for participating in evil. Then it is also necessary to identify certain tendencies in their behavior, promulgated and even demanded by the Auschwitz environment, which greatly facilitated the doubling. This exploration is meant to serve two purposes: First, it can provide new insight into the motivations and actions of Nazi doctors and of Nazis in general. Second, it can raise broader questions about human behavior, about ways in which people, individually and collectively, can embrace various forms of destructiveness and evil, with or without the awareness of doing so. The two purposes, in a very real sense, are one. If there is any truth to the psychological and moral judgments we make about the specific and unique characteristics of Nazi mass murder, we are bound to derive from them *principles* that apply more widely—principles that speak to the extraordinary threat and potential for self-annihilation that now haunt humankind.

Chapter 19

Doubling: The Faustian Bargain

> Not only will you break through the paralysing difficulties of the time—you will break through time itself . . . and dare to be barbaric, twice barbaric indeed.
>
> —THOMAS MANN

> Any of us could be the man who encounters his double.
>
> —FRIEDRICH DURRENMAT

The key to understanding how Nazi doctors came to do the work of Auschwitz is the psychological principle I call "doubling": the division of the self into two functioning wholes, so that a part-self acts as an entire self. An Auschwitz doctor could, through doubling, not only kill and contribute to killing but organize silently, on behalf of that evil project, an entire self-structure (or self-process) encompassing virtually all aspects of his behavior.

Doubling, then, was the psychological vehicle for the Nazi doctor's Faustian bargain with the diabolical environment in exchange for his contribution to the killing; he was offered various psychological and material benefits on behalf of privileged adaptation. Beyond Auschwitz was the larger Faustian temptation offered to German doctors in general: that of becoming the theorists and implementers of a cosmic scheme of racial cure by means of victimization and mass murder.

One is always ethically responsible for Faustian bargains—a responsibility in no way abrogated by the fact that much doubling takes place outside of awareness. In exploring doubling, I engage in psychological probing on behalf of illuminating evil. For the individual Nazi doctor in Auschwitz, doubling was likely to mean a choice for evil.

Generally speaking, doubling involves five characteristics. There is, first, a dialectic between two selves in terms of autonomy and connection. The individual Nazi doctor needed his Auschwitz self to function psychologically in an environment so antithetical to his previous ethical standards. At the same time, he needed his prior self in order to continue to see himself as humane physician, husband, father. The Auschwitz self had to be both autonomous and connected to the prior self that gave rise to it. Second, doubling follows a holistic principle. The Auschwitz self "succeeded" because it was inclusive and could connect with the entire Auschwitz environment: it rendered coherent, and gave form to, various themes and mechanisms, which I shall discuss shortly. Third, doubling has a life-death dimension: the Auschwitz self was perceived by the perpetrator as a form of psychological survival in a death-dominated environment; in other words, we have the paradox of a "killing self" being created on behalf of what one perceives as one's own healing or survival. Fourth, a major function of doubling, as in Auschwitz, is likely to be the avoidance of guilt: the second self tends to be the one performing the "dirty work." And, finally, doubling involves both an unconscious dimension—taking place, as stated, largely outside of awareness—and a significant change in moral consciousness. These five characteristics frame and pervade all else that goes on psychologically in doubling.

For instance, the holistic principle differentiates doubling from the traditional psychoanalytic concept of "splitting." This latter term has had several meanings but tends to suggest a sequestering off of a portion of the self so that the "split off" element ceases to respond to the environment (as in what I have been calling "psychic numbing") or else is in some way at odds with the remainder of the self. Splitting in this sense resembles what Pierre Janet, Freud's nineteenth-century contemporary, originally called "dissociation," and Freud himself tended to equate the two terms. But in regard to sustained forms of adaptation, there has been confusion about how to explain the autonomy of that separated "piece" of the self—confusion over (as one thoughtful commentator has put it) "What splits in splitting?"[1]*

"Splitting" or "dissociation" can thus denote something about Nazi

---

*This writer seemed to react against the idea of a separated-off piece of the self when he ended the article by asking, "Why should we invent a special intrapsychic act of splitting to account for those phenomena as if some internal chopper were at work to produce them?"[2] Janet meant by "dissociation" the hysteric's tendency to "sacrifice" or "abandon" certain psychological functions, so that these become "dissociated" from the rest of the mind and give rise to "automatisms," or segmented-off symptom complexes.[3] Freud spoke, in his early work with Josef Breuer, of "splitting of consciousness," "splitting of the mind," and "splitting of personality" as important mechanisms in hysteria.[4] Edward Glover referred to the psychic components of splitting or dissociation as "ego nuclei."[5] And, beginning with the work of Melanie Klein, splitting has been associated with polarization of "all good" and "all bad" imagery within the self, a process that can be consistent with normal development but, where exaggerated, can become associated with severe personality disorders now spoken of as "borderline states."[6]

doctors' suppression of feeling, or psychic numbing, in relation to their participation in murder.* But to chart their involvement in a continuous routine of killing, over a year or two or more, one needs an explanatory principle that draws upon the entire, functioning self. (The same principle applies in sustained psychiatric disturbance, and my stress on doubling is consistent with the increasing contemporary focus upon the holistic function of the self.)[8]

Doubling is part of the universal potential for what William James called the "divided self": that is, for opposing tendencies in the self. James quoted the nineteenth-century French writer Alphonse Daudet's despairing cry *"Homo duplex, homo duplex!"* in noting his "horrible duality" —as, in the face of his brother Henri's death, Daudet's "first self wept" while his "second self" sat back and somewhat mockingly staged the scene for an imagined theatrical performance.[9] To James and Daudet, the potential for doubling is part of being human, and the process is likely to take place in extremity, in relation to death.

But that "opposing self" can become dangerously unrestrained, as it did in the Nazi doctors. And when it becomes so, as Otto Rank discovered in his extensive studies of the "double" in literature and folklore, that opposing self can become the usurper from within and replace the original self until it "speaks" for the entire person.[10] Rank's work also suggests that the potential for an opposing self, in effect the potential for evil, is *necessary* to the human psyche: the loss of one's shadow or soul or "double" means death.

In general psychological terms, the adaptive potential for doubling is integral to the human psyche and can, at times, be life saving: for a soldier in combat, for instance; or for a victim of brutality such as an Auschwitz inmate, who must also undergo a form of doubling in order to survive. Clearly, the "opposing self" can be life enhancing. But under certain conditions it can embrace evil with an extreme lack of restraint.

The Nazi doctor's situation resembles that of one of Rank's examples (taken from a 1913 German film, *The Student of Prague*): a student fencing champion accepts an evil magician's offer of great wealth and the chance for marriage with his beloved in return for anything the old magician wishes to take from the room; what he takes is the student's mirror image, a frequent representation of the double. That double eventually becomes a killer by making use of the student's fencing skills in a duel with his beloved's suitor, despite the fact that the student (his original self) has promised the woman's father that he will not engage in such a duel. This variation on the Faust legend parallels the Nazi doctor's "bargain" with Auschwitz and the regime: to do the killing, he offered an opposing self (the evolving Auschwitz self)—a self that, in violating his own prior moral standards, met with no effective

---

*Henry V. Dicks invokes this concept in his study of Nazi killers.[7]

resistance and in fact made use of his original skills (in this case, medi-cal-scientific).[11]*

Rank stressed the death symbolism of the double as "symptomatic of the disintegration of the modern personality type." That disintegration leads to a need for "self-perpetuation in one's own image"[13]—what I would call a literalized form of immortality—as compared with "the per-petuation of the self in work reflecting one's personality" or a creative-symbolic form of immortality. Rank saw the Narcissus legend as depicting both the danger of the literalized mode and the necessity of the shift to the creative mode (as embodied by the "artist-hero").† But the Nazi movement encouraged its would-be artist-hero, the physician, to remain, like Narcissus, in thralldom to his own image. Here Mengele comes immediately to mind, his extreme narcissism in the service of his quest for omnipotence, and his exemplification to the point of caricature of the general situation of Nazi doctors in Auschwitz.[15]

The way in which doubling allowed Nazi doctors to avoid guilt was not by the elimination of conscience but by what can be called the *transfer of conscience.* The requirements of conscience were transferred to the Ausch-witz self, which placed it within its own criteria for good (duty, loyalty to group, "improving" Auschwitz conditions, etc.), thereby freeing the orig-inal self from responsibility for actions there. Rank spoke similarly of guilt "which forces the hero no longer to accept the responsibility for certain actions of his ego, but to place it upon another ego, a double, who is either personified by the devil himself or is created by making a diabolical pact"[16]: that is, the Faustian bargain of Nazi doctors mentioned earlier. Rank spoke of a "powerful consciousness of guilt" as initiating the trans-fer;[17] but for most Nazi doctors, the doubling maneuver seemed to fend off that sense of guilt prior to its developing, or to its reaching conscious dimensions.

There is an inevitable connection between death and guilt. Rank equates the opposing self with a "form of evil which represents the perishable and mortal part of the personality."[18] The double is evil in that it represents one's own death. The Auschwitz self of the Nazi doctor similarly assumed the death issue for him but at the same time used its evil project as a way of staving off awareness of his own "perishable and

---

*Rank's viewing of *The Student of Prague,* during a revival in the mid-1920s, was the original stimulus for a lifelong preoccupation with the theme of the double. Rank noted that the screenplay's author, Hanns Heinz Ewers, had drawn heavily on E. T. A. Hoffmann's "Story of the Lost Reflection."[12]

†In his earlier work, Rank followed Freud in connecting the legend with the concept of "narcissism," of libido directed toward one's own self. But Rank gave the impression that he did so uneasily, always stressing the issue of death and immortality as lurking beneath the narcissism. In his later adaptation, he boldly embraced the death theme as the earlier and more fundamental one in the Narcissus legend and spoke somewhat disdainfully of "some modern psychologists [who] claimed to have found a symbolization of their self-love principle" in it.[14] By then he had broken with Freud and established his own intellectual position.

mortal part." It does the "dirty work" for the entire self by rendering that work "proper" and in that way protects the entire self from awareness of its own guilt and its own death.

In doubling, one part of the self "disavows" another part. What is repudiated is not reality itself—the individual Nazi doctor was aware of what he was doing via the Auschwitz self—but the meaning of that reality. The Nazi doctor knew that he selected, but did not interpret selections as murder. One level of disavowal, then, was the Auschwitz self's altering of the meaning of murder; and on another, the repudiation by the original self of *anything* done by the Auschwitz self. From the moment of its formation, the Auschwitz self so violated the Nazi doctor's previous self-concept as to require more or less permanent disavowal. Indeed, disavowal was the life blood of the Auschwitz self.*

Doubling, Splitting, and Evil

Doubling is an active psychological process, a means of *adaptation to extremity.* That is why I use the verb form, as opposed to the more usual noun form, "the double." The adaptation requires a dissolving of "psychic glue"[20] as an alternative to a radical breakdown of the self. In Auschwitz, the pattern was established under the duress of the individual doctor's transition period. At that time the Nazi doctor experienced his own death anxiety as well as such death equivalents as fear of disintegration, separation, and stasis. He needed a functional Auschwitz self to still his anxiety. And that Auschwitz self had to assume hegemony on an everyday basis, reducing expressions of the prior self to odd moments and to contacts with family and friends outside the camp. Nor did most Nazi doctors resist that usurpation as long as they remained in the camp. Rather they welcomed it as the only means of psychological function. If an environment is sufficiently extreme, and one chooses to remain in it, one may be able to do so *only* by means of doubling.

Yet doubling does not include the radical dissociation and sustained separateness characteristic of multiple or "dual personality." In the latter condition, the two selves are more profoundly distinct and autonomous, and tend either not to know about each other or else to see each other as alien. The pattern for dual or multiple personality, moreover, is thought to begin early in childhood, and to solidify and maintain itself more or less indefinitely. Yet in the development of multiple personality, there are likely to be such influences as intense psychic or physical trauma, an atmosphere of extreme ambivalence, and severe conflict and confusion over identifications[21]—all of which can also be instrumental in doubling. Also relevant to both conditions is Janet's principle that "once

---

*Michael Franz Basch speaks of an interference with the "union of affect with percept without, however, blocking the percept from consciousness."[19] In that sense, disavowal resembles psychic numbing, as it alters the *valencing* or emotional charge of the symbolizing process.

baptized"—that is, named or confirmed by someone in authority—a particular self is likely to become more clear and definite.[22] Though never as stable as a self in multiple personality, the Auschwitz self nonetheless underwent a similar baptism when the Nazi doctor conducted his first selections.

A recent writer has employed the metaphor of a tree to delineate the depth of "splitting" in schizophrenia and multiple personality—a metaphor that could be expanded to include doubling. In schizophrenia, the rent in the self is "like the crumbling and breaking of a tree that has deteriorated generally, at least in some important course of the trunk, down toward or to the roots." In multiple personality, that rent is specific and limited, "as in an essentially sound tree that does not split very far down."[23] Doubling takes place still higher on a tree whose roots, trunk, and larger branches have previously experienced no impairment; of the two branches artificially separated, one grows fetid bark and leaves in a way that enables the other to maintain ordinary growth, and the two intertwine sufficiently to merge again should external conditions favor that merging.

Was the doubling of Nazi doctors an antisocial "character disorder"? Not in the classical sense, in that the process tended to be more a form of adaptation than a lifelong pattern. But doubling can include elements considered characteristic of "sociopathic" character impairment: these include a disorder of feeling (swings between numbing and rage), pathological avoidance of a sense of guilt, and resort to violence to overcome "masked depression" (related to repressed guilt and numbing) and maintain a sense of vitality.[24] Similarly, in both situations, destructive or even murderous behavior may cover over feared disintegration of the self.

The disorder in the type of doubling I have described is more focused and temporary and occurs as part of a larger institutional structure which encourages or even demands it. In that sense, Nazi doctors' behavior resembles that of certain terrorists—and members of the Mafia, of "death squads" organized by dictators, or even of delinquent gangs. In all these situations, profound ideological, family, ethnic, and sometimes age-specific ties help shape criminal behavior. Doubling may well be an important psychological mechanism for individuals living within any criminal subculture: the Mafia or "death squad" chief who coldly orders (or himself carries out) the murder of a rival while remaining a loving husband, father, and churchgoer. The doubling is adaptive to the extreme conditions created by the subculture, but additional influences, some of which can begin early in life, always contribute to the process.* That, too, was the case with the Nazi doctors.

In sum, doubling is the psychological means by which one invokes the evil potential of the self. That evil is neither inherent in the self nor foreign to it. To live out the doubling and call forth the evil is a moral

*Robert W. Rieber uses the term "pseudopsychopathy" for what he describes as "selective joint criminal behavior" within the kinds of subculture mentioned here.[25]

choice for which one is responsible, whatever the level of consciousness involved.* By means of doubling, Nazi doctors made a Faustian choice for evil: in the process of doubling, in fact, lies an overall key to human evil.

Varieties of Doubling

While individual Nazi doctors in Auschwitz doubled in different ways, all of them doubled. Ernst B., for instance, limited his doubling; in avoiding selections, he was resisting a full-blown Auschwitz self. Yet his conscious desire to adapt to Auschwitz was an accession to at least a certain amount of doubling: it was he, after all, who said that "one could react like a normal human being in Auschwitz only for the first few hours"; after that, "you were caught and had to go along," which meant that you had to double. His own doubling was evident in his sympathy for Mengele and, at least to some extent, for the most extreme expressions of the Nazi ethos (the image of the Nazis as a "world blessing" and of Jews as the world's "fundamental evil"). And despite the limit to his doubling, he retains aspects of his Auschwitz self to this day in his way of judging Auschwitz behavior.

In contrast, Mengele's embrace of the Auschwitz self gave the impression of a quick adaptive affinity, causing one to wonder whether he required any doubling at all. But doubling was indeed required in a man who befriended children to an unusual degree and then drove some of them personally to the gas chamber; or by a man so "collegial" in his relationship to prisoner doctors and so ruthlessly flamboyant in his conduct of selections. Whatever his affinity for Auschwitz, a man who could be pictured under ordinary conditions as "a slightly sadistic German professor" had to form a new self to become an energetic killer. The point about Mengele's doubling was that his prior self could be readily absorbed into the Auschwitz self; and his continuing allegiance to the Nazi ideology and project probably enabled his Auschwitz self, more than in the case of other Nazi doctors, to remain active over the years after the Second World War.

Wirths's doubling was neither limited (like Dr. B.'s) nor harmonious (like Mengele's): it was both strong and conflicted. We see Auschwitz's chief doctor as a "divided self" because both selves retained their power. Yet his doubling was the most successful of all from the standpoint of the Auschwitz institution and the Nazi project. Even his suicide was a mark of that success: while the Nazi defeat enabled him to equate his Auschwitz self more clearly with evil, he nonetheless retained responsibility to that

---

*James S. Grotstein speaks of the development of "a separate being living within one that has been preconsciously split off and has an independent existence with independent motivation, separate agenda, etc.," and from which can emanate "evil, sadism, and destructiveness" or even "demoniacal possession." He calls this aspect of the self a "mind parasite" (after Colin Wilson) and attributes its development to those elements of the self that have been artificially suppressed and disavowed early in life.[26]

Auschwitz self sufficiently to remain inwardly divided and unable to imagine any possibility of resolution and renewal—either legally, morally, or psychologically.

Within the Auschwitz structure, significant doubling included future goals and even a sense of hope. Styles of doubling varied because each Nazi doctor created his Auschwitz self out of his prior self, with its particular history, and with his own psychological mechanisms. But in all Nazi doctors, prior self and Auschwitz self were connected by the overall Nazi ethos and the general authority of the regime. Doubling was a shared theme among them.

Doubling and Institutions

Indeed, Auschwitz as an *institution*—as an atrocity-producing situation—ran on doubling. An atrocity-producing situation is one so structured externally (in this case, institutionally) that the average person entering it (in this case, as part of the German authority) will commit or become associated with atrocities. Always important to an atrocity-producing situation is its capacity to motivate individuals psychologically toward engaging in atrocity.[27]

In an institution as powerful as Auschwitz, the external environment could set the tone for much of an individual doctor's "internal environment." The demand for doubling was part of the environmental message immediately perceived by Nazi doctors, the implicit command to bring forth a self that could adapt to killing without one's feeling oneself a murderer. Doubling became not just an individual enterprise but a shared psychological process, the group norm, part of the Auschwitz "weather." And that group process was intensified by the general awareness that, whatever went on in other camps, Auschwitz was the great technical center of the Final Solution. One had to double in order that one's life and work there not be interfered with either by the corpses one helped to produce or by those "living dead" (the *Muselmänner*) all around one.

Inevitably, the Auschwitz pressure toward doubling extended to prisoner doctors, the most flagrant examples of whom were those who came to work closely with the Nazis—Dering, Zenkteller, Adam T., and Samuel. Even those prisoner doctors who held strongly to their healing ethos, and underwent minimal doubling, inadvertently contributed to Nazi doctors' doubling simply by working with them, as they had to, and thereby in some degree confirmed a Nazi doctor's Auschwitz self.

Doubling undoubtedly occurred extensively in nonmedical Auschwitz personnel as well. Rudolf Höss told how noncommissioned officers regularly involved in selections "pour[ed] out their hearts" to him about the difficulty of their work (their prior self speaking)—but went on doing that work (their Auschwitz self directing behavior). Höss described the Auschwitz choices: "either to become cruel, to become heartless and no longer to respect human life [that is, to develop a highly functional Auschwitz self] or to be weak and to get to the point of a nervous breakdown [that is, to hold onto one's prior self, which in Auschwitz was nonfunctional]."[28] But in the Nazi doctor, the doubling was particularly stark in that a prior healing self gave rise to a killing self that should have been, but functionally was not, in direct opposition to it. And as in any atrocity-producing situation, Nazi doctors found themselves in a psychological climate where they were virtually certain to choose evil: they were propelled, that is, toward murder.

Doubling—Nazi and Medical

Beyond Auschwitz, there was much in the Nazi movement that promoted doubling. The overall Nazi project, replete with cruelty, required constant doubling in the service of carrying out that cruelty. The doubling could take the form of a gradual process of "slippery slope" compromises: the slow emergence of a functional "Nazi self" via a series of destructive actions, at first agreed to grudgingly, followed by a sequence of assigned tasks each more incriminating, if not more murderous, than the previous ones.

Doubling could also be more dramatic, infused with transcendence, the sense (described by a French fascist who joined the SS) of being someone entering a religious order "who must now divest himself of his past," and of being "reborn into a new European race."[29] That new Nazi self could take on a sense of mystical fusion with the German *Volk*, with "destiny," and with immortalizing powers. Always there was the combination noted earlier of idealism and terror, imagery of destruction and renewal, so that "gods . . . appear as both destroyers and culture-heroes, just as the Führer could appear as front comrade and master builder."[30] Himmler, espccially in his speeches to his SS leaders within their "oath-bound community,"[31] called for the kind of doubling necessary to engage in what he considered to be heroic cruelty, especially in the killing of Jews.

The degree of doubling was not necessarily equivalent to Nazi Party membership; thus, Hochhuth could claim that "the great divide was between Nazis [meaning those with well-developed Nazi selves] and decent people, not between Party members and other Germans."[32] But probably never has a political movement demanded doubling with the intensity and scale of the Nazis.

Doctors as a group may be more susceptible to doubling than others. For example, a former Nazi doctor claimed that the anatomist's insensitivity toward skeletons and corpses accounted for his friend Hirt's grotesque "anthropological" collection of Jewish skulls (see pages 284–87). While hardly a satisfactory explanation, this doctor was referring to a genuine pattern not just of numbing but of medical doubling. That doubling usually begins with the student's encounter with the corpse he or she must dissect, often enough on the first day of medical school. One feels it necessary to develop a "medical self," which enables one not only to be relatively inured to death but to function reasonably efficiently in relation to the many-sided demands of the work. The ideal doctor, to be sure, remains warm and humane by keeping that doubling to a minimum. But few doctors meet that ideal standard. Since studies have suggested that a psychological motivation for entering the medical profession can be the overcoming of an unusually great fear of death, it is possible that this fear in doctors propels them in the direction of doubling when encountering deadly environments. Doctors drawn to the Nazi movement in general, and to SS or concentration-camp medicine in particular, were likely to be those with the greatest previous medical doubling. But even doctors without outstanding Nazi sympathies could well have had a certain experience with doubling and a proclivity for its further manifestations.

Certainly the tendency toward doubling was particularly strong among *Nazi* doctors. Given the heroic vision held out to them—as cultivators of the genes and as physicians to the *Volk,* and as militarized healers combining the life-death power of shaman and general—any cruelty they might perpetrate was all too readily drowned in hubris. And their medical hubris was furthered by their role in the sterilization and "euthanasia" projects within a vision of curing the ills of the Nordic race and the German people.

Doctors who ended up undergoing the extreme doubling necessitated by the "euthanasia" killing centers and the death camps were probably unusually susceptible to doubling. There was, of course, an element of chance in where one was sent, but doctors assigned either to the killing centers or to the death camps tended to be strongly committed to Nazi ideology. They may well have also had greater schizoid tendencies, or been particularly prone to numbing and omnipotence-sadism, all of which also enhance doubling. Since, even under extreme conditions, people have a way of finding and staying in situations they connect with psychologically, we can suspect a certain degree of self-selection there too. In these ways, previous psychological characteristics of a doctor's self had considerable significance—but a significance in respect to tendency or susceptibility, and no more. Considerable doubling occurred in people of the most varied psychological characteristics.

We thus find ourselves returning to the recognition that most of what Nazi doctors did would be within the potential capability—at least under certain conditions—of most doctors and of most people. But once embarked on doubling in Auschwitz, a Nazi doctor did indeed separate himself from other physicians and from other human beings. Doubling was the mechanism by which a doctor, in his actions, moved from the ordinary to the demonic. (I discuss the factors in this process in chapter 20.)

Doubling as German?

Is there something especially German in doubling? Germany, after all, is the land of the *Doppelgänger,* the double as formalized in literature and humor. Otto Rank, while tracing the theme back to Greek mythology and drama, stresses its special prominence in German literary and philosophical romanticism, and refers to the "inner split personality, characteristic of the romantic type."[33] That characterization, not only in literature but in political and social thought, is consistent with such images as the "torn condition" *(Zerrissenheit),* or "cleavage," and the "passages and galleries" of the German soul.[34] Nietzsche asserted that duality in a personal way by depicting himself as both "the antichrist" and "the crucified"; and similar principles of "duality-in-unity" can be traced to earlier German writers and poets such as Hölderlin, Heine, and Kleist.[35]

Indeed, Goethe's treatment of the Faust legend is a story of German doubling:

Two souls, alas, reside within my breast
And each withdraws from and repels its brother.[36]

And the original Faust, that doctor of magic, bears more than a passing resemblance to his Nazi countrymen in Auschwitz. In Goethe's hands, Faust is inwardly divided into a prior self responsible to worldly commitments, including those of love, and a second self characterized by hubris in its quest for the supernatural power of "the higher ancestral places."* In a still earlier version of the legend, Faust acknowledges the hegemony of his evil self by telling a would-be spiritual rescuer, "I have gone further than you think and have pledged myself to the devil with my own blood, to be his in eternity, body and soul."[38] Here his attitude resembles the Auschwitz self's fidelity to evil. And Thomas Mann's specific application of the Faust legend to the Nazi historical experience captures, through a musician protagonist, the diabolical quest of the Auschwitz self for unlimited "creative power": the promise of absolute breakthrough, of

---

*The passage concerning the "two souls" continues:

One with tenacious organs holds in love
And clinging lust the world within its embraces.
The other strongly sweeps this dust above
Into the higher ancestral places.

The historian of German literature Ronald Gray finds patterns of "polarity and synthesis" in various spheres of German culture: Luther's concept of a God who "works by contraries," the Hegelian principle of thesis and antithesis, and the Marxist dialectic emerging from Hegel. In all of these, there is the "fusion of opposites," the rending of the individual as well as the collective self, and the passionate quest for unity.[37] One could almost say that the German apocalyptic tradition—the Wagnerian "twilight of the gods" and the general theme of the death-haunted collective end—may be the "torn condition" extended into the realm of larger human connectedness and disconnectedness.

conquering time and therefore death; if the new self will "dare to be barbaric, twice barbaric indeed."[39]*

Within German psychological and cultural experience, the theme of doubling is powerful and persistent. Moreover, German vulnerability to doubling was undoubtedly intensified by the historical dislocations and fragmentations of cultural symbols following the First World War. Who can deny the Germanic "feel" of so much of the doubling process, as best described by a brilliant product of German culture, Otto Rank?

Yet the first great poet to take up the Faust theme was not Goethe but the English playwright Christopher Marlowe. And there has been a series of celebrated English and American expressions of the general theme of the double, running through Edgar Allan Poe's "William Wilson," Robert Louis Stevenson's *The Strange Case of Dr. Jekyll and Mr. Hyde,* Oscar Wilde's *Picture of Dorian Gray,* and the comic strip *Superman.* Indeed, the theme penetrates the work of writers of all nationalities: for instance, Guy de Maupassant's *Le Horla* and Dostoevski's novel *The Double.* [41]

Clearly, the Nazis took hold of a universal phenomenon, if one given special emphasis by their own culture and history. But they could not have brought about widespread doubling without the existence of certain additional psychological patterns that dominated Auschwitz behavior. These internalized expressions of the environment of the death camp came to characterize the Auschwitz self, and have significance beyond that place and time.

---

*Mann also captures the continuity in doubling by speaking of the "implicit Satanism" in German psychology, and by having the devil make clear to the Faust figure that "we lay upon you nothing new . . . [but] only ingeniously strengthen and exaggerate all that you already are."[40]

Chapter 20

The Auschwitz Self: Psychological Themes in Doubling

> The doctor, . . . if not living in a moral situation
> . . . where limits are very clear, . . . is very danger-
> ous.
>
> —Auschwitz survivor

> He has the capacity to veer with every wind, or,
> stubbornly, to insert himself into some fantastically
> elaborated and irrational social institution only to
> perish with it. [For man is a] fickle, erratic, danger-
> ous creature [whose] restless mind would try all
> paths, all horrors, all betrayals . . . believe all things
> and believe nothing . . . kill for shadowy ideas more
> ferociously than other creatures kill for food, then,
> in a generation or less, forget what bloody dream
> had so oppressed him.
>
> —LOREN EISELEY

The Healing-Killing Paradox

The Nazi doctors' immersion in the healing-killing paradox was crucial
in setting the tone for doubling, as the Auschwitz self had to live by that
paradox. To the extent that one embraces the far reaches of the Nazi
vision of killing Jews in order to heal the Nordic race, the paradox disap-
pears. The Auschwitz self can see itself as living out a commendable
principle of "racial hygiene" and working toward a noble vision of or-

ganic renewal: the creation of a vast "German biotic community" in which one can draw parallels between the vast world-conquering German mission and the smallest physiological intracellular system.[1] Even the term *anus mundi* can become associated with a positive mission involving the principle of "the necessity to sweep clean the world."[2] The healing achieved by killing could also become part of the immortalizing vision, of the *"holiest human right and . . . obligation,"* which is *"to see to it that the blood is preserved pure and, by preserving the best humanity, to create the possibility of a nobler development of these beings."*[3]

The Auschwitz self was the means by which the Nazi doctor could bring to his killing the mana of a shaman, a priest, a magician. For in the case of such an ancient healer, "there is no cleavage between the domain of fantasy in which he acts and the world of affairs wherein his mystic acts are efficacious."[4] In that way the Auschwitz doctor-shaman becomes "loaded up with powers"[5] in his deadly "healing" (see also pages 481–84). He is a recognized healer with special powers; his killing is legitimated by, and at the same time further legitimates, the regime's overall healing-killing reversals. Thus it became quite natural to use a vehicle marked with a red cross to transport gas, gassing personnel, and sometimes victims, to the gas chambers.

Since the healing-killing paradox epitomized the overall function of the Nazi regime, there was some truth in the Nazi image of Auschwitz as the moral equivalent of war. War is the only accepted institution (a highly honored one in the case of the Nazis) in which there is a parallel healing-killing paradox. One has to kill the enemy in order to preserve—to "heal"—one's people, one's military unit, oneself. And if one follows the rules of war, one also heals those among the enemy whom one has not quite killed but merely wounded and captured. The "equivalent of war" image, with its claim to courage and endurance, lends "honor" to the self. A Nazi doctor could thus avoid a war in which his life would really be threatened (that on the Russian front) but participate in a claimed moral equivalent of war in which he faced no such danger. The analogy was furthered by the sea of death he encountered and contributed to in Auschwitz. He could experience a *psychological* equivalent of war, at moments feel himself on "the battlefield of the race war."[6] On this and many other issues, partial conviction could combine with rationalization.

Of the three Nazi doctors discussed in detail, Mengele was most in tune with the healing-killing paradox; Wirths did most to maintain it but was least at ease with it; and Ernst B. was at its periphery and for the most part able to limit his activities to healing. But healing-killing perversions came to define all of their outer and inner reality. We remember, for instance, Dr. B.'s essential agreement with his friend Mengele's insistence that "it would be a sin, a crime" not to utilize the special opportunity Auschwitz presented for research with twins; and B.'s further sympathy for the Nazi doctor subjected to "Auschwitz conditions," having to make instant decisions during selections. His message is that the Auschwitz self, developed in response to the healing-killing paradox, should be everyone's basis for judgment—Mengele's, his own, and even mine.

Ritual Reversals

For the Nazi doctor, the selections process had the ritual function of "carefully staged death immersions culminating in honorable survival and earned rebirth."[7] In Auschwitz the psychological survival of the ordeal of the *anus mundi* of selections enabled him to experience that earned rebirth via the formation of the Auschwitz self. He had solidified his relationship to his Auschwitz group by means of what was called "blood cement" (*Blutkitt*),[8] meaning direct participation in the group's practice of killing— a policy long followed by criminal groups throughout the world. In that way the Auschwitz self was "baptized" by passing a test for "hardness."

Like most functioning rituals, selections became regularized over time, as the Auschwitz self became established and more experienced. Ritual thus heightened the "sense of actuality"[9] of that Auschwitz self, and provided it with the "enactments, materializations, realizations" of its commitment.[10] In buttressing the Auschwitz self, selections served the major ritual function of "overcoming of ambivalence as well as of ambiguity," and of "order perceived and yet also participated in."[11] Selections thus ritualized the practice of murder and the acceptance of evil, both made possible by the increasing immersion of the Auschwitz self in the healing-killing paradox.

Selections also provide a ritual drama. Whether the Auschwitz self entered into that drama with integrated élan (as in the case of Mengele) or with hesitation and conflict (as in the case of many others), participation in that "cultural performance"[12] tended to absorb anxieties and doubts and fuse individual actions with prevailing (Nazi) concepts, as does ritual performance in general. Here Auschwitz epitomized the overall Nazi preoccupation with ritual, much of it having to do with healing and killing. The regime drew much of its power from its ritualization of existence, so that every act it called forth could be seen as having profound mythic significance for the "Third Reich" and the "Aryan race." Even when these were, as in the case of selections, forms of "ritual ignorance,"[13] propounded principles in violation of available knowledge of human behavior (in this case, false racial theories), such ritual could give participants a *feeling* of truth.

The healing-killing paradox so dominated Auschwitz as to create a *world of selections*. The Auschwitz self functioned with the understanding that, when selections were diminished in one place (the medical blocks), they were radically expanded in another (at the ramp). Beyond pragmatic Nazi estimates of "needs" was the psychological principle that atrocity begets atrocity:[14] in order to justify selections, one must keep selecting. A hint why this is so can be found in primitive medicine men, whose "possession of magic . . . is not an entirely comfortable asset" because "its possessor may have to meet the hard condition that once he can use his special talent he must do so, or the power he does not choose to wield may turn against his own life."[15] In psychological terms, we may say that the backed-up power so threatening to its possessor is the potential sense of guilt, which can be fended off only by continuous application of that lethal power outward to an enemy. That same principle was active in the Nazi claim that every single Jew had to be killed, lest those remaining alive or their children kill Germans. The Auschwitz self, then, entered into a vicious circle of killing, threatened guilt and death anxiety, and more killing to fend off those perceived psychological threats.

From the standpoint of maintaining the healing-killing paradox, the doctor's conduct of selections "made it perfect" (in Dr. B.'s phrase) bureaucratically (and therefore psychologically) because it conveyed the idea that "an exact medical judgment had been made." But that very medicalization required the Auschwitz self to take on the physician's self-requirement of "how to carry out the matter [killing] humanely." That principle of "humane killing" could take on considerable power for the Auschwitz self: sending typhus patients or potential carriers to the gas chamber did control that disease, and doing the same to large numbers of weak and sick prisoners did indeed improve the hygienic situation in Auschwitz. If one entered into the healing-killing paradox with a comprehensive Auschwitz self, it could seem to make sense, to "work"; and that in turn buttressed the overall doubling process.

Strong healing tendencies could readily lead to conflict in an SS doctor, to a situation in which his Auschwitz self was less than fully dominant. But, in the great majority of cases, that conflict was sufficiently overcome after the transition period for the doctor to do the work of the camp and for the Auschwitz self to become adequately functional. That was very much Wirths's situation, as we know, and it was true also of men like Rohde, who was said to drink heavily and was described as experiencing "a problem of conscience" to the point of discharging a gun on one occasion out of frustration and anger—but who nonetheless "did exactly the same things as the others," that is, went on doing selections. The healing ethos fights a losing battle if it fights at all, as the Auschwitz self takes over. When telling us how an SS doctor "after a few weeks in this environment . . . thinks, 'Yes,' " B. was describing not a sudden epiphany but rather the end point of a process, brief and intense enough, in which the Auschwitz self progressively took hold.

That is why the Hippocratic oath, though a pledge to remain a healer and to disavow killing or harming those one treats, was all but abandoned in Auschwitz. The oath was perceived as little more than a distant and muted ritual one had performed at medical school graduation, and was readily reversed by the searingly immediate selections ritual, as well as by the array of direct pressures and rewards in the direction of a Hippocrates-free Auschwitz self. Indeed, with the oath to Hitler one essentially excluded the Jews from one's Hippocratic responsibilities.

Ideology and Ethos

Very important to doubling was a Nazi doctor's previous idea structure, his ideology and ethos. Even *ideological fragments*—which were all many doctors held in the way of ideology—could promote the process because they became part of an older, more inclusive image structure, or ethos. "Ethos" includes ideology and is often used to suggest the governing or central principle in a movement, but its earlier meaning is the belief structure, evolved over centuries, of a specific cultural group.

Consider the more or less typical Nazi doctor who sought from the movement a form of national renewal; who laughed at the more extreme claims of Nazi racial theory but was drawn to "scientific racism" with its emphasis on German unity; who considered the Nordic race generally superior, and feared racial mixture; who considered himself a rational rather than a fanatical anti-Semite and was critical of the number and prominence of Jewish doctors in German cities; who had not marched in the streets with the Nazis but came to offer them obedience and service in exchange for rank and a military uniform; who volunteered no great personal sacrifice on behalf of the Nazi cause but respected those who did; and who sought maximum professional and personal success within this newly dominant national movement. Such a doctor, despite a seemingly restrained relationship to ideology, could experience the mystical power of the German-Nazi ethos. He could also respond in some degree to the call of Auschwitz.

One was asked to double in Auschwitz on behalf of revitalization that was *communal* (with doctors the racial mediators between the hero-leader and the larger Aryan community) and *sacred* (claiming its ultimate sanction from the dead of the First World War). Hitler was specific about this, declaring with "icy clarity" his doctrine "of the nothingness . . . of the individual human being and of his continued existence in the visible immortality of the nation";[16] as was Alfred Rosenberg in his insistence that human personality is achieved only insofar as one "is integrated, mind and soul, into an organic succession of thousands of his race."[17]* Here is the powerful lure of immortalizing racial-cultural substance.

In young doctors' response to that lure, enthusiasm for practical Nazi achievements merged with a sense of mythic communal power. Communal ethos was so strong that, even when one was deeply troubled by Nazi policies, one hesitated to oppose them because that meant "you become a traitor and stab your own people in the back." One either adheres to the sacred community or is seen (and sees oneself) as a murderous, cowardly traitor.

---

*Rosenberg added that "the new German style . . . is the style of a marching column, no matter where, or to what end, this marching column may be directed."[18] The marching column perfectly represents the merging of individuals into an aggressively omnipotent, perfectly disciplined community, always ready for violence and always on the move.

The SS was the élite "community within the community," "oath-bound," full of "corps spirit," consistent in its mixture of cruelty and courage. Nazi doctors entering the SS imbibed some of this ethos. Each took the SS oath:

> I swear to you, Adolf Hitler—as the Führer and Chancellor of the Reich—loyalty and bravery. I pledge to you and to my superiors, appointed by you, obedience unto death, so help me God[19]—

and thereby became what one observer called an "ideological fighter," whether or not one wore on one's belt buckle (as did ordinary SS men) the SS slogan: "My honor is loyalty" *(Meine Ehre heisst Treue)*. That idealism, however eroded by Auschwitz corruption, was a prod for SS doctors in their initial adaptation and part of the ideological call to doubling. We recall Dr. B.'s stress on "faith" in Nazi ideology as a "bridge" to the SS community. That faith in the *Gemeinschaft* became a source of murderous action and a crucial support for the Auschwitz self. For that self was a creation not just of the individual but of the mystical "collective will," the Auschwitz version in fact of the "triumph of the will."

Ordeal and Ethos

Whatever their original recalcitrance toward it, Auschwitz doctors became caught up in the Nazi-German principle of killing as a difficult but necessary form of *personal ordeal.* When asked how he could bring himself to do such terrible things, Heinrich Himmler is said to have referred to the "karma" of "the Germanic world as a whole," for which "a man has to sacrifice himself even though it is often very hard for him; he oughtn't to think of himself."[20]* Here the killer claims for himself the ordeal of sacrifice. To perform the prescribed ritual slaughter, he offers both himself and his victims to the immortal Germanic people and its hero-deity, Adolf Hitler.

To his high-ranking SS leaders, and on at least one occasion at Auschwitz, Himmler expressed this ethos of killing as an ennobling ordeal. He raised "frankly" the matter of "the annihilation of the Jewish people" and mocked the weak-hearted, even among Party members, each of whom had "his one decent Jew" he wished to save:

> Of all those who talk this way, not one has seen it happen, not one has been through it. Most of you must know what it means to see a hundred corpses lie side by side, or five hundred, or a thousand. To

---

*Thomas Mann captured this principle in his novel *Doctor Faustus* in describing Georges Sorel's pre–First World War *Reflections on Violence* as a precursor of Nazi ideology. Connecting the fate of truth with that of the individual, and indicating for both "a cheapening, a devaluation," *Reflections on Violence* "opened a mocking abyss between truth and power, truth and life, truth and the community," showing that "precedence belonged far more to the community," as truth was abandoned for "community-forming belief."[21]

have stuck this out and excepting in cases of human weakness—to have
kept our integrity, this is what has made us hard. In our history, this
is an unwritten and never-to-be-written page of glory.[22]

The Auschwitz self could be experienced as a call to such an ordeal and
to the necessary but difficult, even heroic, hardness that entailed. That
hardness was race-centered: "We must be honest, decent, loyal and comradely to members of our own blood, but to nobody else," so that if
"10,000 Russian females fall down from exhaustion digging an anti-tank
ditch . . . [that] interests me only insofar as the anti-tank ditch for Germany
is finished," as Himmler expressed it in the same Posen speech of 4
October 1943. All that was to be done within the immortalizing SS mission
as "a National-Socialist order of men of Nordic stamp . . . [who are] the
forebears of later generations essential to ensure the eternal existence of
the Germanic people of Germany."[23] The "blood cement" of direct
involvement (see page 432) was part of the shared ordeal: one *Einsatzgruppen* staff officer "insisted on principle that all commissioned and noncommissioned officers" under him "participate in the executions" in order to
"overcome" themselves as he had "overcome" himself. He was demanding from all an *Einsatzgruppen* equivalent of the Auschwitz self—or, what
has been aptly termed "heroic action in a criminal cause."[24]

When most of the mass murder of Jews had already been accomplished
(in May 1944), Himmler stressed that only the SS could have done it, that
the killing *"could only be tolerable to and could only be carried out by an organization consisting of the staunchest individuals, of fanatical, deeply committed National
Socialists."*[25] SS officials were always to "carry the burden for our people"
—that is, to maintain an *ordeal readiness* for murder.

The shift from face-to-face killing by the *Einsatzgruppen* to the elaborate
machinery of the gas chambers can be said to have diminished the degree
of the ordeal. But the ordeal remained, as did the demand for ordeal
readiness. Then Nazi doctors' conscious sense was more that of "unpleasant" ramp duty involving strain, fatigue, and hardship (what Karl K.
called *eine Strapaze*), requiring a great deal of alcohol to keep going, which
in turn led to the further unpleasantness of a hangover that ruined the
next day. The mutual toasting over the course of a night was undoubtedly
an effort to lend some nobility to what was a further degrading of a
criminal ritual. But the sense of ordeal was still there, as clearly suggested
by B.'s description, when trying to convince me how difficult Nazi doctors' decisions were in Auschwitz, of the pressure on Nazi doctors at the
moment of selection (*"You* must go there, *you* go there—these alternatives leave no room for discussion"). Wirths's insistence upon doing
selections himself, rather than leaving them to other doctors, was a commitment to personal participation in this ordeal—and probably also an
effort to "overcome" his prior self in favor of an emerging Auschwitz self.

The combination of ordeal and ethos gives us another perspective on
the case of Delmotte (see pages 309–11) and on the effective function

of a precarious Auschwitz self. Initially revolted by selections, Delmotte felt that they violated his strong SS idealism. His being treated gently by his medical superiors and brought slowly around to doing selections was in keeping with Himmler's dictum of allowance for weakness. I suspect that part of the message conveyed to him by Mengele (as designated head of the "rehabilitation team") was that a true SS officer—a member of the special SS community—takes on, when necessary for his Führer and his race, precisely those tasks he finds repellent. That powerful argument and related pressures held for Delmotte's Auschwitz self—the latter also ironically buttressed by "fatherly" support from his prisoner physician-professor-mentor—only for a year or so until the end of the war. Then, with the collapse of the Auschwitz environment, Delmotte's relatively admirable capacity for guilt, associated with the quick emergence of his humane prior self, undoubtedly contributed greatly to his suicide. But the principle of ordeal on behalf of ethos and community maintained the Auschwitz self sufficiently for Delmotte to perform the deadly task for which he was brought to Auschwitz.*

Here was a vicious circle, in which the very conflicts over killing that may have haunted the Auschwitz self contributed to its sense of ordeal, which in turn diminished further its concern about what it was doing to others. And as the overall ethos took hold in any such Nazi environment, a man could act as he did and promote his Auschwitz self because "it was expected that I do this."[29] An incremental tendency might also be present, so that the "ordeal" of the Auschwitz self could gradually be accepted.

Biological Renewal

Nazi doctors were always affected by the unique feature of the revitalization ethos, its focus on biological renewal. They, the medical biologists,

---

*There are psychological parallels between Delmotte's case and that of the far more prestigious Nazi, General Erich von dem Bach-Zelewski, who headed the *Einsatzgruppen* in Central Russia (see page 159). Himmler took a keen interest in the case of his "favorite general," conferring by telephone with Grawitz, whom he severely chastised for failing to convey a full picture of Bach-Zelewski's condition and for what he considered the doctor's poor psychological treatment.[26] Nonetheless, the general recovered sufficiently that a few months later he was back killing Jews as the newly appointed overall chief of anti-partisan formations in Russia. His breakdown had been in early March 1942. In September of that year, he wrote to Himmler recommending himself for the new position as the most experienced higher police leader.[27] Bach-Zelewski had a reputation, even within the SS, for his unusual brutality in such activities as putting down the Warsaw rebellion.

As solicitous as Himmler was of Bach-Zelewski during his illness, the Reichsführer bristled when the general, at the time of his breakdown, asked whether the killing of Jews might be stopped in the East, and replied angrily, "That is a Führer order. The Jews are the disseminators of Bolshevism. . . . If you don't keep your nose out of the Jewish business, you'll see what'll happen to you!"[28] For one who collapsed under his ordeal, sympathetic therapy was the order of the day—until he could resume that ordeal. Sympathy stopped when the policy behind the ordeal was questioned. We may strongly suspect that both Bach-Zelewski and Delmotte internalized the desire to harden themselves by SS standards as a means of recovering from psychological breakdown.

were working toward an "organically indivisible national community," opposition to which was considered "the symptom of an illness which threatens the healthy unity of the . . . national organism."[30] For the image of National Socialism as "nothing but applied biology" was not just one doctor's perception from a single Nazi speech; it was a vision put forward by the movement for building nothing less than a biologically evolved state. Gottfried Benn, one of the few German writers of stature who, at least temporarily, embraced the Nazi cause, welcomed "the emergence of a new biological type, a mutation of history and a people's wish to breed itself." Benn was also a physician concerned with the "vitality" of the German race. There seems to have been a bit of the same in Martin Heidegger—no physician but one of the great philosophers of the modern era—in justifying his early sympathy as the Germans' "will to be ourselves."[31]

The temptation for doctors lay in the fact that their realm (that of biology and cure) was to be the realm of national rejuvenation. Their difficulty lay in the murderous course chosen for that rejuvenation and in the group entrusted with the task of "racial police"—the SS. Doctors joining the SS had little difficulty accepting its racial *requirements*—the establishment of Aryan family roots going back several generations—as part of the principle of SS people embodying the racial ideal. Where they began to have difficulty was when, as members of this exemplary group, they were expected to take part in the killing. For that they needed an Auschwitz self, or an equivalent product of doubling. Its formation was aided by the medical temptation of taking over the entire Nazi ethos—of controlling the controlling image of Nazi life.

The Anti-Semitic Ethos

The anti-Jewish aspect of the Nazi ethos was also biologized, so that the Nazi doctor arriving in Auschwitz brought with him some of the ethos of Jews as the threatening anti-race. That imagery was psychologically helpful to the Auschwitz self, since selections were easier to perform if one viewed as potentially murderous enemies the people one was sending to their deaths.

Different from these draconian, abstract, and primal images of Jews were specific contacts with actual Jewish colleagues. Here resentment and envy concerning the number—and, in many cases, the success and talent of Jewish doctors—led to satisfaction at their being forced out of German medicine (which tended quickly to improve the position of Nazi doctors), along with a guilty awareness of complicity in the mistreatment of men who were, after all, their colleagues. As a doctor who was briefly at Auschwitz put it, "You could always say that Jews were guilty" in connection with the Communist danger and other political difficulties, and declare them to be "arch enemies of Germany," after which "the step to their annihilation is only a millimeter long." The anti-Jewish ethos, that is, was everywhere.

But Jewish doctors one had actually known, sometimes as close colleagues or respected teachers, interfered with the ethos. One former Nazi doctor, for instance, recalled "the great figures [with whom he had studied]—Wasserman, Morganroth—and also Blumenthal, the man from whom I learned most about serology," and told me how the Jews "disappeared" from his institute.* While this doctor pleaded helplessness, and held to his ardent Nazi views, his sense of guilt here was palpable, and the pattern was true for other Nazi doctors as well. There could be parallel tendencies even in Auschwitz: Wirths, for instance, was "correct" and even "gentlemanly" to individual Jewish doctors, helping them and putting them in responsible positions, while at the same time holding to a strongly anti-Jewish Nazi ethos. He kept the faith—on one level by maintaining separate hospital blocks for Jews and non-Jews, and much more malignantly by his active role in the medicalized killing of Jews. In virtually all cases the Auschwitz self sought to block out potentially guilty images of actual Jews in favor of an ideological vision of constructive purpose in eliminating Jews or of "solving" the "Jewish problem." There were conflicts in that combined stance, as we know, but mostly of a kind that did little to interrupt the work of the Auschwitz self.

Deadly Logic and Sacred Science

Highly important to the German-Nazi ethos was the claim to logic, rationality, and science. In Auschwitz that claim had special significance in its very grotesqueness. Consider Ernst B.'s description of "rational" Auschwitz discussions among the doctors concerning the necessity of killing all the Jews—providing a "real" solution to an intractable problem rather than the unfeasible solutions of the past (the Madagascar Plan, ghettos that "leaked," etc. [see pages 205–6]). It was this claim to rational thought that made Dr. B. so irate when I raised the question of possible similarities between Auschwitz attitudes and those of the Jonestown mass suicide-murder of 1978 (see page 330): the latter was a form of craziness and emotionalism, while he and his Auschwitz colleagues carefully considered questions of logic and theory. Here one thinks of Hitler's "ice-cold logic," operating so that (as one scholar put it): "from insane premises to monstrous conclusions Hitler was relentlessly logical" and in this way "derived the conclusion that he who loves the human race must destroy the Jews."[32] This deadly logic has an important relationship

---

*August von Wasserman (1866–1925), serologist, developer of Wasserman reaction for the diagnosis of syphilis, and, for a time, director of the Kaiser Wilhelm Institute in Berlin-Dahlem; Julius Morganroth (1871–1924), bacteriologist, who worked with Paul Ehrlich; and Franz Blumenthal (1878–), leading dermatologist and serologist who worked with Wasserman and emigrated to the United States in 1934 (and therefore was the only one of these doctors to "disappear").

to individual paranoia. In paranoia, ideas, even if delusional or hallucinatory, tend to be logically systematized, and therefore convincing to the afflicted individual and often to others as well. Paranoia is in fact a disease of logic, of logic gone mad because divested of critical restraint of any kind. Certain ideological thinkers carry their ethos to the border of paranoia or across that border, without being psychotic; they can then be considered "paranoid personalities," as could Hitler himself, though in some cases it would be difficult to diagnose any form of mental illness.

Newer theories of paranoia stress underlying fear of annihilation, whether of the individual himself or of humankind in general (end-of-the-world imagery). This imagery is sometimes referred to as "soul murder," the term used by a famous early paranoid patient; and the structure of ideas and symptoms, including at times delusions and hallucinations, can be understood as efforts at regaining life power, efforts at revitalization. The exaggerated logic is part of that effort to hold the self together.* A collective version of this pattern is apparent in what I have said about post–First World War Germany as a whole: a sense of having been militarily and psychically annihilated, subjected to "soul murder." Demagogic leaders (notably Hitler, but there were others) could touch that raw nerve of annihilation and soul murder in ways that attributed it to a specifically evil outside force, the Jews.

The extremity of death-camp logic was an attempt to hold together the Auschwitz community, itself an ultimate manifestation of the German-Nazi ethos of Jewish threat and evil—the whole process paralleling that of the logical extremities resorted to in paranoia in order to hold together the individual self. But there is an important difference as well. Individual paranoid logic tends to form over a lifetime, usually originating in extreme early trauma readily perceived as "soul murder" and also influenced by any inherited vulnerability to paranoid states. The collective experience of and response to perceived soul murder can absorb into its deadly logic adults with varied psychological backgrounds, as occurred with Nazi doctors. We therefore do well to resist the temptation to invoke the clinical term "paranoia," even if we draw a partial model from that condition. Rather, the Nazis' logic lays claim to what I have called a "sacred science" as part of a total ideology, an ideology that has totalized the original social trauma as well as the argument and policy invoked in the name of revitalization.[34]

The Nazi ethos thus came to contain a *sacred biology,* whose logic was taken on and actively promulgated by the Auschwitz self. For the claim of logic and rationality was part of the larger Nazi claim of direct outgrowth from the biological laboratory. To be sure, other movements, Marxism and Soviet Communism, for instance, have also claimed scientific validity. But only the Nazis have seen themselves as products and

---

*The sequence from Freud to contemporary work by Ida Macalpine and Richard H. Hunter and by Harold F. Searles is discussed in *The Broken Connection* and placed within a paradigm of symbolization of life and death.[33]

practitioners of the science of life and life processes—as biologically ordained guides to their own and the world's biological destiny. Whatever their hubris, and whatever the elements of pseudo science and scientism in what they actually did, they identified themselves with the science of their time.

They drew upon that science, however, in an apocalyptic, wildly romantic fashion. Hence the merging of the death-haunted, Wagnerian "twilight of the gods" with the most absolute positivism. Whatever the visionary absurdities in projected killing and healing, the logic of science was always, at least in Nazi eyes, close at hand. This combination, apparently manageable in the abstract, required considerable mental effort when acted upon in places like Auschwitz. That combinatory effort was an important struggle of the Auschwitz self, a struggle made possible by the claim of return to the solid ground of science from the most far-flung, romantic stratosphere. The insistence upon rationality and science was as vehement as it was precarious.

The contribution of the actual scientific tradition to this ethos was exemplified by the quintessentially German figure of Ernst Haeckel, that formidable biologist and convert to Darwinism who combined with ardent advocacy of the *Volk* and romantic nationalism, racial regeneration, and anti-Semitism.* He was to become what Daniel Gasman has called "Germany's major prophet of political biology."[35] Nonscientific visionaries could combine their Haeckel with occultist racial views of a kind that undoubtedly inspired Hitler and other high-ranking Nazis. Haeckel himself moved in the latter direction when he embellished his own anti-Semitism with a claim that Christ's merits derived from the fact that he was only half Jewish.†

Haeckel embraced a widely held nineteenth-century theme (found in the English naturalist Alfred Wallace, though not as specifically in Darwin) that each of the major races of humanity can be considered a separate species. Haeckel believed that varied races of mankind are endowed with differing hereditary characteristics not only of color but, more important, of intelligence, and that external physical characteristics are a sign of innate intellectual and moral capacity. He, for instance, considered "woolly-haired" Negroes to be "incapable of a true inner culture and of a higher mental development." And the "difference between the reason of a Goethe, a Kant, a Lamarck, or a Darwin, and that of the lowest savage . . . is much greater than the graduated difference between the reason of the latter and that of the most 'rational' mammals, the anthropoid apes." Haeckel went so far as to say, concerning these "lower races," that since they are "psychologically nearer to the mammals (apes and

---

*Haeckel was a constantly cited authority for the *Archiv für Rassen- und Gesellschaftsbiologie* (Archive of Racial and Social Biology), which was published from 1904 until 1944, and became a chief organ for the dissemination of eugenics ideas and Nazi pseudo science.

†More precisely, Christ's true father was, according to Haeckel, a "Roman officer who had seduced Mary."[36]

dogs) than to civilized Europeans, we must, therefore, *assign a totally different value to their lives*" (italics added).[37] The Auschwitz self could feel a certain national-scientific tradition behind its harsh, apocalyptic, deadly rationality.

In all these ways, Nazi-German ideology and ethos could create in the Auschwitz self an individual form of belief resembling that of primitive people in witchcraft: "The web [of this belief] is not an external structure in which he is enclosed . . . [but] the texture of his thought and he cannot think that his thought is wrong. Nevertheless, his beliefs are not absolutely set but are variable and fluctuating to allow for different situations and to permit empirical observations and even doubts."[38]

Numbing and Derealization

The Auschwitz self depended upon radically diminished feeling, upon one's not experiencing psychologically what one was doing. I have called that state "psychic numbing," a general category of diminished capacity or inclination to feel. Psychic numbing involves an interruption in psychic action—in the continuous creation and re-creation of images and forms that constitutes the symbolizing or "formative process" characteristic of human mental life. Psychic numbing varies greatly in degree, from everyday blocking of excessive stimuli to extreme manifestations in response to death-saturated environments. But it is probably impossible to kill another human being without numbing oneself toward that victim.[39]

The Auschwitz self also called upon the related mechanism of "derealization," of divesting oneself from the actuality of what one is part of, not experiencing it as "real."* (That absence of actuality in regard to the killing was not inconsistent with an awareness of the killing policy—that is, of the Final Solution.) Still another pattern is that of "disavowal," or the rejection of what one actually perceives and of its meaning. Disavowal and derealization overlap and are both aspects of the overall numbing process. The key function of numbing in the Auschwitz self is the avoidance of feelings of guilt when one is involved in killing. The Auschwitz self can then engage in medicalized killing, an ultimate form of numbed violence.

To be sure, a Nazi doctor arrived at Auschwitz with his psychic numbing well under way. Much feeling had been blunted by his early involvement with Nazi medicine, including its elimination of Jews and use of terror, as well as by his participation in forced sterilization, his knowledge of or relationship to direct medical killing ("euthanasia"), and the information he knew at some level of consciousness about concentration camps and medical experiments held there if not about death camps such

---

*Alexander and Margarete Mitscherlich stress the widespread pattern of derealization among Nazis in general, both during their time in power and afterward.[40]

as Auschwitz. Numbing was fostered not only by this knowledge and culpability but by the admired principle of "the new spirit of German coldness."[41] Moreover, early Nazi achievements furthered that hardness; and it is often the case that success breeds numbing.

In discussing patterns of diminished feeling, Ernst B. told me that it was the "key" to understanding what happened in Auschwitz. In also pointing out that "one could react like a normal human being in Auschwitz only for the first few hours," he was talking about how anyone entering the place was almost immediately enveloped in a blanket of numbing. And there was similar significance to the prisoner doctor Magda V.'s rhetorical question: "I mean, how can you understand the horror of it all?"

Transition to Group Numbing

There has to be a transition from feeling to not feeling—a transition that, in Auschwitz, could be rapid and radical. It began with a built-in barrier toward psychologically experiencing the camp's main activity: killing Jews. The great majority of Jews were murdered upon arrival, without having been admitted to the camp and achieving the all-important status of having a number tattooed on one's arm, which in Auschwitz meant life, however precarious. Numbing toward victims was built in because, in Auschwitz terms, those victims never existed. The large selections brought about that massive non-existence; and the selections themselves became psychologically dissociated from other activities, relegated to a mental area that "didn't count"—that is, both derealized and disavowed. In that sense, there was a kernel of truth to Dr. B.'s claim that selections were psychologically less significant to Nazi doctors than the problems of hunger they encountered from moment to moment.

But only a kernel, since Nazi doctors knew that selections meant killing, and had to do the psychological work of calling forth a numbed Auschwitz self in order to perform them. While Nazi doctors varied in their original will, or willingness, to perform selections, they tended to have to overcome some "block" (as Dr. B. put it) or "scruple" (as Nazi literature has it). With the actual performance of one's first and perhaps second selections, one had, in effect, made a pledge to stay numbed, which meant to live within the restricted feelings of the Auschwitz self.

For this transition, the heavy drinking I have referred to has great significance on several levels. It provided, at the very beginning, an altered state of consciousness within which one "tried on" the threatening Auschwitz realities (the melodramatic, even romanticized declarations of doubts and half opposition described by Dr. B.). In this altered state, conflicts and objections need not have been viewed as serious resistance, need not have been dangerous. One could then explore doubts without making them real: one could derealize both the doubts and the rest of one's new Auschwitz life. At the same time, alcohol was central to a pattern of male bonding through which new doctors were socialized into the Auschwitz community. Men pull together for the "common good," even for what was perceived among Nazi doctors as group survival. Drinking enhanced the meeting of the minds between old-timers, who could offer models of an Auschwitz self to the newcomer seeking entry into the realm of Auschwitz killing. The continuing alcohol-enhanced sharing of group feelings and group numbing gave further shape to the emerging Auschwitz self.

Over time, as drinking was continued especially in connection with selections, it enabled the Auschwitz self to distance that killing activity and reject responsibility for it. Increasingly, the Jews as victims failed to touch the overall psychological processes of the Auschwitz self. Whether a Nazi doctor saw Jews without feeling their presence, or did not see them at all, he no longer experienced them as beings who affected him—that is, as human beings. Much of that transition process occurred within days or even hours, but it tended to become an established pattern by two or three weeks.

The numbing of the Auschwitz self was greatly aided by the diffusion of responsibility. With the medical corpsmen closer to the actual killing, the Auschwitz self of the individual doctor could readily feel "It is not I who kill." He was likely to perceive what he did as a combination of military order ("I am assigned to ramp duty"), designated role ("I am expected to select strong prisoners for work and weaker ones for 'special treatment'"), and desirable attitude ("I am supposed to be disciplined and hard and to overcome 'scruples'"). Moreover since "the Führer decides upon the life and death of any enemy of the state,"[42] responsibility lay with him (or his immediate representatives) alone. As in the case of the participant in direct medical killing ("euthanasia"), the Auschwitz self could feel itself no more than a member of a "team," within which responsibility was so shared, and so offered to higher authorities, as no longer to exist for anyone on that team. And insofar as one felt a residual sense of responsibility, one could reinvoke numbing by means of a spirit of numerical compromise: "We give them ten or fifteen and save five or six."

Numbing could become solidified by this focus on "team play" and "absolute fairness" toward other members of the team. Yet if the "team" did something incriminating, one could stay numbed by asserting one's independence from it. I have in mind one former Nazi doctor's denial of responsibility for the medical experiments done by a team to which he provided materials from his laboratory, even though he showed up on occasion at a concentration camp and looked over experimental charts and subjects. That same doctor also denied responsibility for the "team" (committee) decision to allocate large amounts of Zyklon-B for use in death camps, though he was prominent in the decision-making process, because, whatever other members of the team knew, he had not been informed that the gas would be used for killing. In this last example in particular, we sense that numbing can be willed and clung to in the face of the kind of continual involvement of the self in experiences that would ordinarily produce lots of feeling (see footnote on page 161).

Killing without Killing

The language of the Auschwitz self, and of the Nazis in general, was crucial to the numbing. A leading scholar of the Holocaust told of examining "tens of thousands" of Nazi documents without once encountering the word "killing," until, after many years he finally did discover the word —in reference to an edict concerning dogs.[43]

For what was being done to the Jews, there were different words, words that perpetuated the numbing of the Auschwitz self by rendering murder nonmurderous. For the doctors specifically, these words suggested responsible military-medical behavior: "ramp duty" (*Rampendienst*) or sometimes even "medical ramp duty" (*ärztliche Rampendienst*) or "[prisioners] presenting themselves to a doctor" (*Arztvorstellern*). For what was being done to the Jews in general, there was, of course, the "Final Solution of the Jewish question" (*Endlösung der Judenfrage*), "possible solutions" (*Lösungsmöglichkeiten*), "evacuation" (*Aussiedlung* or *Evakuierung*), "transfer" (*Überstellung*), and "resettlement" (*Umsiedlung*, the German word suggesting removal from a danger area). Even when they spoke of a "gassing *Kommando*" (*Vergasungskommando*), it had the ostensible function of disinfection. The word "selection" (*Selektion*) could imply sorting out the healthy from the sick, or even some form of Darwinian scientific function having to do with "natural selection" (*natürliche Auswahl*), certainly nothing to do with killing.

The Nazi doctor did not literally believe these euphemisms. Even a well-developed Auschwitz self was aware that Jews were not being resettled but killed, and that the "Final Solution" meant killing all of them. But at the same time the language used gave Nazi doctors a discourse in which killing was no longer killing; and need not be experienced, or even perceived, as killing. As they lived increasingly within that language—and they used it with each other—Nazi doctors became imaginatively bound to a psychic realm of derealization, disavowal, and nonfeeling.

As one gradually became habituated to Auschwitz, the Auschwitz self internalized its own requirements. Group support for the adaptation was always present, and life there became "like the weather," except more predictable: part nature, an enveloping reality. When Dr. Magda V. told me, "The thing was, there were never very many Germans around," she was not only commenting on the small number of SS personnel needed to control the camp but also suggesting a sense of automated natural power. As the Auschwitz self enabled a Nazi doctor to go on selecting, with his assistants taking care of all the details and inmates keeping records of all that took place in the camp; as transports arrived and the crematoria smoked; as winter gave way to spring and spring to summer —if the Auschwitz self did not exactly feel that "God is in His heaven," it at least experienced the security of being part of a larger, inexorable flow of human events.

In equating Auschwitz with an ordinary "civilian enterprise" such as a "sewerage project," Dr. B. reflected the intense psychological requirement of the Auschwitz self to hold to that image, to feel nothing more. The attitude resembled that, described by Raul Hilberg, among officials of German railroads responsible for transporting Jews from ghettos to death camps, who both "realize[d] what they were doing" and "coped with it finally in the most ingenious way by not varying their routine and not restructuring their organization, not changing a thing in their correspondence or mode of communications."[44] The Auschwitz self did continuous psychological work to maintain that internal sense of numbed habituation in order to fend off potentially overwhelming images of its relationship to guilt, death, and murder. It could largely succeed, as Dr. B. told me, because dead bodies did not have to be viewed* but "only smelled," and one got used to the smell.

Insofar as it took in some of the actual atrocity, the Auschwitz self may have moved quickly to a resigned, "above the battle" stance: Dr. B.'s view, for example, that it was no different from other destructive events except "for the dimensions . . . and that is clearly a technical question." Or Dr. Otto F.'s insistence, concerning the Nazi era, that one "see the good as well as the bad and . . . evaluate . . . what really happened." The Auschwitz self may have come to view its own survival in the midst of so much death as proof of virtue, of (as Dr. F. went on to say) "having an absolutely white vest," or pure conscience. And that claim to virtue was maintained by clinging to a sense of "status honor" (in Max Weber's term),[46] of good standing within the mores of one's group.

When Ernst B. spoke of the extraordinary "Auschwitz atmosphere" as determining all behavior, he was suggesting the sheer power of the numbed habituation of Auschwitz routine. That power was manifest in the eventual contributions to Auschwitz of both Wirths and Delmotte, whatever their inner conflict and residual humanity.

"A Separate Reality"

Nazi doctors discussing Auschwitz seemed to me to be messengers from another planet. They were describing a realm of experience so extreme, so removed from the imagination of anyone who had not been

---

*As routines became established, an assistant could look through the peephole to confirm that people inside the gas chamber were dead. Or even if the doctor himself looked, he would not necessarily "see" the victims—that is, experience them as human beings. Virtually the only SS personnel in Auschwitz who seemed to experience themselves as killers were some of those most directly involved in the gassing, including medical *Desinfektoren*. Not all "poured out" their hearts to Höss; some exhibited sadism, and just one was "calm and relaxed, unhurried and expressionless" (that is, absolutely numbed).[45] We could say that these men for the most part took over the burden of guilt feelings for Nazi doctors and other higher-ranking Auschwitz officers, including Höss himself.

there, that it was literally a separate reality. That quality—that absolute removal from ordinary experience—provided the Auschwitz self with still another dimension of numbing. Even as part of itself was absorbed in routine, another part could feel the environment to be so distinct from the ordinary that *anything* that happened there simply did not count. One could not believe what one was doing, even as one was doing it. Marianne F. captured this sense in Nazi doctors around her when she observed, "The fact is that if you do something that is totally unbelievable, and you are incapable of believing, you don't believe it. . . . The gas chambers, . . . the houses that the crematoria had, . . . brick houses, windows, curtains, white picket fences. . . . Nobody would have believed that." Part of the schizophrenic situation was the ability to mobilize the Auschwitz self into perverse actions in which it could not itself believe. The feeling was something like: "Anything I do on planet Auschwitz doesn't count on planet Earth." And what one does not believe, whatever the evidence of one's own actions, one does not feel. That is why Dr. Tadeusz S. could say, of Nazi doctors, with bitter irony: "They have no moral problems."

Auschwitz was a staged melodrama in which the authors had so indulged their wildest fantasy as to render it completely absurd, unbelievable to its director (Nazi doctors and other officials), to its actors (inmates) pressed into the melodrama, or to its audience (the local population, the Germans, the world), all the more so since each group within that audience had considerable additional motivation toward disbelief. Otto F., the Nazi doctor who was considerably implicated during his brief stay at Auschwitz, spoke of the whole Nazi era as "a momentary phenomenon, the coming together of the most varied elements, . . . not at all in the mentality of the German people."

For the Auschwitz self, that is, the very bizarreness of its actions—the dimensions of evil it knew—supported its numbed capacity for that very evil.*

Omnipotence and Impotence

The Auschwitz self wavered between the sense of omnipotent control over the lives and deaths of prisoners and the seemingly opposite sense of impotence, of being a powerless cog in a vast machine controlled by unseen others. These polarized feelings were undoubtedly widespread among death-camp personnel. But they had special meaning for doctors, who ordinarily experience both extremes of feeling in everyday confrontations with disease and death and accompanying struggles with their

---

*Hence the statement, made to me directly by Alexander Mitscherlich, to the effect that most Germans of the Nazi generation were incapable of confronting their guilt because its dimensions would be too overwhelming. That is, they could not, then or now, permit themselves to feel.

own death anxiety. The polarity took on grotesque dimensions in Auschwitz, as Nazi doctors called forth feelings of omnipotence and related sadism on the one hand, and of impotence and sometimes masochism on the other, in order to quiet this death anxiety.

It is difficult for most of us to imagine what it means psychologically to experience the degree of power over the lives and deaths of others held by the Auschwitz self. A prisoner doctor tried to make a similar point in speaking of Nazi doctors as "holding a [form of] power superior to that of the Roman emperors." While the omnipotence was supposed to be limited by policies from above—weak prisoners were to be killed and stronger ones preserved—in actuality the mood or whim of the SS doctor could determine the prisoners' fate. That omnipotence was extended to unlimited manipulative use of the bodies of prisoners, especially Jews, in connection with medical experiments: again a cruel caricature of ordinary patterns touching on omnipotence that can be present in authentic medical researchers.

The omnipotence was given still another dimension by the general degradation of prisoners and by their desperate efforts in camp selections to create the appearance of strength: struggling to march or run vigorously when actually close to death from starvation, stuffing their clothes in order to look more robust, or finding something with which to color their cheeks or lips and hide their extreme pallor. Moreover, both omnipotence and degradation become themselves routine, so that the Auschwitz self came to require them for its function.

Death Control

Yet these all-powerful figures seemed fearful. "They were terribly afraid of death [as Tadeusz S. observed]. The greatest murderers were the greatest cowards." And they appeared "petrified" (as Marianne F. put it) of possible infection and went to extremes to avoid potentially contagious inmates.* There is no doubt that the omnipotent stance of the Auschwitz self clearly served the psychological function of warding off its own death anxiety. Having renounced the commitment to healing which can protect one from some of that anxiety, one had constant need for omnipotence.

I have noted repeatedly how omnipotence merged with sadism: Mengele's "special kind of smile" while performing selections undoubtedly included pleasure in others' suffering. But the suffering inflicted with a constant threat of death can be understood as a maximal expression of

---

*The sick people to be avoided were mostly Jews, of course, precisely the agents of alleged "contamination" of the entire Nordic race. The Nazis combined these levels of contamination in their slogan "Jews, lice, typhus!" The avoidance of Jewish patients by a Nazi doctor was both a self-fulfilling prophecy (the Nazis forcing Jews into situations where they developed typhus so that they really became infectious and dangerous) and a newly vivid metaphor which could further cement the Nazi doctor's constellation of omnipotence and impulse to victimize Jews.

domination and control over another human being. From the standpoint of a life-death paradigm, sadism is an aspect of omnipotence, an effort to eradicate one's own vulnerability and susceptibility to pain and death.

There is a similar combination in SS doctors' toying with inmates' feelings; and, in manipulative shows of kindness followed by extreme cruelty and apparent joy, in sending people to their death. Indeed, the Auschwitz self took shape within an omnipotent-sadistic structure and expectation, so much so that avoiding that stance required some form of inner resistance.

It is likely that impulses toward omnipotence in doctors attracted them to the SS and to the concentration-camp system. Here, too, SS doctors varied and formed a kind of continuum according to the degree of those impulses. But the environmental structuring was crucial. That is why it could be said that Mengele, surely at the extreme end of the omnipotence-sadism continuum, would have become under other conditions a relatively ordinary German physician-professor. It can even be argued that a doctor whose omnipotent-sadistic impulses were too great would have had difficulty functioning in Auschwitz because those impulses could have been at odds with the numbing required, and their expression could have interrupted the smooth technology of killing. (Mengele, we recall, was able to harmonize these and other personal tendencies with the requirements of the environment.)

Yet the Auschwitz self became involved in a process of perpetual reinforcement: it responded to encouragement for strong feelings of omnipotence and expressed them as required in relatively structured Auschwitz form; that expression in turn created actual or potential anxiety having to do with death and killing, which then required additional feelings of omnipotence-sadism in order to ward off that anxiety. Hence the apparent increase noted by some prisoner doctors, over time, in the Auschwitz self's expression of omnipotence and sadism.

Auschwitz was the hub of the vast Nazi store of omnipotence and sadism, which included an enormous attraction to death and its borders. For doctors there were the added components of omnipotent tendencies in medicine in general but most especially the vision of National Socialism as "nothing but applied biology" (see pages 129–31). That vision also incorporated the mystical Nazi version of the collective "will," which in much of German philosophy has been viewed as an absolute metaphysical principle and "the agent of a law of nature and of history."[47] Thus believing Nazis saw themselves as "children of the gods,"[48] empowered to destroy and kill on behalf of their higher calling, as men who claimed "spurious attributes of divinity."[49] All Nazis staked some claim to this transcendent state, but doctors could buttress their omnipotence with those bizarre and compelling claims made in the name of biology, evolution, and healing. The Auschwitz self could feel itself to be tapping the power source of nature itself in becoming the engine of the Nazi movement, or nature's engine.

Nature's Engine

That metaphor of "nature's engine" suggests the relationship of omnipotence to the apparently opposite feeling of powerlessness or impotence, of being no more than a tiny cog in someone else's machine. The Auschwitz self could swing from the one emotion to the other, both turning out to be part of the same psychological constellation. The very forces that provided its sense of power over others could cause it to feel itself overwhelmed, threatened, virtually extinguished. For another principle suggested by the observation that "one could react like a normal human being in Auschwitz for only the first few hours" is the extraordinary power of that environment over *any* self that entered it.

Moreover, the Auschwitz self quickly sought that stance of powerlessness (as Dr. B. cited some doctors: "I'm not here because I want to be. . . . I can't change the fact that prisoners come here. I can just try to make the best of it") as a way of renouncing responsibility for what was unsaid: that "prisoners come here" to be murdered. This emotional and moral surrender to the environment had great psychological advantages. The Auschwitz self could feel: "*I* am not responsible for selections. *I* am not responsible for phenol injections. *I* am a victim of the environment no less than the inmates." More than mere retrospective rationalization, this stance of nonresponsibility was still another means of avoiding feelings of guilt at the time. The Auschwitz self permitted the murderous environment to sweep over and into it. It accepted that environment's givens: "Mass murder is the norm, so it is commendable to select and thereby save a few people, or to experiment on prisoners and maim or kill a few here and there since they are in any case destined for death." The Auschwitz self could then become an absolute creature of context, and there is no better way to abnegate moral responsibility of any kind. One can expend considerable psychic energy in seeking and achieving the status of the helpless pawn.

But the more accurate image may be that of environmental *tool.* A tool does not initiate action but plays an important technical role in it by enhancing the skill and efficiency of the wielder. Here, of course, the wielder was the Nazi leadership—ultimately, the Führer himself. But from the standpoint of the Nazi biomedical vision, the Auschwitz self was a tool also of the evolutionary process, of a biological imperative. In this way the biologization of Auschwitz—of Nazi Germany in general—contributed to a doctor's self-abnegation and powerlessness no less than to his omnipotence.

The Auschwitz self could also experience the pleasures of obedience. For just as omnipotence becomes readily associated with sadism, so can powerlessness or impotence be associated with masochism. The fear experienced by the Auschwitz self had to do not only with specific superiors but with threats of being somehow dislodged from its balance of omnipotent power and impotent helplessness. It required that balance for continuously warding off anxiety and, above all, responsibility. The equilibrium tended to be unsteady in the Auschwitz self, as in the case of the shaman for whom "no amount of power . . . seems to be enough" and who lives constantly in "the sense of his relative impotence in the spirit-world."[50]

"Helpless" Omnipotence

This powerlessness associated with omnipotence was in fact cultivated throughout the Nazi movement. Dr. Otto F. epitomized it, declaring that for a student it was "a matter of course" to undergo military training with weapons; as a doctor one underwent *Gleichschaltung* because "you had to," and you had to perform sterilizations also "as it was simply ordered by the university which received its order from the state health offices;" and in Auschwitz "you're just there on the spot and helpless" (although he was actually chief camp doctor, at least briefly). Doctors received commands from the camp commander, Dr. F. explained, but even the latter was trapped by a kind of blackmail held over him by the Nazi regime so that "he suffered badly." Similarly, about sending *Einsatzgruppen* personnel back to duty after successfully treating them, one former Nazi doctor told me that "it was a horrible thing but we couldn't do anything [else]." And concerning cooperation with direct medical killing, or "euthanasia," another doctor remembered thinking, "Well what can be done? First of all we are powerless, we can't change this situation."

But in all those situations, however Nazi doctors felt and wanted to feel powerless, they were also in a stance of omnipotence. Indeed, the entire *Führer* principle rendered one simultaneously a helpless tool (because only the Führer decided all things) and one who shared in the Führer's omnipotence, by serving as the agent (or tool) of the Führer. Since the Führer's will was the court of last resort, it was for everyone else a system of nonresponsibility. And, indeed, even the Führer could be painted as "helpless": because the Jew's evil forced the Führer to act or make war on him; or because psychologically the Führer's sense of helplessness was "projected onto the Jews" along with "the fear of contamination, of impotence . . . [and] the destruction of the male's chief source of identity and power that was being culturally eroded . . . by the modern mass world . . . most particularly and painfully in Germany where a long patriarchal tradition was crumbling traumatically away."[51]

Killers as Doctors: Professional Identity

It is ironic, but psychologically not surprising, that these men struggled, in the midst of their killing function, to hold on to their sense of themselves as doctors. All the more so since, as Dr. B. told us, "medical activity [for Nazi doctors] in Auschwitz consisted only of selecting people for the gas chamber." Among the elements required for the function of a doctor's Auschwitz self was the assertion of medical identity.

Hermann Langbein sensed the importance of that identity in developing a policy of addressing them as "Doctor," instead of by military rank as one was supposed to do, because he noted that it created a softer, more informal tone. The title also confirmed a man's sense of himself as physician and not merely SS officer and thus undoubtedly helped Langbein in his efforts on behalf of the prisoner population, mostly concerning matters in the medical blocks. We know that Nazi doctors' medical identity had been permeated by the Nazi ethos before their arrival in Auschwitz. They were heirs of a great medical tradition with an abiding concern for medical ethics, including long-standing restriction among German doctors on the use of drugs with unknown effects on human subjects and the frequent practice of trying out such drugs on themselves. They were also heirs of considerable medical-political infighting, and of a profession that could encourage to the point of caricature the idea of the physician-scientist who focused exclusively on a disease entity to the point of being oblivious to the humanity of his patient, and whose position, especially if a professor, gave him a claim to unerring wisdom. While individual doctors varied in their relation to this stance—there were, of course, many dedicated healers among them—they had available to them, long before the Nazis, the model of the "medical *Führer.*" This heritage of a great professional tradition in decline—highly uncertain of its standing among the professions[52]—made Nazi doctors especially responsive to promises of professional, no less than personal and national, revitalization.

The Nazis courted, bullied, flattered, threatened, and above all "coordinated" physicians in accordance with their relentless *Gleichschaltung* policy (see pages 33–35). At the same time they expanded the doctor's identity into that of the *militarized medical Führer.* Kurt Blome, who became deputy to Leonardo Conti, chief physician of the Reich, captured the spirit of this medical identity in an autobiographical book, *Arzt im Kampf* ("Physician in Struggle" [1942]), in which he exuberantly equated medical and military power in their battle for life and death.[53] The militarization of medicine began at universities, where, as Dr. Otto F. tells us, "most students became soldiers," as did many professors; and it became a matter of pride for medical students to undergo training with weapons. Many senior Nazi medical leaders had fought in the *Freikorps,* and one could not in Nazi Germany achieve full medical prestige without a prominent military background.

There could be considerable confusion about the new identity. For one thing, many of the medical "old fighters," such as Lolling and Blome, could be looked down upon by other doctors as lacking in medical skills, as more *Nazi* than physician; and they were surely medical versions of the characteristically Nazi "deeply half-educated man" (see pages 492–93). The term was used by Joachim C. Fest for ideologue Alfred Rosenberg.[54]

Nor did *well-*educated Nazi doctors escape that confusion in clinging tenaciously to their medical identity. One former Nazi doctor spent decades, following conviction at Nuremberg (for involvement in experiments) and a long prison sentence, attempting to restore his medical honor; during our interviews, he repeatedly asked that I intervene formally and even legally on his behalf, despite my clear declarations from the beginning that no such action on my part was remotely possible.

For Jews to be made into victims, Jewish doctors had to be divested of their standing as healers (as I have described in chapter 1). Long before Auschwitz, the slogan was put forward in Germany that "a Jewish doctor is no doctor; he is an abortionist and a poisoner."[55] But German doctors became precisely what they had accused Jewish doctors of being—not abortionists but killers of infants and children, certainly "poisoners," and also, in their way, "treaters" or "handlers" of the sick. The further Auschwitz irony (found in other camps as well) was that the only authentic healers were the prisoner doctors, who were, of course, mainly Jewish.

Nazi doctors could make psychological use of that irony by living vicariously, medically speaking, through the prisoner doctors they sponsored and ruled over. The Auschwitz self could take on its own medical identity (furthered by medical hobbies and "scientific" experiments) and thereby become better able to kill.

The Purely Technical

Perhaps the single greatest key to the medical function of the Auschwitz self was the technicizing of everything. That self could divest itself from immediate ethical concerns by concentrating only on the "purely technical" or "purely professional" *(das rein Fachliche)*. Demonstrating "humanity" meant killing with technical efficiency.

For the Auschwitz self there is a logical sequence: a doctor's task is to alleviate suffering and to exert a humane influence in any setting. When the setting is one of mass murder, that means calling forth medical and technical skills to diminish the pain of victims. While the logic depends upon a highly technicized view of medical function, the Auschwitz self can grasp at the pseudo-ethical principle of "humane killing."

That principle was put forward not just by Auschwitz doctors but by the Nazi regime in general. Hitler himself, in his final testament-suicide note, contrasted the painful deaths of "Europe's Aryan peoples" by hunger, battle, or bombing with the "more humane means" by which "the real criminal . . . [had] to atone for his guilt."[56]

The use of poison gas—first carbon monoxide and then Zyklon-B—was the technological achievement permitting "humane killing." Hence, the early advice by Grawitz, chief SS physician, when consulted by Himmler on the matter, in favor of gas chambers—surely the ultimate in such technical-medical consultation.

But these two "humanitarians" were undoubtedly more concerned about the well-being of the killers. The psychological difficulties experienced by the *Einsatzgruppen* in face-to-face killing (see pages 159–62) were also met by a form of medical technicism. The *Wehrmacht* neuropsychiatrist who had treated these psychological difficulties in *Einsatzgruppen* troops, described them to me—the general manifestations of anxiety, including anxiety dreams—in the most detached clinical tones. When I asked him whether *he* had ever experienced anxiety dreams in response to all this killing or to his treating the killers, he answered that he had not: "I never killed anybody"; and, "As doctors . . . we were outsiders." It also became clear that he and his colleagues did not alter their medical approach in any significant way when treating these "killer troops" (as he called them during our interviews), but simply did what they could to relieve symptoms and help the men to return to duty. He would even sometimes gently warn them, "Be careful now, you're complaining but you're well." He was trying to suggest to me that, in doing so, he was considering the interests of the individual killer soldier. But there was no doubt that he was playing the role of the physician suspicious of malingering, who insisted upon holding to strictly medical criteria in decisions concerning sending these men back to duty where they could continue their killing. The extreme medical-psychiatric technicism here has two dimensions: first, the use of one's specialized knowledge for the sake of the command structure of one's military unit, whose function even ordinarily is the killing of enemy soldiers; and the special feature here that the "duty" to which patients were returned had nothing to do with war and its rules but was simply that of murdering Jews. One was returning them to an atrocity-producing situation in the extreme, to a form of duty where atrocity was not only likely in the average case but was precisely one's assignment (see page 15).

The more crude forms of killing in Nazi camps described by Ernst B. as being on the level of a "handicraft" could be seen as intermediate stages in the shift from primitive *Einsatzgruppen* to sophisticated Auschwitz killing. The evidence suggests that the doctors were active at all levels, and that they contributed their professional knowledge all through the improving technological sequence, culminating in what Dr. B. called the "perfection" of Auschwitz. Examples here include doctors' important role in 14f13 connections between "euthanasia" killing and death camps and the early role of doctors in the development of Zyklon-B gas, though we know that the gas itself and its applicability to the killing of human beings were discovered by nonmedical technical experts. The importance of this medical-technological stance to the Auschwitz self is suggested by B.'s statement that when a doctor's specific suggestion for improving the efficiency of the crematorium turned out to be successful, "he was just as pleased about it as [any doctor would be] after a well-performed [surgical] operation." Here professional pride merges into German cultural preoccupation with individual and organizational efficiency. That combination was also reflected in the Auschwitz doctors' resentment of their superiors in Berlin for providing inadequate technical facilities (gas chambers and crematoria) for the professional requirements of the mass killing.

There is always a technical element to medicine and a necessity for a mechanical model of the body. The ordinary doctor, in effect, says (or should say) to the patient: "Allow me to look at your body as a machine, in order to do what I can in the service of your overall health as a human being." But the Nazi doctor held to an absolutized mechanical model extending out into the environment. The machine of the body was subsumed to an encompassing killing machine, and Auschwitz inmates had no standing except as they could be seen as contributing to that larger machine. The Auschwitz self of the Nazi doctor was also part of that environmental machine, charged with maximizing its own as well as the inmate's contribution to it. The extraordinary technical-medical success of the killing machine could create the impression for the Auschwitz self that nature itself was responding—that the project was in harmony with the natural world.

Simply absorbing oneself in medical work, in Auschwitz or elsewhere, was a way that physicians could technicize their relationship to mass murder. When I asked Dr. Otto F. whether, over the course of his extensive medical service with the police and the SS (outside of his brief stay in Auschwitz), he had encountered any atrocities or examples of Nazi mass killing, his answer was that he had been extremely busy setting up hospitals and medical programs so that at times he worked from fourteen to sixteen hours a day. More specific for the Auschwitz self of physicians was Wirths's intensity in seeking actual medical work whenever possible. A nonmedical but parallel example is a statement by Rudolf Höss describing his superhuman efforts to get Auschwitz built and functional and declaring, "I lived only for my work."[57]

"A Doctor Remains a Doctor"

The matter became more complicated for the Auschwitz self when performing something close to a medical act in the very process of killing: for example, examining the degree of muscular emaciation of medical block inmates as a criterion for whether to send them to the gas chamber. Even then, one's momentary sense of functioning as a doctor could have specifically diminished awareness of killing. The same could be true of such medical judgments that overcrowding and pure hygienic conditions required selecting larger numbers of prisoners for the gas chambers: then, too, as absurd as it may seem from the outside, the Auschwitz self could still distance itself from the killing by the sense it was performing a medical function. As a prisoner doctor put it, "A doctor remains always a doctor—a physician who tortures remains a physician all the same," so that as a doctor he must "justify himself to himself."

Justifying oneself to oneself as a doctor was what Ernst B. was doing when he suggested that, while helping people in Auschwitz, he found his medical calling there; and what Wirths was doing in his persistent claim of medical purity. But the truth was, as one survivor phrased it, that no physician in the entire German concentration-camp system "gained distinction for his work *as a doctor.*" The statement accurately suggests that working as part of the Nazi project in the camps meant abnegation of medical responsibility. An important psychological step here is the SS doctor's giving expression to his "holy terror of infection" (in Kogon's words)[58] by absolute avoidance of typhoid and other contagious patients. That meant stepping out of the Hippocratic sphere of the healer. The Auschwitz self could not psychologically afford that interpretation and sought to avoid it by clinging to every possible fragment of remaining medical identity.

An aspect of that struggle was some Nazi doctors' glorification of their role. Dr. Otto F., for instance, told me that "there existed an outstanding medical attitude from the beginning to the end, and of everything published about it so far not one single word is applicable." He went on to present a series of unsubstantiated claims that doctors assigned to Auschwitz had resisted the killing process there, and spoke of a duty that "I owe . . . to my colleagues who fell during the war" to bear witness to their courage in adversity. One could say that he was still promoting the Nazi equation of Auschwitz with service in war, while at the same time expressing actual feelings of a survivor mission, however misguided, in terms of fellow doctors killed during his military service. Significantly, such implicated Nazi doctors never brought up any of the few cases of genuine medical resistance to the Nazis: that of Ewald in opposing direct medical killing, or "euthanasia" (see pages 82–87); or the more quiet resistance to that program by men like Karl Bonhoeffer (see pages 81–82). To do so would have further contrasted genuine resistance with their own behavior. What these doctors sought to do instead was to defend more broadly the good name of German medicine at that time as a means of claiming for themselves a kind of automatic, reflected medical virtue.

The Postwar Self

Most Nazi doctors who worked in camps fled from approaching Allied armies. But others, less identifiable as having been associated with criminal activities, told me proudly of collegial encounters, sometimes even joint medical work, with Allied physicians soon after the surrender. Whatever the accuracy or exaggeration of these accounts, and the possible need of some Allied physicians to see German colleagues as having been less corrupted than was actually the case, what was involved psychologically for Nazi doctors was their intense effort to reconnect with the Hippocratic sphere as a way of claiming they had never left it.

Upon returning to their homes, they continued, for the most part, to try to cast off their Auschwitz or Nazi self and to see themselves (and of course to represent themselves to the world) as essentially decent and moderate postwar German burgher-physicians of a conservative stamp. An incentive for being interviewed was to meet with me as doctor to doctor and thereby reinforce their sense of themselves as healers. They were ambivalent, of course, given their residual doubling and their sense, accurate enough, that I would probe for the Auschwitz or Nazi self. Yet to refuse to see me would be to suggest—to themselves, if not to me— that the Nazi self still loomed large for them and had to be protected. What many of them wanted from me was an opportunity to put forward the healing self and to receive my American, or American-Jewish, confirmation of it. And that healing self tended to be available to them professionally. Even Nazi doctors who had been directly involved in murder could initiate or resume medical practice in their home areas and become conscientious, much-admired physicians.* Hence, the strange three-part odyssey from pre-Nazi physician-healer, to Nazi physician-killer, to post-Nazi physician-healer.

What these doctors could not psychologically do was confront the Nazi or Auschwitz self in its relationship to medicalized killing. Here there was conscious and unconscious collusion on the part of much of the postwar German medical profession. There was, for example, the protection given Heyde by other doctors before he was brought to trial, as well as his strange death (see page 119). And even a man like Ewald who showed considerable courage in resisting direct medical killing, destroyed records that might have implicated other psychiatrists in that destructive project and perhaps raised certain questions about himself as well. But the most striking medical collusion in this respect was the ostracism by the German medical profession of the distinguished psychoanalyst Alexander Mitscherlich because he insisted upon full disclosure of its crimes.†

Precisely because it had not been confronted, the Nazi or Auschwitz self tended to surface at odd moments: Ernst B.'s nostalgia for people's sense of purpose during the Nazi era; and the attempt of several doctors I interviewed to bear witness to the Nazi era in their own way, by covering over crimes of Nazi doctors and preserving the reputation of German medicine. A doctor's inability to confront the Nazi or Auschwitz self left him without moral clarity concerning his contemporary self.

---

*One example was Dr. Kurt Heissmeyer, who conducted cruel medical experiments in the Neuengamme concentration camp on twenty Jewish children taken from Auschwitz. Artificially infected with tuberculosis, they were murdered on Heissmeyer's request so they could not be witnesses. Also murdered were two French doctors, two Dutch orderlies, and twenty-four Russian prisoners of war. After the war, Heissmeyer returned to his home in Magdeburg, now in East Germany, where he was highly regarded as a lung and tuberculosis specialist.[59]

†According to Dr. Mitscherlich, the first report on medical crimes he and his collaborator, Fred Mielke, produced immediately disappeared from bookstores; German physicians arranged to buy up the entire printing in order to prevent the book from being read by anyone else.[60]

The fate of Nazi doctors after the defeat varied enormously. Quite a few killed themselves, probably relatively more than in other professions. Another group was executed after trials under Allied authority in Nuremberg and elsewhere and after later trials under German authority. Many served prison sentences, which were, however, generally considered light for the crimes committed. A few, like Mengele, escaped and were never caught. A considerable number returned to medical practice and continued with it until retirement or natural death—or until, as in a few cases, they were discovered to have been criminals and belatedly tried. Many are practicing now. But the doubling process and the residual Nazi or Auschwitz self has remained with them and significantly affected their attitudes and their lives. For this reason, younger Germans could say to me that there was no hope of salvaging that generation.

A prisoner doctor who struggled painfully to maintain healing principles when there, asked me somewhat rhetorically, "Can Auschwitz be a true reflection of the medical?" He was trying to point to the extremity of conditions behind the profound medical corruption. A German anti-Nazi doctor, in discussing my research, asked, "What are we allowed to do with other people? What is the limit?" A former Nazi doctor who had spent a brief period at a killing center for mental patients, in discussing any future principle of mercy killing, asked, "Who would do it? A doctor? A hangman?" As Nyiszli said, "Among all the criminals and murderers, the most dangerous type is the criminal physician."[61] The doctor's danger, we now see, lies in his capacity to double in a way that brings special power to his killing self even as he continues to anoint himself with medical purity.

The Construction of Meaning

Finally, the Auschwitz self takes on a larger sense of meaning. Its activities take on a logic and purpose and come to seem appropriate to the environment and its overall ethos. What that self becomes is not only acceptable but significant.

Such a sense of significance is an important means of fending off feelings of guilt. More than that, it is part of a universal proclivity toward constructing good motives while participating in evil behavior. That proclivity is one of the remarkable dimensions of human adaptability, of man's capacity (in Loren Eiseley's words) "to veer with every wind, or, stubbornly, to insert himself into some fantastically elaborated and irrational social institution only to perish with it."[62] For no reality is directly or fully given us as human beings. Rather we must inwardly "construct" that reality on the basis of what we inwardly bring to what is "out there." Each such construction, every reality, is influenced by all aspects of one's psyche, as influenced in turn by individual and cultural history and even by species evolution. At the same time, we are meaning-hungry creatures; we live on images of meaning. Auschwitz makes all too clear the principle that the human psyche can create meaning out of anything.

The Force of Routine

The meaning derives partly from *routine* as such. The daily happenings and environmental rhythm at Auschwitz became (as the word's derivation suggests) a *route* or path, a direction of the inner as well as the outer being. To report to an office, to speak to colleagues, to make one's rounds on the medical block, to spend a bit of time at one's research, to confer with camp officials and prisoner functionaries on diet and sanitary procedures, to issue medical and disciplinary orders, to here and there exchange an amusing anecdote or tell a little joke, to conduct selections for an arriving transport, to have meals and evening entertainment with fellow officers—all these came together as a life form, within which the mind could build coherence and significance. The whole vast institution was on the same "route," including coerced activities of prisoner doctors as well as other inmates. It was in that sense a total mission—everyone's —though the nature of the mission may have been kept more hazy than the sense that there was one.

Through the blur of the medical mystification of the "as if" situation, selections themselves took on meanings for the SS doctor: he was saving a few Jews; the "Jewish problem" was being "solved"; he was improving the health of the camp, diminishing the danger of epidemics, lessening the danger of overcrowding.

For the Auschwitz self, the daily routine, including notably selections, was *totalized:* meaning came to lie in the performance of one's daily tasks rather than in the nature or impact of those tasks. Then, however "topsy-turvy" things became in Auschwitz (as one survivor put it), "nothing seemed strange there." Auschwitz could even come to seem a place whose very extremity permitted freer and franker discussion of meaning —as in Dr. B.'s descriptions of spirited discussions with Mengele concerning the pros and cons of the Final Solution. At the same time, by not contesting the Auschwitz project, one maintained one's meaningful organizational ties, one's "status honor." And if one were a prime mover in Auschwitz, as were Wirths or Höss, one derived enormous meaning from one's work. But, even as he killed, every doctor's Auschwitz self could retain some sense of mediating between man and nature and thereby serving life.

The Ultimate Biological Soldier

Nazi ideology lent considerable support to all meaning structures. Underneath the absolute routinization, for instance, the Auschwitz self could have the unspoken sense of being part of a purification process, in which it was carrying out the laws of "the natural history and biology of man."[63] Rather than being a mere anti-Semite like everyone else, the Nazi could see himself in the forefront of what came to be called "biological anti-Judaism." Even if a bit troubled by mass killing, he could see it as part of the necessary combination of destruction and creation always stressed in Nazi imagery. Whatever meaning one gave these events, it was not that of murder, because as a former Nazi doctor said in reference to "euthanasia," "there was a certain . . . sensibility that this couldn't be, . . . [that] one cannot simply murder a mentally ill or . . . old person or an imbecile. Do you understand me?" That "sensibility" was what I have called derealization and disavowal: the meaning within the killing center or within Auschwitz was not that helpless people were being murdered but something else: one was doing one's duty, one was achieving heroic hardness, one was being the ultimate biological soldier.

Blaming the Victim

The meaning structure of the Auschwitz self depended greatly upon the pattern of "blaming the victim."[64] Mengele's insistence that the Gypsies were genetically responsible for their fatal noma tumors, Ernst B.'s disgust with the Gypsies for not distributing their food equitably among themselves, the repeated blame placed on prisoner doctors for the terrible condition of their patients and the frequent deaths among them—all these were psychologically of a piece. The blame could be deadly: a group of Polish prisoner doctors were sent to almost certain death in the punishment *Kommando*, together with their infectious patients, because of a small trachoma outbreak. As Dr. Henri Q. commented, the approach was "at the very least original," did succeed in stopping the trachoma epidemic, and permitted the "innocent Germans" to do their killing. The meaning structure imposed was that the Germans bore no guilt because they had been "forced" by the medical negligence of the prisoner doctors to take stern measures.

The imagery also closely parallels Hitler's own in his famous "warning" issued on 30 January 1939: "If international finance Jewry within Europe and abroad should succeed once more in plunging the peoples into a world war, then the consequence will not be Bolshevization of the world and therewith a victory of Jewry, but on the contrary, the destruction of the Jewish race in Europe."[65] The usual psychological explanation to the effect that Hitler was "projecting" his own intention onto the Jews is true enough. But probably more important was the narrative (or collective meaning experience) Hitler was constructing, in which the designated victims, already identified as the source of the world's "fundamental evil," could now be seen as posing a military threat to the Aryan nation, and therefore as the group responsible for the ensuing bloodbath.

As in the case of the Auschwitz self, Hitler's position was that, because Jews were, biologically and existentially, a permanent locus of evil and a permanent threat, it was *they* who must be blamed for anything done to overcome that threat and extirpate that evil. In other words, because as Jews (and, to a lesser extent, Poles) the prisoner doctors were by definition evil, they were therefore responsible for medical negligence and all other evil in the camp—a position the Auschwitz self could hold while simultaneously depending upon the medical skills of Jewish doctors for maintaining its own professional identity.

When a Nazi doctor became enraged at a tiny mistake made by a prisoner doctor on a medical chart—a pattern all the more remarkable when one considers the extent of falsification throughout Auschwitz documents—that anger had an important psychological function. It was the Auschwitz self's effort to hold to the "as if" situation of a decent medical establishment and to deflect potential guilt by attacking the other rather than confront itself.[66] But blaming the victim can extend to retrospective Auschwitz reflections, such as those of Höss himself. The camp commandant attributed the high mortality rate among Jews to "their psychological state," blamed "Jewish gold" for the "camp's undoing" (extensive corruption), and described Jewish prisoners in Dachau as having "protected themselves in typical fashion by bribing their fellow prisoners." Höss took pains to make clear his opposition to vulgar attitudes in this area, condemning Julius Streicher and his notorious *Der Stürmer* for its "disgusting sensationalism" and pornography as harmful to the cause of "serious anti-Semitism."[67]

Höss suggests once more the Auschwitz self's quest for meaning on the basis of a *story*, within which one can claim to have made every effort to be reasonable and humane in the face of extraordinary provocation, but had to point, however reluctantly, to one's designated victim as the source of evil and threat; which in turn required that one take the matter in hand, as any clear-minded, responsible person would have done. Or more subjectively: "God knows I tried. I did my best with them. But being what they were, they kept spreading their poison and endangered my compatriots and myself, so we were left with no choice."

Blaming the victim is highly important to the doubling process creating the Auschwitz self and to the Nazi doctor's function within the healing-killing paradox.

The Auschwitz Self as Performer

The element of "performance" in the Auschwitz self, especially during selections, had considerable importance for the experience of meaning. Mengele, of course, is the exemplar here, the outstanding player of the Auschwitz game whose "graceful and quick movements" reflected his harmonious sense of meaningful work in the Auschwitz environment. But his relation to meaning, though exaggerated, reflected shared patterns of the Auschwitz self. There was the suggestion, in the flow of omnipotence and of smooth sadism, that this degree of cruel control over inmates was natural and appropriate.

Most meaningful of all was the sense that Mengele did things right: killed without flinching when people had to be killed; insisted upon saving those supposed to be saved, even when they resisted by inadvertently joining the wrong line. Like any talented actor, Mengele inwardly experienced the role and made the drama believable, thereby helping other performers to feel that similar roles could make sense.

Part of the Mengele style of selections performance was Nazi male macho: immaculately clean black SS uniform with riding boots and riding crop, exaggeratedly straight posture with reserved, dignified bearing, together with a slight military swagger and an aura of absolute authority over everyone. Behind that picture, the Auschwitz self nurtured its detached correctness, its readiness to be tested by death (in Auschwitz mainly by inflicting it), and above all, its cult of heroic hardness, always available to dominate or destroy designated others with an absolute absence of either compassion or empathy. While those designated others in Auschwitz and elsewhere were mostly Jews and sometimes Slavs, Gypsies, and non-Aryans in general, they could be close to home as well—political enemies, homosexuals, subordinates, family members, and women (see the first footnote on page 494).

The Auschwitz self medicalized this overall Nazi male ideal and thereby gave it a further claim to ultimate power and symbolic immortality. In this combination, the Auschwitz self made especially clear how far anti-empathic male power can be mobilized to fend off every form of death anxiety, including that associated with fear of homosexuality and of women, and with the erosion of one's ideology and ethos. This brings us to the realm of killing as a specific means of holding back death (which I shall discuss further in the final chapter), a realm always inhabited by a perverse expression of maleness.

Other Sources of Meaning

We know of the Auschwitz self's additional access to meaning through medical "hobbies," including experiments, and through other "medical accomplishments." Both Mengele and Wirths saw Auschwitz as providing an opportunity for scientific breakthrough: the former via his studies of hereditary traits in identical twins, and the latter in his so-called discovery of a dramatic new form of actual disinfection (via Zyklon-B) that could control and prevent typhus epidemics. The idea of scientific breakthrough was equally stirring to the great Auschwitz sterilizers, Schumann and Clauberg, both of whom had the further vision of combining that breakthrough with highly practical achievements in racial politics.

All this suggests that for the Auschwitz self there was sufficient breadth of opportunity to create one's own version of meaning. The substructure of chaos and nihilism made it an environment in which, as several former inmates put it, "everything was possible." One could find meaning in extravagant killing (as did Mengele), in more moderate killing (as did most SS doctors), or in saving lives while living in harmony with the killing (as did B.). We know also that meaning structures could become strained for the Auschwitz self: conflicts over selections on the part of Delmotte and Ernst B. are cases in point. But Auschwitz demonstrated itself to be sufficiently malleable to reassert meaning for both: for B. via avoiding selections (while helping prisoners); and for Delmotte via performing them. For Wirths, Auschwitz provided the opportunity for a moral crusade with improvements for virtually everyone, certainly for the killers. Rohde's impulsive firing of a pistol just after performing selections (and drinking a bit) was also a breakdown of meaning; but here, too, Auschwitz was sufficiently flexible to permit him his expressionist protest as a way of enabling him to continue to select without interruption. Doubts about meaning are inevitable within institutions and movements, religious and secular. They are in fact *necessary* ingredients in that they reveal areas of difficulty and inspire methods of function that depend upon less than total ideological conviction.

For the Auschwitz self, doubt could be inundated by the call of the biological vision as well as the need for elements of ethos and ideology, however fragmentary, that enabled one to survive psychically in that land of death.

In other words the Auschwitz self was highly motivated toward what Mircea Eliade has called "transformation of chaos into cosmos," toward those actions that "organized chaos by giving it forms and norms."[68] In Auschwitz, "cosmos" meant viable ethos, and men desperately sought meaning structures that harmonized self with ethos. Yet one could say of the Auschwitz self developed by doctors what Susanne Langer said about the Inca and sacrificial killing: "Their ethos always had a peculiar frangibility, extremes of royal pomp mingling with equally great extremes of wildness and backwardness . . . most evident in the contrast between . . . their bureaucracies and concepts of order and authority, and the very low level of their religious [or, in the case of the Nazis, ideological] thinking."[69]

The Auschwitz Nazi ethos was rendered "frangible" by its very murderous extremity, yet, as we have observed, was buttressed by the many-sided elements of meaning that could work within that fragility. Again, we find (as does Loren Eiseley in an epigraph to this chapter) that man can make meaning of anything.[70]

Doubling: The Broader Danger

Although doubling can be understood as a pervasive process present in some degree in most if not all lives, we have mainly been talking about a destructive version of it: *victimizer's doubling.* The Germans of the Nazi era came to epitomize this process not because they were inherently more evil than other people, but because they succeeded in making use of this form of doubling for tapping the general human moral and psychological potential for mobilizing evil on a vast scale and channeling it into systematic killing.

While victimizer's doubling can occur in virtually any group, perhaps professionals of various kinds—physicians, psychologists, physicists, biologists, clergy, generals, statesmen, writers, artists—have a special capacity for doubling. In them a prior, humane self can be joined by a "professional self" willing to ally itself with a destructive project, with harming or even killing others.

Consider the situation of the American psychiatrist doing his military service during the Vietnam War. In working with Vietnam veterans, I was surprised by their special animosity toward "chaplains and shrinks." It turned out that many of these veterans had experienced a mixture of revulsion and psychological conflict (the two were difficult to distinguish in the midst of Vietnam combat) and were taken to either a chaplain or a psychiatrist (or the assistant of either), depending upon the orientation of the soldier himself or of his immediate superior. The chaplain or the psychiatrist would attempt to help the GI become strong enough to overcome his difficulties and remain in combat, which in Vietnam meant participating in or witnessing daily atrocities in an atrocity-producing situation. In that way, the chaplain or psychiatrist, quite inadvertently, undermined what the soldier would later come to view as his last remnant of decency in that situation. The professional involved could do that only because he had undergone a form of doubling which gave rise to a "military self" serving the military unit and its combat project. One reason the chaplain or psychiatrist was so susceptible to that doubling was his misplaced confidence in his profession and his professional self: his assumption that, as a member of a healing profession, whatever he did healed. In this case, the military self could come to subsume the professional self. Thus, psychiatrists returning from Vietnam to their American clinical and teaching situations experienced psychological struggles no less severe than those of other Vietnam veterans[71] (see page 454).

Consider also the physicist who is for the most part a humane person devoted to family life and strongly opposed to violence of any kind. He may undergo a form of doubling from which emerges what we can call his "nuclear-weapons self." He may actively involve himself in making the weapons, argue that they are necessary for national security and to combat Soviet weapons, and even become an advocate of their use under certain circumstances as a theorist of limited nuclear war. It is precisely his humane commitment to democracy and family life (his prior self) that enables him to claim similar humanity for his nuclear-weapons self despite its contribution to devices that could slaughter millions of people. He can do what he does because his doubling is part of a functional psychological equilibrium.[72]

In light of the recent record of professionals engaged in mass killing, can this be the century of doubling? Or, given the ever greater potential for professionalization of genocide, will that distinction belong to the twenty-first century? Or, may one ask a little more softly, can we interrupt the process—first, by naming it?

Chapter 21

Genocide

To live means to kill.
　　　　　　　　　　—ERNST JÜNGER

In a dark time the eye begins to see.
　　　　　　　　　　—THEODORE ROETHKE

Doubling facilitates genocide. And while Mann's devil declares that German "happens to be just precisely my favoured language,"[1] we know well enough that the Devil can speak in any tongue. Genocide is a potential act of any nation.

Yet the Nazis did provide the impetus for the legal naming of a very old crime. The word "genocide" was coined (from the Greek *genos*, "race, tribe," and the Latin *cide*, "killing") in 1944, and defined by the United Nations General Assembly in 1946 as "a denial of the right of existence of entire human groups." The Convention on Genocide approved by the U.N. General Assembly in 1948 associated the concept with killing, seriously harming, or interfering with the life continuity (by preventing births or forcibly transferring children) of "a national, ethnical, racial or religious group."[2] Significantly, the original definition of the word by its coiner, Raphael Lemkin, speaks of "an old practice in its modern development," includes long-term actions aimed at "the destruction of essential foundations of the life of national groups," and limits the concept to attempts to destroy groups in their entirety or biological totality.[3]

This book has been mainly about what we call the "Holocaust," a unique expression of Nazi genocide perpetrated against the Jews—unique in dimensions, in bureaucratic organization for annihilation, and in degree of absolute focus on a victim group dispersed throughout the world. Yet it is significant that, in accordance with their biological vision, the Nazis attempted genocide of other groups—Gypsies, Russians, and Poles. Now I shall examine some of the psychohistorical themes of Nazi genocide in order to derive more general principles. I shall refer to other genocides—notably the Turks' annihilation of about one million Armenians in 1915—not with any claim to comprehensiveness but only to suggest wider applicability. These principles could also apply to recent examples of genocide in Cambodia, Bangladesh, Nigeria, Paraguay, and the Soviet Union. Rather than a definitive theory of genocide, I want to suggest a sequence of collective patterns that occur in at least certain forms of genocide.

At the heart of the task is the question: Why *all?* What is the source of the impulse to destroy a human group in its entirety? No conceptual approach can be made to this question without satisfying two fundamental requirements: it must consider a combination of psychological and historical forces, and be sensitive to questions of death and killing and their relationship to individual and collective life. Such an approach must also be sufficiently flexible to connect with a variety of historical events, some of them unforeseen and even unprecedented.

Freudian theory cannot in itself meet these requirements, but those of us who would apply alternative theory are nonetheless children of Freud.[4]* Otto Rank, the early follower of Freud and subsequent dissident, is a key figure here as a major source of the paradigm of death and the continuity of life—or the symbolization of life and death—that I have been employing in this book and in other work over several decades. A central tenet of that model would be that human beings kill in order to assert their own life power. To that tenet may now be added the image of curing a deadly disease, so that genocide may become an absolute form of killing in the name of healing.

The model I propose includes a perception of collective *illness,* a vision of *cure,* and a series of motivations, experiences, and requirements of perpetrators in their quest for that cure.

The Historical "Sickness unto Death"

The perceived illness is a collectively experienced inundation in death imagery, a shared sense of Kierkegaard's "sickness unto death." It is the despairing edge of historical (or psychohistorical) dislocation, of the breakdown of the symbolic forms and sources of meaning previously shared by a particular human group. That collective sense of immersion in death, bodily and spiritually, could not have been greater than that experienced in Germany after the First World War. But the larger dislocation had begun much earlier. The German struggle with what has been called anti-modern despair[6] goes back at least to the last half of the nineteenth century. So much so that Fritz Stern called his 1961 study of

---

*George Kren and others also note the inadequacy of classical Freudian thought for approaching the Holocaust, and look tentatively toward Jung and Wilhelm Reich for more relevant theory. Israel W. Charny suggests the usefulness of Rank's early work, in connection with which he cites Ernest Becker and myself.[5]

pre-Hitler Germanic ideology *The Politics of Cultural Despair.* And he ascribed to a leading creator of that ideology, Paul de Lagarde, the motivation of a "mounting disgust with modernity" which led him to explore over several decades "the causes, the symptoms, and the cure of Germany's spiritual collapse."[7]

Post–First World War confusion, the experience of the Weimar Republic as "an era of dissolution, without guidance," was at least in part a continuation of that earlier process. By then German culture had begun to divide itself into two camps: the artistic and social experimentalists who tried out every variety of new form in a great rush of creativity and excess; and the right-wing political restorationists who "despised . . . precisely this free-floating spirit of experimentation."[8]

Both camps were dealing with an intense experience of loss. There was an immediate sense of disintegration, separation, and stasis; and an ultimate breakdown in larger human connection, in the symbolization of cultural continuity or of collective immortality. Thus one historian could describe the political atmosphere in Germany from 1919 to 1923 as "oppressive with doom, almost eschatological."[9] The atmosphere, that is, was dominated by "last things," by both death and a sense of doom.

The pattern was intensified by the perpetual German cultural sense of "cleavage," or the "torn condition" mentioned previously. Also important is a cultural corollary, what could be called a German immortality hunger: the constant quest for experiences of transcendence and affirmations of ultimate meaning and connectedness. Goethe mocked that immortality hunger when he declared, in 1826, "It is now about twenty years since the whole race of Germans began to 'transcend.' Should they ever wake up to this fact, they will look very odd to themselves."[10]*

Failed Regeneration

But the First World War holds the key to the pre-Nazi, pre-genocidal German perception of collective historical illness. For in that experience we find not only death immersion on an extraordinary scale but a survivor experience so intense as to remain even now difficult to grasp. The First World War for Germany represented still another crucial psychological dimension, the profound experience of *failed regeneration.*

The outbreak of the war was marked by exultation or "war fever"

---

*Here I follow a long-standing principle of a trinity of influences affecting all collective behavior: psychobiological universals (that which is common to all people in all cultures in all eras); cultural emphasis (that which is given particularly intense expression over a long course of cultural experience); and recent historical forces (those currents of a specific, identifiable historical period that act upon the other two parts of the trinity). In this case the psychobiological universal would be susceptibility to death imagery in response to impairments at both proximate and ultimate levels of psychological function; the cultural emphasis would be the perennially "torn condition" of the German self; and the relevant historical forces would be the rapid industrialization and modernization of the latter part of the nineteenth century and the inundation with death and disillusionment in association with the First World War.

among most of the belligerents. But for Germany the situation was quickly transcendent, so that "regardless of social station or political conviction, August 1914 was a sacred experience." Even Stefan Zweig, the Austrian-Jewish writer later associated with intense anti-war sentiment, said at the time, "Each one of us is called upon to cast his infinitesimal self into the glowing mass there to be purified of all selfishness."[11]

Thomas Mann, characteristically convoluted, referred to the war as "brutality for intellectual reasons, an intellectually based will to become worthy of the world, to qualify in the world," and concluded that "Germany's whole virtue and beauty . . . is unfolded only in war."[12] And the related Expressionist literature of the time—whose catchword, *Rausch,* meant "intoxication" or "ecstasy"—had a vision of "war as an Armageddon whose end must mean a rebirth into a better world," the creation of a "New Man," a "union with all mankind," or some related combination of wallowing in death with "a welcome . . . to extinction" and "the mystical union with the cosmos."[13]

Nor were social theorists and intellectual leaders such as Max Weber, Friedrich Meinecke, or even Sigmund Freud immune from the intoxication. Weber pointed with pride at Germans as "people of great culture . . . human beings who live amidst a refined culture, yet who can even stand up to the horrors of war (which is no achievement for a Senegalese!) and then, in spite of it, return basically decent like the majority of our soldiers—this is genuinely humane."[14] (However reluctant one may be to compare Max Weber with Heinrich Himmler, there is a clear parallel here with the latter's orations on the nobility of the German accomplishment in killing so many Jews and remaining "decent.") Meinecke was still more extreme, recalling thirty years and two wars later that "the exultation of the August days of 1914 [was] one of the most precious and unforgettable memories of the highest sort" because it contained within it the anticipation of "an inner renovation of our whole state and culture."[15] And for about two weeks, Freud was "quite carried away . . . excitable, irritable, and made slips of the tongue all day long"; he was disturbed by Austrian defeats but "rejoic[ed] in German victories."[16]

With the defeat, adult Germans were to become the most devastated survivors: of the killing and dying on an unprecedented scale, and of the equally traumatic death of national and social visions, of meaning itself. There were individual breakdowns, notably among artists who served in the war. A prominent example was Max Beckmann who described having experienced no physical wounds but rather "injuries of the soul": grotesque death imagery that subsequently haunted all of his life and art. Other Expressionist artists experienced similar "spiritual wounds," creating "an atmosphere of painful contrivance . . . hysterical abandonment to the wildest hopes and the unlikeliest despair."[17]

But there was also a more brutalized survivor response, as exemplified by Hitler's own sequence: First, his memory of how "those hours [the beginning of the war] seemed like . . . a release . . . [and] I fell down on

my knees and thanked Heaven from an overflowing heart for granting me
the good fortune of being permitted to live at this time." Then his equally
enthusiastic soldiering and apparent willingness to risk his life for that
"release." Then his survivor formulation of the times as *"inwardly sick and
rotten,"* yet "moving toward a great metamorphosis." His subsequent
vision and social action can be understood as an effort to re-create "that
awesome moment [at the beginning of the First World War] to cleanse
it of all impurities, and preserve it, so that this time the goal of 1914
would be reached: to endow Germany with a political foundation fitted
to the scale of the times."[18]

There seem to have been definite parallels in Turkish historical experience prior to their mass murder of Armenians in 1915. Within the Ottoman empire, throughout the latter part of the nineteenth century, there
was an atmosphere of progressive "decay and disintegration," along with
a continuous if losing struggle for spiritual and political unification. The
Turks also experienced humiliating forms of failed regeneration in their
disastrous military enterprises during the 1912 Balkan war (ignominious
defeat at the hands of their former slaves and wards, the Greeks and the
Bulgarians) and their abortive Russian campaign in 1915 as a German
ally. Vahakn N. Dadrian observes that the Turks moved closer to genocide as their perception of their situation proceeded "from the condition
of mere strain, to that of crisis, to a precipitate crisis, and eventually to
the cataclysm of war."[19]

The stage of sickness, then, includes the experience of collective loss
and death immersion; the promise of redemptive revitalization, including
total merging of self with a mystical collectivity; the absolute failure of
that promise, followed by newly intensified experience of collective death
imagery and death equivalents; leading in turn to a hunger for a "cure"
commensurate in its totality with the "sickness."

The Vision of Total Cure

There develops a collective desperation for cure. But whatever vision
is to qualify as a cure must hold out the promise of shared vitality and
renewed confidence in collective immortality. In our century, any such
vision is likely to be bound up with a sense of *nation*, with what we call
"nationalism." The national comes to combine spiritual and biological
connectedness, to provide a blending of the immortal cultural and racial
substance of any particular group. One may thus speak of a "national
organism" in terms both of general biological continuity and of viewing
one's society as similar to a biological organism with "needs for its proper
development." Those needs become "supreme values" that take precedence over everything else because, unless they are pursued, the organism will die.[20]

Isaiah Berlin stresses nationalism as a response to "wounds inflicted upon one society by another," but a response that requires as well "a new vision of life" around which to organize collective experience. In that way images of nationalism could replace "the church or the prince or the rule of law or other sources of ultimate values," could "relieve . . . the pain of the wound to group consciousness, whoever may have inflicted it," and become "incarnations of men's conceptions of themselves as a community, a *Gemeinschaft.*" To ignore nationalism, then, is to ignore "the explosive power generated by the combination of unhealed mental wounds, however caused, with the image of the nation as a society of the living, the dead and those yet unborn."[21]

The Nazis drew upon images of German racial and cultural substance —whether of myths or Teutonic knights or Germanic emperors (Charlemagne and Frederick the Great) or physicians (Paracelsus)—culminating in Hitler's commandment: "Thou shalt have no other God but Germany!"[22]

Hitler and the Nazis provided a vision of cure that focused upon nation but did much more. While it was in one sense an "expressionist shriek,"[23] it was also a powerful message to Germans that, in the face of those who have "deliberately ruined Germany, . . . I will lead you all, every single one of you, to a glorious future."[24] He offered a vision that enabled most Germans to view his accession to power "not as the creation of an authoritarian police state but as the dawn of an era of recuperation and regeneration of German community life."[25] In other words, among the various contemporary visions, Hitler's most powerfully provided the promise of vitality and national immortality—a grandiose promise of cure for the "deadly sickness."

To move in a genocidal direction, that cure must be *total.* It becomes an all-or-none matter, equally absolute in its claim to truth and in its rejection of alternative claims.

The cultural climate of post–First World War Germany was compatible with totalism: a mood of extremity, of "often ludicrous immoderation" in literary and artistic expressionism. Whatever the impressive achievements of the time, many artistic experiments came to be consumed by a death-saturated confusion, within which it was unclear whether brutality was being protested against or joined. A typical Expressionist play might have included any of the following events:

> Skeletons go on parade as soldiers and roll skulls by numbers; a severed head in a sack converses with its former owner; a woman bleats her Dionysiac love to a billy-goat; a father horsewhips his son, a son chases lustfully round the table after his mother, a society is formed for the Brutalization of the Ego. A man earns his living by eating live mice. . . . A bank-cashier stands with arms outstretched in front of a crucifix, his dying gasps accidentally suggesting the words "Ecco Homo."[26]

Many artists struggled against this totalism by opening themselves to pain and death (Max Beckmann's painting from his "spiritual wound" of the First World War) and maintaining a spirit of exploration and play. Other artists felt the lure of the absolute. It was Hans Johst, an Expressionist novelist and playwright and later head of the Nazi Chamber of Literature, who first used the phrase later made famous by Göring: "When I hear the word culture, I draw my revolver."* *That* was the only cure for Germany's disease.

The Dispensing of Existence

Totalistic ideology avoids the sting of death in its claim to invincibility and omnipotence. It puts forward its own claim to immortality and exclusive truth in specific psychological manipulations of the environment I have delineated elsewhere: milieu control (of all communication); mystical manipulation (continuous efforts at behavior control from above while maintaining the appearance of spontaneity from below); demand for purity (constant accusations of guilt and shame in the name of an unrealizable ideal of absolute devotion and self-sacrifice); the cult of confession (ritual self-exposure to the totalistic "owner" of every self); the sacred science (combining deification of the Word with the claim of equally absolute secular scientific authority); loading of the language (into definitive, thought-terminating solutions for the most complex human problems); doctrine over person (so that the evidence of individual experience must be subsumed to or negated by the idea system); and the dispensing of existence (the ultimate and inevitable line drawn between those with a right to exist and those who possess no such right).[28] The last, the dispensing of existence, is the larger principle that encompasses all of the others, whether expressed in merely metaphorical or, as in the case of the Nazis, in directly murderous ways.

Indeed, the Nazi movement brought a new literalism to the dispensing of existence by making the existence of each individual a matter of either harm or benefit to the biological health of the group.

Only this totalized approach can heal the sickness, so that the *Führer* principle, the apex of Nazi totalism, could be embraced not only by the uneducated but by intellectuals who felt keenly their "torn condition"— as by the internationally known economist and economic historian who declared in 1935:

> The art of discussion is gone. Not discussion but decision now dominates the scene. The creation of a political will comes about today by quite another way. It is no longer the indirect way of influencing public opinion but the direct way of the *Führer* principle. This is a fact which

*Johst's original phrase was: "When I hear the word culture, I slip back the safety catch of my revolver."[27]

may be evaluated in different ways. I, for my part, say "Thank God, that this is so!"[29]

The totalized modern state always claims a higher principle—in this case, purification of the world's most valuable race as a means of curing the prevailing human illness. And we recall Werner Best's declaration of the Nazi cure as the "political principle of totalitarianism," within which any alternative ideas must be "ruthlessly dealt with, as the symptom of an illness which threatens the healthy unity of the indivisible national organism" (see page 153).[30]

One renders the body politic total as a means of controlling underlying chaos and formlessness—a principle especially stressed in the creation of an overall, German imperial state—the Reich—from a politically disunited group of regional entities.* Hitler meant it when he contrasted "the saving doctrine of the nothingness and insignificance of the individual human being, and of his continued existence in the visible immortality of the Nation."[32] Rather than be individuals, people—at least those who qualified biologically—could share in this immortalizing power of state and race. One could even come to believe the specific historical totalism in the claim that "all German history . . . must be seen only as the pre-history of National Socialism."[33]

Again, there are suggestions of similar currents in the Turkish situation. The "young Turks" who sought to reform the Ottoman empire spearheaded "a major campaign to change the social structure of Ottoman society as an antidote to internal discord and conflict, and also as a means of recapturing imperial, Panturkic glory." *Their* cure included "an admixture of religious and political ideologies," and "genocide became a means for [bringing about] a radical . . . change in the system."[34]

Totalism in a nation state, then, is most likely to emerge as a cure for a death-haunted "illness"; and victimization, violence, and genocide are potential aspects of that cure.

The Quest for Transcendence

Part of the cure is the experience of transcendence: of a psychic state so intense that time and death disappear. The cure must maintain, or at least evoke periodically, that psychic experience. One's own sense of transcendence merges with the image of the endless life of one's people. In that experience—or promise—of ecstasy, one may be ready to kill, or at least to sanction killing.

*George Weippert, a conservative sociologist, lauded the principle of "totality of power" and of "only one ruler" in the "all-embracing" task of achieving one Reich as "Germany's mission in this world."[31]

Indeed, the transcendence is likely to be related to some such killing, often to war or the expectation of war. Examples here are religious wars of the past and their contemporary expressions, as well as secular analogues of these religious wars. The war fever of 1914 mentioned earlier, with its anticipation of victory and national deliverance, set a standard for Nazi transcendence. And that 1914 moment, in turn, drew upon earlier historical memories. Consider the words of a German "national liberal" upon the return of the victorious (over Austria) Prussian troops to Berlin in 1866: "I feel more attached to the goddess of beauty and the mother of graces than to the powerful god of war, but the trophies of war exercise a magic charm even upon the child of peace. . . . One's spirit goes along with the boundless rows of men who acclaim in the god of the moment —[military] success."[35]

Hitler became an agent of this transcendence, because of both his oratorical-demagogic genius and the German hunger for transcendence. As he invoked principles of " 'honor,' 'fatherland,' *'Volk,'* 'loyalty,' and 'sacrifice,' . . . his German hearers not only took his words in deadly earnest but hung on them as upon the message of a savior."[36] For each of these words represented a transcendent principle, a means of offering the self to an ultimate realm that provided a sense of immortality bordering on omnipotence. Then "the will of the Führer" could become a "cosmic law"[37] because his message of revitalization could invoke the experience of transcendence and place that experience within a structure of thought and a program of action.

Albert Speer described to me the extraordinary impact of hearing Hitler speak for the first time. It was 1930; and Speer, a young architect at the university, seemed, in that time of economic and political duress, to have no future. He had boyhood memories of being part of a voluntary group greeting returning soldiers at the railway station at the end of the First World War ("It was terrible, terrible, awful. [They were] dirty, neglected, really a defeated army") and of experiencing "kind of a mourning about this situation." Now Hitler appeared, addressing a university audience* in measured tones with the simple message that "all can be changed": Germany could become great again, and individual Germans could divest themselves of guilt and loss by embracing this glorious future. Speer was moved to the point of rapture, felt himself to be "drunk" or in an altered state of consciousness, and needed to go off by himself to walk in the woods outside Berlin in order to "absorb" what was happening to him. He was describing a classical experience of transcendence, an ecstatic state of feeling outside oneself and swept up by a larger force that could connect or reconnect one with ultimate spiritual principles. From that day on, he belonged to Hitler and came to share his sphere of omnipotence and power, so that he could describe the whole

---

*Speer said that Hitler had two separate speeches: a simplistic rabble-rousing message for ordinary audiences; and a more careful "historical analysis," no less "rousing," for the educated.

Nazi era as "like a dream." He remained confused by the power Hitler held over him, dating back from that first speech.

Speer was referring to the almost continuous sense of transcendence he and other Germans experienced during the Nazi era. Given Hitler's call for a form of national "redemption," for "a renewed spiritual *Reich* realized in a political framework . . . yet also beyond politics," every small event, indeed every single moment, could be bound up with transcendence, with the messianic purpose of the Thousand-Year Reich. This quality of transcendence associated with the regime could help one avoid awareness of one's corrupt and self-serving behavior, as was surely the case with Speer and others.

The Continuous "High State"

The Nazis were heirs to an extreme form of romantic nationalism, of worship of the "holy, divine Reich" called forth by writers, philosophers, and youth-movement leaders over the previous century. It had to do with "the intimate connection between political reaction and literary romanticism" and included strong elements of Protestant pietism as well as related Catholic religious emotions.[38]

All this combined with specific Nazi ideological omnipotence to contribute to a sense of being those particular "children of the gods" who had the right to kill, in a spirit described by one as: "If you will not be my brother, your head will be dropped off your shoulders."[39] That pattern was exemplified by the "oath-bound community" entered into by SS members, so that they could, in their sense of special mission for the Führer and the race, move toward their killing while psychologically maintaining a "high state."

Transcendence, like everything else, became biologized—as in Ernst Haeckel's "scientific expressionism" (see pages 441–42) and in Fritz Lenz's mystical genetics ("Racial hygienists also want to be workers in God's vineyard"[40]). Moreover, under the Nazis, science was so molded that it not only failed to criticize the false assumptions associated with these high states but itself joined the transcendence. There was even an attempt to create an "Aryan physics" with the claim that "scholarship—like everything else brought forth by men—is conditioned by race and blood."[41]

Goethe's critique more than a century earlier of German "transcendence hunger" was remarkable for his inclusion in that category of not only transcendental philosophy but Newtonian physics. He was probably the first to see that what was later to be called positivism could itself be associated with mysticism and transcendence[42]—a pattern exemplified, for instance, by Josef Mengele. Viewing himself as a scientific revolutionary, Mengele could become "God playing doctor" by embracing the transcendent state made available by a highly romanticized, positivistic, and ultimately genocidal Nazi version of science.

In the case of the Turks, whatever their attitude toward science, they did put forward a mystical vision of pan-Turanianism (or "Turkification") "which alleged a prehistoric mythic unity among Turanian peoples based on racial origin."[43] And one cannot doubt the experience of transcendence of Turkish nationalists in their reversion to fundamentalist Mohammedanism as a call to an anti-Armenian-Christian crusade—all on behalf of a new vision of Ottoman glory.

The experience of transcendence, then, anticipates the genocide, and to a considerable degree prefigures a state of transcendence that can become associated, directly or by proxy, with the killing itself.

Killing as Therapy

The "disease" with which the Nazis were attempting to cope was death itself, death made unmanageable by "the modern necrophilia" of the First World War. Thus Hugo Ball wrote of "death, working systematically, counterfeiting life . . . bestial, monstrous, yet unreal."[44]* One way to deal with a death-saturated historical environment is to embrace death itself as the means of cure. The Nazis did this in a variety of ways: in a romantic worship of death and the creation of "an ancestor cult where the dead were more important than the living"; in an art "deeply tinged with death" (Nordic heroes, for instance) as "a prelude to initiation into the community"; and especially in remobilizing the martyred dead of the First World War in the claim of carrying out for them an immortalizing survivor mission of annihilating enemies of the German state. Hitler, as prophet and savior, came to represent the martyred dead and serve as their link with the new community of the living. The "healing" vanguard was the Waffen SS, whose "supreme duty was to deal out and accept death"; to seek out the most dangerous missions, to seek out death itself if necessary, and to kill with complete hardness. Also part of a vision of healing was the policy of individual SS members serving as models of racial purification.[46] Having met the ultimate test of health and cure, the SS could represent the sacred dead and be licensed to kill without limit.

The "Deadly" Victim

Genocide requires both a specific victim group and certain relationships to that group. While their biological focus enabled the Nazis to extend their genocidal efforts to Gypsies, Russians, and Poles, the Jews remained the central target and the most specific psychological victim of the Nazi genocidal dynamic.

Nazi perpetrators had to see their victims as posing absolute danger,

*Ball was attacking materialism and the machine, and declared that "belief in matter is a belief in death."[45]

as "infecting" the "German national body," and as (in the last three words of Hitler's testament) "deadly Jewish poison." Similarly, *"Kultur-*poisoning Jews" were infiltrating the art world, and the general danger of "inner Judaization" and "racial pollution" was perceived as a fundamental threat to German biological and biosocial continuity and immortality.[47] In addition, Jews—or the concept of "the Jew"—were equated with every form of death-associated degeneracy and decomposition, including homosexuality, urban confusion, liberalism, capitalism, and Marxism. Goebbels could use straight medical imagery in declaring, "Our task here is surgical . . . drastic incisions, or some day Europe will perish of the Jewish disease."[48]

There may also be a universalization of the alleged evil of the victim —as in Hitler's claim, "If . . . the Jew conquers the nations of this world, his crown will become the funeral wreath of humanity, and once again this planet, empty of mankind, will move through the ether as it did thousands of years ago."* The victim will destroy not only the perpetrator, it is claimed, but everyone and everything else. Where the threat is so absolute and so ultimate—where the struggle becomes "fighting between humans and subhumans," in Himmler's phrase—genocide becomes not only appropriate but an urgent necessity. Such a struggle must be "fought to the last man, *until one side or the other is eliminated without trace"* (italics added). Once that genocidal necessity is established, perpetrators can take the more casual tone of Himmler's suggestion that "anti-Semitism is exactly the same as delousing."[50]

In other work I have spoken of rival claims to immortality—to ultimate spiritual power—as a source of victimization. For some Christian groups, Jews are both the originators and the destroyers of the Christian theological mode of immortality, in the sense that Jews are seen as rejectors, betrayers, or murderers of Jesus. To this general pattern the Germans brought a status described by Freud as "badly christened Christians," as people who held tenaciously in the face of their own apparent Christianization to their heathen, pre-Christian feelings and modes of being.[51] This could well have been a source of German vulnerability, over centuries, to threats to their Christian belief system, and ultimately to their sense of immortality.

For instance, during the plagues of the Middle Ages, Jews everywhere in Europe were accused of responsibility for the Black Death, often specifically of having poisoned drinking wells. But although the mortality in Germany was relatively lower than in some other countries, anti-Jewish pogroms arose there with special ferocity, as did the phenomenon of the flagellants, fanatical bands of Christians who beat themselves ritually and mercilessly and also turned violently upon the Jews.[52] More significant

---

*The quotation is from *Mein Kampf.* Eberhard Jäckel points out that, in later editions, the phrase was "appropriately" changed to "millions of years ago."[49] This suggests that Hitler or his sympathetic editors believed in the concept sufficiently to present it in its most "reasonable" form.

for Germany as victimizer is its function as "the land of anti-Semitic myths." The myth of the Wandering Jew, while anticipated earlier, took shape in sixteenth- and early-seventeenth-century Germany: the gaunt, old, white-haired man with a long beard condemned to roam the earth until Jesus' Second Coming for having in his youth mocked him and enthusiastically joined the crowd chanting "Crucify him!" The German term for "Wandering Jew," *der ewige Jude,* means "Eternal Jew"; this is an accursed specter, a figure who can neither live nor die and remains an amalgam of murderer, corpse, and survivor-remnant. He is death-tainted but survives everyone (the Wandering Jew was described as having "buried the Egyptians, the Greeks, and the Romans") and therefore represents the ultimate embodiment of survivor contagion, of a carrier of deadly infection.[53]

The Threatened Community

A second, powerful German cultural emphasis in its historical relation to Jews is its victimization of them on a communal and ultimately biological basis. The situation begins with Jews having not just integrated themselves into modern German culture but having helped to shape it, so that as emancipated Jews gained intellectual respect as Goethe and Kant scholars, they were viewed in another corner of the German mind as "upstarts . . . sons and grandsons of the ghetto,"[54] as a fundamentally alien people all the more threatening because of the depth of their apparent cultural integration.

That tendency to understand the idea of community, or *Gemeinschaft,* in terms of biological romanticism lent itself readily not only to "race mysticism" but to invoking the authority of science to denigrate the Jews. The German coining of the term "anti-Semitism" *(Antisemitismus)* in 1879 was in fact a claim to a scientific position of the necessity of excluding Jews from the threatened German *Gemeinschaft.* And by 1886, Paul de Lagarde, a distinguished professor of oriental studies and a prominent Christian thinker, could denounce Jews as "aliens" and "nothing but carriers of decomposition," and went on in terms with which we are familiar to declare that "with trichinae and bacilli one does not negotiate, . . . they are exterminated as quickly and thoroughly as possible."[55] That medical imagery, and other references to the threat of "blood poisoning" by "the new Judaized Germanness," maintained the claim to science and even to high-minded humanitarianism.[56] Thus one turn-of-the-century educational reformer wished to combine an "organic state" overcoming class differences with a means of freeing Germany from the "Jewish spirit."[57] Even the seemingly mild lament by the historian Treitschke— "The Jews are our misfortune"—was part of a *Gemeinschaft-*centered tract expressing an underlying fear of racial death—a fear verbalized directly by Richard Wagner: "That we Germans especially will perish because of them is certain."[58]

Martin Luther, as "the most German of Germans, the most pious of the pious,"[59] combined communal and theological forms of anti-Semitism. Significantly, he was first a defender of the Jews whom he wished to become "of one heart with us." But when they failed to convert and become part of the Christian-Protestant-German spiritual and biological community, he denounced them as "children of the Devil" who "being foreigners, should possess nothing," and were, moreover, profoundly dangerous: "Know, O adored Christ . . . that aside from the Devil, you have no enemy more venomous, more desperate, more bitter, than a true Jew who truly seeks to be a Jew." For Luther, Jews were an intolerable reminder of flawed German Christian claims to totalized spiritual and communal immortality. By their very existence, Jews subvert those claims ("These dogs mock us and our religions!").[60] To be sure, Luther stood for much else, including the internalization of conscience—what Erik Erikson called "the meaning of meaning it."[61]

But that very achievement deepened the psychological power of his anti-Semitic message. The development of a "Nordic Christianity" four hundred years later could then be said to have "completed Luther's work," with Hitler and Luther "partners in the service of the German people's welfare."[62] The genocidal *principle* of destroying the Jews in the name of healing the Germans is not new.

Thus perceived as an absolute threat to the continuous life of one's own people, the victimized group is seen as the bearer of death and therefore the embodiment of evil. More than merely nonhuman or heathen, it is dangerously anti-man and anti-God (or anti-Christ). Its disease takes the form of infecting others with death taint and deadly weakness: Hitler referred contemptuously to "conscience, this Jewish invention" and to Judeo-Christian compassion for weakness. Only genocide, total elimination of the disease, will protect one from that weakness, and in the very act of genocide one overcomes vestiges of the deadly weakness-disease already in one, such as (in the case of the Nazis) "brotherhood . . . humanity [and] 'pacifism.'"[63] Hence the parallel imagery in genocide: the bearer of deadly disease threatens one's own people with extinction so one must absolutely extinguish him first.

The Genocidal Threshold

There is a threshold in genocide—the step from image to act. The Nazi evidence suggests no single cause or trigger so much as a sequence of events and attitudes and problem solving (dealing with unmanageable ghettos, with rivalries between increasingly dominant SS groups and other Nazi institutions and between individual Nazi leaders) within an increasingly murderous atmosphere ("euthanasia" killing, the expanding concentration-camp system, war fever of early victories, and the pending invasion of Russia). From early 1941, a series of "demoniac orders"[64] came from high Nazi authorities that increasingly articulated a policy to kill not just Jews but *all* Jews. As I suggested in chapter 6, there is evidence that a specific order for the Final Solution was issued by Göring to Heydrich on 31 July 1941 but was actually requested by Heydrich and drafted by Eichmann.[65] Much of the impetus for the order may have come from below the highest levels of Nazi authority, but always as expressions of known desires of Hitler and the people around him. One plausible view is that Hitler, without issuing any such decree under his name, made fully clear to close subordinates that he wanted the threshold crossed, wanted to implement the genocide of Jews. In this combination of drift and deliberation—and it is significant that scholars are uncertain about whether a single order bringing about the Final Solution can be identified[66]—a point is reached at which a collective understanding takes shape that the designated group is to be annihilated. Collective understanding quickly becomes collective will as perpetrators join in the process on the basis of perceptions of what is expected of them, calling forth prior inclination and adaptive doubling. With the Nazis, that genocidal process was probably well under way before the introduction of a systematic plan for the genocide, as reflected in Himmler's discussions with Höss about creating a Jewish death factory in Auschwitz.

That genocidal threshold requires extensive prior ideological imagery of imperative. One has to do this thing, see it through to the end, for the sake of a utopian vision of national harmony, unity, wholeness. When Hitler wrote in *Mein Kampf* that "this world belongs only to the forceful 'whole' man and not to the weak 'half' man," he was speaking for the special virtue of those who are strong, hale and healthy, cured.*

That vision was more fundamental for the Nazis than was any single myth about the Jews (such as that of the world-destroying intent of the Elders of Zion) as a "warrant" for genocide. The warrant is developed more broadly from many sources that feed the image which associates destruction of the entire collectivity of designated victims with the robust revitalization of one's people and race. There is likely to be a prefiguring or rehearsal in the form of a prior, smaller genocidal event: in the case of the Nazis, the direct medical killing or "euthanasia" project. The smaller genocide develops the technology (poison gas), personnel (medical units), and institutional structures (killing centers) for the larger genocidal act. But the prior event does something more: it provides a shared sense, notably among the élite, that it *can be done*; that one can move from relatively amorphous imagery of victimization and triage to the act of total murder; and that it seems to work—a problem is solved, there is a sense of achievement, a movement toward health.

Early perpetrators become a scientific and moral élite and form a spiritual engine of biological necessity. The rest of the population is not deemed ready for full knowledge; there is an ambivalence between se-

---

*Hitler's preceding sentence reads (with his emphasis): *"If the power to fight for one's own health* [he had been speaking of "decay" brought about by prostitution and syphilis] *is no longer present, the fight to live in this world of struggle ends."*[67]

crecy tinged with shame and pride of achievement as the genocidal radius moves outward into an increasingly enveloping system of order and policy, of bureaucratic and technological arrangement. The grand triage is always present: in Himmler's juxtaposition of "annihilation of the Jewish people," with painstaking programs "to select the Nordic-Germanic blood" in order to promote "the creative, heroic and life-preserving qualities of our people."[68] That image of absolute revitalization applied to both genocidal rehearsal and larger act.

Purification and Human Sacrifice

The Nazis tapped mythic relationships between healing and killing that have had ancient expression in shamanism, religious purification, and human sacrifice, and evoked all three in ways that reveal more about their psychological motivation. Thus, the shaman of central and northern Asia, though mainly a healer making use of ecstatic rites, is also a "psychopomp" or conveyor of the souls of the dead to the underworld. Some cultures distinguish "white" shamans, who have relations with the gods, from "black" shamans, who may be involved with "evil spirits" and are consequently dangerous.[69] Generally, the white shaman applies healing magic; and the black shaman, killing magic.

German culture, with its tendency toward death-haunted, apocalyptic historical visions, is more likely than most to seize upon this relationship between killing and healing and between the dead and the living. The Germans developed a particularly strong "cult of the fallen" after the First World War, stressing the continuing contribution of the dead, as soldiers who fight and kill, to the Fatherland. The German War Graves Commission contrasted the sea of flowers and modest acknowledgment of the dead in British, American, and French cemeteries with the German "tragic-heroic" motif and "celebration of heroic sacrifice."[70] But since death had to be conquered, one Nazi educator deplored photographs of the dead and wounded because these "cannot show the joy they felt in making the final sacrifice."[71]

As a sixteenth-century version of a good shaman, the Nazis had available both the historical figure and the mythology of Paracelsus. In one Nazi version, the Swiss-German physician-alchemist overcomes great suffering, severe illness, and despair on behalf of a utopian *völkisch* vision. And in another, he struggles valiantly, his struggles "centered upon the overcoming of death" (see page 31).[72] As biological soldiers, all Nazi physicians were to be in the front line in the struggle to kill death. All Nazi doctors, that is, were to become shamans, many of them black shamans in their ritualistic participation in killing processes in the name of healing the tribe or people.

Genocide is a response to collective fear of pollution and defilement. It depends upon an impulse toward purification resembling that given collective expression in primitive cultures. But it brings to that impulse a modern, much more deadly stress on health and hygiene—for the Nazis, racial hygiene. Mary Douglas has shown that concern with pollution, whether we call it magical or religious, has to do with symbolic systems dealing with the "relation of order to disorder, being to non-being, form to formlessness, life to death."[73] In primitive purification rituals combating defilement, "uncleanness or dirt is that which must not be included if a pattern is to be maintained."[74] And the ultimate issue is death: "Just as the focus of all pollution symbolism is the body, the final problem to which the perspective of pollution leads is bodily disintegration."[75]

Pollution imagery is associated with many forms of victimization involving class and caste as well as color and race. The traditional Japanese group of outcasts bear the name "Eta," whose literal meaning is "full of pollution," "full of filth," or "abundant defilement." The word itself is taboo, as if threatening the speaker with some of the disturbing taint of the outcast group itself. As in the case of many such victimized groups, the Eta have long been associated with despised and defiling occupations, including those connected with slaughter of animals and with handling human waste, animal skins, and corpses—that is, those "centered . . . around blood, death, and dirt."[76]

Jews have also been frequently associated with death and defilement, but in ways even more dangerous to others: accusations of being well poisoners and plague spreaders, of practicing necromancy and in ceremonial drinking of blood or ritual murder of Christian children as sacrifices for a black mass. Jews have also over the course of their history been confined to the same defiling professions in which the Eta engage, as well as forced to associate with money or "usury," the term meaning "lending money with interest" but conveying a sense of dishonesty, ugliness, and taboo very close to defilement. The symbolism of money as "filthy lucre," "evil excrescence," and also "immortal stuff" (mystical and magical) suggests its relation both to feces and death on the one hand, and to an immortalizing mode on the other. But by becoming bound up with what was generally perceived as an illegitimate and tainted mode of immortality, the Jews became further vulnerable to victimization. German Jews could be viewed as élite victims, as in the case of Gerson von Bleichröder, the banker to Bismarck and the "German Rothschild." Both respected and reviled, he became an arch example for the anti-Semites of the 1870s who saw in him "Jewish power [that] had become a mortal menace to German life."[77] Having, by means of earlier victimization, relegated the Jews to this defiled, death-tainted immortality system, the victimizers came to feel nonetheless "out-immortalized" by them. Hence, subsequent German cruelties could be seen as revictimization of the Jews, still in connection with purification.

Nazi genocide can, in fact, be understood as a fierce purification procedure. But purifying principles were subsumed to the modern principle of "medical materialism": that of invoking bodily hygienic explanations for spiritual and psychological matters. The classical retrospective example is the view of Moses as "an enlightened public health administrator, rather than as a spiritual leader" because certain of his precepts enhanced individual bodily health.[78]*

Medical materialism can overlay symbol systems that closely parallel those of primitive purification rituals. But in its concrete focus on the body, on biology, medical materialism lends itself directly to purification projects that kill in the name of healing. Medically oriented purification included getting rid of the incurably ill and hereditarily impaired as well as those considered sexually deviant, notably homosexuals.

In their principle of taking over evolution from nature in order to prevent humanity from being "annihilated by degeneration" (in Lorenz's words [see page 134]), the Nazis were putting forward their sweeping version of biological—one might say evolutionary—purification. Doctors became the professional purifiers, once they themselves had undergone purification (Hitler's stress on the "cleansing" of the medical profession —which meant getting rid of Jews and political opponents—so that it could assume "racial leadership"), the "alert biological soldiers" on guard against anything strange or deficient and therefore defiling with its contagion. Scientific racism and mental hygiene were the medical-materialistic principles by which the Nazis murdered in the name of purification. Above all, one had to "purify the blood," an image that in its full meaning and with its related expressions ("blood and soil," "blood flag," "Order of the Blood," and "thinking with the blood") suggests what one commentator called "the mysterious relationship of organic to inorganic nature."[79] "Purifying the blood" becomes a means of rendering sacred the mystical-immortal Aryan race and community. Paracelsus was again useful here, now as a great purifier of history itself.† As exemplified by Paracelsus, there had been a long-standing German tendency, expressed in various youth and adult movements, toward purification of mind and body. The Nazis called forth that tradition in a violent attack on all that they saw as defiling in urban life, human relations, sexual behavior, and social experiment.

The Nazis also developed the medical-purification method *par excellence*, applied to purification of genes and race—that of selections. The pivotal statement that "National Socialism is nothing but applied biology" could be even more pivotally understood: "National Socialism is nothing but applied biological purification." It was from this standpoint that one Nazi writer declared that the doctor had been "restored to the priesthood and

*The term "medical materialism," used originally by William James, has been developed in the manner used here by Mary Douglas. Norman O. Brown, in personal conversation, told me of a childhood teacher at a church school who impressed his students by declaring that Moses was a "sanitary officer." The teacher considered himself a "modernist" and constantly connected biblical events with scientific principles.

†The reference is to Richard Billinger's *Paracelsus*, as presented in a drama staged at the Salzburg Festival in 1943. Erwin Guido Kolbenheyer had written an influential Paracelsus trilogy in 1925–26, which was taken up by the Nazis; in it Paracelsus seeks virtually to eliminate history by replacing it with a divine form of nature.[80]

to the holiness of his calling"; and that another writer held forth the vision that "physicians could be the true savior of the human race."[81] We have seen this visionary medical materialism associated with various occult ideas, as in the case of Rudolf Hess and Johann S., who was in part a follower of Hess (see pages 129–30). When Dr. S. plunged into personal purification via war, in response to impending defeat and other disillusionments with the Nazi movement, he was, so to speak, attempting to *purify* his purification, to find the simplest (or most pure) expression of life-death confrontation. The purifying impulse, once established, may not easily give way and, when its violence falls into disrepute, can lend itself to alternate forms of killing.

The goal of Nazi purification, like that of primitive peoples, was to "create one single, symbolically consistent universe."[82] Both sought qualities of "wholeness and completeness" as well as "physical perfection," but the Nazis were much more extreme than any primitives in their literalism and in their deadly application of medical materialism and high technology to a totalistic spiritual goal.

For the Nazis were much less at home in their skins than were primitive peoples: as a modern movement seeking by their purification procedures to *restore* a past of perfect harmony that never was, the Nazis' actions inevitably were compensatory and more desperate. Starting from modern forms of collective dislocation and of fragmentation of the self, their purification was bound to fail. It is simply not possible to create, from a modern psychic vantage point, a "primitive, undifferentiated universe" within which a *Führer* principle becomes the source of all judgments about life, death, and killing. Indeed, one suspects that the very impossibility of the project takes it from mere victimization to genocide. For, just as in primitive cultures, "witchcraft . . . is found in a non-structure,"[83] so in modern cultures can genocide be found in the non-achievable ideal of total medical-hygienic purification.

Purification tends to be associated with sacrificial victims, whether in primitive or contemporary religious or secular terms. Genocide can be understood as a quest to make sacrificial victims out of an entire people.

The practice of human sacrifice was pursued not just to appease the gods but to engage in a mutually sustaining exchange of life power. The Aztecs of Mexico, for instance, as late as the fifteenth century and just before the Spanish conquests, pursued as their sacred duty a course of endless warfare in order to obtain prisoners to offer in sacrifice "to preserve the universe from the daily threat of annihilation."[84] But for the gods to provide this service, they in turn had to be nourished by man, "kept alive by life itself, by the magic substance that is found in the blood of man, . . . 'the precious liquid' . . . with which the gods are fed." As in the case of the Nazis, in a very different context, the mass sacrificial killing became part of a vast revitalization project bound up with "national identity and collective zeal" in political matters and "fanaticism . . . [and] tireless dynamism" in military combat.[85]

But the historical differences are important: for the Aztecs, the mass killing was always carried out in ritual fashion as an extension of a long-standing ideology and ethos; while for the Nazis, the killing was carried out through technology and was an unprecedented historical step. Nazi genocide was kept secret, except from the SS inner élite, while Aztec sacrificial killing was open and celebrated.

For the Nazis as for the Aztecs, "human sacrifice was 'an alchemy by which life was made out of death.' " The therapeutic component in both was strong: for the Nazis, therapy to the Aryan race; and for the Aztecs, to gods whose weakened or ailing state, or displeasure at not having been sufficiently nourished, had led to disasters and other untoward events ("The prescription to cure such supernatural ailments was inevitably more sacrifice, requiring new victories to obtain captives").[86] In both cases, whatever the more-than-natural imagery, the therapy was ultimately for the life power of one's own group.

Both groups killed and went on killing in the face of increasing evidence that the killing itself interfered with the survival of the state: with the conduct of the war, in the case of the Nazis; and with the entire social and economic existence of an exhausted empire, in the case of the Aztecs. Both had to continue "killing" death. For it was as true of the Nazi as of the Aztec that each "could insist on offering blood in return for life until his whole religion became an emotional bulwark around the specter of death."[87]

The Nazi perversion of primal human psychological forces was prefigured by Joseph de Maistre, an early-nineteenth-century Catholic reactionary, who was to influence the later development of European fascism:

> from maggots up to man, the universal law is the violent destruction of human beings. The whole earth, continually steeped in blood, is nothing but an immense altar on which every living thing must be sacrificed without end, without restraint, without respite until the consummation of the world, the extinction of evil, the death of death.[88]

In order to extinguish evil and kill death, that is, we require not just violence but violence without end—some form of genocide.[89]

Götterdämmerung *and Self-Genocide*

As it becomes total—that is, genocidal—the violent cure draws upon all facets of the perpetrators' culture.

The Nazis drew upon powerful German cultural impulses toward a unified, fully merged polity, society, and person. The individual self was no longer to be haunted by its own fear of disintegration, or by conflicts over competing alternatives; no longer subject to the German "torn condition." Rather, it was to become part of "a monolithic unit, bound together by blood and fate."[90] In applying that communal cure, the Nazis created something on the order of "racial time" as an ultimate dimension in which took place the cosmic struggle for Aryan health and against Jewish infection—ultimate, because it allegedly determined the outcome of events in conventional historical time (the First World War, Weimar, etc.) In its primal nature and timelessness, "racial time" was a vulgarized counterpart of what Eliade has called "mythic time,"[91] and connected every act of mass murder to a vision of mystical unity.

The violent cure must draw, however selectively, upon existing intellectual tradition. The Nazis found that tradition in Nietzsche, whom they interpreted as advocating war as therapy for weakness and the cultivation of "that deep impersonal hatred, that cold-blooded murderousness coupled with a good conscience, that communal, organizing zest in the destruction of the enemy" as a path to collective health.[92]* Above all, Nietzsche's vision was one of all-consuming illness and cure. The condition, he declared, was "not . . . sickness but *sickliness*," by which he meant perpetual weakness and concern with morality.[93] Nietzsche went on to declare that "one is healthy when . . . one feels that the 'bite' of conscience is like a dog biting on a stone—when one is ashamed of one's remorse," and one can attribute "more *health of soul*" to a criminal who "does not slander his deed after it is done" than to the sinner who "abase[s] himself before the cross."[94]

To be sure, the Nazis said nothing of Nietzsche's repeated mocking of German chauvinism (" 'German' had become an argument. *Deutschland, Deutschland über alles* a principle; the Teutons . . . the 'moral world order' in history"),[95] of anti-Semitism, and of "the morality of races and classes." What mattered was that Nietzsche could bring to a vision of cure what he himself called "the magic power of extremes" and his declaration that "we have to be destroyers."[96]

That one-sided Nietzschean vision was more important to the Nazis than any formal psychological system. They did sponsor scientific-psychological work claiming to demonstrate the role of the Jew as "the anti-type," so constructed biologically and sociologically as to have a "disintegrative" effect on the larger German community.[97] And they had some sympathy for Jungian psychology, particularly at the time of Jung's collaboration with Nazi psychiatry and his insistence on distinctions between the "Aryan" and the Jewish unconscious.[98] But more fundamentally the Nazis rejected introspective psychology because, as Rosenberg insisted, "the Nordic soul is not contemplative and . . . does not lose itself

---

*Nietzsche had nothing to do with the nation- and race-centered "German ideology" long prominent in German intellectual life, and specifically important to the development of Nazi ideology. Such towering independent cultural visionaries who have made militant metaphorical calls for killing in the name of healing are probably necessary to genocidal movements for legitimizing their own literal application of that principle.

in individual psychology, but . . . it willfully experiences cosmic-spiritual laws."[99]

Genocidal projects are likely to seek strong *psychological connections* with such "cosmic-spiritual laws" rather than utilize an exact psychological system or approach. Indeed the Nazis were on guard against the kind of experimentation with the self—what I call Protean man or woman (see page 499)—that psychology is likely to document or even encourage.[100] Moreover, both psychology and experimentation with the self were associated in their eyes with Jewish influence, as well as being antithetical to the monolithic vision of self, people, and polity.*

The proposed cure is impossible to achieve, but genocide can appear, at least for a time, to be approaching that cure and solving important problems. The Nazis, for instance, did solve the problem of the "leaking ghettos" and did enable large numbers of people to internalize the idea of the Reich as a mystical community.[101] Within that mystical frame, the killing of most of the Jews could re-create for Hitler and other Nazis a quality of experience reminiscent of the shared transcendence at the time of the beginning of the First World War. While none of this was enough to render the cure continuously successful, it helped the Nazis in general and Auschwitz doctors in particular to sufficiently overcome conflicts they experienced to be able to continue with their contribution to the killing.

Was the therapeutic killing aimed ultimately at all Germans no less than at all Jews? This is the issue contained in the question of whether Hitler's path, from the beginning, included a *Götterdämmerung*—a "twilight of the gods" or massive self-destruction—of his own people.

Certainly Hitler ordered such a *Götterdämmerung* at the end, the demolition of all industrial, transportation, communications, and supply facilities; and had not Speer and others intervened there would have been death on so massive a scale as to approach self-genocide.[102] Hitler had always totalized the genocidal cure: either the Aryan or the Jewish race would be destroyed. He told Speer that, if the war were lost, the German people too were "lost" so one need not worry about their needs for survival. That is, the cure had failed: they had shown themselves weak and unworthy. In that light, the final words of his testament reasserting the necessity of destroying the Jews was a defense of correct therapy proven not quite good enough. Hitler's own suicide could be understood as part of the necessity he felt for the entire German people to share a similar sacrificial fate, possibly on behalf of future political resurrection.

The perpetrator of genocide kills to cure himself as well as his people. As complete cure eludes him—he can never quite kill them *all* or eliminate the source of the infection—he must use his own people and himself to continue the flow of victims. His vision of cure then becomes still more confused; he may turn his violence inward to act on a deserved fate as a final purification. Now collective suicide (actually the leader taking his

---

*Yet perpetrators of genocide may themselves take on Protean characteristics as they experiment with limitless human manipulation and violence.

people with him in death) has the future-oriented message that the genocidal cure must go on. In the way that "the blood of Christ in the Sacrament was to be replaced by the blood of the German war dead,"[103] the blood of one's own people and of oneself must now supplement that mythic blood bank.

The process may be still more paradoxical: just as one reasserts immortalizing principles in killing oneself, so may the self-genocide of the people, mainly engendered by a leader, seek to assert the immortalization of the whole people. The perpetrating individual or the group, that is, is cured by its own self-destruction. Then there can be no danger of hidden infection, of "inner Judaization." Purification and sacrifice are absolute. Self-destruction may well be the *only* logical outcome of truly committed genocide.

Medical Fundamentalism

If you are curing a sickness, *anything* is permissible. That image of cure lends itself to the restorative myth of state violence and to the literal enactment of that myth. Attitudes associated with modern nationalism—the healing of the wounds of one's own extended biological group or family—can readily move the myth into the territory of genocide. The myth of collective cure can then become associated with a cosmology and even approach a biologically centered state religion. Rites and rituals are established, which increasingly organize the meaning of life for individual people around the struggle to cure the wounded race by assaulting relentlessly the source of its infection. Differing nationalisms may give their own coloration to the process—"Each country develops its own sickness, medicine, and doctor"[104]—but the genocidal reach is associated with the image of killing to cure.

We may then speak of a medical fundamentalism. In all fundamentalisms, and they are usually religious or political, there is the sense of profound threat to what are considered fundamental beliefs and symbols, and a compensatory invocation of a sacred text (the Bible, the Koran, *Mein Kampf*) as a literal guide to every form of action.[105] History stops so that murderous therapy can be applied. While medicine does not provide the sacred text, one can revert to ancient practices of shamans, witch doctors, and tricksters who could be expected to kill in order to heal. For physicians as well as charismatic spiritual physicians, there is a release from Hippocratic restraint. George Santayana wrote in 1915, "The Germans have been groping for four hundred years toward a restoration of their primitive heathenism,"[106] and we may say that they found the means of doing so in their medical fundamentalism.

Susan Sontag has written that "the concept of disease is never innocent," and that "to describe a phenomenon as a cancer is an incitement to violence."[107] Armenians were described as "a canker, a malignance which looks like a small pimple from the outside, which, if not removed by a skillful surgeon's scalpel, will kill the patient."[108] (Similarly, the Ache, an Indian group in Latin America, who are hunted by Paraguayans, are described by the latter as " 'rabid rats'; and rabid rats must be exterminated.")[109] Turkish doctors also played a large part in the genocide of Armenians; and one has been quoted as saying, "My Turkishness prevailed over my medical calling."[110] Turkish leaders also asserted their need to destroy the Armenians as a way of revitalizing their empire, of curing their people.

Here the white-coated doctor replaces the black-robed priest as arbiter of death and immortality. The medical figure, the biological soldier, becomes in fact a biological general in the campaign to kill death.

The task is Sisyphean rather than utopian: no amount of killing can bring about the desired solution. So one keeps trying, keeps killing, commits oneself to the principle of killing not just one's victims but every last one of them. The primal images are those of death, immortality, and murderous cure.

The Agents

Genocide requires two groups of people: a professional élite that formulates and supervises the killing, and professional killers who kill. Well before these groups are enlisted for the actual killing, they are influenced by what can be called an atmosphere of genocide. There seems to be something murderous in the air, stories of mass killing that are both disbelieved and believed. It becomes a kind of "middle knowledge"— something one knows and does not know, or acts upon without clearly knowing, or knows and does not act upon.[111] It is a combination of knowledge and numbing, but the knowledge seeps through.

There may be a period of impasse and confusion, as occurred in Germany in about March 1941, during which the genocidal dynamic takes shape. The killing project comes to be perceived as the only overall "solution" to a series of dilemmas. Initiatives from below (based on perceptions of what the leader or leaders desire) converge with attitudes, orders, and indirect messages from above in a sequence that is unlikely to be traceable to a specific document but that nonetheless takes definite form, is systematically enacted, and involves a vast number of people working in concert as perpetrators. The process is both arcane and secret on the one hand, and ordinary and almost respectable on the other.

The Killing Professionals

Genocidal projects require the active participation of educated professionals—physicians, scientists, engineers, military leaders, lawyers, clergy, university professors and other teachers—who combine to create not only the technology of genocide but much of its ideological rationale, moral climate, and organizational process.

Ironically, these very professional groups, lumped together as "intellectuals," are likely to be a particular object of scorn for the genocidal regime. Rolf Hochhuth, for instance, has spoken of Hitler as the culmination of "a long tradition of contempt for intellectuals, for reason and the things of the mind." Indeed, the regime's leaders were likely to equate this educated group with those who must be victimized: "The moment Goebbels began to equate Jews with intellectuals his hatred of them became homicidal."[112]

Hitler recognized the regime's need for particular professional groups, and its determination to make functionaries of those professionals; he issued a call to healers and thinkers to take leadership in destroying healing and thinking as they had known them. For the principle of annihilation of the mind, orchestrated by the most educated, precedes, accompanies, and motivates genocide throughout.

The susceptibility of professionals to extreme environments, including genocidal ones, is suggested by the sequence now familiar to us in one German profession: from ordinary doctors (before 1933), to Nazi doctors (1933–45), to ordinary doctors (after 1945). Doctors reflect the more general tendency to claim virtue for maintaining under duress the function of a profession, especially a healing profession, even when that duress includes participating in genocide.

Recall the description of Heyde, the psychiatrist in charge of direct medical killing, as "a Nazi who was not really a scientist but who with the help of science became the mouthpiece for the Nazis." When that "help of science" includes a healing claim, professionals can move to the farthest shore of evil. That journey requires the kind of immersion in ideology with its promise of a unified worldview and of knowledge put to passionate purpose, an immersion toward which the educated are especially inclined.

Consider two Nobel Prize winners' embrace of the concept of "Aryan physics," and a great psychoanalyst's insistence upon sharp distinctions between "Aryan" and "Jewish" psychology.[113] Intellectuals can all too readily welcome relief from the burden of thought, as described by Karl Stern in depicting "a peculiar brand of irrationalism" that took hold of German colleagues at the psychiatric institute where he worked—a "mysticism which opposed itself to Reason"— but, we may add, came to do so always in the name of science.[114]

Even members of the victimized group can join in this process of taking science almost anywhere. Otto Weininger, himself a Jew, described Judaism as "the greatest negation," as "the abyss over which Christianity is erected," and as Christ's own "original sin."[115]* Not only is Weininger expressing extraordinary self-hate, but he shows how far psychology and

*Weininger's *Sex and Character*, published in 1903, was said to have been admired by Hitler in its polarity of Aryan attributes and Jewish nonhumanity.[116]

the social sciences in particular can be ideologized in lethal directions, again in the name of science.

While the collective dynamic is working, individual professionals can feel themselves to be doing something earthshaking, "creating something new." The most grotesque violation of reason can be hailed as admirable innovation, especially in the case of scholars of international standing, such as Erich Jaensch (who claimed to "demonstrate" the psychology of the Jewish "anti-type").[117] The dynamism of genocide offers considerable temptation to the professional to become the "spiritual engine" of change, revolution, renewal.

Professionals and intellectuals have additional susceptibilities: to the call of the *Führer* principle as an antidote for isolation and weakness; to romanticized violence and a cult of hardness, as a denial of effeteness, softness, and "scruples"; to the crude and primitive, as a way of disowning sophistication and worldliness. Most of these susceptibilities involve claims to omnipotence in the name of humility, calls to sacrifice in which the sacrificial group is made up of the regime's designated victims. These contradictions can be maintained, lived with, through the professional's special talent for doubling. Only he or she can become a murderous sorcerer while claiming to be a healer, as did the talented Nazi bacteriologist—"in his early thirties . . . very self-assured"—who lectured to high Nazi officials on a bacteriological serum he had prepared, "a drop of [which] . . . would suffice to kill a man . . . and . . . leave no trace," and presented these and other details "as clearly and calmly as though he were addressing a class on the most ordinary matters."[118] One would have to be a professional to engage in the Auschwitz style of medical activity which (in Dr. B.'s words) "consist[ed] . . . only of selecting people for the gas chamber." Worse, one may do these things with the conviction that they are "in accord with the natural history and biology of man," and that one is acting as healer and savior.

The Professional Killers

The second, less educated group is likely to make up the "hit men" on the front line of the killing. They do the shooting or insert the gas pellets and their role, however diminished, is not eliminated in potential nuclear genocide. Rather than formulate principles or technology of killing, they act on these formulations and carry out the work. Limited in opportunities, they are likely to make killing their *only* profession; they become the artisans of killing, or the technologists of mass murder.

They can have most of the susceptibilities of the more educated group, and can certainly embrace ideologies that render mass murder a form of cleansing or healing. But rather than viewing themselves as scientists applying higher knowledge, they draw from a "corps spirit," the sense of shared combat of the most demanding kind. Their hardening is enormously stressed and related to cultural principles of masculinity (or sometimes feminine strength) as well as with a special commitment and self-sacrifice: in Himmler's term, not just ordinary soldiers but "ideological fighters." They are encouraged, and embrace the opportunity, to view their genocidal project as a military operation: one of subduing "partisans," as in the case of the *Einsatzgruppen;* or of "fighting" on the "racial battlefield" against the "dangerous Jewish enemy."

Himmler was not without psychological accuracy when, in speaking of killer troops, he referred to "the road between the two . . . possibilities —either to become too brutal . . . heartless and no longer respect human life, or to become weak and be pushed to the point of a nervous breakdown"; he added that "the road between this Scylla and Charybdis is frightfully narrow." While he was wrong in his conclusion that the road had been taken "without any mental and spiritual harm to our men and our leaders,"[119] he was exploring the limits of the human capacity for numbing and doubling on behalf of mass killing. Nor were numbing and doubling rendered superfluous by the higher technology of Auschwitz killing, as suggested by a drunken Birkenau *Blockführer* who was overheard to say: "Mother, if you knew that your son has become a murderer!"[120]

Genocidal organizers are likely to combine corps spirit with literal mobilization of criminality. The Turks made extensive use of criminals in their genocide against Armenians, and the Nazis did the same in bringing to Auschwitz a large contingent of criminals to help set up and run the camp. Traditional criminality and corps spirit can of course be combined, as they were when the SS adopted a policy of welcoming criminals to its ranks and using them for murderous tasks. The Nazis made extensive use of other outside groups, including ethnic Germans from various parts of Europe, Ukranians, Latvians, and Lithuanians.

Men are drawn to these groups of professional killers by destructive psychological traits that can be considered psychopathic, but also by omnipotence and sadism, aggressiveness and violence, and inclinations toward numbing and doubling that are within an ordinary social range. Such is the potential human store of these traits that they can be all too readily combined with elements of ideology and military discipline to form efficient killing units.

The "Half-Educated Man"

Professionals who kill and professional killers in many ways merge. One link is the "half-educated man" or "half-intellectual" common among the Nazis (see page 452). He can assume prominence in genocide by bringing to the project certain necessary elements: the smattering of knowledge that can enable one to ideologize radically the professional sphere and to embrace wholeheartedly false theories; rage and bitter envy toward those with authentic professional qualifications; and tendencies toward destructive and violent behavior (sometimes full psychopathy) as well as doubling and numbing. These half-educated men abound among both the killing professionals and the professional killers.

As we have learned from Nazi doctors and their assistants, functions can be reversed: killing professionals can murder directly, and professional killers can contribute to planning and technology. Everybody can join the killing. As we evoke images of Dr. Pfannmüller demonstrating to visitors an emaciated infant he was starving to death, of Mengele utilizing scrupulous medical technique as he injected phenol into a victim's heart, or of Klehr performing the same injection without benefit of a medical education—we are hard put to distinguish one killer from another.

Indeed, the two groups are drawn together by the shared secret that is not quite a secret; by a mix of ideology, ethos, corruptibility; and by accumulated evil. Together they constitute a killing élite. They are given special privileges and take on a more-than-natural aura. Even as they kill they can be looked upon as the standard for the endless purification justifying the killing, as the "children of the gods." The SS, for instance, was to constitute the ideal Nordic type as well as to take responsibility for eliminating virtually all others. And should more of one's own people be included in the genocidal project, always a possibility, the élite killers would be expected to survive, or at least be the last to die. On the one hand their taint of death and evil is likely to increase, in their own as well as in others' eyes. But on the other hand they become the carriers of the immortal racial-cultural substance. Only by either dying heroically or endlessly surviving—the two patterns are closely related—can they promote and articulate the immortalizing project they serve.

The Technology of Genocide

One cannot say that any particular level of technology is required for genocide: the Turks killed about one million Armenians by means of shooting, clubbing, beating, slave labor, starvation, and other forms of torture. The Nazis killed millions of Jews by the same crude methods, even without benefit of gas chambers.

Higher technologies render the killing more efficient, in time and numbers, and in easing the psychological burden of the perpetrators. A clear example is the Nazi sequence from face-to-face shooting to fatal injections and carbon monoxide gas chambers to cyanide gas: the sequence, to paraphrase Ernst B., from pre-craftsmanship to craftsmanship to modern technology. The sequence helps eliminate the impediment of empathy, of experiencing one's victims as fellow human beings.

As Auschwitz achieved its peak function of killing more than twenty thousand Jews in one twenty-four-hour period, with their bodies burned either in crematoria or open pits, "the capacity for destruction was approaching the point of being unlimited." Now after years "in constant application of administrative techniques,"[121] the Auschwitz killing system could be described by Dr. B. as "perfect."

In the process of being improved, the technology itself comes increasingly to dominate the perpetrators' field of attention. Thus, the Nazis could reach a state of function in which (again in Dr. B.'s term) "ethics played no part—the word does not exist." The technology helps create a hermetic world in which everyone is motivated to help make things "work." And that preoccupation takes on a sense of everydayness, of normality.

Albert Speer wrote of having "exploited the phenomenon of the technician's often blind devotion to his task. . . . These people were . . . without any scruples about their activities." Speer considered himself to have been the top representative of a technocracy which had without compunction used all its knowledge in an assault on humanity.[122] While Speer to some degree tried to hide behind technology in minimizing his own ideological passion, he rightly stressed the Nazis' success in rendering their most murderous actions into technological problems. The term, "reactionary modernism" is appropriate for the regime's combination of technocracy and pre-modern visions and structures.* The "reactionary" part of the regime's psyche was anti-technological; and precisely that contradiction toward technology and modernism—not so much a contradiction as the most extreme ambivalence—is likely to characterize genocidal regimes.

The rationalized search for a "final solution of the Jewish question" involved the idea of solving a problem in the most conclusive or "final" manner. From top to bottom, each perpetrator's part in solving the problem can thus be looked upon as essentially technical. And the pattern can be insidious: for technology does not require the conceptual level of scientific thought, but tends instead to create a focus on maintenance and function. Those closely related to it—especially when embracing it to avoid perceiving themselves as killers—are likely to model themselves after it. More than that, the very creation of the technology of murder is made possible by those same "manacles" (expressions of the technological mind-set)† increasingly transmitted by modern industrial society. Because it works—or so long as it does—technology can quickly be perceived as part of the natural order of things, an aspect of nature.

Technological distancing and altering of the moral mind-set was illuminatingly demonstrated by the striking correlation between attitude and altitude among American pilots and air crews in Vietnam and Cambodia. B-52 pilots and crews, who bombed at such high altitudes that they

---

*The term is Jeffrey Herf's. He sees Ernst Jünger (see page 127) as a key forerunner of reactionary modernism, and draws upon Klaus Theweleit's study of fascist male fantasy to identify Jünger as the prototypical "martial man" who needs such dichotomies as man/woman, dam/flood, purity/filth, height/depth in order to achieve domination over the feminine both inside and outside himself.[123]

†The phrase "mind-forged manacles" is William Blake's, quoted by William Barrett to suggest our own mental responsibility for these attitudes toward technology.[124]

saw nothing of their victims, tended to speak exclusively of professional skill and performance; those on fighter-bomber missions had glimpses of people below and tended to have at least a slight inclination to explain or rationalize what they did; those who flew helicopter gunships saw everything and could experience the fear, horror, questioning, and guilt that was felt by ground personnel.[125]

This psychological benefit for perpetrators is what makes the high technology of destruction compatible with genocide. The progress is terrifying in connection with present nuclear-weapons stockpiles. Alternating ideological antagonisms between the United States and the Soviet Union are accompanied by embrace of nuclear weapons, even worship of them, by both powers as ultimate sources of "security" and of life-sustaining "power." This pattern of "nuclearism"[126] combines morally blind technicism with awed genuflection before all-powerful objects that can do what in the past only God could do: destroy the world.

No wonder, then, that Americans now take to playing little war games with rifles or individual automatic weapons; or join "survivalists" groups who buy land in isolated places, take regular target practice, and stock up on canned goods in order to ready themselves for the nuclear holocaust. Operating here is deep and violent nostalgia for the days when a man need only master the simplest technology to protect himself and his family, as opposed to the technological genocide that shadows us all.[127]

One reason perpetrators of genocide can enlist many people for their project is that "belief in the decisive role of technique has . . . passed from the philosophers into the culture at large."[128] In connection with evolving Nazi ideas, Theweleit has spoken of "the fascination of the machine" in suggesting how one could "live . . . without having any feelings" and make one's body into a "steel form." That "steel form" enables one to kill promiscuously and without pain.[129]

Genocidal Bureaucracy

Bureaucracy makes possible the entire genocidal sequence: organization, continued function, and distancing, numbing, and doubling of perpetrators.

Bureaucracy helps render genocide unreal. It further diffuses the impact of murderous events that, to begin with, are difficult to believe. In this sense we may say that the bureaucracy *deamplifies* genocide: diminishes the emotional and intellectual tones associated with the killing, primarily for perpetrators but also for bystanders and victims. Central to the process is the dampening of language, the use not only of euphemisms ("resettlement" or "deportation" for killing) but also of certain code terms ("special treatment," for instance) that are specific enough in designating murderous acts to maintain bureaucratic efficiency, even to give them special priority, while contributing to a partial sense that one is not murdering people at all but doing something benign. This deamplification of language—with its attendant numbing, denial, and derealization—may extend to the point of relative silence, thereby maintaining the mixture of part-secrecy and "middle knowledge" likely to surround genocide.

Max Weber, though recognizing the necessity of bureaucracies, was acutely aware of their danger, especially to the mind. He equated bureaucracy with the "inanimate machine" of "mind objectified" and saw the phenomenon of bureaucratic organization as "busy fabricating the shell of bondage which men will perhaps be forced to inhabit some day, as powerless as the fellahs of ancient Egypt."[130] The Nazi genocidal project demonstrated that the human structure can be rendered relatively "inanimate" and "machine"-like, and the mind of bureaucratic perpetrators sufficiently "objectified" that the killing was rarely experienced in human terms, as vital beings murdering other vital beings. An important part of bureaucratic function is its sealing off of perpetrators from outside influences, so that intrabureaucratic concerns become the entire universe of discourse. What can result has been termed "group think," a process by which bureaucracies can make decisions that are disastrous for all concerned and, when viewed retrospectively, wildly inappropriate and irrational. Irving Janis attributes "group think" to the collective need for cohesiveness and unity and to the avoidance of the kind of conflict engendered by dissenting voices.[131] But when the group concerned is a genocidal bureaucracy, there is a powerful impulse, both from without and within, to create absolute barriers of thought and feeling between itself and the outside world. Only then can the strange assumptions of virtue within the group be maintained: ideological ("We are doing this for revitalization of our people"), technical ("What is most efficient is best for everyone"), and therapeutic ("We are healing our race and going about it as humanely as possible").

The genocidal bureaucracy contributes also to collective feelings of inevitability. The elaborateness of the bureaucracy's organization conveys a sense of the inexorable—that one might as well (as perpetrator or victim) go along because nothing can be done. The bureaucracy's structure and function—the murderous flow of its action—becomes itself the rationale, as clarity of cause and effect gives way to a sense not only of inevitability but of necessity.

Ancillary bureaucracies can be all too readily enlisted to carry out the genocide, as in the case of the German railroad organization in transporting Jews to the death camps while holding strictly to its own conventional bureaucratic routine (see page 446).[132]

Under certain circumstances, victims' bureaucracies can be coerced into participating in their own people's victimization (as, for instance, *Judenrat* organizations, and also those prisoner doctors who collaborated closely with the Nazis [see chapter 13]). Perpetrators' bureaucratic deamplification can contribute to that participation of victims, and to victims' own distancing from, and resistance to, the truth about the mass murder of their fellows. (Hence the failure of many Jews in Germany and Europe to recognize the danger they faced, and the relative inactivity of most American Jews despite increasing evidence of Jewish genocide in Europe.)

The combination of relative silence and organizational reach puts the bureaucracy in the best position to plan the details of genocide. That original involvement in planning contributes in turn to the bureaucracy's normalization of a genocidal universe.[133] Mass murder is everywhere but at the same time (through the efforts of the bureaucracy) nowhere. There is only a flow of events to which most people in the environment (as Dr. B. said of Auschwitz doctors) come to say yes. To say no would take one outside that flow, outside of normal social existence, outside of reality. One seeks instead the most "humane" path within the going project.

Yet it is a mistake to speak of bureaucracy as "faceless" and "monolithic." The faces are there, even if hidden and merged into a mass. And the apparent monolith can encompass divergent and contending positions. These conflicts make up part of the dynamic of any bureaucracy, even in totalistic circumstances. People vary considerably in how they function in bureaucracies, and the bureaucracies themselves vary in their relationships to political regimes. Bureaucracies can give rise to initiative for pursuing genocide, even at relatively low levels (as we have seen to be the case with Nazi bureaucrats, including doctors). That initiative is. likely to reflect an individual or a group's keen sense of what is desired by the regime's leaders, to whom bureaucracies, at least totalistic ones, are likely to be closely attuned.

Bureaucratic practice also contributes to the later cover-up of genocide by not only dampening everyone's responses but also serving to hide individual perpetrators. The attempt of German doctors to suppress the truth of their profound involvement in Nazi genocide is a case in point, even if that attempt eventually failed; there were similar patterns in Armenian genocide.

Bureaucracy, then, does much to render into a machine the human killing network and to deamplify the killing process for all concerned: the experience of killing for perpetrators, and the actuality of killing for bystanders and potential victims. But bureaucratic deamplification and hiding should not be confused with nonresponsibility.

The Genocidal Self

No individual self is inherently evil, murderous, genocidal. Yet under certain conditions virtually any self is capable of becoming all of these. A self is not a thing or a person but an inclusive representation or symbolization of an individual organism—as experienced by a particular person and (in related but by no means identical ways) by other people.[134]* To emphasize activity, shift, and change, we may speak of "self-process."

Extreme numbing can, as we have seen, lead to amoral self-process; and numbing and doubling to evil self-process, sometimes with the self losing its capacity to distinguish between good and evil. Yet evil self-process can include struggles of conscience that propel one in the direction of *principled mass killing*. Precisely when the principle called upon takes on a strongly therapeutic tone can self-process move readily toward genocide.

The self's capacity for such action is always influenced by ideological currents in the environment. Again, in terms of self-process, the sequence from ordinary doctor to Nazi doctor to ordinary doctor suggests the extraordinary power of an environment to issue a "call" to genocide. Everything said here about the self's response to that call depends importantly upon idea structures of a collective nature, upon shared mentality rather than any isolated self.

Yet people have differing vulnerabilities to amoral or evil action. Studies of the "authoritarian personality" were inspired by German behavior under the Nazis.[136] And I have suggested the relevance for genocide of certain features of self-process in German culture: tendencies toward guilt and self-condemnation; toward inner divisions of the "torn condition" as inclinations toward doubling and Faustlike behavior; toward all or none commitments or ideological totalism; and toward death-haunted immortality hunger. But Germans have no monopoly on any of these traits or upon evil self-process of the potentially genocidal self. One need only consider the situation in which idealistic young Americans, working in a mental hospital as conscientious objectors to war and violence, reached the point where they "helped to kill"[137] deteriorated mental patients. While their actions were hardly genocidal, these people of notably developed ethical sensitivity were led by their environment to collude in killing.

An Auschwitz survivor went further: On seeing Eichmann and his Israeli prosecutor together on television during the trial, this woman developed the uncomfortable feeling that the two men "had something similar . . . [in] their looks." And although she "reproached" herself and was "very shocked," she could not rid herself of that impression. She was clear about Eichmann's guilt, and made no particular criticism of the prosecutor. Rather, her troubling perception of apparent similarity reflected her inner struggle with the idea that others, her own people, she herself, could, under certain conditions, also be capable of evil behavior.

The self's movement toward genocide is likely to be impelled by a powerful sense of survivor mission, which can include a therapeutic need of its own. One lives through actual or symbolic death immersion of war

---

*Michael Basch speaks of the self as "the symbolic transformation of experience into an overall goal-directed construct."[135]

or collective spiritual trauma (or both, in the case of the Germans with the First World War); one embarks on a desperate quest for meaning and revitalization; above all, one seeks an individual-psychological cure from the death imagery with which one remains afflicted. A decisive psychological issue is the extent to which one can envision self-cure in total elimination of the group one sees as perpetuating the affliction or illness. In any case, the genocidal self is impelled by its own struggle with disintegration: indeed, rage directed at victims can derive partially from a displacement of this death equivalent, from rage at one's own fear of disintegration. Rage can also distance the killer from the act of killing.

Fascist ideology can have particular appeal for the survivor self fighting off disintegration because it holds out, at all levels, a promise of unity, oneness, fusion. It deals with death anxiety, moreover, by glorifying death, even worshiping it. While one's own death as a warrior is idealized, the self mostly escapes death—achieves the death of death—by killing others. There can readily follow a vicious circle in which one kills, needs to go on killing in order to maintain one's cure, and seeks a continuous process of murderous, deathless, therapeutic survival. One can then reach the state of requiring a sense of perpetual survival through the killing of others in order to re-experience endlessly what Elias Canetti has called "the moment of power"[138]—that is, the moment of cure.

Beyond Nazi or Turkish experience, certain characteristics of the contemporary self and its experience of historical dislocation may render it particularly vulnerable to this genocidal direction. I have in mind such characteristics as exacerbated meaning-hunger due to one's loss of symbolic moorings, to confusion about the endless images of possibility to which one is exposed, along with one's intensified struggles with death anxiety having to do with nuclear-weapons imagery of annihilation or even extinction. There can result swings between the Protean style (repeated shifts in the self's involvements and beliefs) and the constricted style (compensatory narrowing of the self's involvements and search for a single path to truth).[139] This compensatory struggle against Protean experiment can take the shape of various forms of social purification and can lead to a collective sequence from dislocation to totalism to victimization to genocide.

Alternatives: The Embodied Self

There are other possibilities. Given life-enhancing environmental conditions, the self can avoid the doubling of the genocidal direction and move instead toward principles of integrity. Our model here can be what I call the "embodied self": a self that includes a measure of unity and awareness of body and person in regard to oneself and others. The infant's perception of its own body is crucial to the early development of a sense of self, and we can speak of a sequence in awareness from body to organism to person in the evolving concept of the "I." With subse-

quent symbolization over the course of childhood and adulthood, intellectual and ethical principles become combined with images of body and
person. Pitfalls along the way are various forms of dissociation and doubling resulting in a "disembodied self" in which these various elements
no longer cohere. Our understanding of the embodied self includes a
continuous symbolic or formative process, with constant creation and
re-creation of images and forms; an awareness of larger social and historical projects around one; and a capacity to confront the idea of one's own
death as related to broader principles of life continuity or larger human
connectedness. A sense of the embodied self enables us to say, with
William Barrett, "We are always more than any machine we may construct."[140]

It must be emphasized that the problem is never merely, or even
primarily, one of individual psychology. Collective currents either press
large numbers of people in the direction of dissociation and disembodi-
ment or, in contrast, encourage or even nurture the more integrated,
embodied self. Individuals nonetheless vary in degrees of what I am
calling embodiment, and therefore in the capacity to avoid the destructive
forms of doubling associated with victimization and genocide.

Prophylaxis against the genocidal directions of the self, therefore, must
always include critical examination of ideologies and institutions in their
interaction with styles of self-process. We have seen this to be true in
special ways for professionals. For instance, the physician with a strong
sense of embodied self has a greater chance to hold on to universal
healing principles in the face of ideological pressures to the contrary. He
or she would be less susceptible than were most Nazi doctors either to
a technicized professional identity ("I am a professional healer and nothing else, in no way responsible for Auschwitz; so I go along with it and
heal when I can") or to an ideologized professional identity ("As a doctor
to the *Volk* and a cultivator of genes, my participation in killing is in the
service of healing the Nordic race"). But if the destructive ideological and
behavioral pressures are sufficiently great, virtually any professional self
may be susceptible to moving in genocidal directions.

The professional does well to prepare for such exigencies by maintaining a balance of what I call advocacy and detachment, of clear ethical
commitment and technical skill. A physician's "calling" would include
commitment under all conditions to Hippocratic principles of healing.
The embodied self requires both constant critical awareness of larger
projects demanding allegiance and equally pervasive empathy, fellow
feeling, toward all other human beings.

Afterword

Bearing Witness

The story is not ended, it has not yet become
history, and the secret life it holds can break out
tomorrow in you or in me.

—GERSHOM SCHOLEM

I complete this book with many different feelings: relief at the idea of Nazi doctors no longer inhabiting my study, uneasiness concerning the limitations of my work, anger toward Nazi killers in general and Nazi doctors in particular, and a certain satisfaction that I have seen the effort through. My mind darts back and forth between the sitting rooms in which I talked to former Nazi doctors and images of Jews lined up for selections at Auschwitz and mental patients being gassed at killing centers. From the beginning I have been on guard against letting the sitting rooms block out the victims.

Yet it was in those sitting rooms that I did a great part of the research, and did it in a way that required me to view medical perpetrators, whatever their relationship to evil, as human beings and nothing else. That meant requiring of myself a form of empathy for Nazi doctors: I had to imagine my way into their situation, not to exonerate but to seek knowledge of human susceptibility to evil. The logic of my position was clear enough: only a measure of empathy, however reservedly offered, could help one grasp the psychological components of the *anti-empathic* evil in which many of these Nazi doctors had engaged.

Yet whatever its logic, it felt strange and uncomfortable to hold out even minimal empathy (and even with full awareness of the clear distinction between empathy and sympathy) for participants in a project so murderous, and one aimed specifically at my own people, at me. If I never fully resolved the matter, I managed it by understanding my empathy to be in the service of a critical rendition of those doctors' psychological actions and experiences. One sometimes enters into another's situation not to help but to expose and evaluate motivations and behavior.

Even then, one is making human contact, avoiding what Erik Erikson has called "pseudospeciation," or seeing other human beings as belonging to a different species.[1] One sympathetic commentator suggested that I could best avoid lapsing into pseudospeciation with Nazi doctors by "insisting on separating the fallible person from the evil deed, retaining our identification with the one while condemning the other." He took this to be a psychological counterpart of Jesus' saying "Love thine enemies." But while I found the suggestion moving, it did not quite capture my sense of the situation. For once a man performs an evil deed he has become part of that deed, and the deed part of him. That deed or deeds has probably required some doubling with the formation of an evil self. And while one must acknowledge that all of us are fallible human beings potentially capable of such evil deeds, we must also underscore the distinction between potential and actual evil.

My discomfort with Nazi doctors undoubtedly had to do with uneasiness about a proper moral stance and perhaps also with fear of contagion. Of course, I was also making contact with much more ordinary, all too human aspects of these doctors. Whatever satisfaction that contact provided was more than mitigated by their virtually complete absence of moral confrontation, of acknowledgment of their own moments of evil or even of the degree to which they had been part of an evil project. While that moral distancing did not prevent me from learning a great deal about their psychological motivation, it did greatly limit any possibility for what could be called a genuine human encounter. It also limited the "affective resonance" between us, and therefore my empathy for them, since empathy is after all a two-way process.

From my side came the problem of how much and for how long to "join" a doctor in his Nazi world. My psychological behavior consisted of altering my sense of self sufficiently to imagine his stance in relation to events being described, while at the same time performing two other maneuvers: bringing the victims into the picture, and holding to an ethical context depending on my own sense of self. That stance is consistent with the contemporary view of empathy as "not to be equated with identification, [and] indeed is in a sense contrasted with it . . . [because] we are empathic with what that person is trying to communicate to us, not with the person or his conduct." Empathy has an important cognitive aspect and can, most simply, be understood as "coming to know." This same observer, Michael Basch, also writes that "empathy involves resonating with the other's unconscious affect and experiencing his experience with him while the empathizer maintains the integrity of his self intact."[2] I came to see this tension concerning empathy as the key to my approach, and perhaps to the study in general.

Whatever empathy I mustered was in the service of something else: bearing witness. While I claim no prerogatives of an actual survivor, that survivorlike impulse comes quickly to anyone who seriously investigates Nazi mass murder. My kind of witness was psychological and moral, and strongly concerned with questions of the human future.

The form of witness too is unusual in that it concerns perpetrators and stems largely from their words, and yet differs radically from the witness most of them wished me to bear. What made it possible for me to bear a different witness were the contributions of victims and survivors. Physician survivors, in the observations and perspective they provided, lent support to my own sense of self and to my way of bearing witness.

What I have tried to chart is a particular sequence of human actions involved in a particular form of mass murder and genocide—that of medicalized killing. My witness is to the fact that doctors killed and did so in the name of healing, and includes questions of how, in what way, and why.

But my witness does not end with the Nazis. I want to extract from what they did whatever can be psychologically useful for us to know now. Nazi doctors doubled in murderous ways; so can others. Doubling provides a connecting principle between the murderous behavior of Nazi doctors and the universal potential for just such behavior. The same is true of the capacity to murder endlessly in the name of national-racial cure. Under certain conditions, just about anyone can join a collective call to eliminate every last one of the alleged group of carriers of the "germ of death."

Yet my conclusion is by no means that "we are all Nazis." We are *not* all Nazis. That accusation eliminates precisely the kind of moral distinctions we need to make. One of these distinctions concerns how, with our universal potential for murder and genocide, we for the most part hold back from such evil. A sensitive healer aghast at discovering her own impulses to slap a patient who had become unruly wrote to me of this "problem of our daily humanity." But we learn from the Nazis not only the crucial distinction between impulse and act, but the critical importance of larger ideological currents in connecting the two in ways that result in mass evil. Those connections and steps are my witness—not the undifferentiated moral condemnation of everybody.

But there is an additional witness I cannot avoid making: the bearing of this study on the nuclear technology of genocide which now haunts us all. The Holocaust we have been examining can help us avoid the next one. We need consider only the possible transfer to the nuclear-weapons threat not only of individual doubling but of all of these genocidal principles: the fear of the "germ of death," of a contagious illness (Soviet communism or American capitalism) threatening the life of the group (the United States or the Soviet Union); a promise of revitalizing cure via an absolutized vision (of American virtue and Soviet evil, or the reverse) that justifies "killing them *all*" and excludes the suicidal dimension of that vision; the mobilization of claims of spiritual altruism and scientific truth, and of opportunities for transcendence, as one presses toward mass killing in the name of healing; the designation of killing professionals and professional killers for the task, along with increasingly perfected technology and high bureaucratic organization that radically deamplify the genocidal actions; and finally, the creation of a widely embraced model of the genocidal self through collective patterns of "nuclearism" (embrace of the weapons out of attraction to their ultimate power and to their high technology), and visions of idealistic purification and ultimate sacrifice extending even to the lure of Armageddon.

Must all this happen? Some of it has already, but the rest need not. Any witness tells of the danger of some form of repetition of what one has observed, in order to encourage steps to prevent that repetition. One listens to what Loren Eiseley called "the dark murmur that rises from the abyss beneath us, and that draws us with uncanny fascination,"[3] and realizes that the murmur is our own, a whisper of danger that must be heard before it becomes a hopeless genocidal scream.

So much stays with me from this work, but I want to end with two images that continue to reverberate within me.

The first is from Auschwitz. I went to the camp a few years ago and was shown the many exhibits maintained there, exhibits that leave nothing to be added concerning the evil human beings can do to other human beings. But the one that left the most profound impression on me was the simplest of all: a room full of shoes, mostly baby shoes.

The second image is from a talk with a Jewish doctor who survived Auschwitz incarceration, told me his story, and became my friend. He described how, at a certain point, he and a few other prisoner doctors were overwhelmed with moribund patients, with suffering people clamoring for relief. They did what they could, dispensed the few aspirin they had, but made a point in the process of offering a few words of reassurance and hope. He found, almost to his surprise, that his words had effect, that "in that situation it really helped." He concluded that by maintaining one's determination to try to heal, even under the most extreme conditions, "I was impressed with how much one could do."

NOTES
ACKNOWLEDGMENTS
INDEX

List of Abbreviations

Anthology. International Auschwitz Committee, *Anthology,* 3 vols. in 7 parts (Warsaw, 1971–72). Collection of articles originally published 1961–67 in Polish journal *Przeglad Lekarski (Medical Review).*

BDC. Berlin Document Center

Hadamar Trial. Earl W. Kintner, ed., *The Hadamar Trial: Trial of Alfons Klein, Adolf Wahlmann, Heinrich Ruoff, Karl Willig, Adolf Merkle, Irmgard Huber, and Philipp Blum* (London: William Hodge, 1949).

Heyde Trial. Trial of Werner Heyde, Gerhard Bohne, and Hans Hefelmann, Generalstaatsanwalt Frankfurt, Js 17/59 (GStA), 4 VU 3/61, Strafkammer des Landgerichts Limburg/Lahn.

JAMA. Journal of the American Medical Association.

Mengele/Haifa. "Wo ist Mengele?," Friedmann archive, Haifa.

Nuremberg Medical Case. Nuernberg Military Tribunals, *United States of America v. Karl Brandt et al., Case I ("The Medical Case"),* 2 vols. (Washington, 1947), and accompanying transcripts (National Archives, Washington).

Wolken transcript. German original of Otto Wolken papers is in the Polish State Auschwitz Museum.

YVAJ. Yad Vashem Archive, Jerusalem.

Notes

(The numbers in brackets refer to the original, complete citation of a particular reference in each chapter. The dates in brackets denote original publication of a title.)

Introduction: "This World Is Not This World"

1. Hannah Arendt, *Eichmann in Jerusalem: A Report on the Banality of Evil* (New York: Viking, 1963).

2. Otto Rank, *Beyond Psychology* (New York: Dover, 1958 [1941]).

3. Robert Jay Lifton, *The Life of the Self: Toward a New Psychology* (New York: Basic Books, 1983 [1976]); *The Broken Connection: On Death and the Continuity of Life* (New York: Basic Books, 1983 [1979]).

4. See Lifton, *Broken Connection* [3], chap. 1.

5. George L. Mosse, *The Crisis of German Ideology: Intellectual Origins of the Third Reich* (New York: Grosset & Dunlap, 1964), p. 4.

6. Robert Jay Lifton, *Revolutionary Immortality: Mao Tse-tung and the Chinese Cultural Revolution* (New York: W.W. Norton, 1971 [1968]).

7. See Raul Hilberg, *The Destruction of the European Jews* (Chicago: Quadrangle, 1967 [1961]); Richard L. Rubenstein, *The Cunning of History: Mass Death and the American Future* (New York: Harper & Row, 1975); Arendt, *Eichmann* [1]. Hilberg's expanded edition of his classic work was too recent to consult fully for this book; see *The Destruction of the European Jews*, 3 vols., rev. and definitive ed. (New York: Holmes & Meier, 1985).

8. Hilberg, *Destruction* [7], p. 256.

9. A slightly different, published version is found in Ella Lingens-Reiner, *Prisoners of Fear* (London: Gollancz, 1948), pp. 1–2.

10. Adolf Hitler, *Mein Kampf* (Boston: Houghton Mifflin, 1943 [1925–26]), p. 435.

11. Ibid., pp. 150, 300–308, 312–13. For scholarly treatments of Hitler's (and earlier) metaphors for the Jews, see Eberhard Jäckel, *Hitler's Weltanschauung: A Blueprint for Power* (Middletown, Conn.: Wesleyan University Press, 1972 [1969]); Rudolph Binion, *Hitler Among the Germans* (New York: Elsevier, 1976); Lucy S. Dawidowicz, *The War Against the Jews, 1933–1945* (New York: Holt, Rinehart & Winston, 1975), pp. 19–21, 55–56; Uriel Tal, *Christians and Jews in Germany: Religion, Politics and Ideology in the Second Reich, 1870–1914* (Ithaca: Cornell University Press, 1975), pp. 259–89.

12. Hans Buchheim, quoted in Helmut Krausnick, "The Persecution of the Jews," in Krausnick et al., *Anatomy of the SS State* (New York: Walker, 1968 [1965]), p. 15.

13. Hilberg, *Destruction* [7], p. 12.

14. J. P. Stern, *Hitler: The Führer and the People* (Glasgow: Fontana/Collins, 1971), p. 70. The celebration of that religious impulse was epitomized by the gigantic Nuremberg rally of 1934, whose theme, "The Triumph of the Will," became the title of Leni Riefenstahl's noted film. Riefenstahl, in an interview with an assistant of mine, made clear that Hitler himself provided that slogan.

15. Mosse, *German Ideology* [5], p. 103.

16. Himmler, quoted in Krausnick, "Persecution" [12], p. 14.

17. George L. Mosse, *Toward the Final Solution: A History of European Racism* (New York: Fertig, 1978), p. 77.

18. Hitler, *Mein Kampf* [10], pp. 397–98.

19. *Nuremberg Medical Case,* especially vol. I, pp. 8–17 (the indictment) and 27–74 (opening statement by Chief Prosecutor Telford Taylor, 9 December 1946); personal interview with James M. McHaney, prosecutor of the Medical Case.

Chapter 1. Sterilization and the Nazi Biomedical Vision

1. Fritz Lenz, *Menschliche Auslese und Rassenhygiene,* vol. II of Erwin Bauer, Eugen Fischer, and Lenz, *Grundriss der menschlichen Erblichkeitslehre und Rassenhygiene* (Munich: J. F. Lehmanns Verlag, 1923), p. 147. See the expanded version of this joint work's third (1927) edition, especially for American readers: *Human Heredity* (New York: Macmillan, 1931). On Davenport and Cold Spring Harbor, see Daniel J. Kevles, *In the Name of Eugenics: Genetics and the Uses of Human Heredity* (New York: Alfred A. Knopf, 1985), pp. 44–56.

2. George L. Mosse, *Toward the Final Solution: A History of European Racism* (New York: Harper & Row, 1978), p. 81.

3. Albert Edward Wiggam, *New Decalogue of Science* (Indianapolis: Bobbs-Merrill, 1923), pp. 25–26.

4. J[acob] P. Landman, *Human Sterilization: The History of the Sexual Sterilization Movement* (New York: Macmillan, 1932), pp. 4–5.

5. Helmut Krausnick, "The Persecution of the Jews," in Krausnick et al., *Anatomy of the SS State* (New York: Walker, 1968 [1965]), pp. 16–17.

6. "Human Sterilization in Germany and the United States," *JAMA* 102 (1934):1501–2; see Kevles, *Eugenics* [1], pp. 113–17.

7. Kevles, *Eugenics* [1], p. 116.

8. Ibid., p. 117.

9. Adolf Hitler, *Mein Kampf* (Boston: Houghton Mifflin, 1943 [1925–26]), pp. 403–4, 257, respectively.

10. *JAMA* 101 (1933):866–67; 102 (1934):630–31, 1501; 103 (1934):849–50. W. W. Peter, "Germany's Sterilization Program," *American Journal of Public Health* 24 (1934):187.

11. *JAMA* 105 (1935):1999.

12. *JAMA* 104 (1935):2109 (Wagner); 101 (1933):867; 106 (1936):1582.

13. *JAMA* 106 (1936):1582.

14. *JAMA* 103 (1934):766–67, 850; 106 (1936):58, 308–9.

15. *JAMA* 104 (1935):2110.

16. *JAMA* 102 (1934):57; 103 (1934):1164; 104 (1935):2110.

17. *JAMA* 104 (1935):1183.

18. *JAMA* 105 (1935):1051.

19. W[alter] von Baeyer, "Die Bestätigung der NS-Ideologie in der Medizin unter besonderer Berücksichtigung der Euthanasie," *Universitätstage* 5 (1966):64; Ernst Klee, *"Euthanasie" im NS-Staat: Die "Vernichtung lebensunwerten Lebens"* (Frankfurt/M.: S. Fischer, 1983), p. 86. Much of my manuscript had been completed when this important book appeared, but I have used it to confirm and supplement information from other sources. Another important recent study is Gisela Bock, "Racism and Sexism in Nazi Germany: Motherhood, Compulsory Sterilization and the State," in *When Biology Became Destiny: Women in Weimar and Nazi Germany,* Renate Bridenthal, Atina Grossmann, and Marion Kaplan, eds. (New York: Monthly Review, 1985), pp. 271–96.

20. *JAMA* 105 (1935):1052–53.

21. Ernst Rüdin, "Zehn Jahre nationalsozialistischer Staat," *Archive für Rassen- und Gesellschaftsbiologie* 36 (1942):321.

22. Robert Wistrich, *Who's Who in Nazi Germany* (New York: Macmillan, 1982), p. 261. See also B. Schultz, "Ernst Rüdin," *Archive für Psychiatrie und Zeitschrift für Neurologie* 190 (1953): 189–95.

23. Judge Goetz and Wagner quoted in *JAMA* 106 (1936):1582; party paper in *JAMA* 105 (1935):1051.

24. Rudolf Ramm, *Ärztliche Rechts- und Standeskunde: Der Arzt als Gesundheitserzieher*, 2d. rev. ed. (Berlin: W. deGruyter, 1943), pp. iv, 43, 79–80.

25. Ibid., pp. 101, 135.

26. Ibid., pp. 154–56.

27. Ibid. See Kurt Blome, *Arzt im Kampf: Erlebnisse und Gedanken* (Leipzig: J. A. Barth, 1942).

28. Bernward J. Gottlieb and Alexander Berg, *Das Antlitz des Germanischen Arztes in vier Jahrhunderten* (Berlin: Rembrandt-Verlag, 1942), pp. 3, 51–52.

29. Joachim Mrugowsky, "Einleitung," Christoph Wilhelm Hufeland, *Das ärztliche Ethos: Christoph Wilhelm Hufelands Vermächtnis einer fünfzigjährigen Erfahrung* (Munich and Berlin: J. F. Lehmann, 1939), pp. 14–15, 22; see pp. 7–40.

30. Hanns Löhr, *Über die Stellung und Bedeutung der Heilkunde im nationalsozialistischen Staate* (1935), quoted in George L. Mosse, ed., *Nazi Culture: Intellectual, Cultural and Social Life in the Third Reich* (New York: Grosset & Dunlap, 1968), p. 229.

31. Ernst Grawitz, ed., *Hippokrates: Gedanken ärztlicher Ethik aus dem Corpus Hippocraticum*, vol. I: *Ewiges Arzttum* (Prague, Amsterdam, Berlin, and Vienna: Volk und Reich Verlag, 1942), p. 5.

32. Werner Leibbrandt, 27 January 1947, *Nuremberg Medical Case*, vol. II, p. 81.

33. Ramm, *Ärztliche Standeskunde* [24], p. 19. On the Nazis' related elevation of pain, see Michael H. Kater, "Medizinische Fakultäten und Medizinstudenten: Eine Skizze," in Fridolf Kudlien, ed., *Ärzte im Nationalsozialismus* (Cologne: Kiepenheuer & Witsch, 1985), p. 93.

34. *Nuremberg Medical Case*, vol. I, p. 58.

35. Ramm, *Ärztliche Standeskunde* [24], pp. 80–83.

36. Mrugowsky, "Einleitung" [29], pp. 9–10, 14.

37. George L. Mosse, *Masses and Man: Nationalist and Fascist Perceptions of Reality* (New York: Fertig, 1980), p. 81.

38. Quoted in Karl Dietrich Bracher, *The German Dictatorship: The Origins, Structure and Effects of National Socialism* (New York: Praeger, 1970 [1969]), p. 232.

39. See Kater, "Medizinische Fakultäten" [33], pp. 82–92.

40. Michael H. Kater, "Hitlerjugend und Schule im Dritten Reich," *Historische Zeitschrift* 228 (1979):609–10.

41. Michael H. Kater, *The Nazi Party: A Social Profile of Members and Leaders, 1919–1945* (Cambridge, Mass.: Harvard University Press, 1983), pp. 112, 134–35.

42. Bracher, *Dictatorship* [38], pp. 247–48.

43. Wistrich, *Who's Who* [22], p. 330.

44. Heinrich Class, quoted in Lucy S. Dawidowicz, *The War Against the Jews, 1933–1945* (New York: Holt, Rinehart & Winston, 1975), p. 36.

45. Alfred D. Low, *Jews in the Eyes of Germans: From the Enlightenment to Imperial Germany* (Philadelphia: Institute for the Study of Human Issues, 1979), pp. 371–72.

46. Ibid., p. 371.

47. Kater, *Nazi Party* [41], p. 342 n. 180; Kater, "Medizinische Fakultäten" [33], pp. 94–95.

48. Heinrich Lammers, quoted in Geoffrey Cocks, *Psychotherapy in the Third Reich: The Göring Institute* (New York and Oxford: Oxford University Press, 1985), p. 91.

49. Opening statement by Chief Prosecutor Telford Taylor, 9 December 1946, *Nuremberg Medical Case*, vol. I, p. 57.

50. *JAMA* 100 (1933): 1877.

51. Taylor's statement [49], vol. I, pp. 57–58.

52. Bracher, *Dictatorship* [38], pp. 268–69.

53. See Kater, "Medizinische Fakultäten" [33], pp. 94–104.

54. See Kater, "Hitlerjugend" [40] and *Nazi Party* [41], pp. 97–100.

55. *JAMA* 107 (1936):979–80. On Laughlin, see Kevles, *Eugenics* [1], pp. 102–4, 118. For Kennedy's views, see "The Problem of Social Control of the Congenital Defective: Education, Sterilization, Euthanasia," *American Journal of Psychiatry* 99 (1942):13–16.

56. *JAMA* 110 (1938):298.

57. Kater, "Medizinische Fakultäten" [33], pp. 94–104; Leo Alexander, "The Medical School Curriculum in War-Time Germany," Combined Intelligence Objectives Sub-Committee, Item 24 (Medical), File No. XXVII–71.

58. Karl Saller, *Die Rassenlehre des Nationalsozialismus im Wissenschaft und Propaganda* (Darmstadt: Progress-Verlag, 1961); *JAMA* 104 (1935): 2010.

59. Richard Hanser, *A Noble Treason: Students Against Hitler* (New York: Putnam, 1970), pp. 187, 22, 117, respectively.

60. *JAMA* 112 (1939): 1982.

61. *JAMA* 106 (1936): 1214–15; 113 (1939): 2163.

62. On the nature movement," see Cocks, *Psychotherapy* [48], pp. 138–43; Kater, "Medizinische Fakultäten" [33], pp. 91–93; *JAMA* 103(1934):1164–65 ("house of health"); 112 (1939):1740.

63. Stephan Leibfried and Florian Tennstedt, *Berufsverbote und Sozialpolitik, 1933: Die Auswirkungen der nationalsozialistischen Machtergreifung auf die Krankenkassenverwaltung und die Kassenärzte* (Bremen: Universität Bremen, 1981), pp. 67–76, 210–13; Cocks, *Psychotherapy* [48], pp. 87–89.

64. Dr. M. Stämmler, "Das Judentum in der Medizin," *Ärzteblatt für Norddeutschland* (1938), quoted in Leibfried and Tennstedt, *Berufsverbote* [63], pp. 307–12.

65. Interior Minister Wilhelm Frick, quoted in *JAMA* 105 (1935):1998; see 106 (1936): 136.

66. Kater, *Nazi Party* [41], pp. 112–14, 134–37; *JAMA* 106 (1936):1214–15. On the Nuremberg laws and related legislation, see Raul Hilberg, *The Destruction of the European Jews* (Chicago: Quadrangle, 1967 [1961]), pp. 42–53, and Helmut Krausnick, "The Persecution of the Jews," in Krausnick et al., *Anatomy of the SS State* (Chicago: Walker, 1968 [1965]), pp. 23–43.

67. Jan Sehn, "Carl Claubergs verbrecherische Unfruchtbarmachungs-Versuche an Häftlings-Frauen in den Nazi-Konzentrationslagern," *Hefte von Auschwitz* 2 (1959):3–31.

68. Larry V. Thompson, "*Lebensborn* and the Eugenics Policy of the *Reichsführer*-SS," *Central European History* 4 (1971):55.

69. Marc Hillel and Clarissa Henry, *Of Pure Blood* (New York: McGraw-Hill, 1976 [1975]), pp. 55, 116–26, 191–203.

70. Alexander Mitscherlich and Fred Mielke, *The Death Doctors* (London: Elek Books, 1949), p. 17.

71. Ernst Mann [Gerhard Hoffmann], *Die Erlösung der Menschheit vom Elend* (Weimar: F. Fink, 1922), p. 39.

Chapter 2. "Euthanasia": Direct Medical Killing

1. See Foster Kennedy, "The Problem of Social Control of the Congenital Defective: Education, Sterilization, Euthanasia," *American Journal of Psychiatry* 99 (1942):13–16. Kennedy was rebutted by Leo Kanner, the leading American child psychiatrist of the time, who did, however, favor sterilization. "Exoneration of the Feebleminded," *American Journal of Psychiatry* 99 (1942):17–22.

2. Adolf Jost, *Das Recht auf den Tod: Sociale Studie* (Göttingen: Dieterich'sche Verlagsbuchhandlung, 1895); Klaus Dörner, "Nationalsozialismus und Lebensvernichtung," *Vierteljahrshefte für Zeitgeschichte* 15 (1967):123–24. On the intellectual background, see Amnon Amir, "Euthanasia in Nazi Germany" (unpublished dissertation, State University of New York, Albany, 1977).

3. Karl Binding and Alfred Hoche, *Die Freigabe der Vernichtung lebensunwerten Lebens: Ihr Mass und ihre Form* (Leipzig: F. Meiner, 1920). On Binding and Hoche, see Ernst Klee, "*Euthana-*

sie" im NS-Staat: Die "Vernichtung lebensunwerten Lebens" (Frankfurt/M.: S. Fischer, 1983), pp. 19–25.

4. Binding, "Rechtliche Ausführung," in *Freigabe* [3], pp. 16–37.

5. Hoche, "Ärztliche Bemerkungen," in *Freigabe* [3], pp. 46–47, 54–58.

6. Ibid., pp. 61–62.

7. Dörner, "Lebensvernichtung" [2], p. 129.

8. Adolf Dorner, *Lehrbuch der Mathematik für höhere Schulen* (1935, rev. ed. 1936), quoted in Heyde Trial, pp. 33–36.

9. Walter Schultze, quoted in Klee, *"Euthanasie"* [3], p. 47.

10. Ibid., pp. 76–77, 163–65.

11. Erwin Leiser, *Nazi Cinema* (New York: Macmillan, 1974 [1968]), pp. 89–94, 143–45. On Unger, see Klee, *"Euthanasie"* [3], pp. 79, 342–43. Helmut Unger's novel was *Sendung und Gewissen* (Berlin: Brunnen Verlag, 1935).

12. Leiser, *Cinema* [11], pp. 146–49; Heinz Höhne, *The Order of the Death's Head: The Story of Hitler's S.S.* (New York: Coward-McCann, 1969 [1966]), pp. 423–27.

13. Testimony of Professor Böhm, 12 July 1961, Heyde Trial, pp. 41–42. Also named in the 1936 discussions were Dr. Walter Gross of the Office of Racial Politics and Minister-Director Walter Schultze.

14. Testimony of Otto Mauthe, 20 December 1961, Heyde Trial, pp. 42–43.

15. Brandt testimony, 4 February 1947, *Nuremberg Medical Case,* transcript, pp. 2409–10, and vol. I, p. 894; also in Heyde Trial, pp. 51–52. See also Lothar Gruchmann, "Euthanasie und Justiz im Dritten Reich," *Vierteljahrshefte für Zeitgeschichte* 20 (1972):238–39, on general euthanasia requests involving the incurably ill during 1938–39; in the absence of a law they were directed to Hitler's Chancellery.

16. Brandt testimony [15]. See also Hans Hefelmann's account, 31 August and 7–14 November 1960, Heyde Trial, pp. 48–51, 53–54; and Gruchmann, "Euthanasie und Justiz" [15], pp. 240–41.

17. Brandt transcript [15], p. 2410.

18. Heyde Trial, pp. 53–54.

19. Secret order, 18 August 1939, "re: duty to report malformed, etc. newborns," quoted fully in Klee, *"Euthanasie"* [3], pp. 80–81.

20. Heyde Trial, pp. 53–54.

21. Ibid., pp. 66–72.

22. Hefelmann testimony, 7–14 November 1960, Heyde Trial, p. 66.

23. On the questionnaires and experts, see Heyde Trial, pp. 74–177.

24. Hefelmann testimony, 7–9 December 1960, Heyde Trial, p. 149.

25. Heyde Trial, p. 117.

26. Ibid., pp. 116–77; the centers are listed on pp. 128–31.

27. Heinze testimony, 27 September 1961, Heyde Trial, pp. 150–51.

28. Sample letter to parents, 30 September 1941, Heyde Trial, p. 111; see pp. 100–116.

29. Testimony of Dr. Valentin Faltlhauser, 22–23 April 1948; and Nurse Mina Wörle, 7 May 1948 (Kaufbeuren asylum), Heyde Trial, pp. 143–47.

30. Hefelmann testimony, 7–14 November 1960, Heyde Trial, p. 123.

31. On the broadening of categories, see Heyde Trial, pp. 82–90, 131–34.

32. Ibid., pp. 165–72.

33. Lehner testimony, cited in Klee, *"Euthanasie"* [3], pp. 88–89.

34. Lammers testimony, 7 February 1947, *Nuremberg Medical Case,* transcript, pp. 2687–88; Heyde Trial, pp. 178–79, dates the events "July at the latest."

35. Heyde Trial, p. 203; see pp. 201–6. See also Doc. 630–PS, *Nuremberg Medical Case,* vol. I, p. 893; Brandt testimony, 4 February 1947, transcript, pp. 2407–8.

36. Brandt testimony [35], p. 2407.

37. Hermann Pfannmüller, quoted in Gerhard Schmidt, *Selektion in der Heilanstalt 1939–1945* (Stuttgart: Evangelisches Verlagsanstalt, 1965), p. 34; see pp. 34–35.

38. Alice Platen-Hallermund, *Die Tötung Geisteskranker in Deutschland* (Frankfurt/M.: Verlag der Frankfurter Hefte, 1948), p. 18; Gruchmann, "Euthanasie" [15], p. 241.

39. Heyde Trial, p. 180.

40. Hefelmann testimony, 31 August 1960, in ibid., pp. 187–90, 319–20; Klee, *"Euthanasie"* [3], p. 83.

41. Gruchmann, "Euthanasie und Justiz" [15], pp. 277–78.

42. Mennecke testimony, 2 December 1946, Heyde Trial, pp. 307–13.

43. Dr. Walter Schmidt, quoted in Alexander Mitscherlich and Fred Mielke, *Doctors of Infamy: The Story of the Nazi Medical Crimes* (New York: Henry Schuman, 1949 [1947]), p. 94.

44. Mennecke testimony, 2 December 1946, Heyde Trial, p. 313. See also Heyde Trial, pp. 196, on secrecy; pp. 197, 313, on de Crinis; and passim, pp. 193–201, 307–13.

45. Professor Dr. Kranz in *NS-Volksdienst,* quoted in Pastor Paul Braune's protest against "euthanasia," Heyde Trial, p. 496.

46. On the RAG as camouflage, see Heyde Trial, pp. 226–32; on the questionnaires, see Heyde Trial, pp. 207–24.

47. Ewald testimony, 24 March 1960, Heyde Trial, pp. 215–16.

48. Mennecke testimony on a fall 1940 Tiergarten meeting, 2 December 1946, Heyde Trial, pp. 312, 318; see pp. 224, 343–46.

49. Heyde Trial, pp. 324–32; see pp. 321–23, 333, on similar actions.

50. Ibid., pp. 217–21, 346–49.

51. Ibid., pp. 350–58.

52. Ibid., pp. 372–76.

53. Ibid., pp. 376–78, 407–9.

54. Testimony by August Becker, 21 April 1960, Heyde Trial, p. 295.

55. Heyde Trial, p. 380.

56. Heyde testimony, 12 October–22 December 1961, Heyde Trial, pp. 292–93.

57. Becker testimony, 21 April 1960, Heyde Trial, pp. 293–95.

58. Brandt testimony (English translation), Nuremberg, 1 October 1945 (National Archives).

59. Heyde Trial, pp. 388–89, 255–56, 268–69, 306 (respectively); Helmut Ehrhardt, *Euthanasie und die Vernichtung "lebensunwerten" Lebens* (Stuttgart: Ferdinand Enke Verlag, 1965), p. 35; Klee, *"Euthanasie"* [3], pp. 226–32. For a discussion of the age of members and leaders of the Nazi party, see Michael Kater, *The Nazi Party: A Social Profile of Members and Leaders, 1919–1945* (Cambridge, Mass.: Harvard University Press, 1983), pp. 139–48.

60. Ullrich testimony, 4–27 September 1961, Heyde Trial, p. 388.

61. Testimony of Hans Bodo Gorgass, 15 August 1960, Heyde Trial, pp. 383–84.

62. Heyde Trial, pp. 447–48.

63. Testimony of Paul Reuter, 14–15 March 1946, Heyde Trial, p. 391.

64. Trial commentary, Heyde Trial, p. 391.

65. Ernst Klee, "Tot und seziert: Bilder eines Albums und die Schrecken der Euthanasie," *Die Zeit,* 5 October 1984.

66. Testimony of Benedikt Härtls, 9 March 1946, Heyde Trial, p. 394.

67. Heyde Trial, pp. 396–99; see also pp. 399–406.

68. Klee, "Tot und seziert" [65], pp. 409–16; Klee, *"Euthanasie"* [3], p. 344.

69. Gerhard Bohne testimony, 10 September 1959, Heyde Trial, p. 417.

70. Mitscherlich and Mielke, *Doctors* [43], p. 105; Florian Zehethofer, "Das Euthanasieproblem im Dritten Reich am Beispiel Schloss Hartheim (1938–1945)," *Oberösterreichische Heimatsblätter* 32 (1978):55; Heyde Trial, pp. 360–68.

71. Klee, *"Euthanasie"* [3], pp. 343–44.

72. On the "euthanasia" project's public relations efforts, see Klee, *"Euthanasie"* [3], pp. 76–77, 163–65, 342–44.

73. Wolfgang Scheffler, *Judenverfolgung im Dritten Reich 1933–1945* (Berlin: Colloquium Verlag, 1960), p. 35.

74. On the formulation of the Final Solution, see Lucy S. Dawidowicz, *The War Against the Jews, 1933–1945* (New York: Holt, Rinehart & Winston, 1975), pp. 70–128; Gerald Fleming, *Hitler and the Final Solution* (Berkeley: University of California Press, 1984 [1982]); Raul Hilberg, *The Destruction of the European Jews* (Chicago: Quadrangle, 1967 [1961]), pp. 257–66.

75. Heyde Trial commentary, p. 451.
76. Klee, *"Euthanasie"* [3], pp. 258–60.
77. Hermann Pfannmüller, quoted in Schmidt, *Selektion* [37], p. 68.
78. Ibid., p. 67.
79. Klee, *"Euthanasie"* [3], pp. 261–63.
80. On Lublin, see Hilberg, *Destruction* [74], pp. 136–38, 292.
81. Klee, *"Euthanasie"* [3], pp. 260–61; Fleming, *Final Solution* [74], pp. 26–27. In personal correspondence (9 November 1985), Ernst Klee confirmed ("with great probability") the fictional nature of the Chelm/Cholm address. Henry Friedlander (letter of 16 December 1985) has also given me information on this question.
82. Klee, *"Euthanasie"* [3], pp. 95–98, 112–14, 367–79; Hilberg, *Destruction* [74], pp. 177–256.
83. Klee, *"Euthanasie"* [3], pp. 401–16.
84. Ibid., pp. 367–79; Christopher R. Browning, *Fateful Months: Essays on the Emergence of the Final Solution* (New York: Holmes & Meier, 1985), chap. 1.

Chapter 3. Resistance to Direct Medical Killing

1. Helmut Ehrhardt, *Euthanasie und Vernichtung "lebensunwerten" Lebens* (Stuttgart: Ferdinand Enke Verlag, 1965), p. 37. Ehrhardt may have exaggerated the extent of this silent resistance, but it clearly existed.
2. Gerhard Schmidt, *Selektion in der Heilanstalt 1939–1945* (Stuttgart: Evangelisches Verlagswerk, 1965), pp. 54–55.
3. L. Schlaich to Hans Frank, 6 September 1940 (copy to Lammers), *Nuremberg Medical Case*, vol. I, pp. 854–55.
4. Geoffrey Cocks, *Psychotherapy in the Third Reich: The Göring Institute* (New York: Oxford University Press, 1985), p. 172; Eberhard Bethge, *Dietrich Bonhoeffer: Man of Vision, Man of Courage* (New York: Harper & Row, 1970 [1967]), pp. 592–93.
5. Bethge, *Bonhoeffer* [4], p. 212; see Cocks, *Psychotherapy* [4], pp. 105–6.
6. Bethge, *Bonhoeffer* [4], p. 212.
7. Ewald testimony, 3 June 1960, Heyde Trial, pp. 553–56. See Ernst Klee, *"Euthanasie" im NS-Staat: Die "Vernichtung lebensunwerten Lebens"* (Frankfurt/M.: S. Fischer, 1983), pp. 224, 274–75.
8. Ewald testimony [7], pp. 554–56.
9. See Cocks, *Psychotherapy* [4]. See also Rose Spiegel, "Survival, Psychoanalysis and the Third Reich," *Journal of the American Academy of Psychoanalysis* 13 (1985): 521–36; Arthur H. Finer, "Psychoanalysis During the Nazi Regime," *Journal of the American Academy of Psychoanalysis* 13 (1985):537–50; Rose Spiegel, G. Chrazanowsky, and Arthur H. Finer, "On Psychoanalysis and the Third Reich," *Contemporary Psychoanalysis* 11 (1975):477–510.
10. Ewald memorandum (copy, n.d.), Heyde Trial, pp. 554–61.
11. Ibid., pp. 561–64.
12. Ibid., pp. 564–65. For the resultant correspondence, see pp. 567–72.
13. "Gutachten über . . . Dr. Ewald" (Hochschulgruppe Göttingen des NSD-Dozentenbundes), 9 January 1939 (BDC: Ewald).
14. Ibid. See also Kreisleiter Göttingen to Gauleitung South Hanover-Braunschweig, 8 March 1939 (BDC: Ewald).
15. Kreisleiter to Gauleitung [14].
16. Kreisleiter Göttingen to Schatzrat Friese (Hanover), 21 March 1938 (BDC: Ewald).
17. Ortsgruppenleiter Mengershausen to Kreisleiter Dr. Gengler (Göttingen), 23 September 1938; Kreisleiter Göttingen to Ewald, 6 October 1938; Ewald to Kreisleitung Göttingen, 8 October 1938 (BDC: Ewald).
18. Ewald to Heyde and Conti, 21 August 1940 (BDC: Ewald).
19. Roger Manvell and Heinrich Fraenkel, *The Canaris Conspiracy: The Secret Resistance to*

Hitler in the German Army (New York: David McKay, 1969), p. 33; Peter Hoffmann, *The History of the German Resistance, 1933–1945* (Cambridge, Mass.: MIT Press, 1977), p. 91.

20. Klee, *"Euthanasie"* [7], p. 223.

21. For biographical information on Ewald, see Klee, *"Euthanasie"* [7], pp. 216–17.

22. Fredric Wertham, *A Sign for Cain: An Exploration of Human Violence* (New York: Macmillan, 1966), pp. 178–79.

23. Eyewitness testimony by chief nurse, 5 June 1946; testimony (second-hand through Götz) of business manager, 6 June 1946, Heyde Trial, pp. 336–39.

24. Boeckh to Reich Interior Minister, 7 November 1940, Heyde Trial, pp. 328–32. See Klee, *"Euthanasie"* [7], pp. 244–47.

25. Klee, *"Euthanasie"* [7], pp. 247–48.

26. Ibid., pp. 216–19.

27. Schmidt, *Selektion* [2], pp. 82–93.

28. Lothar Kreyssig to Justice Minister Gürtner, 8 July 1940, quoted in Klee, *"Euthanasie"* [7], p. 209. See Philippe Aziz, *Doctors of Death* (Geneva: Ferni Publishers, 1976), vol. IV, p. 107.

29. Von Löwis, quoted in Aziz, *Doctors of Death* [28], pp. 100–104; see also p. 116 on Himmler's attitudes.

30. Secret report of Absberg Ortsgruppenleiter, 24 January 1941; Gendarmerieposten Absberg to Landrat Gunzenhausen, 24 February 1941; secret report of Gaustabsamt Sel/Pf. to SS-Sturmbahnführer Friedrich (Nuremberg), copy to Hefelmann, 1 March 1941, Heyde Trial, pp. 360–68.

31. Church President Ernst Wilm's expert statement to Frankfurt court on Protestant reactions to "euthanasia," 3 January 1963, Generalstaatsanwaltschaft Frankfurt/M.: JS 20/61, vol. I, 3 (44); Klee, *"Euthanasie"* [7], p. 284.

32. Klee, *"Euthanasie"* [7], pp. 201–2; see pp. 35, 48, 62, 201–5.

33. Ibid., pp. 201–16, 278–89, 320–26, 421–24. See also Annaliese Hochmuth, "Der Widerstand Bethels gegen die Tötung psychisch Kranker, eine Dokumentation," in Klaus Dörner et al., eds., *Der Krieg gegen die psychisch Kranken: Nach "Holocaust": Erkennen—Trauern —Begegnen* (Rehburg-Loccum: Psychiatrie-Verlag, 1980), pp. 160–62. (The chronology in Hochmuth is not altogether clear.)

34. Klee, *"Euthanasie"* [7], p. 34.

35. Ibid., p. 39.

36. Ibid., pp. 210–11.

37. Braune, "Denkschrift, *Betrifft:* Planwirtschaftliche Verlegung von Insassen der Heil- und Pflegeanstalten" ("Vertraulich"), 9 July 1940, Heyde Trial, pp. 496–501.

38. Ibid., pp. 506–7.

39. Ibid., pp. 510–12.

40. Klee, *"Euthanasie"* [7], p. 340–41, 355; Lothar Gruchmann, "Euthanasie und Justiz im Dritten Reich," *Vierteljahrshefte für Zeitgeschichte* 20 (1972): 244.

41. Braune, "Denkschrift" [37], pp. 513–14.

42. Klee, *"Euthanasie"* [7], pp. 221–23.

43. Ibid., pp. 337–38.

44. Aziz, *Doctors of Death* [28], vol. IV, pp. 92–95. See Klee, *"Euthanasie"* [7], pp. 334–35.

45. Aziz, *Doctors of Death* [28], vol. IV, pp. 94–95. Galen's sermon of 3 August 1941 is printed in Dörner, ed., *Krieg* [33], pp. 112–24; see pp. 124–28.

46. Aziz, *Doctors of Death* [28], vol. IV, pp. 95–96.

47. Ibid., p. 97.

48. Klee, *"Euthanasie"* [7], p. 335.

49. Ibid., pp. 335–37; Raul Hilberg, *The Destruction of the European Jews* (Chicago: Quadrangle, 1967 [1961]), pp. 299–300.

50. Aziz, *Doctors of Death* [28], vol. IV, pp. 98–99.

51. Himmler to Brack and Bouhler, 19 December 1940, Heyde Trial, pp. 577–78. Himmler was responding to the letter by von Löwis [29].

52. Hefelmann testimony, 6–15 September 1960, Heyde Trial, pp. 681–82; see also p. 680.

53. Klee, *"Euthanasie"* [7], p. 340.
54. Ibid., p. 341.

Chapter 4. "Wild Euthanasia": The Doctors Take Over

1. Ernst Klee, *"Euthanasie" im NS-Staat: Die "Vernichtung lebensunwerten Lebens"* (Frankfurt/M.: S. Fischer, 1983), p. 440.
2. Friedrich Mennecke, quoted in Alexander Mitscherlich and Fred Mielke, *Doctors of Infamy: The Story of the Nazi Medical Crimes* (New York: Henry Schuman, 1949), p. 116.
3. See the case of Emma E. in Gerhard Schmidt, *Selektion in der Heilanstalt 1939–1945* (Stuttgart: Evangelisches Verlagswerk, 1965), pp. 121–24.
4. Heyde Trial, pp. 83–86; Klee, *"Euthanasie"* [1], pp. 379–89.
5. Mitscherlich and Mielke, *Doctors* [2], p. 116.
6. Klee, *"Euthanasie"* [1], pp. 291–93, 341–42, 351; Eugen Kogon et al., *Nationalsozialistische Massentötungen durch Giftgas: Eine Dokumentation* (Frankfurt/M.: S. Fischer, 1983), p. 59.
7. Klee, *"Euthanasie"* [1], pp. 329–30.
8. Ibid., pp. 429–30.
9. Ibid.
10. Schmidt, *Selektion* [3], pp. 129–31.
11. Ibid., pp. 131–32.
12. Klee, *"Euthanasie"* [1], p. 430.
13. Schmidt, *Selektion* [3], pp. 130–32.
14. Ibid., pp. 132–45.
15. Testimony of Dr. Hans Gorgass at Hadamar Trial, Frankfurt, February–March, 1947 (4 KLs 7/47, Landgericht Frankfurt). This was the second trial of Hadamar personnel, held in a German court rather than under British occupation authority, and involving Gorgass as well as Wahlmann.
16. Klee, *"Euthanasie"* [1], p. 336.
17. Ibid., p. 170.
18. *Hadamar Trial,* especially pp. 162–63, 174–87.
19. Weimar testimony in 1947 Hadamar Trial [15].
20. Wahlmann testimony, 12 October 1945, *Hadamar Trial,* pp. 162–63.
21. Testimony of Heinrich Ruoff, 12 October 1945, *Hadamar Trial,* p. 176.
22. Testimony of Irmgard Huber, 11 October 1945, *Hadamar Trial,* p. 119.
23. Wahlmann testimony, 12 October 1945, *Hadamar Trial,* p. 163; see pp. 162, 247.
24. Ibid., p. 167.
25. Klee, *"Euthanasie"* [1], pp. 446–54.

Chapter 5. Participants

1. Michael H. Kater, "Medizinische Fakultäten und Medizinstudenten: Eine Skizze," in Fridolf Kudlien, ed., *Ärzte im Nationalsozialismus* (Cologne: Kiepenheuer & Witsch, 1985), p. 123.
2. See Hans Buchheim, "Command and Compliance," in Helmut Krausnick et al., *Anatomy of the SS State* (New York: Walker, 1968 [1965]), p. 373.
3. Sigmund Freud, *Standard Edition of the Works of Sigmund Freud,* James Strachey, ed. (London: Hogarth Press, 1955 [1923]), vol. XIV, p. 27n.
4. Philippe Aziz, *Doctors of Death* (Geneva: Ferni Publishers, 1976), vol. IV, p. 26.
5. Ibid., pp. 14, 17.
6. On Morell, ibid., pp. 48–52; Alan Bullock, *Hitler: A Study in Tyranny* (rev. ed.; New York: Harper & Row, 1962), pp. 718, 766; and Albert Speer, *Inside the Third Reich: Memoirs* (New York: Macmillan, 1970), pp. 104–5.

7. Aziz, *Doctors of Death* [4], vol. I, p. 33.

8. See Speer, *Inside* [6], pp. 330–32, 465–66, 576–77.

9. Aziz, *Doctors of Death* [4], vol. IV, p. 14. Aziz claims to have interviewed a "Hans Kressler" in 1973. Contemporary documents referred to a Knauer infant.

10. See Ernst Klee, *"Euthanasie" im NS-Staat: Die "Vernichtung lebensunwerten Lebens"* (Frankfurt/M.: S. Fischer, 1983), pp. 321–28, 424.

11. "Affidavit of Eduard Woermann, 18 January 1947, concerning discussions of Karl Brandt and Pastor Bodelschwingh on Euthanasia," *Nuremberg Medical Case*, vol. I, p. 873.

12. François Bayle, *Croix gammée contre caducée: Les expériences humaines en Allemagne pendant la deuxième guerre mondiale* (Neustadt [Palatinat]: Commission Scientifique Française des Crimes de Guerre, 1950), pp. 62–64.

13. Aziz, *Doctors of Death* [4], vol. I, p. 16.

14. Ibid., p. 248.

15. Ibid., p. 252.

16. Heyde, "Lebenslauf," (autobiography), 1 January 1939, Heyde Trial, pp. 5–6; see also pp. 1–4. On Heyde's intelligence work, see Walter Schellenberg, *The Labyrinth: Memoirs* (New York: Harper, 1956), pp. 87, 91–92.

17. Schellenberg, *Labyrinth* [16], p. 92.

18. Klee, *"Euthanasie"* [10], p. 414.

19. Pfannmüller, quoted in Gerhard Schmidt, *Selektion in der Heilanstalt 1939–1945* (Stuttgart: Evangelisches Verlagsanstalt, 1965), p. 18.

20. Pfannmüller testimony, 27–28 June 1960, Heyde Trial, p. 224; Hermann Langbein, *Im Namen des deutschen Volkes: Zwischenbilanz der Prozesse wegen national-sozialistischen Verbrechen* (Vienna: Europa Verlag, 1963), pp. 73, 170–71.

21. Geoffrey Cocks, *Psychotherapy in the Third Reich: The Göring Institute* (New York: Oxford University Press, 1985), p. 97.

22. Ibid., pp. 171–74. Stabsführer des Sicherheitshauptamtes Taubert to Reichsführer-SS, 6 February 1936; Oberführer Glatzel to SS-Personelkanzlei, 14 February 1939 (BDC: de Crinis). On the camouflaging of SS members involved in T4, see the testimony of Dr. Werner Kirchert, 2 May 1960, Heyde Trial, pp. 227–29. On the intelligence mission, see Schellenberg, *Labyrinth* [16], pp. 67–73.

23. Schellenberg, *Labyrinth* [16], pp. 338, 387–88; Cocks, *Psychotherapy* [21], pp. 214–15; Gerhard Jaeckel, *Die Charité: Die Geschichte des berühmtesten deutschen Krankenhauses* (Bayreuth: Hestia, 1963), pp. 377–85.

24. Cocks, *Psychotherapy* [21], p. 286 n. 93.

25. Jaeckel, *Charité* [23], p. 385.

26. "Walter Ritter von Baeyer," in *Psychiatrie in Selbstdarstellungen,* ed. Ludwig J. Pongratz (Berne, Stuttgart and Vienna: Hans Haber, 1977), p. 16; Klee, *"Euthanasie"* [10], p. 203.

27. Klaus Dörner, "Nationalsozialismus und Lebensvernichtung," *Vierteljahrshefte für Zeitgeschichte* 152 (1967):134.

28. "Baeyer" [26], p. 16; personal communication.

29. Klee, *"Euthanasie"* [10], pp. 396–401; Benno Müller-Hill, *Tödliche Wissenschaft: Die Aussonderung von Juden, Zigeunern und Geisteskranken 1933–1945* (Reinbek b. Hamburg: Rowohlt, 1983), pp. 69–71, 169–74; documents on Schmidt's research in BDC: Schmidt. On the use of T4 brains, see also Leo Alexander, "Neuropathology and Neurophysiology, Including Electroencephalography, in Wartime Germany," Combined Intelligence Objectives Sub-Committee, Item 24, Medical (1945), pp. 14–22.

30. Heyde Trial, pp. 339–411.

31. Ibid., pp. 396–405.

32. Eberl to Lonauer, 16 July 1940, Heyde Trial, pp. 404–5.

33. Ibid., pp. 466–67.

34. Eberl to Reich Committee, 10 September 1940, Heyde Trial, p. 483. See Klee, *"Euthanasie"* [10], p. 397, quoting Brandt on the "flight" of good physicians from psychiatry.

35. Ibid., pp. 376–77; Adalbert Rückerl, ed., *NS-Vernichtungslager im Spiegel deutscher Strafprozesse* (Munich: DTV, 1977), pp. 208–9, 295; Eugen Kogon et al., *Nationalsozialistische*

Massentötungen durch Giftgas: Eine Dokumentation (Frankfurt/M.: S. Fischer, 1983), pp. 162, 180–82.

36. George L. Mosse, *Toward the Final Solution: A History of European Racism* (New York: Harper & Row, 1978), p. 87.

37. Daniel Gasman, *The Scientific Origins of National Socialism: Social Darwinism in Ernst Haeckel and the German Monist League* (New York: Elsevier, 1971), p. 160. See George L. Mosse, *The Crisis of German Ideology: Intellectual Origins of the Third Reich* (New York: Grosset & Dunlap, 1964), p. 4.

38. See Robert G. L. Waite, *Vanguard of Nazism: The Free Corps Movement in Postwar Germany, 1918–1923* (Cambridge, Mass.: Harvard University Press, 1952), pp. 26–28. Quoted phrase is from a 1939 "semiofficial history" of German noncommissioned officers by a Count von Ledebur.

39. Ibid., p. 281.

40. Jeffrey Herf, "Reactionary Modernism: The Reconciliation of Technology and Unreason in Weimar Germany and the Third Reich" (unpublished dissertation, Brandeis University, 1980), pp. 74–88; published with some revisions as *Reactionary Modernism: Technology, Culture and Politics in Weimar and the Third Reich* (Cambridge: Cambridge University Press, 1985), p. 63.

41. Mosse, *Final Solution* [36], p. 106.

42. Herf, "Reactionary Modernism" [40], pp. 101–19.

43. See Herf, *Reactionary Modernism* [40], pp. 42–43.

44. Ibid., pp. 101–2, 107.

45. Robert Wistrich, *Who's Who in Nazi Germany* (New York: Macmillan, 1982), p. 329.

46. Theodore N. Kaufman, *Germany Must Perish!* (Newark: Argyle Press, 1941).

47. Leonard L. Heston and Renate Heston, *The Medical Casebook of Adolf Hitler* (New York: Stein & Day, 1982), pp. 113–15, 73–103, suggest amphetamine toxicity; Dr. F. C. Redlich questions this diagnosis (personal communication, 1984).

48. George L. Mosse, "Death, Time and History," *Masses and Man: Nationalist and Fascist Perceptions of Reality* (New York: Fertig, 1980), p. 73.

49. Frank Rector, *The Nazi Extermination of Homosexuals* (New York: Stein & Day, 1981).

50. Rolf Hochhuth, *A German Love Story* (Boston: Little, Brown, 1980 [1978]), pp. 143–44.

Chapter 6. Bringing "Euthanasia" to the Camps: Action Special Treatment 14f13

1. Mennecke testimony, 17 January 1947, *Nuremberg Medical Case*, vol. I, p. 832. Mennecke claimed that these early visits were not part of 14f13, but rather were general examinations of the insane.

2. Amnon Amir, "Euthanasia in Nazi Germany" (unpublished dissertation, State University of New York, Albany, 1977), pp. 297–301.

3. Ibid., p. 300; Hans-Günther Seraphim, expert testimony on "Special Treatment" and 14f13 (10 May 1960), *Generalstaatsanwaltschaft* Frankfurt/M., JS 20/61, vol. I/3 (44).

4. Eugen Kogon et al., *Nationalsozialistische Massentötungen durch Giftgas: Eine Dokumentation* (Frankfurt/M.: S. Fischer, 1983), p. 66.

5. Nitsche testimony, 2 May 1947, Heyde Trial, p. 611.

6. Ernst Klee, *"Euthanasie" im NS-Staat: Die "Vernichtung lebensunwerten Lebens"* (Frankfurt/M.: S. Fischer, 1983), pp. 345–47; Kogon, *Massentötungen* [4], pp. 66–71; Heyde Trial, pp. 606–12.

7. Klee, *"Euthanasie"* [6], pp. 349–50.

8. Friedrich Mennecke to his wife, 24 November 1941, Heyde Trial, p. 639. See also Amir, "Euthanasia" [2], pp. 305–6.

9. Heyde Trial, pp. 646–48; Klee, *"Euthanasie"* [6], p. 348, reproduces one of these photos with handwritten diagnosis.

10. Klaus Dörner, "Nationalsozialismus und Lebensvernichtung," *Vierteljahrshefte für Zeitgeschichte* 15 (1967):145.

11. Seraphim, "Special Treatment" [3]; Heyde Trial, pp. 604–9.

12. Seraphim, "Special Treatment" [3].

13. Heyde Trial, pp. 603–12.

14. Amir, "Euthanasia" [2], pp. 305–307.

15. Seraphim, "Special Treatment" [3].

16. Langbein, *Menschen in Auschwitz* (Vienna: Europaverlag, 1972), p. 114.

17. Klee, *"Euthanasie"* [6], pp. 352–55; Kogon, *Massentötungen* [4], pp. 77–78.

18. Amir, "Euthanasia" [2], p. 305.

19. See, for example, Mennecke's letter of 25 November 1941 in Heyde Trial, p. 623. Mennecke's letters to his wife are found in Heyde Trial, pp. 613–46, and are published in Hermann Langbein, *Wir haben es getan: Selbstporträts in Tagebüchern und Briefen, 1939–1945* (Vienna: Europaverlag, 1964), pp. 24–30.

20. Morgen's 1944 report on camp corruption, quoted in Seraphim, "Special Treatment" [3].

21. Kogon, *Massentötungen* [4], pp. 76–77; Klee, *"Euthanasie"* [6], pp. 354–55.

22. SS documents, especially "Lebenslauf" (autobiography), 13 June 1937 (BDC: Mennecke).

23. Klee, *"Euthanasie"* [6], pp. 120–21.

24. Mennecke to investigative judge, 2 November 1946, in Langbein, *Wir haben* [19], p. 19.

25. The photo, without Steinmeyer, is reprinted in Klee, *"Euthanasie"* [6], p. 226. Mennecke to Director of Lohr hospital, 20 October 1940, in Langbein, *Wir haben* [19], p. 20.

26. Langbein, *Wir haben* [19], pp. 38–39.

27. Klee, *"Euthanasie"* [6], pp. 340–41, 355; Lothar Gruchmann, "Euthanasie und Justiz im Dritten Reich," *Vierteljahrshefte für Zeitgeschichte* 20 (1972):244.

28. Florian Zehethofer, "Das Euthanasieproblem im Dritten Reich am Beispiel Schloss Hartheim (1938–1945)," *Oberösterreichische Heimatsblätter* 32 (1978):58–60.

29. Klee, *"Euthanasie"* [6], pp. 372–73.

30. On the transition from T4 to mass killing in the East, see Zehethofer, "Hartheim" [28], pp. 55–56; Christopher R. Browning, *Fateful Months: Essays on the Emergence of the Final Solution* (New York: Holmes & Meier, 1985), chaps. 1 and 3; Gitta Sereny, *Into That Darkness: From Mercy Killing to Mass Murder* (New York: McGraw Hill, 1974); Adalbert Rückerl, *NS-Vernichtungslager im Spiegel deutscher Strafprozesse* (Munich: DTV, 1977); Raul Hilberg *The Destruction of the European Jews*, rev. and definitive ed. (New York: Holmes & Meier, 1985), vol. III, pp. 872–73, 894–95; and the studies by Yves Ternon and Socrate Helman, *Le Massacre des aliénés: Des théoriciens nazis aux praticiéns SS* (Paris: Casterman, 1971); *Les Médicins allemands et le national-socialisme* (Paris: Casterman, 1973), and *Histoire médicin SS* (Paris: Casterman, 1970).

31. Konrad Lorenz, "Durch Domestikation verursachte Störungen arteigenen Verhaltens," in *Zeitschrift für angewandte Psychologie und Charakterkunde* (Journal of Applied Psychology and the Science of Character) 59 (1940): 66, 71.

32. Discussions with Raul Hilberg and Yehuda Bauer have greatly contributed to my understanding of this evolving mentality.

Introduction to Part II

1. Diary entry (5 September 1942) and testimony (Krakow, 18 August 1947), in "Kremers Tagebuch," *Hefte von Auschwitz* 13 (1971): 42, 107n.36. English in *KL Auschwitz Seen by the SS* (New York: Fertig, 1984), p. 215.

2. Ibid.; Antoni Kepínski, " 'Anus mundi,' " in *Anthology*, I, 2:2.

3. The discussion of these medical and nonmedical activities is based on interviews with Nazi doctors and with prisoner doctors, and on the following major sources: Rudolf Höss, *Commandant of Auschwitz: The Autobiography of Rudolf Hoess* (Cleveland: World, 1959) and "Die nichtärztliche Tätigkeit der SS-Ärzte im K.L. Auschwitz" ("The Nonmedical Activity of SS-Doctors in Auschwitz"), [photo of 1947 ms. (trial document)], in *Hefte von Auschwitz* 2 (1959):81–84; Bernd Naumann, *Auschwitz: A Report on the Proceedings Against Robert Karl Ludwig Mulka and Others Before the Court of Frankfurt* (New York: Pantheon, 1966 [1965]); Hermann Langbein, *Menschen in Auschwitz* (Vienna: Europaverlag, 1972) and *Der Auschwitz-Prozess: Eine Dokumentation*, 2 vols. (Frankfurt/M.: Europäische Verlagsanstalt, 1965), as well as the articles in the *Anthology* series (1971) and many of those in the journal *Hefte von Auschwitz* (from 1959 on), published by the Polish State Auschwitz Museum.

4. Majdanek bore some resemblance to Auschwitz regarding this policy but on a considerably smaller scale. See Adalbert Rückerl, *NS-Vernichtungslager im Spiegel deutscher Strafprozesse* (Munich: DTV, 1977), pp. 28–29; Josef Marszalek, *Majdanek* (Hamburg, 1982); Raul Hilberg, *The Destruction of the European Jews*, rev. and definitive ed. (New York: Holmes & Meier, 1985), vol. III, pp. 899, 1219.

5. Transcript of judgment in Frankfurt Auschwitz trial, 19–20 August 1965 (4 Ks 2/63), p. 74; Raul Hilberg, *The Destruction of the European Jews* (Chicago: Quadrangle, 1967 [1961]), pp. 150–51.

6. Jean-François Steiner, *Treblinka* (New York: Simon & Schuster, 1967 [1966]), p. 110.

Chapter 7. The Auschwitz Institution

1. See Hans Mommsen, "The Reichstag Fire and Its Political Consequences," in Hajo Holborn, ed., *Republic to Reich: The Making of the Nazi Revolution* (New York: Pantheon, 1972), pp. 129–222.

2. Martin Broszat, "The Concentration Camps 1933–45," in Helmut Krausnick et al., *Anatomy of the SS State* (New York: Walker, 1968 [1965]), p. 430; see pp. 400–420, 429–30.

3. Ibid., pp. 431–35 (on Eicke); Rudolf Höss, *Commandant of Auschwitz: The Autobiography of Rudolf Hoess* (Cleveland: World, 1959), pp. 83–94.

4. Broszat, "Camps" [2], pp. 450–52; Ota Kraus and Erich Kulka, *The Death Factory: Document on Auschwitz* (Oxford: Pergamon, 1966), pp. 36–40, 283; Tadeusz Iwaszko, "Die Häftlinge," in *Auschwitz: Geschichte und Wirklichkeit des Vernichtungslagers* (Reinbek bei Hamburg: Rowohlt Taschenbuch Verlag, 1980 [1978]), pp. 59–66; Wolken transcript, pp. 214–15; personal communication from Helen Tichauer (known as "Zippi aus der Schreibstube"), a former prisoner working in the Women's Camp Office at Auschwitz-Birkenau, responsible among others for the production and distribution of badges.

5. Broszat, "Camps" [2], pp. 426–27.

6. Eugen Kogon, *The Theory and Practice of Hell* (New York: Berkley Books, 1980 [1950]), pp. 142, 149.

7. Ibid., pp. 145–51.

8. Broszat, "Camps" [2], p. 430.

9. Kogon, *Theory and Practice* [6], p. 150.

10. Ibid., p. 146.

11. Benjamin B. Ferencz, *Less Than Slaves: Jewish Forced Labor and the Quest for Compensation* (Cambridge, Mass.: Harvard University Press, 1979).

12. Höss, *Commandant* [3], p. 83.

13. Broszat, "Camps" [2], p. 481; Raul Hilberg, *The Destruction of the European Jews* (Chicago: Quadrangle, 1967 [1961]), pp. 181–85.

14. Joseph Borkin, *The Crime and Punishment of I. G. Farben* (New York: Free Press, 1978), pp. 115–27.

15. Hilberg, *Destruction* [13], pp. 596–600.

16. Höss, *Commandant* [3], p. 146.

17. Hilberg, *Destruction* [13], p. 596.

18. Lucy S. Dawidowicz, *The War Against the Jews, 1933–1945* (New York: Holt, Rinehart & Winston, 1975), pp. 134–35; Hilberg, *Destruction* [13], pp. 555–74; Gerald Fleming, *Hitler and the Final Solution* (Berkeley: University of California Press, 1985 [1982]), pp. 24–25.

19. Höss, *Commandant* [3], pp. 205–6.

20. Ibid., p. 205; see Hilberg, *Destruction* [13], pp. 563–64.

21. Höss, *Commandant* [3], p. 206.

22. Hilberg, *Destruction* [13], p. 262; see also pp. 257–62.

23. Ibid., p. 265; see pp. 262–66.

24. For a useful discussion of the historiography of the Final Solution and Hitler's role in it, see Saul Friedländer's introduction to Fleming, *Final Solution* [18], pp. vii–xxxvi. Fleming argues that Hitler's order was implicit and known, though of course not written down. See also Christopher R. Browning, *Fateful Months: Essays on the Emergence of the Final Solution* (New York: Holmes & Meier, 1985), chap. 1.

25. Höss, *Commandant* [3], p. 163.

26. Ernst Klee, *"Euthanasie" im NS-Staat: Die "Vernichtung lebensunwerten Lebens"* (Frankfurt/M.: S. Fischer, 1983), pp. 368–69; Hilberg, *Destruction* [13], pp. 218–19.

27. Hilberg, *Destruction* [13], p. 646.

28. Heinz Höhne, *The Order of the Death's Head: The Story of Hitler's S.S.* (New York: Coward, McCann, 1970 [1967], p. 363.

29. Höss, *Commandant* [3], p. 206.

30. Ibid., pp. 206–7.

31. Ibid., pp. 207–8.

32. Ibid., p. 162; personal communication from Erich Kulka and Yehuda Bauer.

33. Ibid., p. 211.

34. Ibid., p. 221.

35. Hilberg, *Destruction* [13], pp. 567–71; Borkin, *Farben* [14], pp. 122–23.

36. Borkin, *Farben* [14], p. 123; Hilberg, *Destruction* [13], pp. 570–72.

37. Pierre Joffroy, *A Spy for God: The Ordeal of Kurt Gerstein* (New York: Harcourt, Brace, Jovanovich, 1971), pp. 207–9. See also Saul Friedländer, *Kurt Gerstein: The Ambiguity of Good* (New York: Alfred A. Knopf, 1969).

38. Hilberg gives an appreciably higher estimate of the amount of Zyklon-B used at Auschwitz in *Destruction* [13], pp. 570–71.

39. Höss, *Commandant* [3], pp. 162–63.

40. Ibid., p. 163.

41. Ibid.

42. Friedrich Entress, quoted in Hilberg, *Destruction* [13], p. 555.

Chapter 8. Selections on the Ramp

1. Wolken transcript, p. 125.

2. Ibid., p. 177.

3. YVAJ: 03/1202 (Yehuda Bauer).

4. Loet Van Duin (pseud.), "The Other Side of the Moon: The Life of a Young Physician from Holland in Auschwitz" (unpublished manuscript, 1980).

5. Mengele/Haifa: 7 (Joshua Rosenblum).

6. Ibid.

7. Konrad Morgen, quoted in Hermann Langbein, *Menschen in Auschwitz* (Vienna: Europaverlag, 1972), p. 336.

8. Rosenblum transcript [5].

9. Ibid.

10. Raul Hilberg, *The Destruction of the European Jews* (Chicago: Quadrangle, 1967 [1961]), p. 629.

11. Langbein, *Menschen* [7], pp. 420–21.

12. Rudolf Höss, *Commandant of Auschwitz: The Autobiography of Rudolf Hoess* (Cleveland: World, 1959), p. 171.

13. Ibid., p. 212.

14. Ibid., pp. 212–13; see pp. 176–79.

15. Hermann Langbein, quoted in Bernd Naumann, *Auschwitz: A Report on the Proceedings Against Robert Karl Ludwig Mulka and Others Before the Court at Frankfurt* (New York: Praeger, 1966 [1965]), pp. 102–3.

16. "Kremers Tagebuch," *Hefte von Auschwitz* 13 (1971): 41 (diary entry, 2 September 1942); also in *KL Auschwitz Seen By the SS* (New York: Fertig, 1984), p. 214.

Chapter 9. Selections in the Camp

1. F. K. Kaul, *Ärzte in Auschwitz* ([E.] Berlin: VEB Verlag Volk und Gesundheit, 1968), pp. 160–61.

2. See Raul Hilberg, *The Destruction of the European Jews* (Chicago: Quadrangle, 1967 [1961]), pp. 557, 586–88.

3. Wolken transcript, p. 38.

4. Ibid., p. 228.

5. Ibid., pp. 265–66; also P IIIh Auschwitz 562 (Wiener Library, London).

6. Mengele/Haifa: 25 (Magdalena Wertesz).

7. Wolken transcript, p. 229.

8. Filip Müller, *Sonderkommando: Three Years in the Gas Chambers at Auschwitz* (London: Routledge & Kegan Paul, 1979), pp. 108–9, 115–16.

9. Ibid., p. 116.

10. Wladyslaw Fejkiel, "Health Service in the Auschwitz I Concentration Camp/Main Camp," *Anthology* II, 1:5–8.

11. Ibid., p. 15.

12. Joseph Borkin, *The Crime and Punishment of I. G. Farben* (New York: Free Press, 1978), pp. 117–19, 124.

13. Ibid., p. 126.

14. Benjamin B. Ferencz, *Less Than Slaves: Jewish Forced Labor and the Quest for Compensation* (Cambridge, Mass.: Harvard University Press, 1979), p. 22.

15. Borkin, *Farben* [12], pp. 124–25.

16. Farben-Auschwitz weekly report, cited in Borkin, *Farben* [12], p. 119.

17. Kaul, *Ärzte* [1], pp. 160–61.

18. *Témoinages Strasbourgeois: De l'Université aux camps de concentration* (Paris: Les Belles Lettres, 1954 [1947]), p. 463.

19. Judgment against Josef Klehr in Auschwitz Trial transcript, 19–20 August 1965 (4 Ks 2/63), pp. 584–86.

20. Hermann Langbein, *Der Auschwitz-Prozess: Eine Dokumentation* (Frankfurt/M.: Europäische Verlagsanstalt, 1965), pp. 583–90.

21. YVAJ: P IIIh Auschwitz 126 (Dr. Lucie Adelsberger).

22. Ibid.

Chapter 10. Socialization to Killing

1. Hermann Langbein, *Der Auschwitz-Prozess: Eine Dokumentation* (Frankfurt/M.: Europäische Verlagsanstalt, 1965), vol. I, p. 144.

2. Hermann Langbein, *Menschen in Auschwitz* (Vienna: Europaverlag, 1972), p. 377; see pp. 406–10.

3. Bernd Naumann, *Auschwitz: A Report on the Proceedings Against Robert Karl Ludwig Mulka and Others Before the Court at Frankfurt* (New York: Pantheon, 1966 [1965]), p. 62.

4. Ibid., pp. 63–66; Langbein, *Menschen* [2], pp. 402–3.

5. Langbein, *Menschen* [2], pp. 460–63; Raul Hilberg, *The Destruction of the European Jews* (Chicago: Quadrangle, 1967 [1961]), pp. 579–80.

6. Fritz Stern, *Gold and Iron: Bismarck, Bleichröder and the Building of the German Empire* (New York: Alfred A. Knopf, 1977), p. 512.

7. Deposition by Miklos Nyiszli, 28 July 1945 before the Budapest Commission for the welfare of deported Hungarian Jews.

8. Olga Lengyel, *Five Chimneys: The Story of Auschwitz* (Chicago: Ziff-Davis, 1947), p. 62.

Chapter 11. Prisoner Doctors: The Agony of Selections

1. Désiré Haffner, "Pathological Aspects of the Concentration Camp at Auschwitz-Birkenau" (Tours: Imprimerie Union Coopérative, 1946 mimeo), p. 21.

2. Loet Van Duin (pseud.), "The Other Side of the Moon: The Life of a Young Physician from Holland in Auschwitz" (unpublished ms., 1980).

3. Ibid.

4. Ibid.

5. Elie A. Cohen, *The Abyss: A Confession* (New York: W. W. Norton, 1973 [1971]), pp. 88–89.

6. Wolken transcript, p. 126.

7. Olga Lengyel, *Five Chimneys: The Story of Auschwitz* (Chicago: Ziff-Davis, 1947), pp. 99–101.

8. Cohen, *Abyss* [5], p. 100.

Chapter 12. Prisoner Doctors: Struggles to Heal

1. Olga Lengyel, *Five Chimneys: The Story of Auschwitz* (Chicago: Ziff-Davis, 1947), pp. 89–94.

2. On Rohde and women, see Hermann Langbein, *Menschen in Auschwitz* (Vienna: Europaverlag, 1972), pp. 400–401.

3. F. K. Kaul, *Ärzte in Auschwitz* ([E.] Berlin: VEB Verlag Volk und Gesundheit, 1968), pp. 212–18.

Chapter 13. Prisoner Doctors: Collaboration with Nazi Doctors

1. Mavis M. Hill and L. Norman Williams, *Auschwitz in England: A Record of a Libel Action* (New York: Stein & Day, 1965); Hermann Langbein, *Menschen in Auschwitz* (Vienna: Europaverlag, 1972), pp. 255–57.

2. Langbein, *Menschen* [1], p. 255.

3. Samuel Steinberg, quoted in Langbein, *Menschen* [1], pp. 255–56; Dering in Hill and Williams, *Auschwitz in England* [1], p. 63.

4. Langbein, *Menschen* [1], p. 256.

5. Ibid., p. 257.

6. Hill and Williams, *Auschwitz in England* [1], p. 53; see pp. 16–18, 54, 69. Leon Uris, *Exodus* (New York: Doubleday, 1958), p. 146; in later printings of the book, the passage on Dehring (as spelled in the novel) omits the controversial number and stresses his status as prisoner.

7. Langbein, *Menschen* [1], p. 257; Hill and Williams, *Auschwitz in England* [1], pp. 25, 269–71.

8. On Samuel, see Langbein, *Menschen* [1], pp. 262–64.

9. Ibid., p. 263.

10. Ibid., p. 264.

Chapter 14. Killing with Syringes: Phenol Injections

1. Stanislaw Klodziński, "Phenol in the Auschwitz-Birkenau Concentration Camp," *Anthology* I, 2:100.

2. Hermann Langbein, *Menschen in Auschwitz* (Vienna: Europaverlag, 1972), pp. 47–48.

3. Klodziński testimony in Hermann Langbein, *Der Auschwitz-Prozess: Eine Dokumentation* (Frankfurt/M.: Europäische Verlagsanstalt, 1965), vol. II, p. 579.

4. Fejkiel deposition. Similar stories are frequent: see, for example, Miklos Nyiszli, *Auschwitz: A Doctor's Eyewitness Account* (New York: Frederick Fell, 1960), chap. 8.

5. Klodziński, "Phenol" [1], p. 113; see Klodziński's testimony which says 30 to 40, and Czeslaw Sowul's testimony, which says 80, in Langbein, *Auschwitz-Prozess* [3], vol. II, p. 767; for 120 children killed, see Bernd Naumann, *Auschwitz: A Report on the Proceedings Against Robert Karl Ludwig Mulka and Others Before the Court at Frankfurt* (New York: Praeger, 1966 [1965]), pp. 152, 185.

6. Schuler testimony, 20 July 1945, *Nuremberg Medical Case*, vol. I, p. 687; see pp. 684–94.

7. Hoven affidavit, 24 October 1946, *Nuremberg Medical Case*, vol. I, pp. 685–86. See Eugen Kogon, *The Theory and Practice of Hell* (New York: Berkley Books, 1980 [1950]), pp. 155–63.

8. Klodziński testimony, in Langbein, *Auschwitz-Prozess* [3], vol. II, p. 584.

9. Langbein, *Menschen* [2], pp. 48–51.

10. Wladyslaw Fejkiel notes the role of German military defeats in improving health care in "Health Service in Auschwitz I Concentration Camp/Main Camp," *Anthology*, II, 1:21–22.

11. Miklos Nyiszli, *Auschwitz: A Doctor's Eyewitness Account* (New York: Frederick Fell, 1960), pp. 53–56.

12. Klodziński, "Phenol" [1], pp. 103–4.

13. Ibid., pp. 109–10.

14. Klodziński testimony in Langbein, *Auschwitz-Prozess* [3], vol. II, p. 584.

15. Witness, Fabian, quoted in Naumann, *Auschwitz* [5], p. 291.

16. Klodziński, "Phenol" [1], pp. 104–5.

17. Witness Weiss, quoted in Naumann, *Auschwitz* [5], p. 295.

18. Ibid., pp. 191–92.

19. Langbein, *Menschen* [2], pp. 379–80.

20. Langbein, quoted in Mavis M. Hill and L. Norman Williams, *Auschwitz in England: A Record of a Libel Action* (New York: Stein & Day, 1965), p. 155; on Entress, see also Langbein, *Menschen* [2], pp. 377–79.

21. Langbein, *Menschen* [2], p. 378.

22. Ibid.

23. Ibid.

24. Ibid., pp. 377–78.

25. Ibid., pp. 212–13.

26. Ibid., p. 213.

27. Ibid.

28. Ibid.

29. Dr. Emil de Martini, quoted in Naumann, *Auschwitz* [5], p. 157.

30. Dr. Johann Kremer, quoted in Naumann, *Auschwitz* [5], p. 161.

31. Dr. Tadeusz Paczula, quoted in Langbein, *Menschen* [2], p. 440.

32. Ibid., pp. 441–42.

33. Stanislaw Glowa, quoted in Naumann, *Auschwitz* [5], p. 184; see also pp. 137, 152, 162.

34. Paczula, quoted in Langbein, *Menschen* [2], p. 441.

35. Josef Farber, quoted in Langbein, *Auschwitz-Prozess* [3], vol. II, p. 759.

36. Farber, quoted in Naumann, *Auschwitz* [5], p. 264.

37. Ibid., p. 410, see pp. 412–13, 425; Langbein, *Menschen* [2], p. 440; Langbein, *Auschwitz-Prozess* [3], pp. 894–96.

38. Naumann, *Auschwitz* [5], p. 410

39. Karl Lill, quoted in Langbein, *Menschen* [2], pp. 440–41.

40. Stanislaw Glowa, quoted in Naumann, *Auschwitz* [5], p. 183.

41. Glowa, quoted in ibid., pp. 185–86. See the testimonies of Tadeusz Holuj, Ota Fabian, and Ludwig Wörl in Langbein, *Menschen* [2], pp. 483–84.

42. Langbein, *Menschen* [2], p. 483; testimonies of Glowacki and Klodziński in Langbein, *Auschwitz-Prozess* [3], vol. II, pp. 766, 768.

43. Naumann, *Auschwitz* [5], pp. 412–13, 421–22.

Chapter 15. The Experimental Impulse

1. Unpublished testimony from Mme. Kleinova, M.D. (Prague), regarding her stay on Block 10.

2. Adelaide Hautval, "Survey of the Experiments Performed in the Women's Camps at Auschwitz and Ravensbrouck" (unpublished testimony) and personal communication.

3. On prostitution at Auschwitz, see Hermann Langbein, *Menschen in Auschwitz* (Vienna: Europaverlag, 1972), pp. 454–55.

4. Jan Sehn, "Carl Claubergs verbrecherische Unfruchtbarmachungs-Versuche an Häftlings-Frauen in den Nazi-Konzentrationslagern," *Hefte von Auschwitz* 2 (1959):3–31 (see p. 16 on the formalin formula). Höss quoted in F. K. Kaul, *Ärzte in Auschwitz* ([E.] Berlin: Verlag Volk und Gesundheit, 1968), pp. 277–78.

5. Kaul, *Ärzte* [4], p. 278.

6. PIIIh (Auschwitz) 863 (Wiener Library, London).

7. Sehn, "Claubergs Unfruchtbarmachungs-Versuche" [4], p. 15.

8. BDC: Clauberg.

9. Sehn, "Claubergs Unfruchtbarmachungs-Versuche" [4], pp. 15–16. See also Raul Hilberg, *The Destruction of the European Jews* (Chicago: Quadrangle, 1967 [1961]), pp. 605–6.

10. Clauberg to Himmler, 30 May 1942 (NO–211), *Nuremberg Medical Case*, vol. I, pp. 724–27.

11. Brandt to Clauberg, 10 July 1942 (NO–213), *Nuremberg Medical Case*, vol. I, p. 729.

12. Pokorny to Himmler, October 1941 (NO–35), *Nuremberg Medical Case*, vol. I, pp. 713–14.

13. Pokorny acquittal, *Nuremberg Medical Case*, vol. II, p. 294.

14. Clauberg to Himmler, 7 June 1943 (NO–212), *Nuremberg Medical Case*, vol. I, pp. 730–32.

15. Langbein, *Menschen* [3], p. 386.

16. Sehn, "Claubergs Unfruchtbarmachungs-Versuche" [4], p. 26.

17. PIIIh (Auschwitz) 659 (Wiener Library, London).

18. Philippe Aziz, *Doctors of Death* (Geneva: Ferni, 1976), vol. II, p. 236, see also pp. 175, 235–37; Sehn, "Claubergs Unfruchtbarmachungs-Versuche" [4], pp. 14, 26–27.

19. Aziz, *Doctors* [18], vol. II, pp. 240–41.

20. Sehn, "Claubergs Unfruchtbarmachungs-Versuche" [4], pp. 31–32.

21. For Clauberg's own stress on his abnormally short stature, see Langbein, *Menschen* [3], p. 387.

22. Brack to Himmler, 28 March 1941 (NO–203), *Nuremberg Medical Case*, vol. I, p. 720.

23. G. M. Gilbert, quoted in Joachim C. Fest, *The Face of the Third Reich: Portraits of the Nazi Leadership* (New York: Pantheon, 1970 [1963]), p. 121.

24. Michael H. Kater, *Das "Ahnenerbe" der SS, 1935–1945: Ein Beitrag zur Kulturpolitik des Dritten Reiches* (Stuttgart: Deutsche Verlags-Anstalt, 1974), pp. 17–24, 47–53, 227–64.

25. Willi Frischaur, *Himmler: The Evil Genius of the Third Reich* (Boston: Beacon Press, 1953), p. 28.

26. Fest, *Face* [23], pp. 116, 122.

27. Brack testimony, May 1947, *Nuremberg Medical Case*, vol. I, pp. 732–33.

28. Brack to Himmler, 23 June 1942 (NO–205), *Nuremberg Medical Case*, vol. I, pp. 721–22; Himmler to Brack (countersigned by Brandt), 11 August 1942 (NO–206), *Nuremberg Medical Case*, vol. I, p. 722.

29. Stanislaw Klodziński, " 'Sterilization' and Castration with the Help of X-Rays in the Concentration Camps: The Crimes of Horst Schumann," *Anthology*, I, 2:61.

30. Ibid., pp. 59–63.

31. Hautval, "Survey" [2].

32. Mavis M. Hill and L. Norman Williams, *Auschwitz in England: A Record of a Libel Action* (New York: Stein & Day, 1965), pp. 149–51, 178.

33. Désiré Haffner (original manuscript).

34. See Aziz, *Doctors of Death* [18], vol. II, pp. 183–85.

35. Hill and Williams, *Auschwitz in England* [32], pp. 18–19; Klodziński, " 'Sterilization' " [29], pp. 64–65.

36. Hill and Williams, *Auschwitz in England* [32], pp. 18–19.

37. Aziz, *Doctors* [18], vol. II, pp. 229–30.

38. Ibid., pp. 228–35.

39. Ibid., p. 235.

40. René Marx, in *Témoinages Strasbourgeois: De l'Université aux camps de concentration* (Paris: Les Belles Lettres, 1954 [1947]), pp. 251–62.

41. Hilberg, *Destruction* [9], pp. 608–9; Jochen von Lang (with Claus Sibyll), ed., *Eichmann Interrogated: Transcripts of the Israeli Police* (New York: Farrar, Straus & Giroux, 1983), pp. 167–75.

42. Alexander Mitscherlich and Fred Mielke, *Doctors of Infamy: The Story of the Nazi Medical Crimes* (New York: Henry Schumann, 1949), pp. 81–89; Hilberg, *Destruction* [9], pp. 608–9; Kater, *Ahnenerbe* [24], pp. 245–55.

43. See Eugen Kogon, *Theory and Practice of Hell* (New York: Berkley Books, 1980 [1950], pp. 155–67; Mitscherlich and Mielke, *Doctors* [42], pp. 4–89; Kater, *Ahnenerbe* [24], passim.

44. Kater, *Ahnenerbe* [24], pp. 245–55; see note 41 above.

45. Mitscherlich and Mielke, *Doctors* [42], pp. 88–89; *Nuremberg Medical Case*, vol. I, pp. 738–59.

46. On Hirt, see also Aziz, *Doctors* [18], vol. III, pp. 193–255; Frederick Kasten, "The Bizarre Case of Nazi Anatomy Professor August Hirt," paper presented at the 1985 meeting of the American Historical Association.

47. Langbein, *Menschen* [3], p. 398.

48. Jan Olbrycht, "The Nazi Health Office Actively Participated with the S. S. Administration in Auschwitz," *Anthology*, I, 1:188–89; Wladyslaw Fejkiel testimony in Bernd Naumann, *Auschwitz: A Report on the Proceedings Against Robert Karl Ludwig Mulka and Others Before the Court at Frankfurt* (New York: Praeger, 1966 [1965]), p. 155; testimonies by Olbrycht and Klodziński in Hermann Langbein, *Der Auschwitz-Prozess: Eine Dokumentation* (Frankfurt/M.: Europäische Verlagsanstalt, 1965), vol. II, pp. 676–77.

49. *Nuremberg Medical Case*, vol. I, pp. 684–95; Hilberg, *Destruction* [9], pp. 569–70, 602.

50. Stanislaw Klodziński, "Criminal Pharmacological Experiments on Inmates of the Concentration Camp in Auschwitz," *Anthology*, I,2: 15–43; see also Jan Mikulski, "Pharmakologische Experimente im Konzentrationslager Auschwitz-Birkenau," *Hefte von Auschwitz* 10 (1967): 3–18; Olga Lengyel, *Five Chimneys: The Story of Auschwitz* (Chicago; Ziff-Davis, 1947), pp. 4, 175.

51. Langbein, *Menschen* [3], p. 389.

52. Testimony before Polish Supreme Court, in Jan Sehn, "The Case of the Auschwitz S. S. Physician J. P. Kremer," *Anthology* I, 1:233.

53. "Kremers Tagebuch," *Hefte von Auschwitz* 13 (1971):42, 49.

54. Sehn, "Case" [52], pp. 211–14; "Tagebuch" [53], pp. 56–58 (3 and 4 December 1942;13 January 1943), 64 (10 June 1943), 69–72 (26 December 1943; 24 February 1944).

55. "Tagebuch" [53], p. 70 (26 December 1943).

56. Langbein, *Menschen* [3], p. 389; Karwowski testimony in Langbein, *Auschwitz-Prozess* [48], vol. II, p. 578; Olbrycht, "Nazi Health Office" [48], pp. 187–88.

57. Testimony of "Mr. Stern, Attorney in Paris," "The Horrors of Auschwitz" (unpublished manuscript).

58. Heinz Schumann and Heinrich Kühnreich, eds., *SS im Einsatz: Eine Dokumentation über das Verbrechen der SS* (7th, rev. ed. [E.] Berlin: Deutscher Militärverlag, 1964), p. 349.

59. Mengele/Haifa: 35 (Sarah Honigsmann).

60. Olbrycht, "Nazi Health Office" [48], p. 186.

61. YVAJ: 2039 (Dr. Aharon Beilin).

62. Langbein, *Menschen* [3], pp. 381–82.

63. L. Simonius, "On Behalf of Victims of Pseudo-Medical Experiments," *International Review of the Red Cross, Geneva* (January 1973), p. 13; Internationaler Suchdienst Arolsen, "Pseudo-medizinische Versuche im KL Auschwitz-Monowitz: Elektroschock-Behandlungsversuche," 15 February 1973.

64. Georges Wellers and Robert Waitz, "Recherches sur la dénutrition prolongée dans les camps de déportation," *Revue Canadienne de Biologie* 6 (1947).

65. Günther Schwarberg, *The Murders at Bullenhuser Damm: The SS Doctor and the Children* (Bloomington: Indiana University Press, 1984 [1980]).

66. Agriculture Minister Walther Darré, quoted in Robert Cecil, *The Myth of the Master Race: Alfred Rosenberg and Nazi Ideology* (New York: Dodd, Mead, 1972), p. 144.

Chapter 16. "A Human Being in an SS Uniform": Ernst B.

1. See Hermann Langbein, *Menschen in Auschwitz* (Vienna: Europaverlag, 1972), p. 357.

2. Ibid., pp. 56–60.

3. Hans Buchheim, "Command and Compliance," in Helmut Krausnick et al., *Anatomy of the SS State* (New York: Walker, 1968 [1965]), p. 373. Buchheim here discusses the acceptable reasons for avoiding orders in the Nazi environment.

Chapter 17. Dr. Auschwitz: Josef Mengele

1. Ernst Schnabel, *Anne Frank: A Portrait in Courage* (New York: Harcourt, Brace, 1958).

2. Ira Levin, *The Boys from Brazil* (New York: Random House, 1976); Rolf Hochhuth, *The Deputy* (New York: Grove Press, 1964 [1963]), pp. 31–32.

3. "The Search for Dr. Mengele," interview by Harry Reasoner, *60 Minutes*, 11 March 1979.

4. Hermann Langbein, *Menschen in Auschwitz* (Vienna: Europaverlag, 1972), pp. 384–85.

5. Helmut von Verschuer, quoted in Benno Müller-Hill, *Tödliche Wissenschaft: Die Aussonderung von Juden, Zigeunern und Geisteskranken 1933–1945* (Reinbek bei Hamburg: Rowohlt, 1984), p. 129.

6. Josef Mengele, "Rassenmorphologische Untersuchung des vorderen Unterkieferabschnittes bei vier rassischen Gruppen" (University of Munich, 1935), published in *Morphologisches Jahrbuch* 79 (1937):60–117.

7. Josef Mengele, "Sippenuntersuchungen bei Lippen-Kiefer-Gaumenspalte," *Zeitschrift für menschliche Vererbungs- und Konstitutionslehre* 23 (1938).

8. Josef Mengele, "Zur Vererbung der Ohrfisteln," *Der Erbarzt* 8 (1940):59–60.

9. Langbein, *Menschen* [4], p. 385.

10. Ibid., p. 384; Müller-Hill, *Wissenschaft* [5], p. 72.

11. Deposition of Klaus Dylewski, [n.d.] for Frankfurt Mengele trial.

12. "Beurteilung des SS Hauptsturmführers (R) Dr. Josef Mengele," 19 August 1949 (BDC: Mengele).

13. Testimony of Arie Fuks, in Bernd Naumann, *Auschwitz: A Report on the Proceedings Against Robert Karl Ludwig Mulka and Others Before the Court at Frankfurt* (New York: Pantheon, 1966 [1965]), p. 272.

14. Olga Lengyel, *Five Chimneys: The Story of Auschwitz* (Chicago: Ziff-Davis, 1947), p. 144.

15. Wieslaw Kielar, *Anus Mundi: 1,500 Days in Auschwitz/Birkenau* (New York: Times Books, 1970), p. 180.

16. Efraim Stiebelmann, quoted in Langbein, *Menschen* [4], p. 143. The same dismissal is cited by Margaret R. Englander in "A Mother's Story," part IV of "Mengele of Auschwitz" (with Flora Rheta Schreiber), New York *Times* Syndicate, 4 May 1975.

17. Mengele/Haifa: 27 (Tova Gruenberger, née Weiss); 14 (Emil Herzel).

18. Englander, "Mother's Story" [16].

19. Lengyel, *Five Chimneys* [14], pp. 144–45.

20. Ibid.

21. Gisella Perl, *I Was a Doctor in Auschwitz* (New York: International Universities Press, 1948), pp. 120–21.

22. Lengyel, *Five Chimneys* [14], p. 145.

23. Englander, "Mother's Story" [16].

24. Mengele/Haifa: 5 (Aluka Scendefi, née Agnes Weiss).

25. Mengele/Haifa: 32 (anonymous).

26. Arrest warrant, Amtsgericht Freiburg/Br., 5 June 1959 (YVAJ).

27. *JAMA* 106 (25 January 1936):308.

28. Ibid.

29. Deposition by Arpad Hajdu (Budapest), 4 May 1972, for Frankfurt Mengele trial.

30. Miklos Nyiszli, *Auschwitz: A Doctor's Eyewitness Account* (New York: Frederick Fell, 1960), pp. 39–40.

31. Deposition by Miklos Nyiszli, 28 July 1945, before the Budapest Commission for the Welfare of Deported Hungarian Jews.

32. Nyiszli, *Auschwitz* [30], p. 59.

33. Mengele/Haifa: 29 (Zivi Ernst Spiegel).

34. A copy of the film is available at the Auschwitz Museum.

35. Müller-Hill, *Wissenschaft* [5], p. 129.

36. Ibid.

37. Nyiszli, *Auschwitz* [30], p. 60.

38. Nyiszli deposition [31].

39. Nyiszli, *Auschwitz* [30], pp. 64–65.

40. Langbein, *Menschen* [4], p. 383.

41. Englander, "Mother's Story" [16].

42. Loet Van Duin (pseud.), "The Other Side of the Moon: The Life of a Young Physician from Holland in Auschwitz" (unpublished manuscript, 1980).

43. Lengyel, *Five Chimneys* [14], p. 174.

44. Nyiszli, *Auschwitz* [30], pp. 138–39.

45. Perl, *Doctor* [21], p. 122.

46. Nyiszli, *Auschwitz* [30], pp. 33, 171.

47. Mengele, "Rassenmorphologische Untersuchung" [6], p. 61.

48. Nyiszli, *Auschwitz* [30], p. 171.

49. Ibid., p. 133.

50. Horst von Glasenapp, personal communication, 7 August 1980.

51. Nyiszli, *Auschwitz* [30], p. 137.

52. Ibid., p. 222.

53. Lengyel, *Five Chimneys* [14], pp. 145–46.

54. Ibid., p. 146.

55. Ibid.

56. Nyiszli deposition [31].

57. Hochhuth, *The Deputy* [2], p. 32.

58. Lengyel, *Five Chimneys* [14], p. 144.

59. On the German reaction to the NBC film *Holocaust,* shown in the United States in 1978 and in West Germany and many other countries the next year, see Peter Märthesheimer and Ivo Frenzel, *Im Kreuzfeuer: Der Fernsehfilm "Holocaust"* (Frankfurt/M.: Fischer Taschenbuch Verlag, 1979) and Klaus Dörner et al., eds., *Der Krieg gegen die psychisch Kranken: Nach "Holocaust"* (Rehburg-Loccum: Psychiatrie-Verlag, 1980).

60. See the series "Der Fall Mengele," based on Mengele's discovered notebooks and his son's recollections in *BUNTE* (20 June–28 July 1985). See also Robert Jay Lifton, "What Made This Man? Mengele," *New York Times Magazine* (25 July 1985), pp. 16–25. "Definitive proof" that the exhumed skeleton was Mengele's was established in March 1986 by means of dental records (*New York Times,* 28 March 1986, p. A8).

Chapter 18. Healing-Killing Conflict: Eduard Wirths

1. Hermann Langbein, *Menschen in Auschwitz* (Vienna: Europaverlag, 1972), pp. 411–12.

2. Ibid., p. 432.

3. Documentary produced by Rolf Orthel and Hans Fels, first shown on Dutch television on 18 April 1975 (communication from Hermann Langbein).

4. Fragebogen zum Verlobungs- und Heiratsgesuch (SS marriage application), 10 November 1936; Wirths to Himmler, 12 November 1936 (regarding marriage permission); SS promotion document, July 1944 (BDC: Wirths).

5. For biographical information, see also Langbein, *Menschen* [1], pp. 422–24.

6. Langbein, *Menschen* [1], pp. 413–14.

7. Ibid., pp. 48–49.

8. Ibid., pp. 49–51.

9. Ibid., pp. 417–18.

10. Ibid., pp. 56–58.

11. Ibid., p. 413.

12. Ibid., p. 415.

13. This self-image is reflected in Wirth's apologia, written in British captivity during the summer of 1945.

14. Langbein, *Menschen* [1], p. 426.

15. Ibid., pp. 426–27.

16. Karl Lill to Albert Wirths, 2 February 1946; Lill to Wirth's wife, 2 December 1976. On the evacuation, see Langbein, *Menschen* [1] p. 431.

17. Langbein, *Menschen* [1], pp. 427–28.

18. Ibid., pp. 428–30.

19. Höss, quoted in Langbein, *Menschen* [1], pp. 413–14.

20. Hermann Langbein, *Die Stärkeren: Ein Bericht* (Vienna: Stern, 1949), p. 100.

21. On the typhus experiments, see Langbein, *Menschen* [1], pp. 428–30.

22. Ibid., pp. 426–27 (on joining the SS); see Langbein's discussion of his half-Jewishness, p. 19.

23. Ibid., pp. 413–14.

24. Ibid., p. 420; Langbein in documentary [3].

25. Bernd Naumann, *Auschwitz: A Report on the Proceedings Against Robert Karl Mulka and Others Before the Court at Frankfurt* (New York: Praeger, 1966 [1965]), pp. 62–66; Langbein, *Menschen* [1], pp. 485–86.

26. Documentary [3].

27. Wirths to his wife, 7 September 1942.

28. Ibid.

29. Ibid.

30. Wirths to his wife, 23 July 1943.

31. Wirths to his wife, 24 August, 22 September 1943.

32. Wirths to his wife, 22 September 1943.

33. Wirths to his wife, 22 September, 24 August 1943, 29 November 1944.

34. Wirths to his wife, 24 August 1943.

35. Wirths to his wife, 22 September 1943.

36. Documentary [3].

37. Wirths to his wife, 26–27 November, 17–18 December 1944.

38. Wirths to his wife, 17 December 1944, 5 January 1945.

39. Wirths to his wife, 26–27 November, 17–18 December 1944, 1 and 5 January 1945.

40. Wirths to his wife, 14 January, 24 May, 5 and 15 July 1945.

41. Wirths to his wife, 19 December 1944.

42. "Kremers Tagebuch," *Hefte von Auschwitz* 13 (1971):52 (4 November 1942).

43. Wirths to his wife, 29 November 1944.

44. Wirths to his wife, 2 January 1945.

45. Wirths to his wife, 14 January 1945.

46. Documentary [3].

47. Wirths to his wife, 7 September 1942; Wirths apologia [13]. On the end of big selections and the demolition of Auschwitz as the Russian troops approached, see Raul Hilberg, *The Destruction of the European Jews* (Chicago: Quadrangle, 1967 [1961]), p. 631; Miklos Nyiszli, *Auschwitz: A Doctor's Eyewitness Account* (New York: Frederick Fell, 1960), pp. 190–200.

48. Wirths to his wife, 29 November 1944; Wirths to his parents, 13 December 1944. Passages to parents quoted in Langbein, *Menschen* [1], pp. 421–22.

49. Wirths to his wife, 23 July 1943.

50. Wirths to his wife, 24 August 1943.

51. Wirths to his wife, 24 July 1945, 1 January 1945.

52. Wirths to his wife, 27 November 1944.

53. Filip Müller (with Helmut Freitag), *Sonderkommando: Three Years in the Gas Chambers at Auschwitz* (London: Routledge & Kegan Paul, 1979), p. 160.

54. Wirths to his wife, 26 and 29 November, 17 December 1944, 5 January 1945.

55. Langbein, *Menschen* [1], pp. 430–31.

56. See ibid., pp. 424–25.

57. Wirths apologia [13].

58. Wirths to his wife, 13 January 1945.

59. Wirths apologia [13].

60. Ibid.

61. Wirths to his wife, 23 July 1943.

62. Wirths apologia; Langbein, *Menschen* [1], p. 431.

63. Wirths apologia.

64. Wirths apologia [13].

65. Wirths to his parents, 13 December 1944; first phrase in Langbein, *Menschen* [1], pp. 421–22.

66. Wirths to his wife, 24 May 1945.

67. Ibid.

68. Wirths to his wife, 24 May and 5 July 1945.

69. Wirths to his wife, 15 July 1945.

70. Ibid.

71. Wirths apologia [13]; military evaluation of SS-Hauptsturmführer Dr. Eduard Wirths, 3 July 1944; Lolling's professional evaluation of Wirths, 5 July 1944 (BDC: Wirths).

72. Wirths's notes on Nietzsche's views on God, from Friedrich Würzbach, ed., *Nietzsche: Sein Leben in Selbstzeugnissen, Briefen und Berichten* (Berlin: Propyläen Verlag, 1942), pp. 44–45 (written on back of airplane schedules).

73. Leslie H. Farber, *The Ways of the Will: Essays toward a Psychology and Psychopathology of Will* (New York: Basic Books, 1966), see chap. 4.

74. Karl Lill to Albert Wirths, 2 December 1946.

75. Langbein, *Menschen* [1], p. 428.

76. Lill to Albert Wirths, 2 December 1946; Lill to Wirths's wife, 2 December 1976.

77. Ibid.

78. Documentary [3].

79. Albert Wirths to the chairman of the Frankfurt Auschwitz trial, 12 September 1964.

Chapter 19. Doubling: The Faustian Bargain

1. Paul W. Pruyser, "What Splits in Splitting?," *Bulletin of the Menninger Clinic* 39 (1975): 1–46.

2. Ibid., p. 46. See also Jeffrey Lustman, "On Splitting," in Kurt Eissler et al., eds., *The Psychoanalytic Study of the Child*, vol. 19 (1977), pp. 19–54; Charles Rycroft, *A Critical Dictionary of Psychoanalysis* (New York: Basic Books, 1968), pp. 156–57.

3. See Pierre Janet, *The Major Symptoms of Hysteria* (New York: Macmillan, 1907) and *Psychological Healing* (New York: Macmillan, 1923). See also Leston Havens, *Approaches to the Mind* (Boston: Little, Brown, 1973), pp. 34–62; and Henri F. Ellenberger, *The Discovery of the Unconscious* (New York: Basic Books, 1970), pp. 364–417.

4. Sigmund Freud and Josef Breuer, *Studies on Hysteria*, in *Standard Edition of the Works of Sigmund Freud*, James Strachey, ed. (London: Hogarth Press, 1955 [1893–95], vol. II, pp. 3–305.

5. Edward Glover, *On the Early Development of Mind: Selected Papers on Psychoanalysis* (New York: International Universities Press, 1956 [1943]), vol. I., pp. 307–23.

6. Melanie Klein, "Notes on Some Schizoid Mechanisms," *International Journal of Psychoanalysis* 27 (1946):99–110; and Otto F. Kernberg, "The Syndrome," in *Borderline Conditions and Pathological Narcissism* (New York: Jason Aronson, 1973), pp. 3–47.

7. Henry V. Dicks, *Licensed Mass Murder: A Socio-Psychological Study of Some SS Killers* (New York: Basic Books, 1972).

8. See, for example, Erik H. Erikson, *Identity: Youth and Crisis* (New York: W. W. Norton, 1968); Heinz Kohut, *The Restoration of the Self* (New York: International Universities Press, 1977); Henry Guntrip, *Psychoanalytic Theory, Therapy and the Self* (New York: Basic Books, 1971); and Robert Jay Lifton, *The Broken Connection: On Death and the Continuity of Life* (New York: Basic Books, 1983 [1979]).

9. William James, *The Varieties of Religious Experience: A Study in Human Nature* (New York: Collier, 1961 [1902]), p. 144.

10. Rank's two major studies of this phenomenon are *The Double: A Psychoanalytic Study* (Chapel Hill: University of North Carolina Press, 1971 [1925]); and "The Double as Immortal Self," in *Beyond Psychology* (New York: Dover, 1958 [1941]), pp. 62–101.

11. Rank, *Double* [10], pp. 3–9; Rank, *Beyond Psychology* [10], pp. 67–69. On "Der Student von Prag," see Siegfried Kracauer, *From Caligari to Hitler: A Psychological History of the German Film* (Princeton: Princeton University Press, 1947), pp. 28–30.

12. E. T. A. Hoffmann, "Story of the Lost Reflection," in J. M. Cohen, ed., *Eight Tales of Hoffmann* (London, 1952).

13. Rank, *Beyond Psychology* [10], p. 98.

14. Ibid.

15. On Rank's "artist-hero," see Rank, *Beyond Psychology* [10], pp. 97–101.

16. Rank, *Double* [10], p. 76.

17. Ibid.

18. Rank, *Beyond Psychology* [10], p. 82.

19. Michael Franz Basch, "The Perception of Reality and the Disavowal of Meaning," *Annual of Psychoanalysis*, 11 (New York: International Universities Press, 1982): 147.

20. Ralph D. Allison, "When the Psychic Glue Dissolves," *HYPNOS–NYTT* (December 1977).

21. The first two influences are described in George B. Greaves, "Multiple Personality: 165 Years After Mary Reynolds," *Journal of Nervous and Mental Disease* 168 (1977): 577–96. Freud emphasized the third in *The Ego and the Id*, in the *Standard Edition of the Works of Sigmund Freud*, James Strachey, ed. (London: Hogarth Press, 1955 [1923]), vol. XIX, pp. 30–31.

22. Ellenberger, *Unconscious* [3], pp. 394–400.

23. Margaretta K. Bowers et al., "Theory of Multiple Personality," *International Journal of Clinical and Experimental Hypnosis* 19 (1971):60.

24. See Lifton, *Broken Connection* [8], pp. 407–9; and Charles H. King, "The Ego and the Integration of Violence in Homicidal Youth," *American Journal of Orthopsychiatry* 45 (1975): 142.

25. Robert W. Rieber, "The Psychopathy of Everyday Life" (unpublished manuscript).

26. James S. Grotstein, "The Soul in Torment: An Older and Newer View of Psychopathology," *Bulletin of the National Council of Catholic Psychologists* 25 (1979):36–52.

27. See Robert Jay Lifton, *Home From the War: Vietnam Veterans, Neither Victims Nor Executioners* (New York: Basic Books, 1984 [1973]).

28. Rudolf Höss, quoted in Karl Buchheim, "Command and Compliance," in Helmut Krausnick et al., *Anatomy of the SS State* (New York: Walker, 1968 [1965]), p. 374.

29. Christian de La Mazière, *The Captive Dreamer* (New York: Saturday Review Press, 1974), pp. 14, 34.

30. John H. Hanson, "Nazi Aesthetics," *The Psychohistory Review* 9 (1981):276.

31. Sociologist Werner Picht, quoted in Heinz Höhne, *The Order of the Death's Head: The Story of Hitler's S. S.* (New York: Coward-McCann, 1970 [1966]), pp. 460–61.

32. Rolf Hochhuth, *A German Love Story* (Boston: Little, Brown, 1980 [1978]), p. 220.

33. Rank, *Beyond Psychology* [10], p. 68.

34. Koppel S. Pinson, *Modern Germany: Its History and Civilization* (2nd ed.; New York: Macmillan, 1966), pp. 1–3 (last phrase is from Nietzsche's *Beyond Good and Evil*).

35. Ronald Gray, *The German Tradition in Literature, 1871–1945* (Cambridge: Cambridge University Press, 1965), pp. 3, 79.

36. *Faust*, quoted in Pinson, *Germany* [34], p. 3.

37. Gray, *Tradition* [35], pp. 1–3.

38. Walter Kaufmann, *Goethe's Faust* (New York: Doubleday, 1961), p. 17.

39. Thomas Mann, *Doctor Faustus: The Life of the German Composer Adrian Leverkühn as Told by a Friend* (New York: Alfred A. Knopf, 1948 [1947]), p. 243.

40. Ibid., pp. 249, 308.

41. Rank, *Double* [10]; see also Robert Rogers, *A Psychoanalytic Study of the Double in Literature* (Detroit: Wayne State University Press, 1970).

Chapter 20. The Auschwitz Self: Psychological Themes in Doubling

1. Paul Brohmer, "The New Biology: Training in Racial Citizenship" (1933), in George L. Mosse, ed., *Nazi Culture: Intellectual, Cultural and Social Life in the Third Reich* (New York: Grosset & Dunlap, 1968), pp. 81–90.

2. Antoni Kepiński, "'Anus mundi,'" *Anthology* I, 2:2.

3. Adolf Hitler, *Mein Kampf* (Boston: Houghton Mifflin, 1943 [1925–26]), p. 402.

4. Susanne K. Langer, *Mind: An Essay on Human Feeling*, vol. III (Baltimore: Johns Hopkins University Press, 1982), p. 70.

5. Ibid., p. 83.

6. See Hitler, *Mein Kampf* [3], pp. 398–407.

7. Robert Jay Lifton, *The Broken Connection: On Death and the Continuity of Life* (New York: Basic Books, 1983 [1979]), p. 74.

8. Leo Alexander, introduction to Alexander Mitscherlich and Fred Mielke, *Doctors of*

Infamy: The Story of the Nazi Medical Crimes (New York: Henry Schumann, 1949 [1947]), p. xxxii.

9. Erik H. Erikson, "Ontogeny of Ritualization in Man," *Philosophical Transactions of the Royal Society of London* 251 (series B [1966]):343.

10. Clifford Geertz, *The Interpretations of Culture: Selected Essays* (New York: Basic Books, 1973), p. 114.

11. Erikson, "Ontogeny" [9], pp. 339, 345.

12. M. Singer, quoted in Geertz, *Interpretations* [10], p. 113.

13. Dorothea Lee, quoted in Langer, *Mind* [4], p. 59.

14. Robert Jay Lifton, *Home From the War: Vietnam Veterans, Neither Victims Nor Executioners* (New York: Basic Books, 1984 [1973]), chaps. 2, 5 and 6.

15. Langer, *Mind* [4], p. 79.

16. Hermann Rauschning, *Hitler Speaks: A Series of Political Conversations with Adolf Hitler on his Real Aims* (London: T. Butterworth, 1939), p. 222.

17. Robert C. Cecil, *The Myth of the Master Race: Alfred Rosenberg and Nazi Ideology* (New York: Dodd, Mead, 1972), p. 147.

18. Ibid.

19. Heinz Höhne, *The Order of the Death's Head: The Story of Hitler's S.S.* (New York: Coward-McCann, 1970 [1966]), p. 147.

20. Himmler, quoted in Felix Kersten, *The Memoirs of Doctor Felix Kersten*, Herma Briffault, ed. (Garden City, N. Y.: Doubleday, 1947), p. 151.

21. Thomas Mann, *Doctor Faustus: The Life of the German Composer Adrian Leverkühn as Told by a Friend* (New York: Alfred A. Knopf, 1948 [1947]), pp. 366–67.

22. Himmler, quoted in Lucy S. Dawidowicz, *The War Against the Jews, 1933–1945* (New York: Holt, Rinehart & Winston, 1975), p. 149.

23. Himmler, quoted in Roger Manvell and Heinrich Fraenkel, *Heinrich Himmler* (London: Heinemann, 1965), pp. 135–36.

24. Karl Hennicke, describing his superior officer, in Raul Hilberg, *The Destruction of the European Jews* (Chicago: Quadrangle, 1967 [1961]), p. 215; Hans Buchheim, "Command and Compliance," in Helmut Krausnick et al., *Anatomy of the SS State* (New York: Walker, 1968 [1965]), p. 328 ("criminal cause").

25. Himmler (May 1944), quoted in Buchheim, "Command and Compliance" [24], p. 366.

26. Hilberg, *Destruction* [24], pp. 215–16; Höhne, *Death's Head* [19], p. 363.

27. Hilberg, *Destruction* [24], p. 243; Höhne, *Death's Head* [19], pp. 544–45.

28. Höhne, *Death's Head* [19], p. 363.

29. See Buchheim, "Command and Compliance" [24], pp. 334–43.

30. Werner Best, quoted in Martin Broszat, "The Concentration Camps," in Krausnick et al., *Anatomy* [24], p. 427.

31. Ronald Gray, *The German Tradition in Literature, 1871–1945* (Cambridge: Cambridge University Press, 1965), pp. 81–82 (on Benn and Heidegger).

32. James H. McRandle, *The Track of the Wolf: Essays on National Socialism and Its Leader, Adolf Hitler* (Evanston, Ill.: Northwestern University Press, 1965), p. 125, credits Hannah Arendt for the term "ice-cold logic." She, however, noted that Hitler, himself, "loved" to refer to the " 'ice-coldness' of human logic" ("Ideologie und Terror," in *Offener Horizont: Festschrift für Karl Jaspers* [Munich: Piper, 1953], p. 244).

33. Lifton, *Broken Connection* [7], pp. 222–38. See also, Daniel Schreber, *Memoirs of My Nervous Illness*, Ida Macalpine and Richard A. Hunter, eds. (London: William Dawson, 1955); and Harold F. Searles, *Collected Papers on Schizophrenia and Related Subjects* (New York: International Universities Press, 1965).

34. Robert Jay Lifton, *Thought Reform and the Psychology of Totalism: A Study of "Brainwashing" in China* (New York: W. W. Norton, 1963), pp. 427–29.

35. Daniel Gasman, *The Scientific Origins of National Socialism: Social Darwinism in Ernst Haeckel and the German Monist League* (New York: Elsevier, 1971), p. 150.

36. Ibid., p. 157.

37. Ibid., pp. 39–40.

38. E. E. Evans-Pritchard, "The Logic of African Science and Witchcraft," in Max Marwick, ed., *Witchcraft and Sorcery: Selected Readings* (Baltimore: Penguin, 1970), p. 327.

39. On psychic numbing and numbed violence, see Robert Jay Lifton, *Death in Life: Survivors of Hiroshima* (New York: Basic Books, 1983 [1968]); Lifton, *Home from the War* [14]; Lifton, *The Life of the Self: Toward a New Psychology* (New York: Basic Books, 1983 [1976]); and Lifton, *Broken Connection* [7].

40. Alexander and Margarete Mitscherlich, *The Inability to Mourn* (New York: Grove Press, 1975 [1967]).

41. See the letter from a friend in the *Luftwaffe* in Friedrich Percyval Reck-Malleczewen, *Diary of a Man in Despair* (New York: Macmillan, 1970), p. 89. On the related idea of "hardness," see Buchheim "Command and Compliance" [24], pp. 334–43.

42. On the understanding of "It is the Führer's wish," see Gerald Fleming, *Hitler and the Final Solution* (Berkeley: University of California Press, 1984 [1982]), especially pp. 126–39.

43. Raul Hilberg, "Confronting the Moral Implications of the Holocaust," *Social Education* 42 (1978):275; Hilberg, *Destruction* [24], p. 216.

44. Hilberg, "Moral Implications" [43], p. 273.

45. Höss, quoted in Buchheim, "Command and Compliance," [24], p. 374.

46. Fred E. Katz, "A Sociological Perspective to the Holocaust," *Modern Judaism* 2 (1982): 280.

47. J. P. Stern, *Hitler: The Führer and the People* (Glasgow: Fontana/Collins, 1971), pp. 70–71.

48. Quotation from a letter from a friend in the *Luftwaffe*, in Reck-Malleczewen, *Diary* [41], p. 87.

49. Cecil, *Myth* [17], pp. 2–3.

50. Langer, *Mind* [4], pp. 79–80.

51. Geoffrey Cocks, "Psyche and Swastika: 'Neue Deutsche Seelenheilkunde' 1935–1945" (Ph.D. dissertation, University of California, Los Angeles, 1975), pp. 332–33.

52. Michael Kater, "Professionalization and Socialization of Physicians in Wilhelmine and Weimar Germany," *Journal of Contemporary History* 20 (1985):677–701.

53. Kurt Blome, *Arzt im Kampf: Erlebnisse und Gedanken* (Leipzig: J. A. Barth, 1942).

54. Joachim C. Fest, *The Face of the Third Reich: Portraits of the Nazi Leadership* (New York: Pantheon, 1970 [1963]), p. 542.

55. Stephan Leibfried and Florian Tennstedt, *Berufsverbote und Sozialpolitik, 1933: Die Auswirkungen der nationalsozialistischen Machtergreifung auf die Krankenkassenverwaltung und die Kassenärzte* (Bremen: Universität Bremen, 1981).

56. Hilberg, *Destruction* [24], p. 635.

57. Rudolf Höss, *Commandant of Auschwitz: The Autobiography of Rudolf Hoess* (Cleveland: World, 1959 [1951]), p. 121.

58. Eugen Kogon, *The Theory and Practice of Hell* (New York: Berkley Books, 1980 [1950]), p. 150.

59. See Günther Schwarberg, *The Murders at Büllenhuser Damm* (Bloomington: Indiana University Press, 1984 [1980]).

60. Alexander Mitscherlich, personal communication.

61. Miklos Nyiszli, quoted in Léon Poliakov, *Auschwitz* (Paris: Renée Julliard, 1964), p. 115.

62. Loren Eiseley, "Man, the Lethal Factor" (unpublished manuscript).

63. Professor Franz Hamburger, in a talk inaugurating the Nazi-controlled Viennese Medical Society, reported in *JAMA* 112 (1939):1982.

64. See William Ryan, *Blaming the Victim*, rev. ed. (New York: Vintage, 1976).

65. Hitler in a speech to the Reichstag, 30 January 1939, quoted in Dawidowicz, *War Against the Jews* [22], p. 106.

66. Lifton, *Broken Connection* [7], pp. 302–34.

67. Höss, *Commandant* [57], pp. 142–46.

68. See Mircea Eliade, *The Sacred and the Profane: The Nature of Religion* (New York: Harcourt, Brace, 1959 [1957]), pp. 29–32.

69. Langer, *Mind* [4], p. 181.

70. Eiseley, "Lethal Factor" [62], quoted in Lifton, *Broken Connection* [7], pp. 292, 297.

71. Lifton, *Home* [14], chap. 6.

72. Steven Kull, "Nuclear Nonsense," *Foreign Policy* 20 (spring 1985):28–52.

Chapter 21. Genocide

1. Thomas Mann, *Doctor Faustus: The Life of the German Composer Adrian Leverkühn, As Told by a Friend* (New York: Alfred A. Knopf, 1948 [1947]), p. 223.

2. Leo Kuper, *Genocide: Its Political Use in the Twentieth Century* (New Haven: Yale University Press, 1981), pp. 19–23, 210–14.

3. Ibid., p. 22.

4. Robert Jay Lifton, *The Broken Connection: On Death and the Continuity of Life* (New York: Basic Books, 1983 [1979]).

5. George M. Kren, "Psychohistory, Psychobiography and the Holocaust," *Journal of Psychohistory* 13 (1984): 40–45; Israel W. Charny, "A Contribution to the Psychology of Genocide: Sacrificing Others to the Death We Fear Ourselves," *Israel Yearbook on Human Rights* 10 (1980): 98, 102–3. See also Charny (with Chanon Rapaport), *How Can We Commit the Unthinkable?: Genocide, The Human Cancer* (Boulder, Col.: Westview Press, 1982).

6. Theodore H. von Laue, "Adolf Hitler: Expressionist and Counterrevolutionary" (unpublished manuscript).

7. Fritz Stern, *The Politics of Cultural Despair: A Study in the Rise of the Germanic Ideology* (Berkeley: University of California Press, 1961), p. 33.

8. See John H. Hanson, "Nazi Aesthetics," *The Psychohistory Review* 9 (1981): 251–81.

9. Robert C. Cecil, *The Myth of the Master Race: Alfred Rosenberg and Nazi Ideology* (New York: Dodd, Mead, 1972), p. 93.

10. Goethe, *Art and Antiquity*, quoted in Erich Heller, *The Disinherited Mind: Essays in Modern German Literature and Thought* (3rd ed.; New York: Barnes & Noble, 1971), p. 101. On collective behavior, see Robert Jay Lifton, "On Psychohistory," in Lifton and Eric Olson, eds., *Explorations in Psychohistory: The Wellfleet Papers* (New York: Simon & Schuster, 1974), pp. 21–41.

11. Von Laue, "Hitler" [6].

12. Thomas Mann, *Frederick and the Great Coalition* (1915), quoted in Ronald Gray, *The German Tradition in Literature, 1871–1945* (Cambridge: Cambridge University Press, 1965), pp. 39–40.

13. Ibid., pp. 48–49.

14. Weber, letter of April 1915, quoted in Gray, *German Tradition* [12], p. 37.

15. Meinecke, quoted in Von Laue, *Hitler* [6].

16. Ernst Jones, *The Life and Work of Sigmund Freud* (New York: Basic Books, 1955), vol. II, pp. 171–72.

17. Gray, *Tradition* [12], p. 49; Hilton Kramer, "Rediscovering the Art of Max Beckmann," *New York Times Magazine*, 19 August 1984, pp. 28–34.

18. Hitler, *Mein Kampf* (Boston: Houghton Mifflin, 1943 [1925–26]), pp. 161, 435.

19. Vahakn N. Dadrian, "The Role of Turkish Physicians in the World War I Genocide of Ottoman Armenians," *Holocaust and Genocide Studies* 1 (1986, forthcoming); Dadrian, "The Common Features of the Armenian and Jewish Cases of Genocide: A Comparative Victimological Perspective," in Israel Drapkin and Emilio Viano, *Victimology: A New Focus*, vol. IV (Lexington, Mass.: D. C. Heath, 1974), pp. 99–120. See also, Helen Fein, *Accounting for Genocide: Victim—and Survivors—of the Holocaust* (New York: Free Press, 1979), pp. 10–18.

20. Isaiah Berlin, "Nationalism: Past Neglect and Present Power," *Partisan Review* 46 (1979):337–58.

21. Ibid.

22. Martin Bormann to Alfred Rosenberg (22 February 1940), quoted in Koppel S. Pinson, *Modern Germany: Its History and Civilization* (2nd ed.; New York: Macmillan, 1966), p. 497.

23. Von Laue, "Hitler" [6].

24. Nationalist politician Hans Schlange-Schoeningen (1948), quoted in Pinson, *Germany* [22], p. 500.

25. Reich President's secretary (under Ebert, Hindenburg, and Hitler) Otto Meissner, quoted in Pinson, *Germany* [22], p. 500.

26. Gray, *Tradition* [12], pp. 48–49.

27. Robert Wistrich, *Who's Who in Nazi Germany* (New York: Macmillan, 1982), p. 162.

28. Robert Jay Lifton, *Thought Reform and the Psychology of Totalism: A Study of "Brainwashing" in China* (New York: W. W. Norton, 1963), chap. 22.

29. Werner Sombart, quoted in Pinson, *Germany* [22], p. 502.

30. Werner Best, quoted in Martin Broszat, "The Concentration Camps 1933–45," in Helmut Krausnick et al., *Anatomy of the SS State* (New York: Walker, 1968 [1965]), pp. 426–27.

31. George Weippert, *The Reich as German Mission* (1934), quoted in Karl Dietrich Bracher, *The German Dictatorship* (New York: Praeger, 1970 [1969]), p. 251.

32. Hitler, *Mein Kampf* [18], p. 442–51.

33. Professor Walter Frank (1936), quoted in Cecil, *Myth* [9], p. 150.

34. See Dadrian, "Turkish Physicians" and "Common Features" [19].

35. Gustav Mevissen, quoted in Pinson, *Germany* [22], pp. 139–40.

36. Ibid., pp. 483–84.

37. Friedrich Percyval Reck-Malleczewen, *Diary of a Man in Despair* (New York: Macmillan, 1970 [1966]), p. 65.

38. On the idea of the *Reich*, see Uriel Tal, " 'Political Faith' of Nazism Prior to the Holocaust," 1978 annual lecture of the Jacob and Shoshona Schreiber Chair of Contemporary Jewish History, Tel Aviv University, 1978, p. 24, and "Nazism as a Political Faith," *Jerusalem Quarterly* 15 (1980):70–90.

39. Letter from a friend in the *Luftwaffe*, quoted in Reck-Malleczewen, *Diary* [37], pp. 87–89.

40. Fritz Lenz, *Menschliche Auslese und Rassenhygiene* (Munich: J. F. Lehmanns Verlag, 1923), p. 337.

41. Nobel laureate in physics Philipp Lenard, quoted in Alan D. Beyerchen, *Scientists Under Hitler: Politics and the Physics Community in the Third Reich* (New Haven: Yale University Press, 1977), p. 131.

42. Heller, *Disinherited Mind* [10], pp. 101–4.

43. Dadrian, "Turkish Physicians" [19].

44. Hugo Ball, quoted in John H. Hanson, "Psychohistorical Perspectives on the European Avant-garde" (unpublished manuscript).

45. Ibid.

46. Hanson, "Nazi Aesthetics" [8], p. 252 (on the ancestor cult). On the Waffen-SS, see Heinz Höhne, *The Order of the Death's Head: The Story of Hitler's S.S.* (New York: Coward McCann, 1970 [1967]), p. 461; see also chap. 16.

47. Hanson, "Nazi Aesthetics" [8], pp. 260–61.

48. Goebbels, quoted in Rolf Hochhuth, *A German Love Story* (Boston: Little, Brown, 1980 [1978]), p. 18.

49. Hitler, quoted in Eberhard Jäckel, *Hitler's Weltanschauung: A Blueprint for Power* (Middletown, Conn.: Wesleyan University Press, 1972 [1969]), pp. 54, 131n17.

50. Himmler, quoted in Hans Buchheim, "Command and Compliance," in Krausnick et al., *Anatomy* [30], p. 338.

51. I discuss this concept of religious victimization in *The Broken Connection* [4], pp. 314–15.

52. Robert S. Gottfried, *The Black Death: Natural and Human Disaster in Medieval Europe* (New York: Simon & Schuster, 1979), pp. 52–53, 68–69, 73–74.

53. Adolf Leschnitzer, *The Magic Background of Modern Anti-Semitism: An Analysis of the German-Jewish Relationship* (New York: International Universities Press, 1969 [1956], pp. 99, 112–20, 221n7. See also Jäckel, *Weltanschauung* [49]; Rudolph Binion, *Hitler Among the Germans* (New York: Elsevier, 1976); Vanberto Morais, *A Short History of Anti-Semitism* (New York: W. W. Norton, 1976).

54. Hermann Glaser, *The Cultural Roots of National Socialism* (London: Croom, Helm, 1978), p. 79.

55. Ibid., pp. 220, 225–26; Paul de Lagarde, quoted in Stern, *Cultural Despair* [7], pp. 62–63.

56. Glaser, *Roots* [54], p. 226.

57. Hermann Lietz, quoted in G[eorge] L. Mosse, "The Mystical Origins of National Socialism," *Journal of the History of Ideas* 22 (1961): 94–95.

58. Glaser, *Roots* [54], p. 224.

59. Ibid., pp. 126–27.

60. Léon Poliakov, *The History of Anti-Semitism: From the Time of Christ to the Court Jew* (New York: Vanguard, 1965), pp. 216–26.

61. Erik Erikson, *Young Man Luther: A Study in Psychoanalysis and History* (New York: W. W. Norton, 1958), chap. 6.

62. W. Beumelburg, quoted in Glaser, *Roots* [54], p. 197.

63. Ibid., pp. 221–22.

64. Testimony of Werner Leibbrandt, *Nuremberg Medical Case*, vol. I, p. 81.

65. Raul Hilberg, *The Destruction of the European Jews* (Chicago: Quadrangle, 1967 [1961]), pp. 262–63.

66. Personal conversations with Raul Hilberg and Yehuda Bauer. For good recent discussions, see Saul Friedländer, "Introduction," Gerald Fleming, *Hitler and the Final Solution* (Berkeley: University of California Press, 1984 [1982]), pp. vii–xxxiii; and Christopher R. Browning, *Fateful Months: Essays on the Emergence of the Final Solution* (New York: Holmes & Meier, 1985).

67. Hitler, *Mein Kampf* [18], p. 257.

68. See Buchheim, "Command and Compliance" [50], p. 362; Höhne, *Death's Head* [46], pp. 309–29.

69. Mircea Eliade, *Shamanism: Archaic Techniques of Ecstasy* (Princeton: Princeton University Press, 1972 [1951]), pp. 184–89. See also Norman Cohn, *Warrant for Genocide: The Myth of the Jewish World-Conspiracy and the Protocols of the Elders of Zion* (Chico, Cal.: Scholars Press, 1981 [1967]).

70. George L. Mosse, "War and the Appropriation of Nature," in Volker R. Berghahn and Martin Kitchen, eds., *Germany in the Age of Total War* (Totowa, N. J.: Barnes & Noble, 1981), p. 107.

71. Alfred Baeumler, quoted in George L. Mosse, "Friendship and Nationhood: About the Promise and Failure of German Nationalism," *Journal of Contemporary History* 17 (1982):363.

72. George L. Mosse, "Death, Time and History," *Masses and Man: Nationalist and Fascist Perceptions of Reality* (New York: Howard Fertig, 1980), pp. 71–73.

73. Mary Douglas, *Purity and Danger: An Analysis of Concepts of Pollution and Decay* (London: Routledge & Kegan Paul, 1978 [1966]), pp. 5, 13–18, 59.

74. Ibid., pp. 34–35.

75. Ibid., p. 173.

76. Lifton, *Broken Connection* [4], pp. 305–6.

77. Fritz Stern, *Gold and Iron: Bismarck, Bleichröder and the Building of the German Empire* (New York: Alfred A. Knopf, 1977), p. xviii.

78. Douglas, *Purity* [73], p. 29.

79. James H. McRandle, *The Track of the Wolf: Essays on National Socialism and Its Leader, Adolf Hitler* (Evanston, Ill.: Northwestern University Press, 1965), pp. 134, 137.

80. Mosse, "Death, Time" [72], p. 72.

81. Hanns Löhr, *Über die Stellung und Bedeutung der Heilkunde im nationalsozialistischen Staate* (*1935*), in George L. Mosse, ed., *Nazi Culture: Intellectual, Cultural and Social Life in the Third Reich* (New York: Grosset & Dunlap, 1966), p. 234.

82. Douglas, *Purity* [73], p. 69.

83. Ibid., p. 102.

84. Geoffrey W. Conrad and Arthur A. Demarest, *Religion and Empire: The Dynamics of Aztec and Inca Expansionism* (Cambridge, England: Cambridge University Press, 1984), pp. 38, 41. (Latter quotation from Miguel León-Portilla.)

85. Ibid., p. 41.

86. Ibid., p. 44.

87. Susanne K. Langer, *Mind: An Essay on Human Feeling*, vol. III (Baltimore: Johns Hopkins University Press, 1982), p. 193. See also Jacques Soustelle, *The Daily Life of the Aztecs: On the Eve of the Spanish Conquest* (New York: Macmillan, 1962), pp. 98–99.

88. Joseph de Maistre, "The Saint Petersburg Dialogues," *The Work of Joseph de Maistre*, Jack Lively, ed. (New York: Macmillan, 1965), p. 253.

89. On these and related issues, see Hyam Maccoby, *The Sacred Executioner: Human Sacrifice and the Legacy of Guilt* (New York: Thames & Hudson, 1982); Norman O. Brown, *Closing Time* (New York: Random House, 1973), p. 35 ff.; Walter Burkert, *Homo Necans: The Anthropology of Ancient Greek Sacrificial Ritual and Myth* (Berkeley: University of California Press, 1984); and the review by Robert Parker, *Times Literary Supplement*, 15 June 1984, p. 654.

90. Glaser, *Roots* [54], p. 79.

91. McRandle, *Track of the Wolf* [79], p. 135; Eliade, *Shamanism* [69], p. 99.

92. Nietzsche, *Human, All Too Human*, quoted in Gray, *Tradition* [12], p. 23. See Hans Kohn, *The Mind of Germany* (New York: Charles Scribner, 1960), pp. 217–21.

93. Nietzsche, *The Will to Power*, Walter Kaufman, ed. (New York: Vintage, 1968), p.29.

94. Ibid., p. 135.

95. "The Case of Wagner," in Walter Kaufman, ed., *Basic Writings of Nietzsche* (New York: Modern Library, 1968), p. 775.

96. Nietzsche, *Will* [93], p. 224.

97. David P. Boder, "Nazi Science," in *Twentieth Century Psychology*, Philip Lawrence Harriman, ed. (New York: Philosophical Library, 1946), pp. 11–22.

98. Geoffrey Cocks, *Psychotherapy in the Third Reich: The Göring Institute* (New York: Oxford University Press, 1985), pp. 127–35.

99. Rosenberg, quoted in Hanson, "Nazi Aesthetics" [8], p. 274.

100. Robert Jay Lifton, "Protean Man," *Archives of General Psychiatry* 24 (1971):298–304; Lifton, *Broken Connection* [4], pp. 29, 129, 296–97, 393–94; Lifton, *Boundaries: Psychological Man in Revolution* (New York: Vintage, 1971 [1970]).

101. On the mystical community, see Glaser, *Roots* [54], p. 97; Tal, " 'Political Faith' " [38]; McRandle, *Track of the Wolf* [79], pp. 136–37.

102. See Albert Speer, *Inside the Third Reich: Memoirs* (New York: Macmillan, 1970), pp. 444–60.

103. Cecil, *Myth* [9], p. 94.

104. Bernward J. Gottlieb and Alexander Berg, *Das Antlitz des Germanischen Arztes in vier Jahrzehnten* (Berlin: Rembrandt-Verlag, 1942), p. 3.

105. See Lifton, *Broken Connection* [4], pp. 340–41; Lifton and Richard Falk, *Indefensible Weapons: The Political and Psychological Case Against Nuclearism* (New York: Basic Books, 1982).

106. George Santayana, quoted in Pinson, *Germany* [22], p. 4n.

107. Susan Sontag, "Disease as Political Metaphor," *New York Review of Books*, 23 February 1978, pp. 29–35.

108. A Young Turk activist, quoted in Kuper, *Genocide* [2], p. 91.

109. Eric Wolf, quoted in Kuper, *Genocide* [2], p. 40.

110. Dadrian, "Turkish Physicians" [19].

111. Avery Weisman and Thomas Hackett, "Predilection to Death: Death and Dying as a Psychiatric Problem," *Psychosomatic Medicine* 33 (1961).

112. Rolf Hochhuth, *A German Love Story* (Boston: Little, Brown, 1980 [1978]), pp. 157–60.

113. Beyerchen, *Scientists* [41], pp. 79–167; Cocks, *Psychotherapy* [98], pp. 127–35.

114. Karl Stern, *The Pillar of Fire* (New York: Harcourt, Brace, 1951), p. 153.

115. Otto Weininger, *Sex and Character*, 6th rev. ed. (New York: Putnam's, 1906), p. 328; see chap. 8.

116. Benno Müller-Hill, *Tödliche Wissenschaft: Die Aussonderung von Juden, Zigeunern und Geisteskranken 1933–1945* (Reinbek b. Hamburg: Rowohlt, 1983), p. 90.

117. Boder, "Nazi Science," [97], pp. 13–22.

118. Walter Schellenberg, *The Labyrinth: Memoirs* (New York: Harper, 1956), p. 170.

119. Himmler, quoted in Hermann Langbein, *Menschen in Auschwitz* (Vienna: Europaverlag, 1974), p. 320.

120. On alcohol and numbing, see Langbein, *Menschen* [119], pp. 337–38.

121. Hilberg, *Destruction* [65], p. 629.

122. Speer, *Inside* [102], pp. 212, 524.

123. Jeffrey Herf, *Reactionary Modernism: Technology, Culture, and Politics in Weimar and the Third Reich* (Cambridge, England: Cambridge University Press, 1984), p. 71; Klaus Theweleit, *Männerphantasien*, 2 vols. (Reinbek b. Hamburg: Rowohlt, 1980 [1977]).

124. William Barrett, *The Illusion of Technique: A Search for Meaning in a Technological Civilization* (New York: Anchor Press, 1978), p. xiv. See also Jacques Ellul, *The Technological Society* (New York: Alfred A. Knopf, 1964) and *The Technological System* (New York: Continuum, 1980).

125. Robert Jay Lifton, *Home From the War: Vietnam Veterans, Neither Victims Nor Executioners* (New York: Basic Books, 1984 [1973]), p. 349.

126. Lifton, *Broken Connection* [4], pp. 369–87; Lifton and Falk, *Indefensible Weapons* [105].

127. For an elegant critique of these attitudes–from within, so to speak–by three members of Computer Professionals for Social Responsibility, see Reid Simmons, Karen Solomon, and Dan Carnese, "Peril of 'Intelligent' Weapons," *Boston Globe*, 29 July 1984, p. 39.

128. Barrett, *Illusion* [124], p. 8.

129. Herf, *Modernism* [123], pp. 71–72.

130. Max Weber, quoted in Martin Green, *The von Richthofen Sisters: The Triumphant and the Tragic Modes of Love* (New York: Basic Books, 1974), p. 152.

131. Irving L. Janis, *Group Think: A Psychological Study of Foreign-Policy Decisions and Fiascos* (Boston: Houghton Mifflin, 1972).

132. Raul Hilberg, "Confronting the Moral Implications of the Holocaust," *Social Education* 42 (1978):272–76; Raul Hilberg, *The Destruction of the European Jews*, rev. and definitive ed. (New York: Holmes & Meier, 1985), vol. III, pp. 407–16.

133. Alan Rosenberg, "The Genocidal Universe: A Framework for Understanding the Holocaust," *European Judaism* 13 (1979):29–34.

134. See Lifton, *Broken Connection* [4], p. 38.

135. Michael Basch, "The Concept of 'Self,'" in *Developmental Approaches to the Self*, Benjamin Lee and Gil Noam, eds., (New York: Plenum Press, 1983), pp. 7–58, especially p. 52.

136. Theodore W. Adorno, et al., *The Authoritarian Personality* (New York: Harper, 1952). David C. McClelland makes the point that the relatively great German submissiveness to authority stems from "an excess of the virtuous emphasis on self-discipline for the common good" ("The United States and Germany: A Comparative Study of National Character," in McClelland *The Roots of Consciousness* [Princeton: Van Nostrand, 1964], pp. 62–92).

137. Harold Orlans, "An American Death Camp," *Politics* 5 (1948):162–67.

138. Elias Canetti, *Crowds and Power* (New York: Viking, 1962), p. 443, see pp. 227–30.

139. Lifton, "Protean Man" [100]; Lifton, *Broken Connection* [4]; Lifton, *Boundaries* [100].
140. Barrett, *Illusion* [124], pp. 101–6.

Afterword

1. Erik H. Erikson, "Evolutionary and Developmental Considerations," in Lester Grinspoon, ed., *The Long Darkness: Psychological and Moral Perspectives on Nuclear Winter* (New Haven: Yale University Press, forthcoming).
2. Michael Franz Basch, "Empathetic Understanding: A Review of the Concept and Some Theoretical Considerations," *Journal of the American Psychoanalytic Association* 31 (1983): 101–26; and personal communication.
3. Loren Eiseley, "Man, the Lethal Factor" (unpublished manuscript).

Acknowledgments

My greatest debt is to survivors of Nazi death camps, many of whom I interviewed but only a few of whom I name here. It is they who carry within them the terrible truths we must all reckon with, and their contribution to my work, and to my life, has been inestimable.

I am especially grateful to Leo Eitinger, who spared himself nothing in teaching me about Auschwitz and much more; to Raul Hilberg, for constant advice, information, and perspective, as well as the kind of close, knowledgeable reading of the manuscript that few authors are privileged to receive; and to Elie Wiesel, for strong support and wise counsel throughout the work.

For valuable discussions and various forms of help with arrangements in the United States and different parts of the world: Erwin H. Ackerknecht, Leo Alexander (who made available to me many of his early materials), Amnon Amir (who sent me his dissertation on Nazi "euthanasia"), Rudolph Binion (who made available his research materials), Vahakn N. Dadrian (who provided writings and information on the Turkish genocide of Armenians), Lucy Dawidowicz, Peter Demetz, Karl Deutsch, Richard Falk, Leslie Farber, Erich Goldhagen, Michael H. Kater, Robert M. W. Kempner, Heinz Kohut, Ruth Lidz, Theodore Lidz, Franklin H. Littell, Peter Loewenberg, James M. McHaney (who made available materials from the Nuremberg Medical Trial), Margaret Mead, Alexander Mitscherlich (who conveyed to me everything he could concerning his invaluable early exposé of Nazi medical crimes), Marguerite Mitscherlich, George Mosse, Fritz Redlich, Fritz Stern, Albert J. Stunkard, Uriel Tal, Telford Taylor, Lionel Tiger, and Henry Turner.

Members of the Wellfleet psychohistory group with whom I have shared much of the work include Norman Birnbaum, Margaret Brenman-Gibson, Peter Brooks, Harvey Cox, Erik Erikson (opening up new dimensions in our dialogue of thirty years), Kai Erikson, Robert Holt, Gerald Holton, Hillel Levine, John E. Mack, Charles Strozier, Francis Winters, and Daniel Yankelovich.

In Germany, Horst von Glasenapp provided important early materials and many additional forms of help during the research phase. Paul Matussek offered crucial support with arrangements and an appointment as Fellow at the Forschungsstelle für Psychopathologie und Psychotherapie in der Max-Planck-Gesellschaft in Munich, which he directs. Fritz Friedmann provided extraordinary intellectual and personal hospitality at the Amerika-Institut at Munich University, which he then headed. Others in Germany were: Walter Ritter von Baeyer, Wanda von Baeyer, Martin Broszat, Helmut Coper, Otto Creutzfeldt, Peter Durr, Elisabeth Fetscher, Iring Fetscher, Lothar Gruchmann, Warner Jochmann, Jurgen Habermas, Helmut Handzik, Horst W. Hartwich, Walter Huder, Uwe Henrik Peters, Adalbert Rückerl, Wolfgang Scheffler, Gerhardt Schmidt, Helm P. Stierlin, Satu Stierlin, George Tabori, and Carl S. von Weizäcker.

In Israel: Yehuda Bauer, Shamai Davidson, Sidra Ezrahi, Yaron Ezrahi, Saul Friedländer, Yisrael Gutman, Hillel Klein, Lilli Kopecky, Erich Kulka, and Jacob Lorch.

In Poland: Adam Szymusik, chairman of the Department of Psychiatry, Medical Academy, Krakow, welcomed me in his department and facilitated arrangements there. Others in Poland: Józef Bogusz, Stanislaw Klodziński, and Maria Orwid.

In Austria, Friedrich Hacker, director of the Institut für Konfliktforschung in Vienna, helped greatly with arrangements. Others in Austria: Alois Hauer (unique in being a former Nazi doctor who served the anti-Nazi underground in a Norwegian camp), Friedrich Heer, Rolf Hochhuth, Edith Kramer, Hermann Langbein (who provided much information and many introductions), Ella Lingens-Reiner, Harald Leupold-Löwenthal, Erich Stern, Josef Toch, and Simon Wiesenthal.

In England: H. D. Adler, Norman Cohn, Gerald Fleming, John Fox, Albert Friedlander, James Joll, Peter Reddaway, Gitta Sereny, and Robert Wistrich.

In France: Roger Errera, Arthur Hartman, Donna Hartman, Adelaide Hautval, Socrate Helman, Serge Klarsfeld, Samuel Pisar, Léon Poliakov, Yves Ternon, and Georges Wellers.

In Holland: Jan Bastiaans, Elie Cohen, Louis de Jong, and Eduard de Wind.

In Australia: Ena Hronsky and Issy Pilowsky.

In Italy: Robert A. Graham.

In Switzerland: Erwin Leiser (who screened Nazi film for me).

Extraordinary research assistance was provided me, over the years spanning the study, in different parts of the world and in relation to the many phases of the work, by the following admirable and dedicated people: Henry Abramovitz, Janet Beizer, Johannes Borger, Andrzej Branny, Christiane Clemm, Rudolph Dolzer, Brigitte Fleischmann, Amy Hackett, Anne Halliwell, Lisa Kaufman, Erich Kramer, Waltraut Lehmann, Annegrette Lösch, Robert Luchs, Rosalyn Manowitz, Eric Markusen, Randi Morrau Markusen, Noel Mathews, Micheline Nilsen, William Patch, Cathrin Pichler, Jean Rainwater, Susannah Rubenstein, Solange Salem, Matthias K. Scheer, Gunther Sommerfeld, Kitty Weinberger, Steven Wolfe, and Katharina Zimmer.

I received valuable assistance from many libraries and archival collections. In the United States: Yale University and Columbia University libraries, New York Public Library at 42nd Street, and the Library of the New York Academy of Medicine; the YIVO Institute for Jewish Research (Dina Abramowicz, librarian), the Jewish Labor Bund archives (Hillel Kempinski), and the National Archives (Robert Wolfe). In Germany: The Institut für Zeitgeschichte in Munich; the Ludwigsburg Zentralstelle der Landesjustizverwaltungen; and the Berlin Document Center (Diana K. Kendall and Daniel P. Simon). In Austria: the Dokumentationszentrum des Widerstandes, Vienna (Erwin Steiner, director). In Israel: the Yad Vashem Holocaust Research Center (Yitzhak Arad, Livia Rothkirchen, Hadassah Modlinger, and Danuta Dabrowska); and the Haifa Institute of Documentation for the Investigation of Nazi War Crimes (Tuvia Friedman, director). In Poland: the Main Committee for the Investigation of Nazi Crimes in Poland (Czeslaw Pilichowski, director); and the Auschwitz Museum (which provided valuable original Auschwitz documents—Kasamierz Smoleń, director, and Tadeusz Iwaszko). In London: the Wiener Library (Gita Johnson).

Lily B. Finn, my assistant at Yale for twenty-two years, did more to coordinate the various strands of the research than I or she can possibly recall, and then typed the entire manuscript, put it on a word processor, and saw through the revisions to the end. Lucy M. Silva, my new assistant at John Jay College/City University, did a very great deal to enable me to complete the work.

John J. Simon made the initial phone call that set the project in motion, and was a partner in dialogue during the early stages of the research. Jane Isay, with rare brilliance and generosity, edited and helped shape the original manuscript. Jo Ann Miller provided editorial advice, and she and Martin Kessler made possible the extraordinary support for the enterprise by Basic Books. Phoebe Hoss provided later manuscript editing remarkable in being as imaginative as it was meticulous. Linda Carbone sensitively guided the manuscript through production.

This study has not been easy on my family. My wife, Betty Jean Lifton, has struggled with it no less than I have, provided balance with her work on a *good* doctor, Janusz Korczak, all the while infusing me with the needed combinations of love and courage. Our children, Natasha and Kenneth Jay, have endured the pain of the project and at the same time made clear to their father that they understand its necessity and meaning.

This work was made possible through the assistance of a research grant from the National Endowment for the Humanities, supplemented by grants from the Humanities Division of The Rockefeller Foundation, the New-Land Foundation, the Foundations' Fund for Research in Psychiatry, the John Simon Guggenheim Memorial Foundation, the Josiah Macy Jr. Foundation, the Holocaust Survivors Memorial Foundation, and the May W. Wise Philanthropic Fund.

Grateful acknowledgment is made to the following sources for their permission to reprint:

Unpublished Manuscripts and Dissertations

Excerpt from "Euthanasia in Nazi Germany" by Amnon Amir (Ph.D. diss., State University of New York at Albany, 1977).

Excerpt from "Psyche and Swastika: 'Neue Deutsche Seelenheilkunde' 1935–1945" by Geoffrey Cocks (Ph.D. diss., University of California at Los Angeles, 1975).

Passages from "The Role of Turkish Physicians in the World War I Genocide of Ottoman Armenians" by Vahakn N. Dadrian. Used with permission of Vahakn N. Dadrian. *Holocaust and Genocide Studies* 1, no. 2 (Sept. 1986), Pergamon Press.

Passages from "Man, the Lethal Factor" by Loren Eiseley.

Excerpt from "Psycho historical Perspectives on the European Avant-garde" by John H. Hanson. Used with permission of John H. Hanson.

Passages from "The Other Side of the Moon: The Life of a Young Physician from Holland in Auschwitz" by Loet Van Duin (pseud.). Used with permission of Loet Van Duin (pseud.).

Passages from "Adolf Hitler: Expressionist and Counterrevolutionary" by Theodore H. von Laue. Used with permission of Theodore H. von Laue.

Published Works

Line from "In a Dark Time" from *The Collected Poems of Theodore Roethke* by Theodore Roethke. "In a Dark Time" copyright © 1960 by Beatrice Roethke as Administratrix of the Estate of Theodore Roethke. Reprinted by permission of Doubleday & Company, Inc.

Lines from "Speak You Also," by Paul Celan, reprinted from *Paul Celan: Poems,* selected, translated and introduced by Michael Hamburger, by permission of Persea Books, Inc., 225 Lafayette Street, New York, New York, and Michael Hamburger. Copyright © 1980 by Michael Hamburger.

Passages from *Menschen in Auschwitz* by Hermann Langbein (Vienna: Europaverlag, 1972). Reprinted by permission of Europa Verlag.

Passages from Rudolf Höss: *Commandant of Auschwitz, The Autobiography of Rudolf Hoess* by Rudolf Höss (Cleveland: World, 1959). Translated from the German by Constantine FitzGibbon with an introduction by Lord Russell of Liverpool (London: George Weidenfeld & Nicolson, Ltd., 1959). Reprinted by permission of George Weidenfeld & Nicolson, Ltd.

Passages from *Doctors of Death,* by Phillippe Aziz (Geneva: Ferni Publishers, 1976).

Passages from *Five Chimneys: The Story of Auschwitz* by Olga Lengyel (Chicago: Ziff-Davis, 1947).

Passages from *"Euthanasie" im NS-Staat: Die Vernichtung lebensunwerten Lebens* by Ernst Klee (Frankfurt/M: S. Fischer Verlag, 1983). Used by permission of S. Fischer Verlag.

Index